# Fire Service First Responder

## FIRST EDITION

VALIDATED BY
THE INTERNATIONAL FIRE SERVICE TRAINING ASSOCIATION

PUBLISHED BY
FIRE PROTECTION PUBLICATIONS
OKLAHOMA STATE UNIVERSITY

Cover Photo Courtesy of: George F. Braun
Gainesville, Florida Fire Department

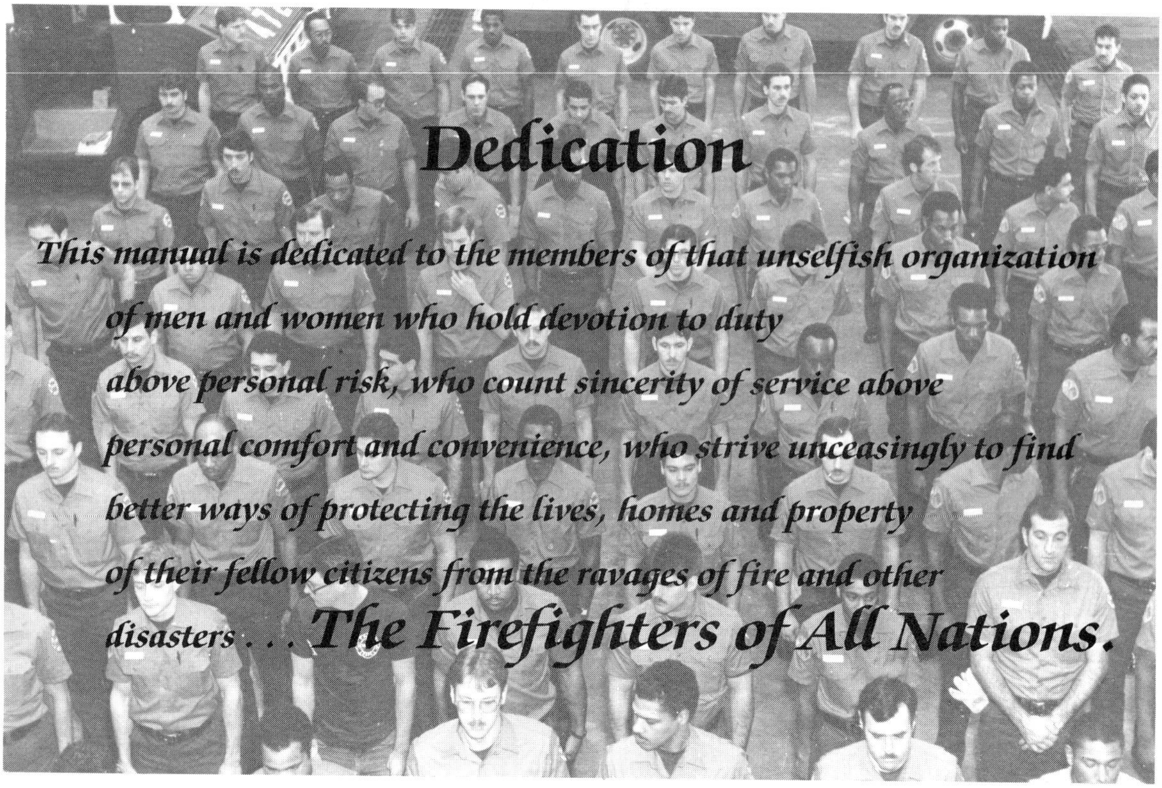

# Dedication

*This manual is dedicated to the members of that unselfish organization of men and women who hold devotion to duty above personal risk, who count sincerity of service above personal comfort and convenience, who strive unceasingly to find better ways of protecting the lives, homes and property of their fellow citizens from the ravages of fire and other disasters . . .* ***The Firefighters of All Nations.***

Dear Firefighter:

The International Fire Service Training Association (IFSTA) is an organization that exists for the purpose of serving firefighters' training needs. IFSTA is a member of the Joint Council of National Fire Organizations. Fire Protection Publications is the publisher of IFSTA materials. Fire Protection Publications staff members participate in the National Fire Protection Association and the International Society of Fire Service Instructors.

If you need additional information concerning these organizations or assistance with manual orders, contact:

Customer Services
Fire Protection Publications
Oklahoma State University
Stillwater, OK 74078-0118
(800) 654-4055
(405) 624-5723 in Alaska and Oklahoma

For assistance with training materials, recommended material for inclusion in a manual, or questions on manual content, contact:

Technical Services
Fire Protection Publications
Oklahoma State University
Stillwater, OK 74078-0118
(405) 624-6832




*ISBN 0-87939-070-0*
*Library of Congress 86-83301*
*First Edition*
*Printed in the United States of America*

# Table of Contents

# List of Tables

# THE INTERNATIONAL FIRE SERVICE TRAINING ASSOCIATION

The International Fire Service Training Association is an educational alliance organized to develop training material for the fire service. The annual meeting of its membership consists of a workshop conference which has several objectives —

... to develop training material for publication
... to validate training material for publication
... to check proposed rough drafts for errors
... to add new techniques and developments
... to delete obsolete and outmoded methods
... to upgrade the fire service through training

This training association was formed in November 1934, when the Western Actuarial Bureau sponsored a conference in Kansas City, Missouri, to determine how all agencies that were interested in publishing fire service training material could coordinate their efforts. Four states were represented at this conference and it was decided that, since the representatives from Oklahoma had done some pioneering in fire training manual development, other interested states should join forces with them. This merger made it possible to develop nationally recognized training material which was broader in scope than material published by an individual state agency. This merger further made possible a reduction in publication costs, since it enabled each state to benefit from the economy of relatively large printing orders. These savings would not be possible if each individual state developed and published its own training material.

From the original four states, the adoption list has grown to forty-four American States; six Canadian Provinces; the British Territory of Bermuda; the Australian State of Queensland; the International Civil Aviation Organization Training Centre in Beirut, Lebanon; the Department of National Defence of Canada; the Department of the Army of the United States; the Department of the Navy of the United States; the United States Air Force; the United States Bureau of Indian Affairs; The United States General Services Administration; and the National Aeronautics and Space Administration (NASA). Representatives from the various adopting agencies serve as a voluntary group of individuals who govern policies, recommend procedures, and validate material before it is published. Most of the representatives are members of other international fire protection organizations and this meeting brings together individuals from several related and allied fields, such as:

... key fire department executives and drillmasters,
... educators from colleges and universities,
... representatives from governmental agencies,
... delegates of firefighter associations and organizations, and
... engineers from the fire insurance industry.

This unique feature provides a close relationship between the International Fire Service Training Association and other fire protection agencies, which helps to correlate the efforts of all concerned.

The publications of the International Fire Service Training Association are compatible with the National Fire Protection Association's Standard 1001, "Fire Fighter Professional Qualifications (1981)," and the International Association of Fire Fighters/International Association of Fire Chiefs "National Apprenticeship and Training Standards for the Fire Fighter." The standards are an effort to attain professional status through progressive training. The NFPA and IAFF/IAFC Standards were prepared in cooperation with the Joint Council of National Fire Service Organizations of which IFSTA is a member.

The International Fire Service Training Association meets each July at Oklahoma State University, Stillwater, Oklahoma. Fire Protection Publications at Oklahoma State University publishes all IFSTA training manuals and texts. This department is responsible to the executive board of the association. While most of the IFSTA training manuals can be used for self-instruction, they are best suited to group work under a qualified instructor.

# Preface

**Fire Service First Responder** is designed to assist the member of the fire service who is receiving instruction in a U.S. Department of Transportation Emergency Medical Services First Responder Training Course. Where appropriate, chapters are referenced to objectives in the First Responder Course. Because this manual is intended for use by members of the fire service, chapters are also referenced to the Emergency Medical Care section of NFPA 1001, *Fire Fighter Professional Qualifications* for levels I and II.

Bear in mind that guidelines for assessment and treatment may differ from area to area. The first responder should follow the guidelines set forth in his or her local jurisdiction.

A manual of this scope and complexity would be impossible to produce without the assistance of many expert individuals. Acknowledgements and grateful thanks are extended to the members of the validating committee, who assisted with the final draft of this manual:

*Chairman*
Max Thomas
Director (Retired)
Fire Service Training
University of Kansas
Lawrence, Kansas

*Vice-Chairman*
Jerry Simmons
Arkansas Fire Academy
East Camden, Arkansas

*Secretary*
Glenn Pribbenow
Fire Service Training Specialist
Oklahoma State University
Stillwater, Oklahoma

*Liaison*
Scott Tyler
Research Technician
Fire Protection Publications
Stillwater, Oklahoma

Steve Nuyen
Fire Chief
Yerington-Mason Valley Fire Department
Yerington, Nevada

Pat Harris
Milwaukee Fire Department
Milwaukee, Wisconsin

Robert Weldon
EMT Vocational Specialist
Okla. State Department of Vocational and Technical Education
Oklahoma City, Oklahoma

Tom Noonan
Deputy Fire Chief
Tiogue Fire Department
Coventry, Rhode Island

Gene Duncan
Asst. Fire Chief (Retired)
Stillwater Fire Department
Stillwater, Oklahoma

Bart Lewis
Fire Chief
Apple Valley Fire Protection District
Apple Valley, California

Special thanks are extended to the following individuals for their expert advice and assistance:

Betty Lack, R.N., Baptist Medical Burn Center, Oklahoma City, Oklahoma.

NancySue Hudson, Assoc. Director for Advanced and Intermediate Training, Dept. of Emergency Medical Training, University of Kansas Medical Center, Lawrence, Kansas.

Phil Davis, California State Fire Marshal's Office, Sacramento, California.

Russell Strickland, Maryland Fire and Rescue Institute, College Park, Maryland.

Vicky Cleary, R.N., Hoag Memorial Hospital, Newport Beach, California.

Sherry York, Dyna Industries, Inc., Carlsbad, California.

Henry Heimlich, M.D., The Heimlich Institute, Xavier University, Cincinnati, Ohio.

Dawn Graham, Armstrong Industries, Northbrook, Illinois.

Members of the Stillwater Fire Department, under the direction of Chief Jim Smith, for assisting with photographs: Dale Parrish, Bill Mizel, Tom Low, Tom Oosting, Chris Neal, and Jerry Stroup.

Additional thanks are due to OSU Fire Service Training Specialists Gary Courtney and Glenn Pribbenow, both of whom were always willing to answer questions, explain procedures, and lend resource materials.

Very special thanks to several staff members whose skills and dedication improved the depth and quality of this manual immeasurably. Suzanne Goodwin's outstanding technical writing skills are reflected throughout the manual. Paramedic David Hiscott provided technical review and Robert Fleischner spent many hours taking and developing nearly all the photographs in the manual. Artists John Dickey and Mike McDonald provided all of the original artwork. Phototypesetters Karen Murphy and Desa Porter typed and patiently retyped; Production Coordinator Don Davis made it all look beautiful.

Gratitude is also extended to the following members of the Fire Protection Publications staff who made final publication of the manual possible:

Lynne C. Murnane, Senior Publications Editor
David W. England, Senior Publications Editor
Mike Wieder, Associate Editor
Suzanne Goodwin, Technical Writer
Carol Smith, Publications Specialist
Cindy Brakhage, Unit Assistant
Rhonda Wiley-Jones, Instructional Developer
Don Davis, Coordinator, Publications Production
Ann Moffat, Graphic Designer
Mike McDonald, Graphic Artist
Karen Murphy, Phototypesetter Operator II
Desa Porter, Phototypesetter Operator II
Terri Jo Gaines, Senior Clerk Typist
Scott A. Stookey, Senior Research Technician
David Hiscott, Research Technician
Jeff Windham, Research Technician
Roger McKim, Research Technician
Robert Price, Research Technician
Brett Lacey, Research Technician
Robert Fleischner, Photographer and Technical Writing Intern
Terri Wheeler, Technical Writing Intern
John Robinson, Technical Writing Intern

Gene P. Carlson
Editor

# Glossary

## A

**ABANDONMENT** — Termination of a first responder-patient relationship by the first responder without consent of the patient and without care to the patient by qualified medical providers.

**ABC's** — Airway, Breathing, and Circulation; the first three steps in the examination of any patient; basic life support.

**ABDOMINAL CAVITY** — The large body cavity below the diaphragm and above the pelvis.

**ABORTION** — Premature expulsion of the products of conception from the uterus; abortion can occur naturally or can be artificially induced.

**ABRASION** — An injury consisting of the loss of a partial thickness of skin from rubbing or scraping on a hard, rough surface; also called a brush burn, friction burn.

**ABSENCE SEIZURE** — A type of seizure characterized by a momentary loss of awareness; also known as petit mal seizure.

**ACUTE** — Having rapid onset, severe symptoms, and a relatively short duration.

**ACUTE ABDOMEN** — Severe pain, tenderness, and muscular rigidity caused by inflammation, infection, or obstruction of an organ within the abdominal cavity.

**ACUTE MYOCARDIAL INFARCTION** — The acute phase of a heart attack, where blockage of a coronary artery produces a number of signs and symptoms, particularly chest pain, nausea, heavy sweating, anxiety, and pallor.

**ADAM'S APPLE** — The projection on the front of the neck formed by the thyroid cartilage of the larynx.

**ADDICTION** — The state of being strongly dependent upon some agent; drugs, tobacco, for example.

**ADJUNCT** — An accessory or auxiliary agent; an oral airway is an airway adjunct.

**ADVANCED LIFE SUPPORT** — Basic life support plus the use of invasive procedures or drugs.

**AGGRAVATE** — To worsen; to make worse.

**AIR** — The gaseous mixture that composes the Earth's atmosphere; composed of approximately 21 percent oxygen, 79 percent nitrogen, plus trace gases.

**ALLERGIC REACTION** — A local or general reaction to an allergen, usually characterized by hives, tissue swelling, or difficulty breathing.

**ALVEOLI** — Air cells of the lungs.

**AMPUTATION** — Complete removal of an appendage.

**ANAPHYLAXIS (Anaphylactic Shock)** — Severe allergic reaction characterized by hives, itching, difficulty breathing, possible circulatory collapse.

**ANATOMY** — The structure of the body, or the study of body structure.

**ANGINA PECTORIS** — A spasmodic pain in the chest caused by insufficient blood supply to the heart; aggravated by exercise or tension and relieved by rest or medication.

**ANTERIOR** — Situated in front of, or in the forward part of; in anatomy, used in reference to the belly surface of the body.

**ANUS** — The outlet of the rectum lying in the fold between the buttocks.

**ANXIETY** — A feeling of apprehension, uncertainty, and fear.

**AORTA** — The largest artery in the body; originates at the left ventricle.

**APGAR SCORE** — A method developed by Dr. Virginia Apgar for assessing the newborn infant at 1 minute of age by designating a score of 0, 1, or 2 for the following: A = appearance; P = pulse rate; G = grimace; A = activity; and R = respiration.

**APNEA** — Cessation of breathing; the absence of respiration.

**APPENDICITIS** — Condition in which the appendix becomes swollen and infected; characterized by sharp pain in lower right abdomen.

**ARREST** — Sudden cessation or stoppage.

**ARRHYTHMIA** — Any disturbance in the rhythm of the heart.

**ARTERIOSCLEROSIS** — A generic name for several conditions that cause the walls of the arteries to become thickened, hard, and inelastic.

**ARTERY** — A blood vessel that carries blood away from the heart.

**ARTICULATION** — Joining of bones, a joint; touching of one part with another.

**ARTIFICIAL RESPIRATION** — Movement of air into and out of the lungs by artificial means; also known as rescue breathing.

**ASPHYXIA** — Suffocation.

**ASPIRATE** — To inhale foreign material into the lungs.

**ASTHMA** — A condition marked by attacks of labored breathing, wheezing, a sense of constriction in the chest, and coughing or gasping.

**ATHEROSCLEROSIS** — A common form of arteriosclerosis characterized by fat deposits in the walls of the arteries.

**ATRIUM** — Upper chamber of the left or right side of the heart.

**AUTONOMIC NERVOUS SYSTEM** — Part of the nervous system concerned with the regulation of body functions not controlled by conscious thought.

## B

**BAG-VALVE MASK** — A portable artificial ventilation unit consisting of a face mask, one-way valve, and an inflatable bag, can be used on a non-breathing or breathing patient.

**BANDAGE** — A material used to hold a dressing in place.

**BASAL SKULL FRACTURE** — A fracture involving the base of the cranium.

**BASIC LIFE SUPPORT** — Maintenance of the ABC's (airway, breathing, and circulation) without adjunctive equipment.

**BATTERY** — The intentional and unauthorized touching of a person without his or her consent.

**BATTLE'S SIGN** — Purplish discoloration above the bone behind the ear indicating a skull fracture.

**BILE** — A fluid secreted by the liver that is concentrated and stored in the gallbladder.

**BIOLOGICAL DEATH** — A condition present when irreversible brain damage has occurred, usually 4 to 10 minutes after cardiac arrest.

**BIRTH CANAL** — The canal through which the fetus passes during childbirth; composed of the cervix, vagina, and vulva.

**BLADDER** — A membranous sac that stores urine.

**BLANCH** — To become white or pale.

**BLOOD** — The fluid that circulates through the heart, arteries, veins, and capillaries, carrying nutrients and oxygen to the body cells, and removing waste products such as carbon dioxide for excretion.

**BLOOD PRESSURE** — The pressure exerted by the flow of blood against the arterial walls.

**BLOOD VOLUME** — The total amount of blood in the heart and blood vessels.

**BP** — Abbreviation for blood pressure.

**BRACHIAL ARTERY** — The main artery of the upper arm.

**BRADYCARDIA** — An abnormally slow heart rate, usually any rate less than 60 beats per minute.

**BRAIN** — A soft, large mass of nerve tissue that is contained within the cranium.

**BRAIN STEM** — The stemlike portion of the brain that connects the brain with the spinal cord.

**BREECH DELIVERY** — Delivery of a fetus with some part of the body other than the head appearing first; usually the buttocks appear first in a breech birth.

**BRONCHUS** — One of the two main branches of the trachea that lead to the right and left lungs.

**BRUISE** — An injury that does not break the skin but causes rupture of small underlying blood vessels with resulting tissue discoloration; a contusion.

**BURN** — Tissue injury caused by heat, electrical current, or chemicals.

**BURN CENTER** — A medical facility especially designed, equipped, and staffed to treat severely burned patients.

## C

**CANNULA** — A tube used to enter a duct or cavity. A nasal cannula is often used to administer supplemental oxygen.

**CAPILLARIES** — Tiny blood vessels in the body's tissues in which the exchange of oxygen and carbon dioxide takes place.

**CARBON DIOXIDE** — $CO_2$; a colorless and odorless gas that neither supports combustion nor burns; a waste product of aerobic metabolism.

**CARBON MONOXIDE** — CO; a colorless, odorless, and dangerous gas formed by the incomplete combustion of carbon; it combines more than 200 times as quickly with hemoglobin than oxygen.

**CARDIAC ARREST** — The sudden cessation of the heartbeat.

**CARDIOPULMONARY RESUSCITATION (CPR)** — The application of rescue breathing and external cardiac compression in patients with cardiac arrest to provide an adequate circulation to support life.

**CAROTID ARTERY** — The principal artery of the neck, easily felt on either side of the trachea.

**CARTILAGE** — Tough, elastic tissue that lines the joints of large bones and separates the vertebrae, providing structure and cushioning.

**CAVITY** — A hollow or space, especially a space within the body or one of its organs. For example, the abdominal cavity is bounded by the abdominal walls, the diaphragm, and the pelvis.

**CELL** — A small cavity or compartment.

**CELSIUS SCALE** — The temperature scale in which the freezing point of water is zero degrees and the boiling point at sea level is 100 degrees, also known as Centigrade Scale.

**CENTRAL NERVOUS SYSTEM** — The portion of the nervous system consisting of the brain and spinal cord.

**CENTRAL NEUROGENIC HYPERVENTILATION** — An abnormal pattern of breathing seen in severe illness or injury involving the brain; characterized by very heavy, rapid breathing.

**CEREBELLUM** — The large posterior portion of the brain just below the cerebrum.

**CEREBROSPINAL FLUID** — A clear, watery fluid surrounding the meninges that protects the brain and spinal cord.

**CEREBROVASCULAR ACCIDENT (CVA) (See also Stroke)** — A hemorrhage or blood clot within a blood vessel in the brain.

**CEREBRUM** — The largest part of the brain; it controls major body functions, including movement, sensation, thinking, and emotions.

**CERVICAL COLLAR** — A device used to immobilize and support the neck.

**CERVICAL SPINE** — The first seven bones of the vertebral column, located in the neck.

**CERVIX** — The lower portion, or neck, of the uterus.

**CHEYNE-STOKES RESPIRATION** — An abnormal breathing pattern characterized by rhythmic increase and decrease in depth of ventilations, with regularly recurring periods during which breathing stops.

**CHIEF COMPLAINT** — The problem for which a patient seeks help, stated in a word or short phrase.

**CHILLS** — A sensation of cold, with convulsive shaking of the body.

**CHRONIC** — Of long duration, or recurring over a period of time.

**CHRONIC OBSTRUCTIVE PULMONARY DISEASE (COPD)** — A term for several diseases that result in obstructive problems in the airways.

**CIRCULATORY SYSTEM** — The body system consisting of the heart and blood vessels.

**CLAVICLE** — The collarbone; attaches to the uppermost part of the sternum, and joins the scapula to form the point of the shoulder.

**CLINICAL DEATH** — A term that refers to the lack of signs of life, when there is no pulse and no blood pressure; occurs immediately after the onset of cardiac arrest.

**CLOSED FRACTURE** — A fracture in which there is no break in the overlying skin.

**CLOT** — A semisolid mass of fibrin and cells.

**COCCYX** — The lowest part of the spine; composed of four small, fused vertebrae; also called the tailbone.

**COFFEE GROUNDS VOMITUS** — A vomitus having the appearance and consistency of coffee grounds; indicates slow bleeding in the stomach.

**COLON** — The large intestine.

**COMMUNICABLE DISEASE** — A disease that is transmissible from one person to another.

**COMPOUND FRACTURE** — An open fracture; a fracture in which there is an open wound of the skin and soft tissues.

**COMPRESS** — A folded cloth or pad used for applying pressure to stop hemorrhage or as a wet dressing.

**CONGESTIVE HEART FAILURE** — Excessive fluid in the lungs or tissues caused by the failure of the heart to effectively pump blood.

**CONJUNCTIVA** — The delicate membrane that lines the eyelids and covers the exposed surface of the eyeball.

**CONSENT** — An agreement by patients to accept treatment offered as explained by medical personnel.

**CONSTRICT** — To be made smaller by drawing together or squeezing.

**CONTUSION** — A bruise; an injury that causes a hemorrhage beneath the skin but does not break the skin.

**CONVULSION** — A violent involuntary contraction or series of contractions of the voluntary muscles; a seizure.

**COON'S EYES** — Bruising around both eyes seen with skull fracture.

**CORE TEMPERATURE** — A body temperature measured in deep structures, such as the lungs or liver.

**CORNEA** — The transparent structure covering the pupil.

**CORONARY ARTERIES** — The blood vessels that supply blood to the walls of the heart.

**CPR** — Abbreviation for cardiopulmonary resuscitation.

**CRAMP** — A painful spasm, usually of a muscle; a gripping pain in the abdominal area.

**CRANIUM** — Skull; the portion of the skull enclosing the brain.

**CREPITUS** — A grating sound heard when the fractured ends of a bone rub together.

**CROUP** — A common viral infection seen in small children, characterized by spasm of the larynx and resulting upper airway obstruction.

**CROWNING** — The condition where the presenting part of a baby, usually the head, first bulges out of the vaginal opening.

**CVA** — Abbreviation for cerebrovascular accident, also known as stroke.

**CYANOSIS** — A blueness of the skin due to insufficient oxygen in the blood.

## D

**DECEREBRATE POSTURE** — A posture assumed by a patient with severe brain injury characterized by extension and internal rotation of the arms and extension of the legs.

**DECONTAMINATE** — To remove a foreign substance that could cause harm; frequently used to describe removal of radioactive material from person, clothing, or area.

**DECORTICATE POSTURE** — The posture assumed by patients with a severe brain injury; characterized by tightly flexed arms, clenched fists, and slightly extended legs.

**DEFIBRILLATION** — The application of direct current electrical shock to terminate ventricular fibrillation. Administered by paramedics and some EMTs.

**DELIRIUM TREMENS** — DT's, a form of insanity, often temporary, caused by alcohol poisoning; characterized by sweating, tremor, great excitement, hallucinations, anxiety, and mental distress; usually occurs during withdrawal from alcohol.

**DEMAND VALVE UNIT** — An intermittent, positive pressure breathing unit used to assist or control ventilation.

**DEPRESSION** — A mental state characterized by feelings of dejection or worthlessness. Patient experiences insomnia, listlessness, and perhaps suicidal thoughts.

**DERMIS** — The inner layers of skin; contains the hair follicles, sweat glands, nerves, and blood vessels.

**DIABETES MELLITUS** — A systemic disease caused by lack of production of insulin, leading to an inability to metabolize carbohydrates and an increase in blood sugar.

**DIABETIC KETOACIDOSIS** — A condition that results when there is too much sugar in the blood and not enough insulin to metabolize it. The body then metabolizes fats, causing acid waste products to build up in the blood.

**DIAPHORESIS** — Profuse perspiration.

**DIAPHRAGM** — The flat group of muscles and tendons that separate the abdominal and thoracic cavities.

**DIGESTION** — The process by which food is converted into simple chemical substances that can be absorbed by the intestines.

**DILATED PUPIL** — A pupil enlarged beyond its normal size.

**DISC** — The cartilaginous pad between the vertebrae that separates and cushions them.

**DISLOCATION** — The state of being misaligned; the condition that results when the surfaces of two bones are no longer in proper contact.

**DISTAL** — Located away from the trunk of the body.

**DISTENTION** — The state of being inflated or enlarged, particularly of the abdomen.

**DISTORTION** — The state of being twisted out of normal or natural shape or position.

**DRESSING** — A protective covering for a wound; used to stop bleeding and to prevent contamination of the wound.

**DROPLET CONTACT** — A means of transmitting a communicable disease indirectly by spray droplets from an infected person's coughing or sneezing.

**DYSCONJUGATE GAZE** — A condition in which the two eyes are not aligned, but stare in different directions.

**DYSPNEA** — Painful or difficult breathing; usually used to mean rapid, shallow respirations.

## E

**ECCHYMOSIS** — Blood under the skin causing a black and blue mark; bruise.

**ECLAMPSIA** — A toxic condition of pregnancy, associated with high blood pressure, edema, convulsions, and possible coma.

**ECTOPIC PREGNANCY** — A pregnancy in which the fetus is implanted elsewhere than in the uterus such as in the fallopian tube or abdominal cavity.

**EDEMA** — A condition in which fluid escapes into the body tissues and causes local or generalized swelling.

**EMBOLISM** — The sudden blocking of an artery or vein by a clot or foreign material which has been carried by the blood.

**EMETIC** — An agent that causes vomiting.

**EMPHYSEMA** — A condition of the lungs in which there is destruction of the alveoli, resulting in labored breathing and increased susceptibility to infection.

**ENVENOMATION** — The poisonous effects caused by the bites, stings, or deposits of insects, spiders, snakes, or other poison-carrying animals.

**EPIDERMIS** — The outermost layer of skin; made up of durable waterproof cells and containing sensory nerve endings.

**EPIGLOTTIS** — An elastic cartilage located at the roof of the tongue that folds over the glottis to prevent food from entering the trachea during swallowing.

**EPIGLOTTITIS** — A bacterial infection occurring in children, marked by swelling of the epiglottis, high fever, pain on swallowing, and drooling; airway obstruction can result with great rapidity.

**EPILEPSY** — A chronic brain disorder marked by seizures; usually associated with alteration of consciousness, abnormal motor behavior, psychic or sensory disturbances.

**EPISTAXIS** — Nosebleed.

**ESOPHAGUS** — The portion of the digestive tract that lies between the throat and the stomach.

**EVISCERATION** — Protrusion of the intestines through an opening or wound.

**EXHALATION** — The act of breathing out; expiration.

## F

**FAHRENHEIT SCALE** — The temperature scale in which the freezing point is 32 degrees and the boiling point at sea level is 212 degrees.

**FAINTING** — A momentary loss of consciousness caused by insufficient blood supply to the brain; syncope.

**FALLOPIAN TUBES** — Paired structures of the female reproductive system that conduct eggs from the ovaries to the uterus.

**FEBRILE CONVULSIONS** — Convulsions brought on by fever; occur most often in children.

**FEMORAL ARTERY** — The principal artery of the thigh; pulse may be felt in the groin area.

**FEMUR** — The bone that extends from the pelvis to the knee; the longest and largest bone of the body; the thigh bone.

**FETUS** — An unborn child after the second month of pregnancy.

**FIBRILLATION** — Rapid, ineffective contraction of the heart.

**FIBULA** — The smaller of the two bones of the lower leg.

**FIRST-DEGREE BURN** — A burn affecting only the outer skin layers; characterized by redness and pain.

**FLAIL CHEST** — A condition in which several ribs are broken, each in at least two places.

**FLOATING RIBS** — The two lowest pairs of ribs, so called because they are connected only to vertebrae in the back.

**FRACTURE** — A break or rupture in a bone.

**FROSTBITE** — Local freezing and tissue damage due to prolonged exposure to extreme cold.

**FROSTNIP** — Superficial tissue damage caused by freezing; limited in scope and does not destroy the full thickness of skin.

**FUSED JOINT** — Bones joined to form a rigid structure, as in the skull.

## G

**GALLBLADDER** — The sac located just beneath the liver that concentrates and stores bile.

**GAMMA RAYS** — Electromagnetic radiation emitted from radioactive substances; similar to x-rays.

**GANGRENE** — Local tissue death as the result of an injury or inadequate blood supply; often caused by frostbite.

**GENITOURINARY SYSTEM** — The system that includes all the organs involved in reproduction and in the formation of voiding of urine.

**GLUCOSE** — A simple sugar.

**GRAND MAL** — See tonic-clonic seizure.

## H

**HEART** — A hollow muscular organ that receives the blood from the veins, sends it through the lungs to be oxygenated, then pumps it to the arteries.

**HEART ATTACK** — See Acute Myocardial Infarction.

**HEAT CRAMPS** — A heat illness resulting from prolonged exposure to high temperatures; characterized by excessive sweating, muscle cramps in the abdomen and legs, faintness, dizziness, and exhaustion.

**HEAT EXHAUSTION** — Heat illness caused by exposure to excessive heat; symptoms include weakness, cold and clammy skin, heavy perspiration, rapid, shallow breathing, weak pulse, dizziness, sometimes unconsciousness.

**HEAT STROKE (Sunstroke)** — Heat illness caused by heat exposure, resulting in failure of the body's heat-regulating mechanism; symptoms include high fever of 105 - 106°F; dry, red, hot skin; rapid, strong pulse; and deep breaths, convulsions; coma; possible death.

**HEMATOMA** — A localized collection of blood in an organ, tissue, or space as a result of injury or a broken blood vessel.

**HEMORRHAGE** — Profuse discharge of blood.

**HIVES** — Red or white raised patches on the skin, often attended by severe itching; a characteristic reaction in allergic responses.

**HUMERUS** — The bone of the upper arm.

**HYPERGLYCEMIA** — Excessive sugar in the blood due to lack of insulin to metabolize the sugar; also known as diabetic ketoacidosis.

**HYPERTENSION** — High blood pressure; higher blood pressure than normal.

**HYPOGLYCEMIA** — Condition in which the level of sugar in the blood is abnormally low; can be life-threatening.

**HYPOTENSION** — Low blood pressure; lower blood pressure than normal.

**HYPOTHERMIA** — Abnormally low body temperature.

**HYPOVOLEMIC SHOCK** — Shock caused by loss of blood.

## I

**ILIUM** — One of the two large bones that form the winged portion of the pelvic girdle.

**IMMOBILIZATION** — To hold a part firmly in place, as with a splint.

**IMPALED OBJECT** — An object that has caused a puncture wound and remains embedded in the wound.

**INFERIOR** — Near the feet; below.

**INGESTION** — Taking in food or other substances through the mouth.

**INHALATION** — The drawing of air or other substances into the lungs.

**INSULIN** — Hormone produced by the pancreas; its function is to regulate the level of sugar in the blood.

**INTERCOSTAL MUSCLES** — Muscles between the ribs.

**INTESTINE** — The portion of the digestive tube that extends from the stomach to the anus.

**INVOLUNTARY MUSCLE** — A muscle that acts without voluntary control.

**IPECAC SYRUP** — A medication used to induce vomiting.

**IRIS** — The colored portion of the eye that surrounds the pupil.

**ISCHIUM** — One of the two bones that form the lower portion of the pelvic girdle.

## J

**JOINT** — The point at which two or more bones come together.

**JUGULAR VEIN** — Large vein on either side of the neck.

## K

**KIDNEYS** — Paired organs located toward the rear wall of the abdominal cavity; their function is to filter blood and produce urine.

**KUSSMAUL'S RESPIRATION** — Deep, rapid, respirations characteristic of hyperglycemia, or diabetic ketoacidosis, that result as the body tries to eliminate excess carbon dioxide.

## L

**LABOR** — The muscular contractions of the uterus designed to expel the fetus from the mother.

**LACERATION** — A jagged tear or wound.

**LARGE INTESTINE** — Hollow structure of the gastrointestinal tract located just below the stomach.

**LARYNGECTOMEE** — A person who has undergone a total or partial surgical removal of the larynx.

**LARYNGECTOMY** — The surgical removal of the larynx.

**LARYNGOSPASM** — A severe constriction of the vocal cords, often in response to allergy or drowning.

**LARYNX** — The organ of voice production.

**LATERAL** — Toward the side of the body.

**LENS** — The portion of the eye that focuses light rays onto the retina.

**LIGAMENT** — A tough band of fibrous tissue that connects bone to bone or that supports any organ.

**LIMB PRESENTATION** — A delivery in which the presenting part of a fetus is an arm or a leg.

**LIVER** — Large solid organ of the abdominal cavity located just below the diaphragm, it secretes bile and performs many important bodily functions.

**LOG ROLL** — A method for placing a patient on a backboard by turning the patient as a unit, first onto the side, then on the back.

**LOWER AIRWAY** — The portion of the respiratory system below the epiglottis.

**LUMBAR SPINE** — The portion of the spinal column formed by the five vertebrae extending from just below the ribs to the pelvis; the lower back.

**LUNGS** — The paired organs of respiration that lie in the chest.

## M

**MANDIBLE** — The lower jaw bone.

**MAST** — Abbreviation for medical antishock trousers, or military antishock trousers; used to counteract the effects of heavy blood loss.

**MAXILLA** — The upper jaw bone.

**MEDIAL** — Toward the midline of the body.

**MEDULLA OBLONGATA** — The small posterior portion of the brain continuous with the spinal cord; contains the centers for respiratory control, heartbeat, and other major control centers.

**MEMBRANE** — A thin sheath or layer of pliable tissue that covers a part; the lining of a cavity.

**METABOLISM** — The conversion of food into energy and waste products.

**METACARPAL BONES** — The five bones of the hand extending from the wrist to the fingers.

**METATARSAL BONES** — The five bones of the foot extending from the ankles to the toes.

**MISCARRIAGE** — A lay term for a premature expulsion of a fetus from the uterus, that occurs naturally.

**MOTOR NERVES** — Nerves that carry impulses from the brain to the muscles.

**MUCOUS MEMBRANE** — A membrane that lines many organs of the body and contains mucus-secreting glands.

**MUCUS** — A slippery secretion that lubricates and protects various body structures.

**MULTIPARA** — A woman who has previously given birth.

**MUSCLE** — A tissue composed of elongated cells that has the ability to contract when stimulated, thus causing bones and joints to move.

## N

**NASAL CANNULA** — A small tubular prong that fits into the patient's nostril to provide supplemental oxygen; usually there are two, one for each nostril.

**NAUSEA** — An unpleasant sensation often resulting in vomiting.

**NERVOUS SYSTEM** — The brain, spinal cord, and nerve branches from the central, peripheral, and autonomic systems.

**NEUROGENIC SHOCK** — Failure of the circulatory system to fill enlarged blood vessels resulting from an injury to the nervous system.

**NITROGLYCERIN** — A drug used in the treatment of angina pectoris, usually taken under the tongue.

## O

**OCCLUSIVE DRESSING** — A watertight dressing for a wound.

**ORBITS** — The bony cavities in the skull that hold the eyeballs.

**ORAL AIRWAY** — A device inserted in the patient's upper airway in order to keep the tongue from blocking the airway.

**OVARIES** — Paired female reproductive organs located in the lower portion of the abdominal cavity.

**OXYGEN** — A colorless, odorless, tasteless gas essential to life and comprising 21 percent of the atmosphere; chemical formula: $O_2$.

**OXYGEN MASK** — A device that fits over a patient's nose and mouth; used to administer supplemental oxygen.

## P

**PALLOR** — A paleness of the skin.

**PALPATE** — To examine by feeling and pressing with the palms and the fingers.

**PANCREAS** — Digestive organ of the abdominal cavity; secretes insulin and other important digestive juices.

**PARADOXICAL MOVEMENT** — The motion of an injured section of a flail chest; opposite to the normal movement of the chest wall.

**PARALYSIS** — A loss of the ability to move a body part.

**PATELLA** — "Floating" bone supported by the tendon of the quadriceps muscle; kneecap.

**PELVIC CAVITY** — The lowermost portion of the abdominal cavity containing the rectum, urinary bladder, and, in the female, the internal sex organs.

**PELVIS** — The large bony ring formed by the sacrum and the two hip bones.

**PENIS** — The male organ of urinary discharge and copulation.

**PERFUSION** — The act of pouring through or into; the process of supplying oxygen and nutrients to the body's cells.

**PERIPHERAL NERVOUS SYSTEM** — The portion of the nervous system consisting of the nerves outside the brain and the spinal column.

**PHALANGES** — The bones of the fingers or toes.

**PHARYNX** — The portion of the airway between the nasal cavity and the larynx.

**PHOBIA** — An abnormal and persistent fear of a specific object or situation.

**PLACENTA** — A vascular organ attached to the uterine wall that supplies oxygen and nutrients to the fetus; also called the afterbirth.

**PLACENTA PREVIA** — Location of the placenta close to the opening of the uterus, rather than high in the uterus as it should be.

**PLASMA** — The fluid portion of the blood.

**PLATELETS** — Cellular components of the blood that promote clotting.

**PLEURA** — A continuous membrane that lines the outer surface of the lungs and the internal surface of the thoracic cavity.

**PNEUMONIA** — An acute infectious disease of the lungs.

**PNEUMOTHORAX** — An accumulation of air in the pleural cavity, usually after a wound or injury that penetrates the chest wall or lacerates the lung.

**POPLITEAL ARTERY** — The continuation of the femoral artery in the area behind the knee joint.

**POSTERIOR** — At or toward the back.

**PREECLAMPSIA** — The condition that precedes eclampsia, or toxemia of pregnancy, characterized by high blood pressure, edema, and headache.

**PRESENTING PART** — The part of the baby that emerges first during delivery.

**PRESSURE POINT** — One of several places on the body where blood flow to that area can be restricted by pressing the artery against an underlying bone.

**PRIAPISM** — A persistent erection of the penis due to spinal cord injury.

**PRIMIPARA** — A woman who is about to give birth for the first time.

**PROLAPSED CORD** — A delivery in which the umbilical cord appears at the vaginal opening before the head of the infant.

**PRONE** — A position of lying face down.

**PROXIMAL** — Located near the trunk of the body.

**PSYCHOMOTOR SEIZURE** — A seizure characterized by an altered personality state; in some patients, psychomotor seizures result in unexplained attacks of rage or stereotyped behavior.

**PUBIS** — One of two bones that form the anterior portion of the pelvic girdle.

**PULMONARY ARTERY** — The major artery leading from the right ventricle to the lungs.

**PULMONARY EMBOLISM** — Obstruction of the pulmonary arteries by foreign substance or blood clot.

**PULMONARY VEINS** — The veins that carry oxygenated blood from the lungs to the left atrium.

**PULSE** — Rhythmic throbbing caused by expansion and contraction of arterial walls as blood passes through them.

**PUNCTURE WOUND** — An open wound caused when an ice pick, knife, or other pointed object pierces the skin.

**PUPIL** — The small opening in the center of the iris.

## Q

**QUADRANT** — One of the four quarters of the abdomen.

## R

**RADIAL ARTERY** — One of the major arteries of the forearm; the pulse can be felt at the base of the thumb.

**RADIUS** — The bone on the thumb side of the forearm.

**RAPE** — Sexual intercourse by force.

**RED BLOOD CELLS** — Cellular components of the blood that transport oxygen from the lungs to body tissues and carbon dioxide from the tissues to the lungs.

**REPRODUCTIVE SYSTEM** — The body system that includes all the organs necessary for reproduction.

**RESPIRATION** — The act of breathing; the exchange of oxygen and carbon dioxide in the tissues and lungs.

**RESPIRATORY ARREST** — The cessation of breathing.

**RESUSCITATION** — The act of reviving an unconscious patient.

**RETINA** — The lining of the back of the eye that receives visual images and transmits them to the brain.

**RIB CAGE** — The skeletal framework of the chest; composed of the sternum, the ribs, and the thoracic vertebrae.

**RIGHT HEART FAILURE** — The failure of the right ventricle to pump blood effectively, causing back-up of blood into the veins.

## S

**SACRUM** — The portion of the spinal column just below the lumbar spine formed by five vertebrae fused with the pelvis.

**SCAPULA** — The shoulder blade.

**SCLERA** — The white portion of the eyeball.

**SECOND-DEGREE BURN** — A burn penetrating beneath the superficial skin layers, producing edema and blisters.

**SEIZURES** — Intense, involuntary muscular contractions caused by abnormal electrical impulses in the brain.

**SEMINAL VESICLES** — Storage area for sperm and seminal fluid in the male reproductive system.

**SENSORY NERVES** — Nerves that conduct impulses from the skin and other sensory organs to the brain.

**SHOCK** — Failure of the circulatory system to provide sufficient blood to all parts of the body; results in depression of bodily functions and eventually death if not controlled.

**SIGN** — Evidence of illness or injury that can be observed by others.

**SIMPLE FRACTURE** — A fracture in which the skin overlying the broken bone is intact.

**SKELETON** — The hard, bony structure that forms the main support of the body.

**SKIN** — The outer covering of the body, and the largest organ of the body; consisting of the dermis and the epidermis; contains various sensory and regulatory mechanisms.

**SKULL** — The bony structure surrounding the brain; consists of the cranial bones, the facial bones, and the teeth.

**SMALL INTESTINE** — The portion of the intestine between the stomach and colon.

**SPHYGMOMANOMETER** — A device for measuring blood pressure.

**SPINAL COLUMN** — Flexible bony structure that supports the central part of the body and encloses the spinal cord.

**SPINAL CORD** — The part of the central nervous system contained within the spinal column, extending from the base of the brain to the coccyx.

**SPLEEN** — Solid organ of the abdominal cavity.

**SPLINT** — Any support used to immobilize a fracture or to restrict movement of a part.

**STATUS ASTHMATICUS** — A severe, prolonged asthmatic attack that cannot be broken with epinephrine.

**STATUS EPILEPTICUS** — The occurrence of two or more seizures without a period of complete consciousness between them.

**STERNUM** — The breast bone.

**STILLBIRTH** — The birth of a dead fetus.

**STOMA** — A small opening, especially an artificially created opening.

**STOMACH** — Hollow digestive organ of the abdominal cavity.

**STROKE** — A hemorrhage or blood clot within a blood vessel in the brain; also known as cerebrovascular accident.

**SUBCUTANEOUS LAYER** — Bottom layer of skin consisting of fatty tissues that insulate the body and store excess calories.

**SUCKING CHEST WOUND** — A wound in which the chest wall is penetrated, causing air to accumulate in the pleural cavity.

**SUDDEN INFANT DEATH SYNDROME (SIDS)** — A sudden, unexplained death of an infant within the first six months of life; crib death.

**SUPERIOR** — Near the head, above.

**SUPINE** — Lying horizontal in a face-upward position.

**SUPINE HYPOTENSIVE SYNDROME** — Condition during pregnancy or delivery in which the weight of the uterus pressing the inferior vena cava against the spine diminishes the flow of blood returning to the heart. To remedy, turn the woman on her side.

**SYMPHYSIS PUBIS** — The juncture of the two pubic bones.

**SYMPTOM** — A sensation or awareness of disturbance of bodily function as reported by the patient.

**SYNCOPE** — Fainting; a brief period of unconsciousness.

## T

**TARSALS** — The seven bones of the ankle.

**TEMPORAL ARTERY** — The artery located on either side of the face above and in front of the upper portion of the ear; supplies blood to the scalp.

**TENDONS** — Tough bands of inelastic tissue that connect muscles to bones.

**TESTICLES** — Paired glands of the male reproductive system that manufacture male hormones and seminal fluid.

**THIRD-DEGREE BURN** — A full-thickness burn destroying all skin layers and underlying tissue; has a charred or white, leathery appearance; insensitive.

**THORACIC SPINE** — The portion of the spinal column to which the ribs are attached.

**THORAX** — The portion of the body between the neck and the diaphragm; the chest.

**THREADY PULSE** — A pulse that is very weak, characteristic of a person in shock.

**TIBIA** — The larger bone of the lower leg; shin bone.

**TONIC-CLONIC SEIZURE**— A generalized seizure characterized by loss of consciousness; severe muscle contractions; and, sometimes, tongue biting, loss of bladder control, and mental confusion; also known as grand mal seizure.

**TOURNIQUET** — Any wide, flat material wrapped around a limb and tightened to stop bleeding; used only for severe, life-threatening hemorrhage that cannot be controlled by other means.

**TOXEMIA OF PREGNANCY** — See Eclampsia.

**TRACHEA** — Tubular structure of the respiratory system descending from the pharynx to the bronchi.

**TRACTION** — The act of exerting a pulling force.

**TRANSIENT ISCHEMIC ATTACK (TIA)** — Temporary blockage of an artery in the brain.

**TRIAGE** — A system used for sorting patients to determine the order in which they will receive medical attention.

## U

**UMBILICAL CORD** — A flexible cord connecting the fetus to the placenta.

**UPPER AIRWAY** — The portion of the respiratory system above the epiglottis.

**URETERS** — Paired tubes that conduct urine from the kidneys to the bladder.

**URINARY BLADDER** — Hollow organ of the urinary system that serves as a storage place for urine until it is discharged from the body.

**UTERUS** — Muscular, pear-shaped organ of the female reproductive system.

## V

**VAGINA** — Muscular, tubular structure of the female reproductive system extending from the uterus to the vulva.

**VAS DEFERENS** — Seminal duct extending from the testicles to the seminal vesicles in the male reproductive system.

**VEIN** — Any blood vessel that carries blood from the tissues to the heart.

**VENA CAVA** — The largest vein in the body.

**VENTRICLE** — Lower chamber of the left or right side of the heart.

**VERTEBRA** — Any one of the 33 bones of the spinal column.

**VITAL SIGNS** — Indicators of a patient's condition that reflect temperature, pulse, respirations, and blood pressure.

**VITREOUS FLUID** — A jellylike, transparent substance filling the inside of the eyeball.

**VULVA** — The external female genitalia.

## W

**WHEEZING** — Breathing noisily and with difficulty.

**WINDPIPE** — The trachea.

**WOMB** — The uterus.

## X-Y-Z

**XIPHOID PROCESS** — The flexible cartilage at the lower tip of the sternum.

# 1

# Introduction

**U.S. DEPARTMENT OF TRANSPORTATION**
**First Responder Training Course**

**Objectives:**

- State the three major roles and responsibilities of the first responder.
- Describe all applicable legal aspects related to providing emergency care as a first responder.

# Chapter 1
# Introduction

## THE FIRST RESPONDER

The fire service has traditionally responded to rescue calls as well as report of fire. Today that rescue role has expanded tremendously; the public expects the fire department to respond to calls of emergency illness or injury as well. Firefighters have emerged as an integral part of the emergency medical system. This system is designed to stabilize a patient and provide life support until the patient reaches the hospital. The faster trained help can be summoned, the better the patient's chances for survival.

As the role of the fire department in emergency medical services has expanded, so have the medical skills possessed by firefighters. The needs and resources of a community dictate whether it will require firefighters trained in basic or advanced life support techniques. But all departments that are part of an EMS system will train firefighters at least to the level of first responder.

The first responder is likely to be one of the first persons to arrive at a medical emergency scene. The care and treatment provided by a firefighter trained as a first responder may make the difference between the patient living or dying. A first responder is also able to provide valuable information and assistance to other members of the emergency medical system, such as EMTs and paramedics.

The skills, knowledge, and abilities of the first responder extend far beyond first aid. The first responder is trained in evaluating and treating patients with serious injuries or illnesses, and is competent in using a variety of medical equipment and supplies.

The emergency medical care rendered by the first responder includes treatment for both injuries and illnesses. Some examples of treatment are controlling bleeding, treating shock and burns, dealing with diabetic states, and administering cardiopulmonary resuscitation. Providing emotional support to a family member of a seriously injured person or to someone involved in an accident may also be necessary. Whatever the problem, the first responder will be the one to administer care to the patient until additional help arrives.

## THE EMS SYSTEM

The goal of an EMS system is to provide organized, rapid, quality care to persons suffering from sudden injury or illness. The fire service is most often concerned with providing either all or a portion of the care that the patient receives between the time of the incident and arrival at a medical facility. Other elements of the EMS system such as private ambulance services, hospital emergency room personnel, municipal safety officers, and law enforcement personnel provide additional services necessary to maintain EMS as a system.

The EMS system has six links in its part of the chain: communications, transportation, training,

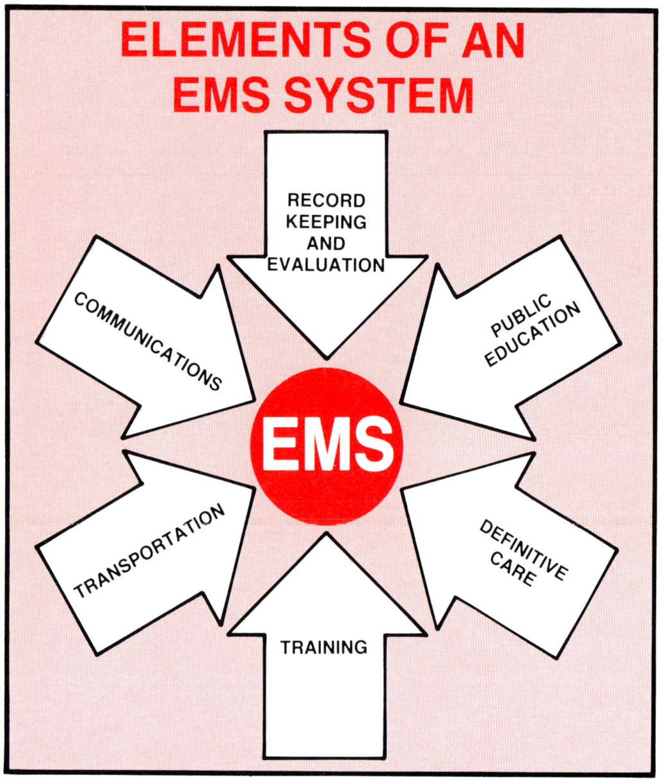


**Figure 1.1** An emergency medical system is composed of many parts; all must work together smoothly to provide quality care for the patient.

definitive care, public education, and record keeping and evaluation (Figure 1.1).

- Communications includes citizens to EMS, dispatcher to EMS team, and EMT/paramedic to doctor.
- Transportation has two elements: getting the properly trained personnel and equipment to the scene of an emergency, and getting the patient to the medical facility equipped to give the best care. The first responder usually does not transport patients, but has an important role in summoning additional equipment and personnel to the scene.
- Training covers all aspects of professional training and education for members of the EMS team.
- Definitive care refers to the medical facility that will take care of the patient, such as a burn center, poison center, or general hospital. The first responder should know the location of each facility in the area and how long it takes to get there.
- Public education involves letting the public know how the EMS system works and how to work with the EMS system more efficiently.
- Record keeping and evaluation help determine how efficient the EMS system is and how it can be improved. Complete records are also vital in case the first responder becomes a witness or defendent in a lawsuit.

## EQUIPMENT AND SUPPLIES FOR THE FIRST RESPONDER

The equipment carried by the first responder is only that needed to help stabilize and comfort the patient until other emergency medical personnel arrive. The minimum equipment needed is as follows:

EMERGENCY MEDICAL CARE EQUIPMENT

- Triangular bandages
- Roller-type bandages
- Universal dressings/gauze pads
- Occlusive dressing
- Adhesive tape
- Bandage shears
- Eye protector (paper cup or cone)
- Stick (for impaled object/tourniquet)
- Blanket
- Pillow
- Penlight
- Upper extremity splint (set)
- Lower extremity splint (set)
- Oxygen equipment and masks*
- Bag-valve-mask resuscitator*
- Oropharyngeal airways (adult and child)*
- Cervical collars*
- Stethoscope*
- Sphygmomanometer*
- Short and long spine boards*

*If personnel are trained to use this equipment.

CAR TOOLS AND MISCELLANEOUS EQUIPMENT

- Jack
- Jack handle
- Cribbing
- Pliers
- Ropes or chains
- Halligan bar, pry axe, or crash axe
- Screwdriver
- Hammer
- Knife

## ROLES AND RESPONSIBILITIES OF THE FIRST RESPONDER

The three major goals of the first responder with respect to patient care are

1. Gaining access to the patient using simple tools
2. Providing emergency care with minimal equipment
3. Lifting and moving the patient if such movement is required

At an emergency scene, the first responder's primary responsibility is to the patient; all activities are performed with this goal in mind. However, as the first-arriving unit on the scene, first responders may be called upon to handle any or all of the following duties to ensure the safety of the patient, other emergency responders, and others at the scene.

- Protect involved parties from approaching passing traffic.
- Avoid any unnecessary blockage of the roadway. Stopped traffic, especially on high-speed highways, can lead to additional accidents.
- Summon appropriate help, such as EMTs, additional fire department units, police, rescue groups, power company.
- Gain access to the patient, using simple hand tools if needed.
- Provide treatment for the patient.
- Lift or move the patient, if needed, without causing additional injuries.
- Stabilize or improve the patient's condition until other emergency specialists arrive.

When emergency medical technicians arrive, the first responder will relinquish the patient(s) to their care, assisting as necessary. Therefore, the first responder must be knowledgeable about more advanced lifesaving procedures performed by EMTs and paramedics in order to provide competent assistance.

## PROFESSIONAL APPEARANCE AND BEHAVIOR

As with any encounter, the first impression is a lasting one. Physical and personal appearance will make a strong impression on the public and patients. Numerous statistical studies have shown that a first responder who is neat and well groomed promotes in the patient's mind the belief that the first responder is competent and professional. Conversely, a slovenly appearance leads the patient to doubt the first responder's capabilities. High health care standards depend on cleanliness and sanitation, so be sure that the emergency vehicle and emergency care equipment are clean and presentable for public inspection at all times (Figure 1.2).

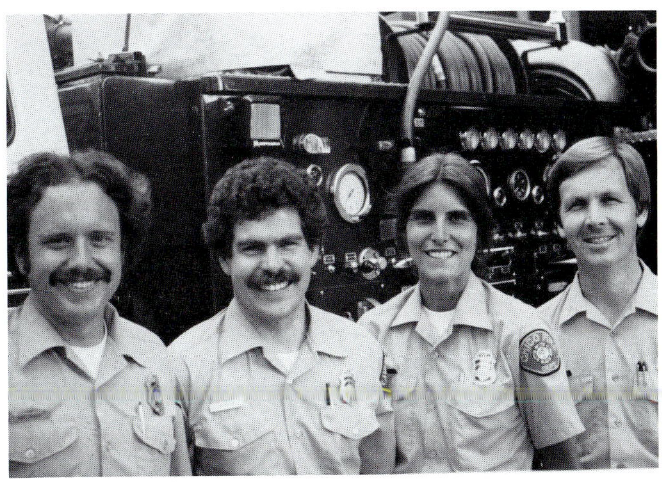

**Figure 1.2** Patients will have more confidence in first responders who are neat and well-groomed. *Courtesy of Chico, California Fire Department.*

Professional behavior is just as important as a professional appearance. Professional behavior consists of speaking politely, showing concern for the patient and family, and helping each patient to the best of one's abilities, even the obnoxious or rude patients. Since establishing trust is crucial when working with patients, displaying a manner that is kind, positive, and professional will make the patient and family much more likely to communicate in a helpful way. Conversely, a hostile, sarcastic, or indifferent manner will only cause other people to behave the same way. Swearing, making jokes or disparaging remarks about the patient, family, or surroundings are unprofessional and will only create hostility. Such unprofessional behavior can only have a negative effect on the care given to the patient and may upset the family so much that they decide to take legal action. Keep negative opinions unsaid and let off steam in private if necessary.

## LEGAL ISSUES CONCERNING EMERGENCY MEDICAL CARE

### Duty to Act

Being trained as a first responder does not obligate an individual to stop and give help at an emergency. However, employees whose job includes being dispatched on emergency medical calls have a duty to provide assistance to the best of their abilities and training.

### Abandonment

Once emergency aid is begun, the first responder is legally required to remain and continue treatment until another person trained in emergency medical procedures arrives and takes over. Any attempts by the first responder to discontinue treatment and leave or "abandon" the patient are grounds for legal action under the laws concerning abandonment.

### Standard of Care

Standards of care have been developed to ensure quality care for an individual who is injured or suddenly taken ill. These standards spell out actions that should or should not be taken by personnel at all levels of an EMS system. The elements that make up a standard of care include the following:

- Actions expected by a certain type of individual. For example, the first responder is expected to provide the level and type of care that a reasonable person with the same amount of training would be expected to provide given the same equipment and circumstances.
- Standards imposed by law. These include statutes, ordinances, case law, or administrative orders.
- Professional or institutional standards. These standards are published recommendations or specific rules of procedure developed by organizations and societies involved in emergency work (such as rules for administering CPR published by the American Heart Association).

It is important to know exactly what the local standards of care are and what statutes or orders pertain to the local community.

### Good Samaritan Laws

Many states have implemented "Good Samaritan" laws to protect physicians and other emergency personnel from legal actions that arise from emergency treatment outside of a medical facility. The typical Good Samaritan law requires that persons responding to an emergency do all that they can within their abilities to sustain life and to prevent further injury.

Good Samaritan legislation does not protect an individual from responsibility for negligence or from failure to provide the proper standard of care. The most likely reasons for a lawsuit are

- Failing to provide care
- Giving improper care
- Abusing or mistreating a patient
- Giving care above the level of training
- Forcing care on a competent adult who has refused treatment
- Violating laws that deal with the operation of an emergency vehicle, such as driving recklessly

The best ways to guard against the possibility of a lawsuit are to follow established procedures and protocols, to give care to the best of one's ability, and to maintain skills through continuing education.

## Consent

Anyone who treats a patient must obtain that person's consent. Obtaining consent is necessary because it is illegal to force a competent adult to accept treatment and is grounds for a lawsuit. Become familiar with state and local laws that cover consent for adults, children (minors), and special categories such as mentally ill or violent persons.

There are three levels of consent: voluntary, involuntary, and implied. The best form of consent is voluntary, or expressed. Expressed consent means that the patient gives verbal or physical agreement to treatment. Involuntary consent arises from the legal system. patients in the custody of the law, or such persons as the mentally ill who are in the custody of the State and are being treated by court order. The last level of consent is implied, which arises when the patient is unable to communicate the wish for treatment. The legal system assumes that such a person, say someone who is unconscious, would give consent for treatment if able to do so.

## Adult Consent

Every conscious, competent adult must give consent for treatment. The patient consents to treatment by requesting help and by responding to questions. Consent must be informed; the patient must understand what is to be done and the reasons why. Consent is implied when the patient is unconscious, disoriented, or too severely injured to make a clear decision.

## Consent for Minors or Mentally Incompetent

Generally, a parent or legal guardian has the right to give consent for treating a minor (usually someone under the age of 18) or an adult who has been declared mentally incompetent. If the patient appears to be suffering from a life-threatening condition and no parent or guardian is available, begin emergency treatment. Hospital personnel can obtain permission to proceed with further treatment if necessary.

## Right to Refuse Treatment

An adult who is conscious and in a competent state has the right to refuse treatment. This refusal can be for any reason, and may include religious reasons or objection to particular medical treatment. If the patient truly seems to be suffering from a life-threatening condition, make every effort to persuade the person to consent to treatment. If the patient still refuses treatment, document the refusal on the patient care form and have the patient sign it. It is also useful to have an impartial observer. The patient care form should contain a complete description of the patient's condition, the number of times consent was requested, and the patient's responses. DO NOT try to restrain the individual or try to provide treatment.

Very rarely, a parent may refuse permission - usually on moral, ethical, or religious grounds to treat a seriously ill child. If this happens, make every effort to convince the parent of the seriousness of the problem and the necessity for treatment. If this is unsuccessful, summon the police and make every effort to have the court juvenile authorities order the child's treatment. These procedures vary from state to state, so become familiar with the regulations put forth by your state's district attorney or attorney general.

Occasionally, on examination a child may appear to have been abused. Almost all states require that any reasonable suspicions that a child has been physically, emotionally, or mentally abused be reported to the proper authorities.

Psychiatric emergencies present difficult problems of consent and often require police assistance. If the patient refuses consent for treatment, do not intervene unless that person is about to do life-threatening harm to him/herself or others. Under most conditions, a police officer is the only person with the authority to restrain and transport a person against that individual's will. The violent patient may have to be restrained by police officers to prevent harm to emergency health care workers and others. Each EMS system should have procedures for dealing with psychiatric emergencies based on local laws and policies. For more information on dealing with behavioral emergencies, see Chapter 11, Behavioral Emergencies.

## STRESS

The job of a firefighter is a stressful one. The firefighter must often endure long hours of relative inactivity, yet be ready for intense, all-out effort at the sound of an alarm. Not knowing exactly what awaits at the emergency, coupled with the dangers of fire fighting, adds to the stress commonly experienced by the firefighter.

Emergency medical calls add another level of stress. EMS calls usually outnumber fire calls by at least three to one. People are extremely unpredictable, and first responders can, and do, encounter people who are hostile, psychologically disturbed, burned, bleeding, vomiting, or severely injured. The circumstances at the emergency scene can also contribute to the stress of a medical call. First responders may encounter people who speak little or no English, hysterical relatives, angry crowds, and unpleasant or dangerous surroundings. Furthermore, any emergency call is more stressful if the patient is a child.

Administrative and political matters, such as long hours, low pay, lack of departmental support, and fear of lawsuits may also add to job stress and dissatisfaction. People naturally have other sources of stress that are not related to their jobs, but that affect their job performance: family relations, finances, and health matters, to name a few.

All these sources of stress, if not vented or managed properly, can contribute to a condition known as *burnout*. Burnout manifests itself in a number of ways:

- Poor attitude toward work
- Increased illness, resulting in loss of time from work
- Constant complaining
- Arguing with coworkers
- Expressing disgust or showing anger toward patients
- Lack of interest in maintaining or increasing job skills
- Depression
- Insomnia
- Substance abuse: drinking, drug use

The firefighter first responder who is suffering from burnout will become a danger to both him or herself and to patients if appropriate action is not taken to alleviate stress. Two stress relievers - someone to talk to and regular exercise - are particularly effective. Firefighters who can vent their feelings and frustrations without fear of punishment may experience a significant reduction in stress. Exercise is very beneficial: physical activity is a well-known stress reliever. A reduction in work hours or temporary shift to a station with lighter duties may be helpful. Professional counseling should be encouraged if necessary. If firefighters have participated in an especially large or horrifying incident, counseling should be looked at as a necessity, not an option. Nightmares, flashbacks, and other psychological problems are normal after such incidents, and professional assistance is needed to help individuals cope with their feelings. Professional assistance may also be useful in teaching firefighters stress reduction techniques and the value of following a balanced diet and health maintenance program. Substance abuse, of course, has no place either on the fireground or at an emergency medical call, so individuals whose stress manifests itself in this way must be referred to a drug or alcohol treatment center.

# 2

# Overview of the Human Body

**NFPA STANDARD 1001**
**EMERGENCY MEDICAL CARE**
**Fire Fighter II**

**4-4.12** The fire fighter shall identify the anatomical process of breathing.



**U.S. DEPARTMENT OF TRANSPORTATION**
**First Responder Training Course**

**Objectives:**

- Starting with the head and working to the feet, identify the major body components, cavities and organs.
- Given the name of each body system, identify its function.
- Given two or more body parts, describe their relationship using the terminology of topographic anatomy.
- State the time in which brain cells will die without oxygen.
- Identify the control center for breathing.
- Identify and describe the function of each of the components of the respiratory system, and describe how air travels through the system to exchange oxygen and waste gases with the body.
- Explain how the diaphragm, rib muscles and pleura operate to permit breathing.

# Chapter 2
# Overview of the Human Body

Familiarity with the human body and its systems is essential to emergency medical care work. A working knowledge of body functions and medical terminology is necessary to conduct a patient examination, provide appropriate emergency medical care, communicate with other emergency care providers and members of the medical community, and to keep accurate reports of medical calls.

The major body systems are

- Skeletal system
- Muscular system (also referred to as the musculoskeletal system)
- Nervous system
- Respiratory system
- Circulatory system
- Digestive system
- Genitourinary system

In addition, the body has several major cavities: the cranial cavity, thoracic (chest) cavity, abdominal cavity, and pelvic cavity. These cavities contain the organs that carry on the processes vital to life, such as breathing, circulation, and digestion.

## TOPOGRAPHIC ANATOMY

Topographic anatomy is a way of describing the relationship of one part of the body to another. This system helps to describe locations and indicate directions on the body. Using standard topographical terms allows any other member of the emergency care team to understand exactly which parts of the body are being described.

Left and right always refer to the *patient's* left or right. If you were to visualize the patient standing in front of you, facing you, the patient's left side would be your right, and his or her right side would be your left side. If you were to draw a vertical line down the middle of the patient's body, locations nearer to the line are called medial, while locations farther from the line are called lateral (Figure 2.1).

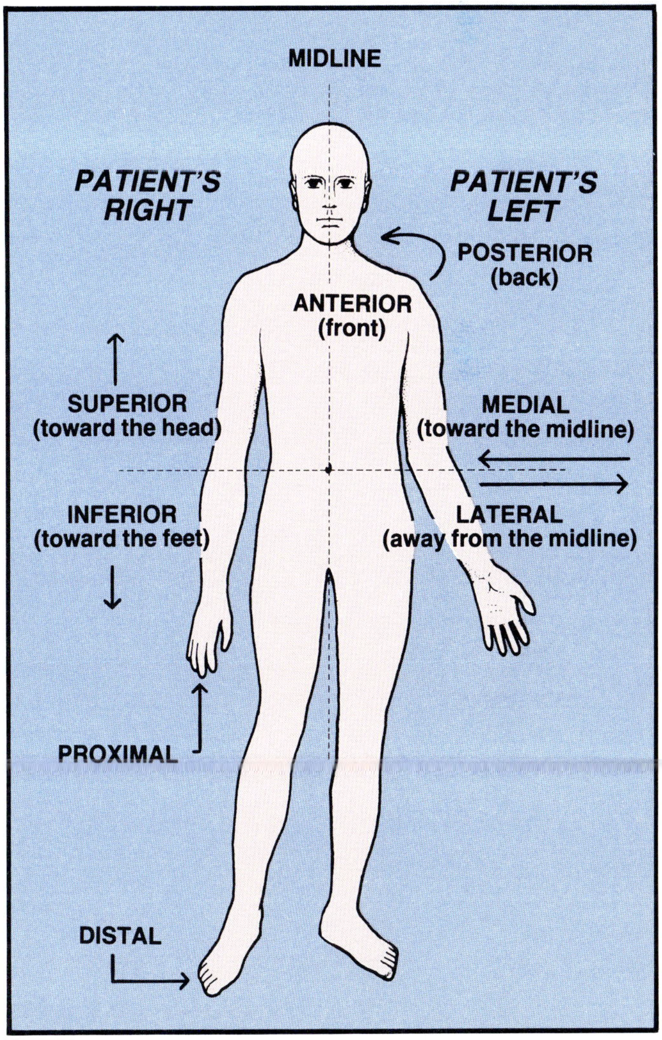


**Figure 2.1** The use of standard topographical terms allows members of the emergency care team to avoid confusion when describing parts of the body.

If you were to draw an imaginary horizontal line through the patient's midsection, those parts of the body that are closer to the head are called superior. The parts nearer to the feet are called inferior.

Anterior and posterior simply mean front and back. The patient's front is the anterior surface, and the patient's back is the posterior surface. These terms may also be used relative to one another, for example, indicating that something is anterior or posterior to something else.

Proximal and distal describe locations relative to places where the arms and legs are joined to the body. A part that is nearer to the point of attachment is said to be proximal, while a part that is farther from the point of attachment is said to be distal.

## SKELETAL SYSTEM

The skeletal system, which is composed of 206 bones, is the supporting framework for the human body (Figure 2.2). The skeleton protects vital organs and serves as the foundation to which muscles, flesh, and tendons are attached. Bones are classified according to their shape as either long, short, flat, or irregular. The femur (upper leg bone) is an example of a long bone, while the bones of the hands are short bones. The sternum (breastbone) is a flat bone and the vertebrae (spinal column) are irregular bones.

### Skull

The skull is composed of 22 bones, eight of which are closely fused to form the upper portion, or cranium (brain case) (Figure 2.3). All bones are

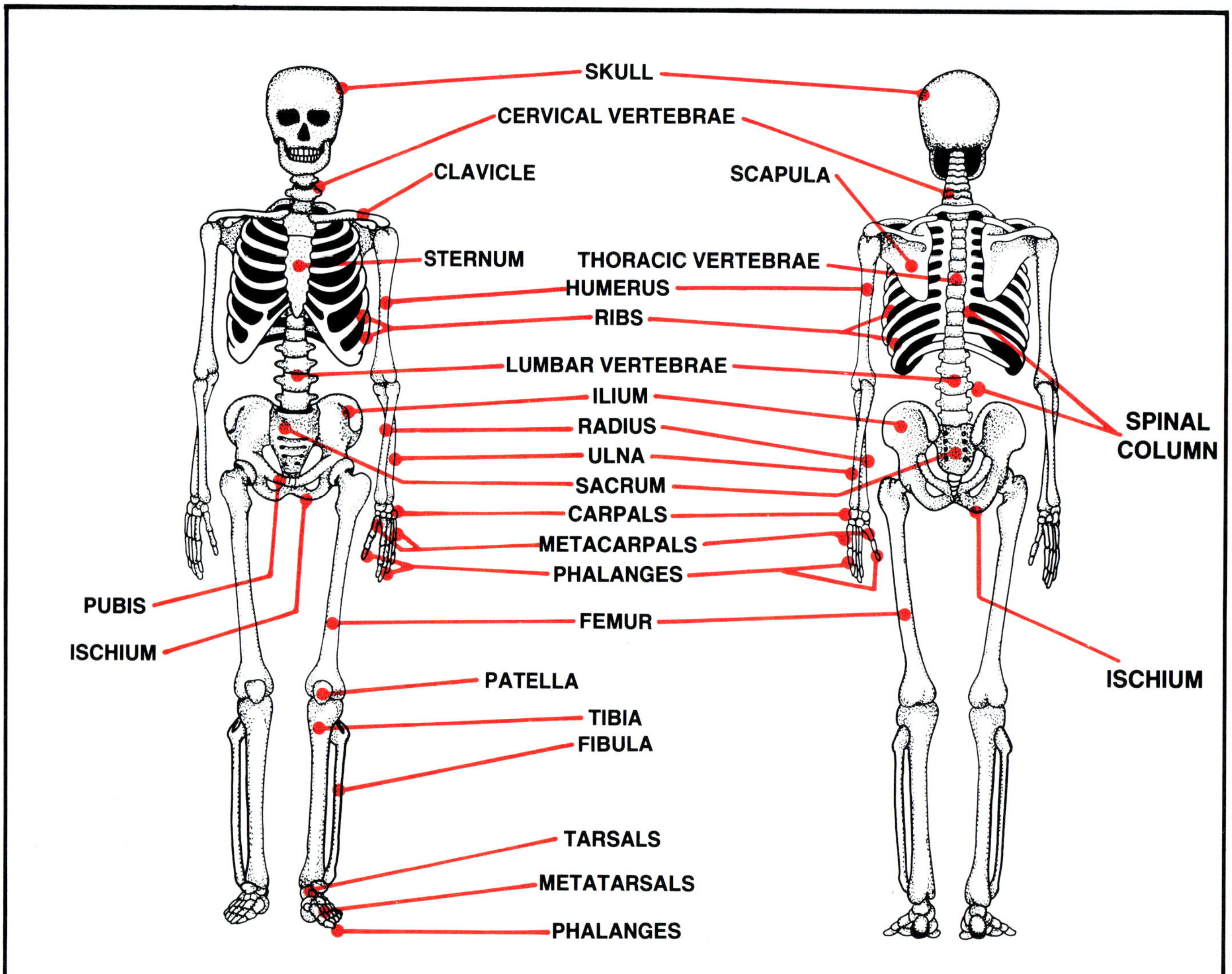


**Figure 2.2** The skeleton forms the frame for the human body.

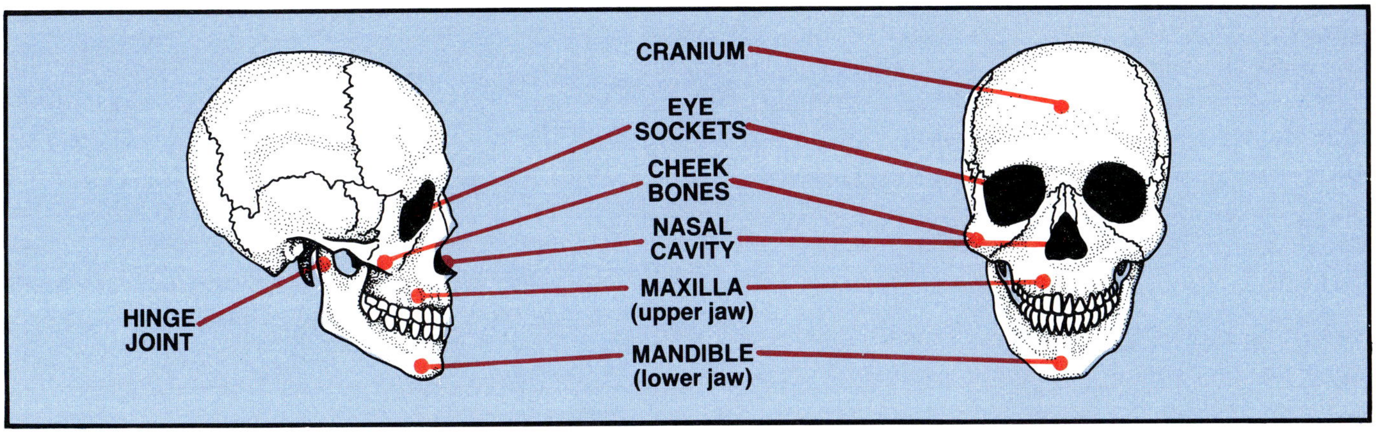


**Figure 2.3** The skull is composed of 22 bones: 8 bones are fused to form the brain case, and the other 14 bones form the face and jaw.

not fully developed at birth, however: the bones of an infant's skull are not fused because the skull must expand and contract during the birth process (see Chapter 15, Emergency Childbirth). As the child ages the bones grow together to form a very sturdy and strong brain case. The other 14 bones of the skull form the face and jaw. These facial bones include bony sockets for the eyes, nasal bones, cheekbones, maxilla (upper jaw), and mandible (lower jaw). The mandible is attached to the skull by a hinge joint just below each ear and is thc only movable structure in the skull.

## Spinal Column

The spinal column is a flexible bony structure that supports the central part of the body and encloses the spinal cord, giving it rigid protection. The brain connects with the spinal cord through a large opening at the base of the skull in the center of the upper neck. The spinal column also serves as a point of attachment and support for the skull, ribs, and pelvis. The spinal column is composed of 33 bones, known as vertebrae (Figure 2.4). Each vertebra is separated from the others by a cartilage disc that cushions the motion of the spinal column.

The spine is divided into five sections:

*Cervical spine* (neck) - formed by the first seven vertebrae

*Thoracic spine* (upper back) - the next twelve vertebrae

*Lumbar spine* - the next five vertebrae

*Sacrum* - five vertebrae, part of the pelvis; they are fused to form the sacrum and they anchor the spinal cord in a fused joint

*Coccyx* (tailbone) - the last four vertebrae, also fused

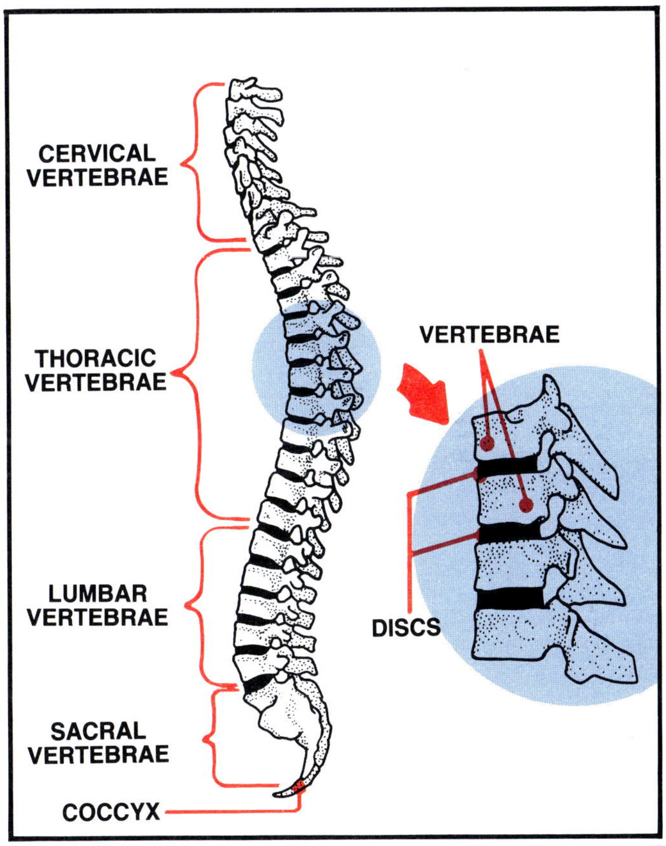


**Figure 2.4** The 33 bones that make up the spinal column are known as vertebrae.

## Shoulder Girdle (Pectoral Girdle)

The shoulder girdle is composed of two bony, muscular rings on either side of the upper part of the thorax (rib cage). It serves as a base for the attachment of the upper extremities. This bony part consists principally of the scapula (shoulder blade)

and the clavicle (collar bone) (Figure 2.5). The shoulder blade is held to the rib cage by large muscles near the back side. The upper, outward part of the shoulder blade forms a socket to which the humerus (upper arm bone) is connected. Because most of the attachment from the scapula to the chest is muscle, the scapula moves quite freely.

The clavicle is a long, slender bone extending from the top of the sternum (breastbone) to the shoulder blade near the shoulder joint. Its purpose is mainly to support the shoulder blade and arm. In a sense, the clavicle acts as a support for the entire shoulder.

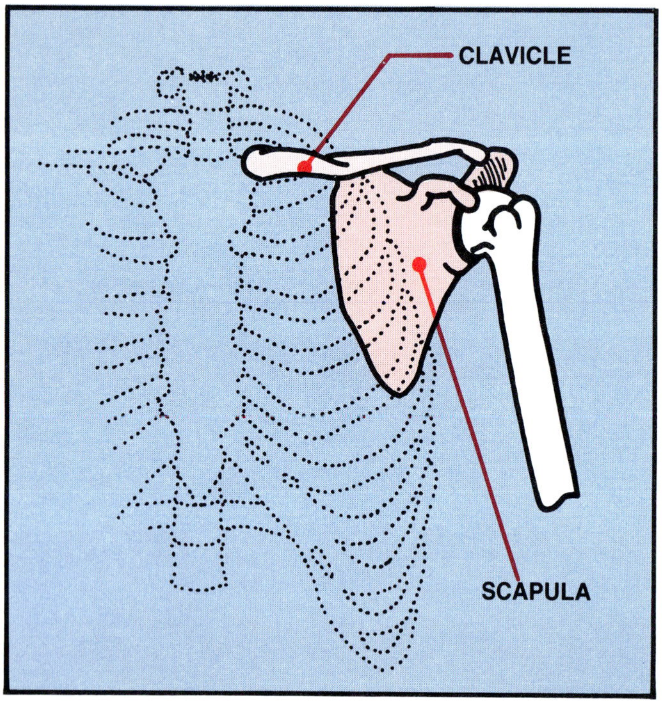


**Figure 2.5** The shoulder girdle serves as a base for the attachment of the upper extremities.

## Upper Extremities

The upper extremities extend from the shoulders to the fingertips and are divided into three parts: the upper arm, the forearm, and the hand. The upper arm extends from the shoulder to the elbow and has only one bone, the humerus. The top portion of the humerus is shaped like a ball and fits against the shallow pocket of the scapula to form the shoulder joint. The bottom portion of the humerus forms the upper half of the hinged elbow joint. The forearm, which extends from the elbow to the wrist, is composed of two bones, the radius and ulna (Figure 2.6). The radius is located on the thumb side of the forearm and the ulna is located on the little finger side. The upper end of the ulna forms the elbow joint and narrows at the wrist to serve as an axis, or pivot, for the hand. The upper part of the radius is rounded, while the lower part helps form the wrist joint.

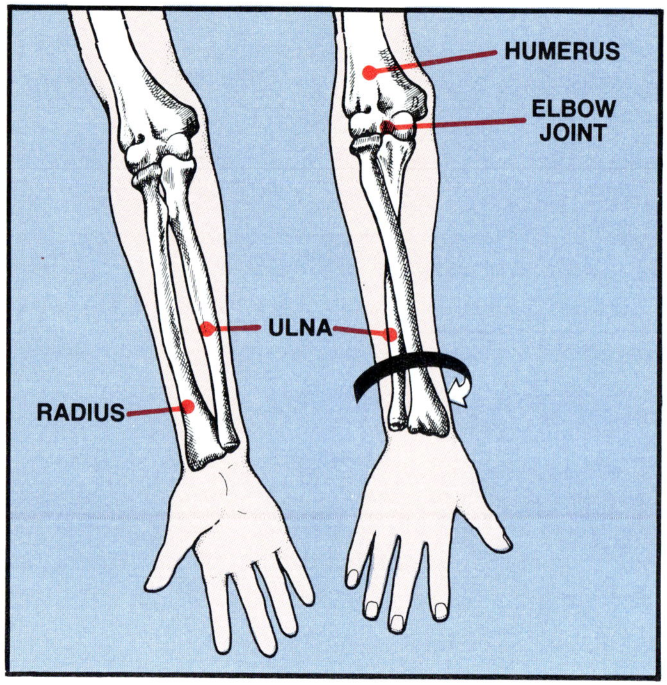


**Figure 2.6** The forearm is composed of two bones, the radius and the ulna.

The forearm articulates (joins) with the hand at the wrist. The bones of the hand are divided into three separate groups: carpals, metacarpals, and phalanges. The carpals are the eight small wrist bones. There are five metacarpals (hand bones); the one in the thumb has the most flexion (ability to bend) and rotation. Each finger has three bones (phalanges) but the thumbs have only two bones other than the metacarpal (Figure 2.7).

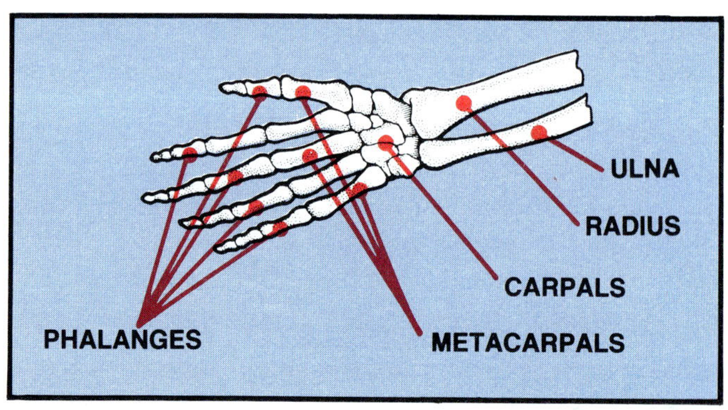


**Figure 2.7** The bones of the hand are divided into three groups: carpals (the wrist), metacarpals (the hand), and phalanges (the fingers).

## Thorax (Rib Cage)

The thorax, or rib cage, is composed of twelve pairs of ribs that are attached to, and suspended from, the twelve vertebrae in the back (Figure 2.8). All of the ribs are attached to a thoracic vertebra in the back and curve around to the front to form the rib cage. The sternum (breastbone) forms the middle part of the front of the rib cage. The sternum narrows at its lower end into a flexible, cartilaginous projection known as the xiphoid process. The first ten ribs are attached to the sternum by strips of cartilage. The lower two pairs of ribs are called "floating" ribs because they are connected only to vertebrae in the back. The thorax protects the heart, lungs, great blood vessels, and esophagus.

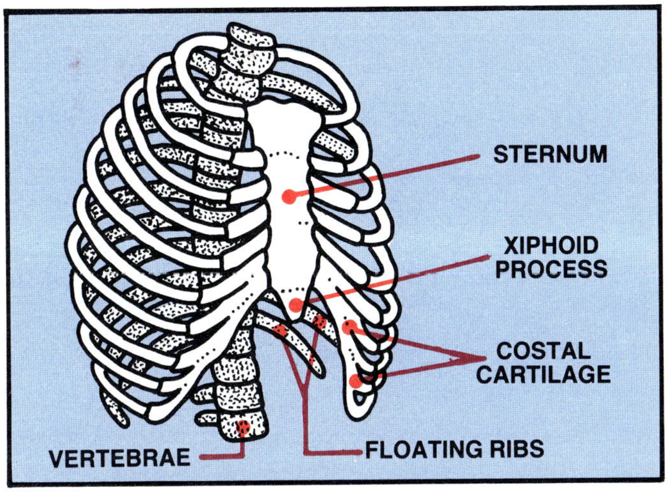


**Figure 2.8** The rib cage is composed of 12 pairs of ribs. The ribs protect the heart, lungs, great blood vessels, and esophagus.

## Pelvis (Pelvic Girdle)

The pelvis is a large bony ring formed by the sacrum (lower five vertebrae) and the two hip bones (Figure 2.9). Each wing-shaped hip bone actually consists of three smaller bones that are fused together: the ilium, the ischium, and the pubis. Each hip bone joins with the sacrum through a broad, strong joint called the sacroiliac joint. The three bones meet on each side of the pelvis and form a socket; the upper end of the femur (thigh bone) inserts into this socket. The two hip bones join in the front at the symphysis pubis. Besides providing support for the upper body, the pelvic girdle protects those organs and structures contained within the pelvic cavity, including the bladder, rectum, and in the female, the uterus and vagina.

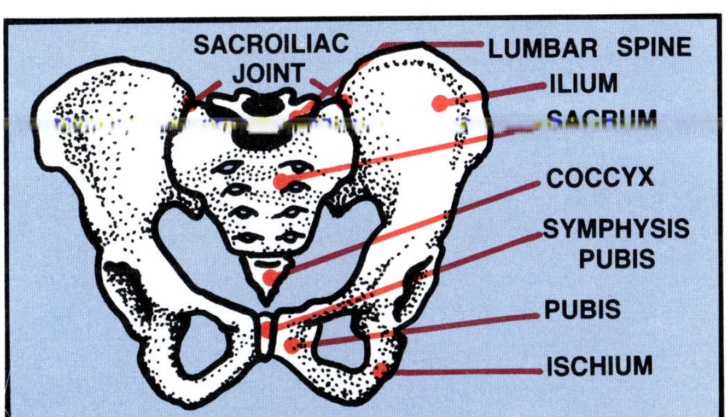


**Figure 2.9** The pelvis provides support for the upper body and protects the organs that lie within the pelvic cavity.

## Lower Extremities

The lower extremities are divided into three parts: the upper leg (thigh), lower leg, and the foot (Figure 2.10). The bone from the hip to the knee is

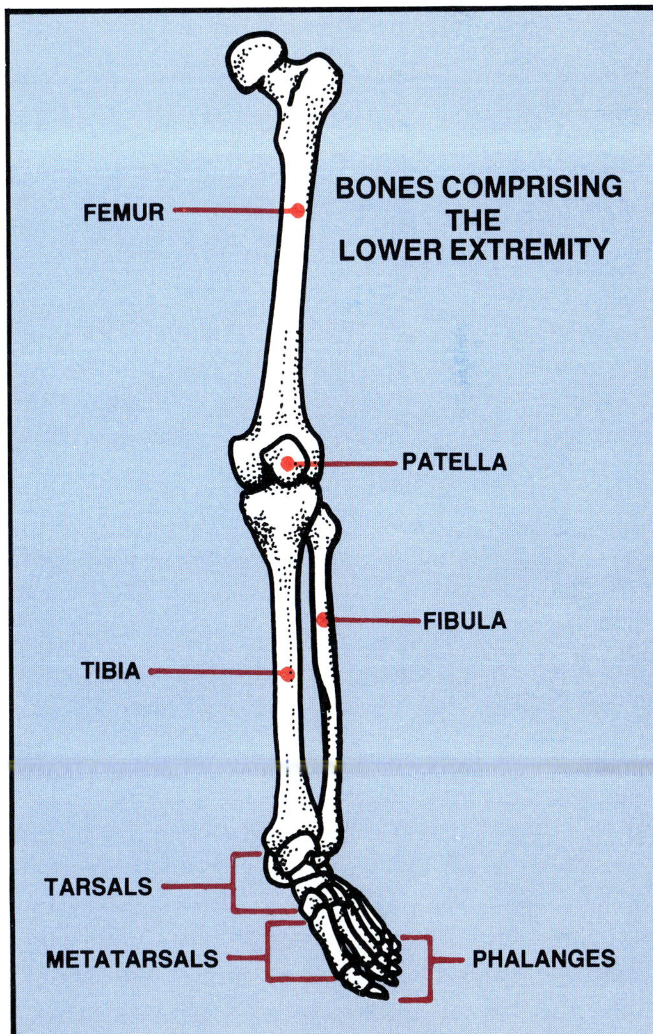


**Figure 2.10** The lower extremities are divided into three parts: the thigh bone (femur), the lower leg (tibia and fibula), and the foot.

called the femur (thigh bone). The femur is the longest, heaviest, and strongest bone of the human skeleton. The head of the femur is shaped like a ball and fits into the hip socket. The lower end of the femur expands into a broadened base to form the upper portion of the knee joint.

At the joint of the knee, where the femur joins the lower leg, there is a floating bone known as the patella (kneecap), which lies within the tendon of the quadriceps muscle. The patella protects the knee joint.

The lower leg contains two bones called the tibia and the fibula. The tibia (shin bone) is the larger of the two and is broad at its upper end to complete the knee joint with the femur. The fibula is considerably smaller and rests against the knee joint; it is attached to the knee by a ligament (Figure 2.11). The fibula forms the outer portion (little toe side) of the ankle joint at its lower end.

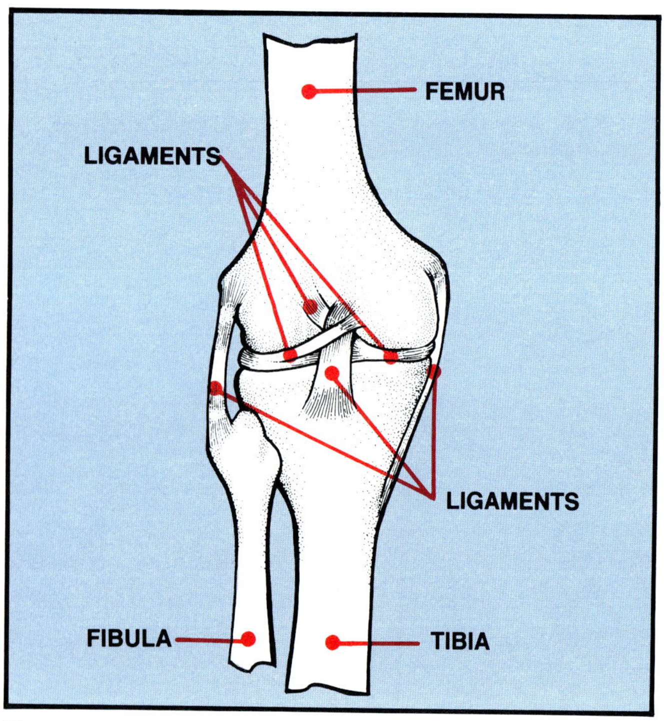


**Figure 2.11** Ligaments are tough, fibrous bands that help join bones. Shown is the ligament that attaches the fibula (the smaller of the two lower leg bones) to the knee.

The ankle joint connects the lower leg to the foot. The bones of the foot resemble the hand and finger bones but have different names. The tarsal bones are the main ankle bones, the metatarsals are the foot bones, and the phalanges are the toe bones.

## Joints

When two or more bones contact each other they articulate, or form, a joint. There are three types of joints: fused (immovable), slightly movable, and freely movable (Figure 2.12). Fused joints can be found in the skull, hip, and coccyx. Slightly movable joints are found in the spinal column and ribs. Freely movable joints are found in the knees, elbows, and fingers (hinge joints), shoulders and

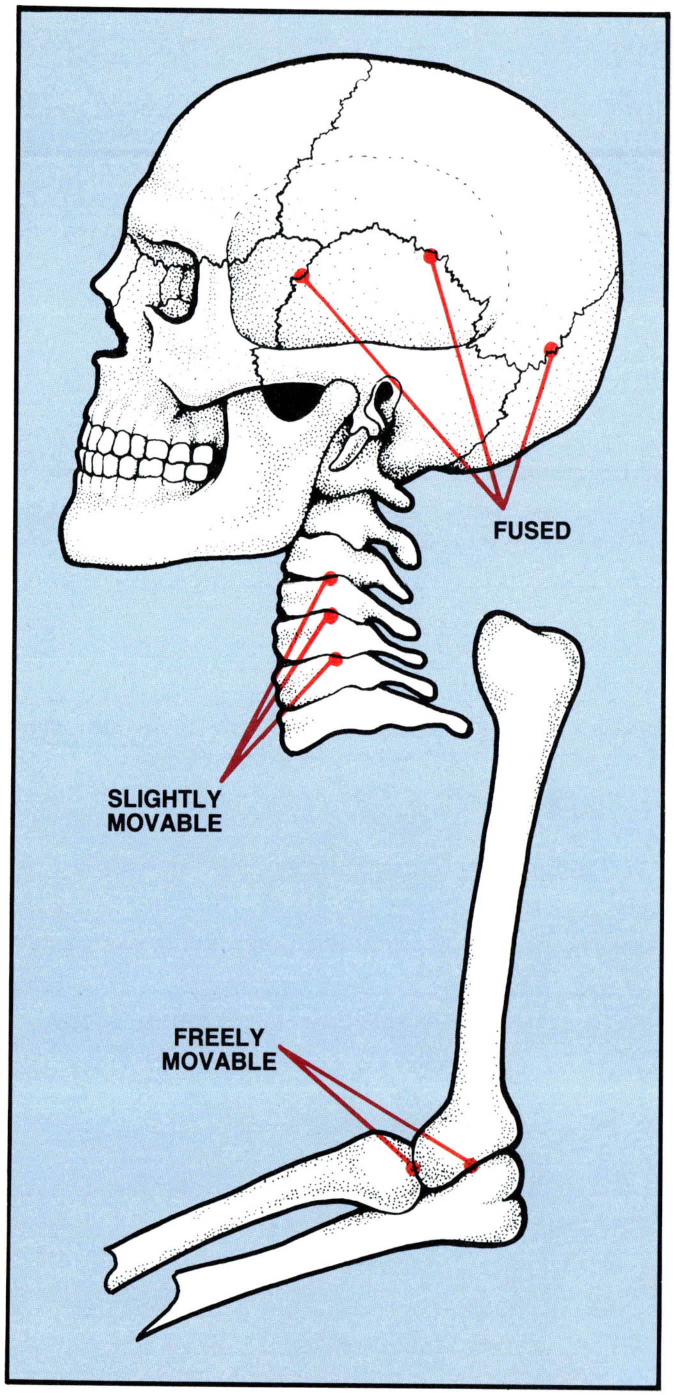


**Figure 2.12** The three types of joints are illustrated. They are fused (immovable), slightly movable, and freely movable.

hips (ball and socket joints). The movable surfaces are covered with a lubricated layer of cartilage and the entire joint is bound by ligaments, which extend from one bone to the other.

Ligaments, tendons, and cartilage work to connect and cushion joints. Ligaments are tough fibrous bands that help join bones, especially in the area of movable joints (see Figure 2.11). Tendons are strong, cord-like tissues that attach muscles to bones. Tendons are inelastic but transmit the force of contraction or extension of the muscles to move a body part. Cartilage is a tough but pliant material that serves as another connective tissue. Cartilage is found at various body sites, especially at the joints of the large bones and between the vertebrae. Cartilage is mainly found in areas where it is necessary to have strength combined with a certain amount of elasticity. Because it is compressible tissue, cartilage serves to cushion bumps and jolts.

## Muscles

Muscle is a special kind of tissue that has the ability to contract, or shorten. By contracting and relaxing, muscles provide the force that allows us to walk, that pushes our blood through the blood vessels, and that propels our food through the gastrointestinal tract.

All controlled movement of the body is a result of muscle action and all muscles are controlled by the nervous system. There are three types of muscles: voluntary, involuntary, and cardiac. Voluntary muscles can be controlled, such as those in the arms and legs. Involuntary muscles are not under the control of the individual's will; they are found in the walls of such hollow organs as the stomach and intestines. Contractions of these muscles help the organs empty their contents. The cardiac muscle is a special type of involuntary muscle. Because it has the ability to contract without any external stimuli, this muscle keeps the dual pumps of the heart functioning automatically to maintain blood circulation.

A muscle has an origin, where it attaches to a stationary bone, and an insertion, where it is attached by a tendon to a movable bone. The muscle usually crosses a joint so that when it contracts, or shortens, it causes the joint to move. Muscles usually work in pairs; one extends a bone, and the other flexes the same bone (Figure 2.13).

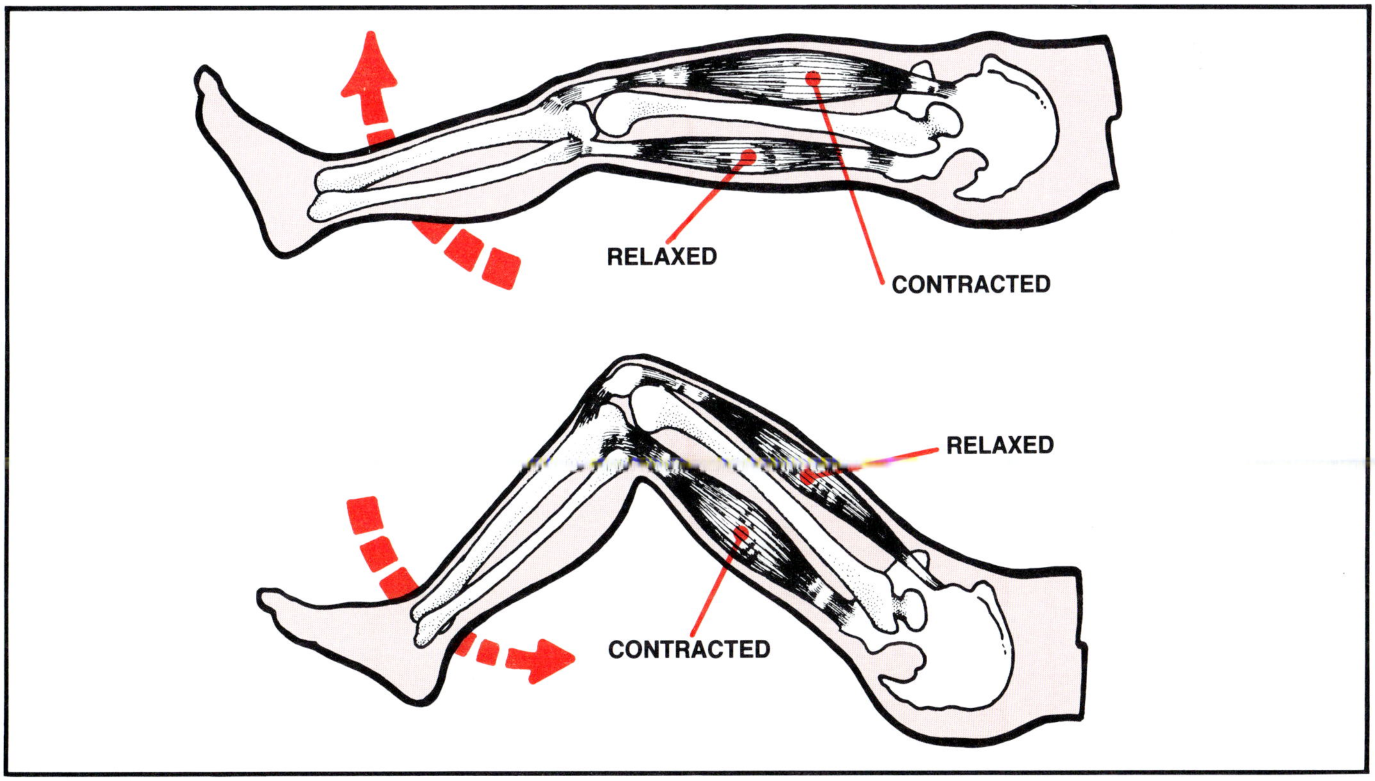


**Figure 2.13** Muscles are usually in pairs to help effect movement. As one extends a bone, the other flexes the same bone.

## NERVOUS SYSTEM

The nervous system consists of the brain, spinal cord, and innumerable peripheral nerves that supply the various body parts. The nervous system has two parts: (1) the central nervous system, which is composed of the brain and spinal cord, and (2) the peripheral nervous system, which is composed of sensory and motor nerves.

### Central Nervous System

The brain is the controlling organ of the body and is the center of consciousness. It controls emotions, judgments, memory, and all of the other qualities that make each person unique. The brain enables an individual to perceive himself or herself, others, and the environment.

The brain occupies all of the space within the cranium, as shown in Figure 2.14. Brain tissue is made up of many different types of cells, each of which has a specific function. Some cells *receive* sensations or stimuli from the environment, while other brain cells *transmit* impulses to cause muscles and organs to act.

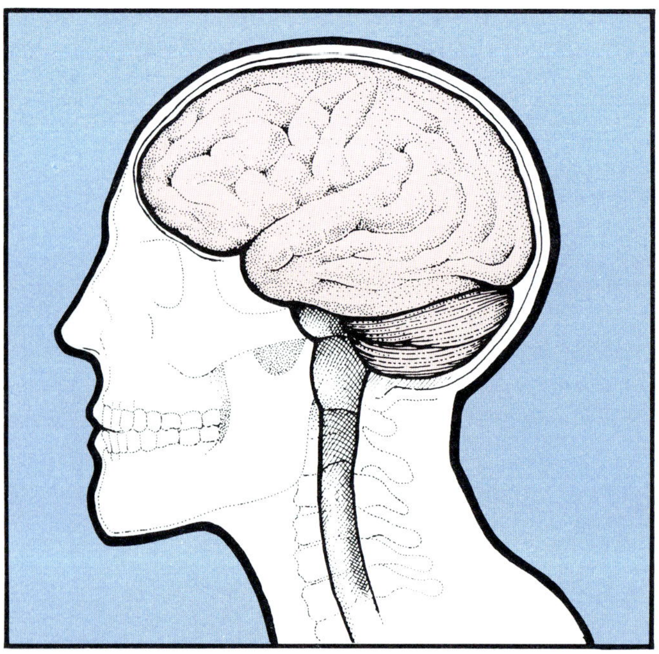

**Figure 2.14** The brain occupies all of the space within the cranium.

Certain areas of the brain control specific functions. There is a sensory area for receiving sensation, another area serving the physical senses (hearing, seeing, and so on), while still another area controls emotional responses (Figure 2.15).

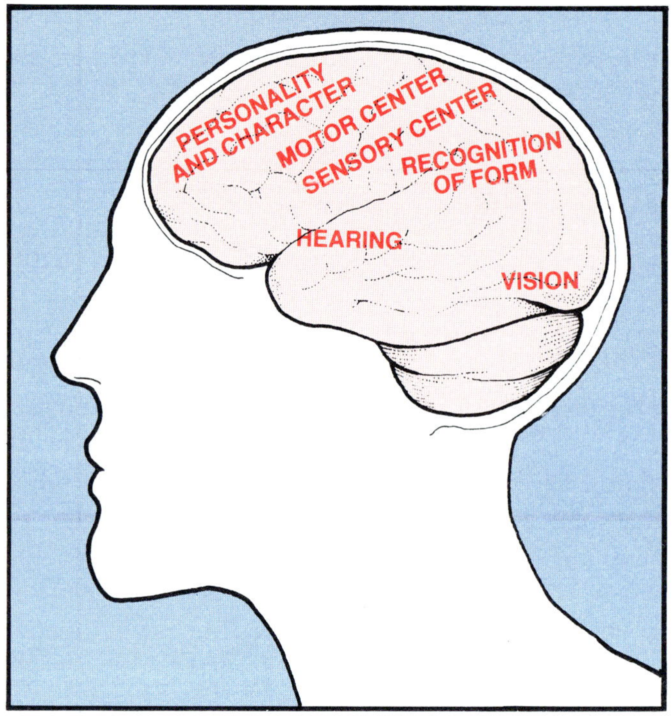


**Figure 2.15** Different body functions are controlled by specialized areas of the brain.

All specialized areas of the brain are connected by a complex network of nerve fibers. Conducting fibers further extend downward from the brain through the skull's base to form the spinal cord (Figure 2.16).

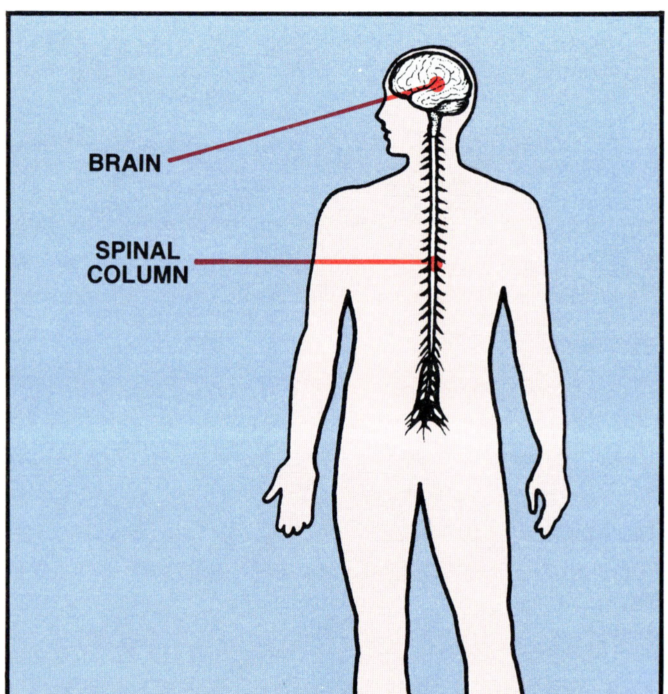


**Figure 2.16** The spinal cord is actually an extension of the nerve fibers of the brain.

The brain has three parts: the cerebrum, the cerebellum, and the medulla oblongata (see Figure 2.17). The cerebrum is the largest part of the brain and is divided into two halves, or hemispheres. The nerves that control movement in these hemispheres are located on the opposite sides of the part of the body they control; for example, the left side of the brain controls movement on the right side of the body. The cerebellum lies beneath the cerebrum and controls balance and muscle coordination. The medulla oblongata forms the uppermost portion of the spinal cord.

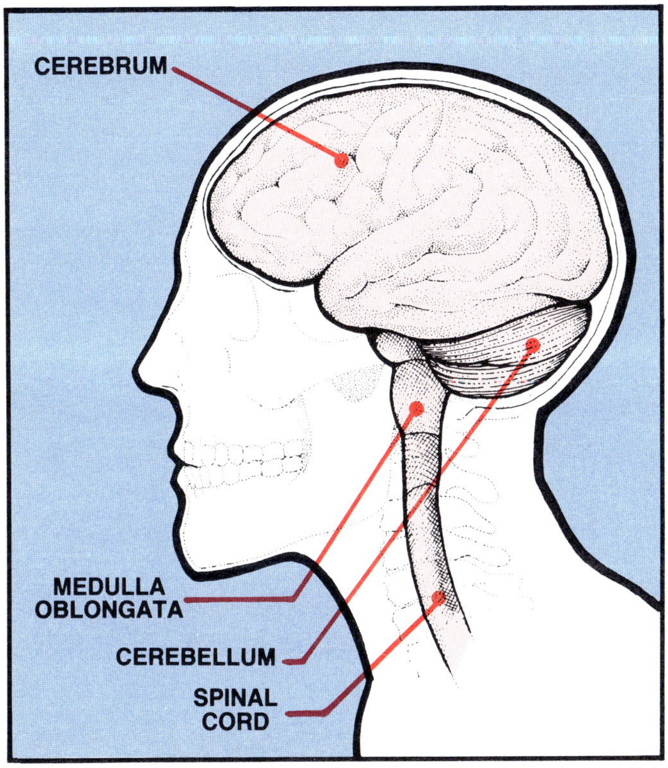


**Figure 2.17** The three main parts of the brain are the cerebrum, the cerebellum, and the medulla oblongata.

## THE SPINAL CORD

The spinal cord is actually a continuation of the brain; it extends from the base of the brain through the center of the spinal column. The nerves that branch off from the spinal cord form the peripheral nervous system, which receives messages from all parts of the body and transmits them to the brain for processing (Figure 2.18).

The peripheral nervous system is made up of both sensory and motor nerves, which transmit their messages as electrical impulses. Sensory nerves conduct impulses from the skin and other sensory organs to the brain. These sensations include cold, heat, pressure, direction, motion, and pain. Most impulses received by the sensory nerves travel to the spinal cord and then to the brain, but some impulses travel directly to the brain. Motor nerves, on the other hand, conduct messages from the brain to the muscles, causing the muscles to contract or relax.

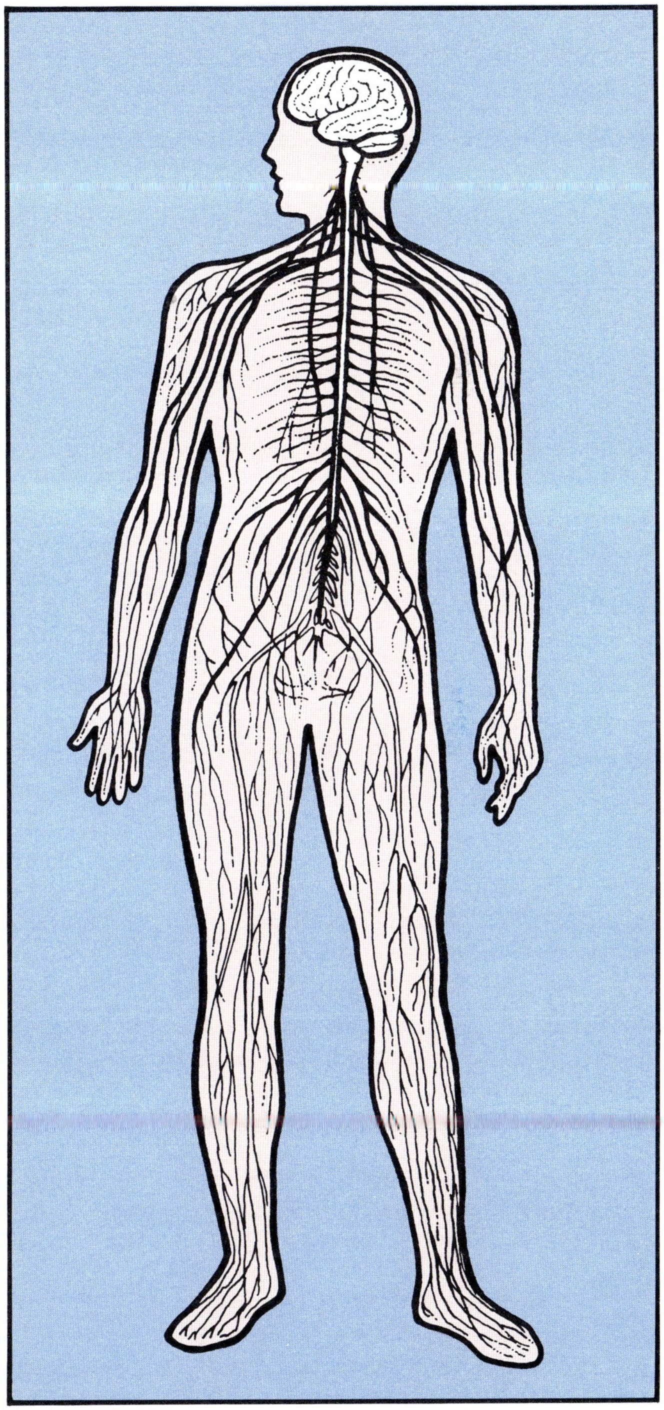

**Figure 2.18** The peripheral nervous system receives messages from all parts of the body and transmits them to the brain.

Because the tissues of the brain and spinal cord are soft and susceptible to injury, they have hard protective coverings. The brain, for example, is completely enclosed in the cranium (skull case). Likewise, bony vertebrae protect the spinal cord (Figure 2.19). The brain and spinal cord are also protected by three layers of tissue and a liquid called cerebrospinal fluid.

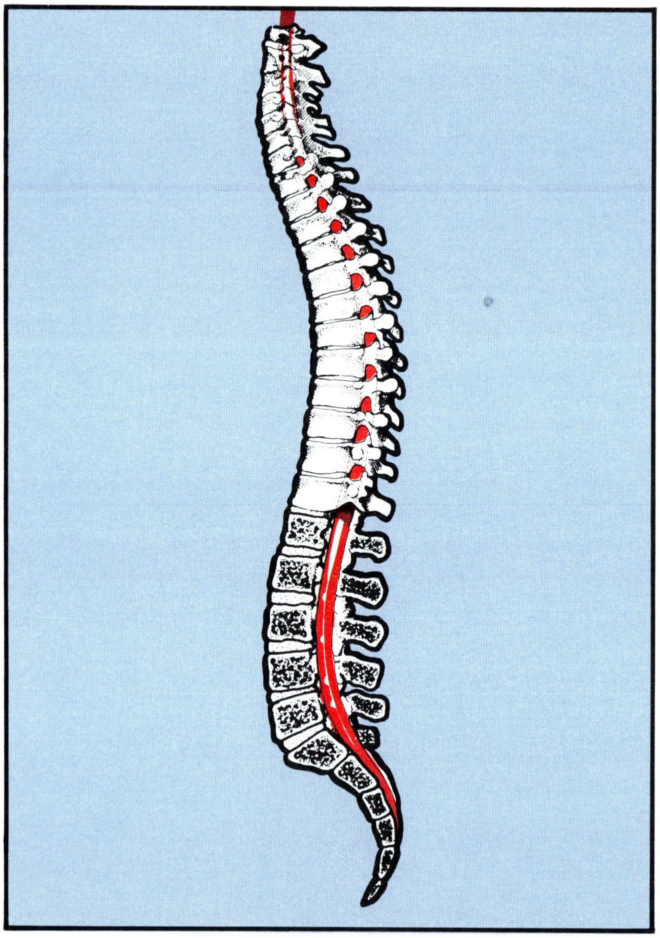

**Figure 2.19** The delicate spinal cord is protected by the bony vertebrae.

The three layers of tissue that suspend the brain and spinal cord within the skull and spinal column are collectively called the meninges. The outer layer is a tough, leather-like tissue called the dura mater. The middle layer (arachnoid mater) and inner layer (pia mater) are filmy, vascular layers.

Cerebrospinal fluid (CSF) is a clear, colorless fluid that fills the spaces between the dura mater and the spinal cord and brain. It gives shock protection to the brain and spinal cord and is a source of nourishment for some of the brain's cells.

### Actions of the Nervous System

The nervous system has two distinct sets of nerve pathways that make up the voluntary and involuntary nervous systems. Reactions that are the result of impulses from the involuntary nervous system cannot be controlled by human will. Automatic or involuntary functions include such processes as digestion, the dilation and constriction of blood vessels, and breathing. Muscles in the walls of the arteries and the heart also function automatically.

The second pathway of nerves, the voluntary nervous system, responds to human will. For example, when someone decides to pick up a magazine, the voluntary nervous system is triggered into action. Impulses that are stimulated by conscious thought travel through the voluntary nerve pathways to the skeletal muscles, causing them to react and enabling the person to pick up the magazine.

## THE RESPIRATORY SYSTEM

The respiratory system supplies the blood with oxygen and removes the gases the blood accumulates in its circulation throughout the body. The respiratory system is generally divided into two parts: the upper airway and the lower airway. The structures of the upper airway include the mouth, nose, pharynx, epiglottis, and larynx. The structures of the lower airway are the trachea, bronchi (left bronchus and right bronchus), lungs, capillaries, and alveoli.

### The Upper Airway

Air enters the respiratory system through the nose and mouth (Figure 2.20). The nose filters, humidifies, and adjusts the temperature of the incoming air. The mouth and nasal passages merge to form a common passage at the back of the mouth called the pharynx (throat). Just below the junction of the mouth and nasal passages, the pharynx divides into two other passageways, the esophagus and the trachea. The esophagus conducts food and liquid from the throat to the stomach, while the trachea conducts air from the throat to the lungs. The epiglottis, a thin flap at the beginning of the trachea, closes automatically when food or liquid passes the opening, thus preventing foreign mate-

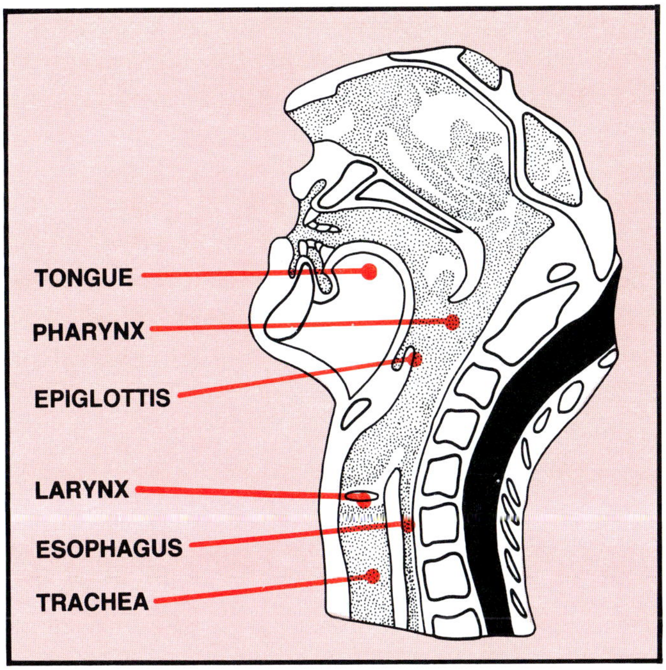


**Figure 2.20** The structures of the upper airway are shown.

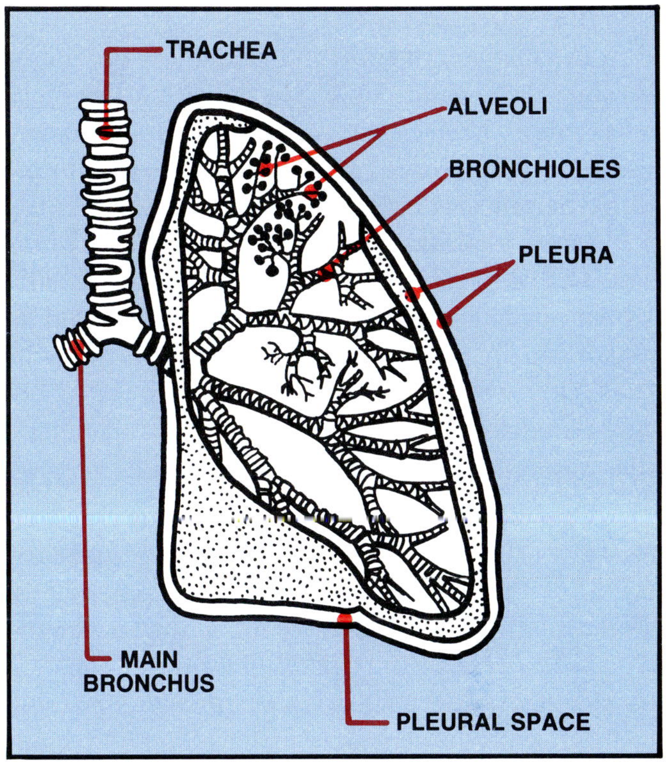


**Figure 2.21** The lower airway is composed of the structures of the respiratory system that lie below the epiglottis.

rial from entering the lungs. If a small amount of food or liquid does slip past the epiglottis, strong gag and cough reflexes work to forcefully expel the foreign matter. Beneath the epiglottis lies the larynx, or "voice box." The larynx contains the vocal cords, which produce sound as air passes over them. The Adam's apple forms the front of the larynx; it can easily be felt as a bump in the middle of the neck.

## The Lower Airway

The structures of the respiratory system that lie below the epiglottis compose the lower airway (Figure 2.21). Just below the larynx lies the trachea, a cartilaginous tube about five inches (127 mm) long that leads to the chest cavity. The trachea branches into two smaller tubes, the left bronchus and right bronchus. The bronchi branch into smaller and smaller air passageways that end in millions of tiny air sacs called alveoli. The alveoli are connected to the lung capillaries, and it is here that the exchange of oxygen and carbon dioxide takes place (Figure 2.22).

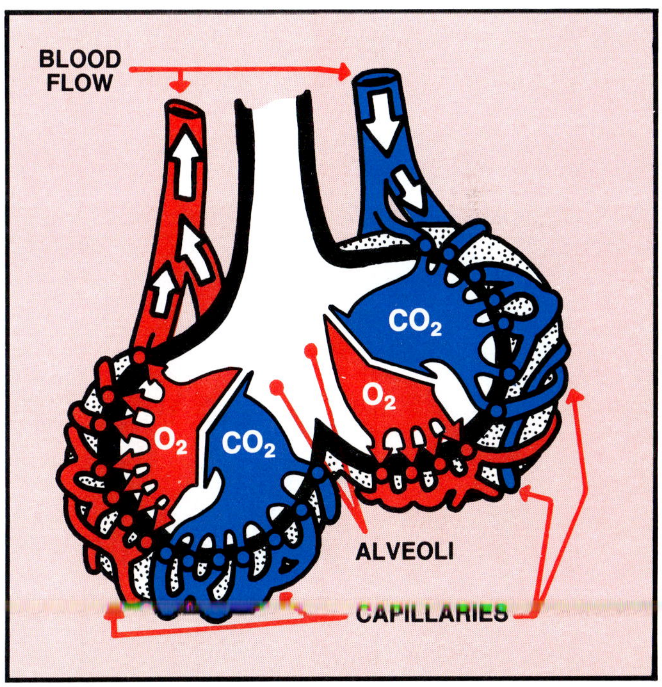


**Figure 2.22** It is within the tiny alveoli that the exchange of gases (oxygen and carbon dioxide) takes place.

The lungs are suspended within the rib cage by the trachea, blood vessels, and ligaments. Both lungs are enclosed by a double membrane called the pleura. Between the pleura is a "space" filled with lubricating fluids that allows the lungs to move in the chest cavity without friction. One pleural layer actually lines the lungs, while the other lines the chest cavity. Between the layers there exists a negative pressure that makes breathing possible.

### The Breathing Process

The movement of air into and out of the lungs essentially depends upon the negative pressure within the chest cavity and the combined movements of the diaphragm and the intercostal muscles (the muscles between the ribs). The pressure within the pleural space is lower than the air pressure within the lungs, that is, within the alveoli. Under normal circumstances, the lungs are held in expansion by this negative pressure. When the chest cavity expands during inhalation, the negative pressure draws the lungs outward and causes the lungs to expand further.

The diaphragm, a muscular structure that separates the chest cavity from the abdominal cavity, allows the chest cavity to expand from below, while the intercostal muscles allow the chest cavity to expand from the front and from the sides. In its relaxed position the diaphragm is dome-shapped, but when it contracts, it flattens and moves downward. The diaphragm contracts during inhalation, the rib cage expands, and this expansion of the chest cavity causes the pressure within the alveoli to become negative with respect to the surrounding atmosphere; consequently, air is drawn into the lungs from the surrounding atmosphere. During exhalation the diaphragm relaxes, the intercostal muscles contract, and air moves out of the lungs (Figure 2.23).

## THE CIRCULATORY SYSTEM

The circulatory system circulates blood throughout the body and removes waste products from body tissues. The circulatory system has three parts: a circulating fluid (blood), a pump (the heart), and a closed network of tubes (arteries and veins).

### The Fluid

Blood delivers a constant supply of oxygen and nourishment to all of the body's tissues and carries waste materials to the lungs, skin, and kidneys to be eliminated from the body. Blood consists of both liquid and cellular components. Plasma, the liquid portion of the blood, makes up about half of the blood's volume. Red blood cells, white blood cells, and platelets make up the other half.

The amount of blood in the body varies from person to person and even varies in the same person on different days. Normally, however, one-

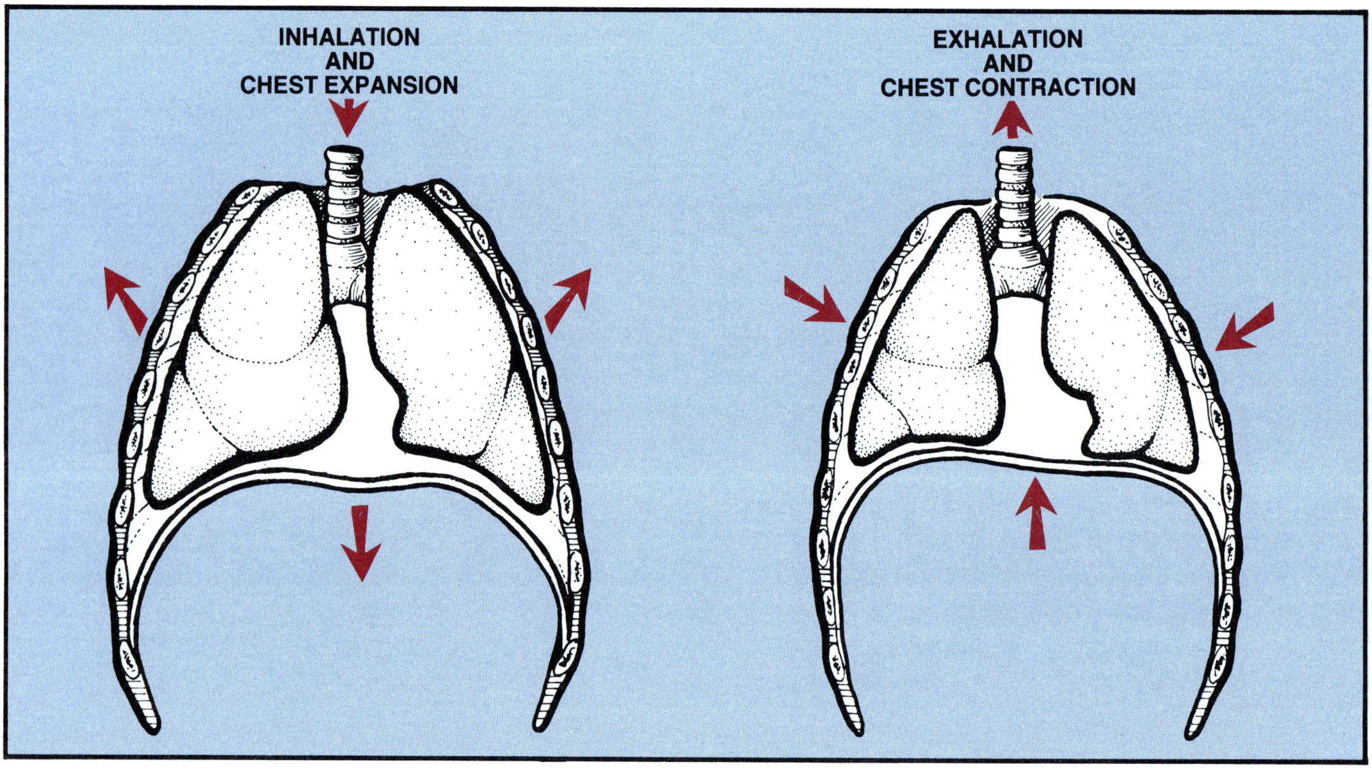


**Figure 2.23** During inhalation, the diaphragm contracts and the chest expands as the lungs fill with air. During exhalation, the diaphragm relaxes, the chest contracts, and air moves out of the lungs.

twelfth to one-fifteenth of the body weight is blood. A person who weighs 150 pounds (68 kg) has about 10 to 12 pints (4.7 L to 5.68 L) of blood.

Red blood cells are produced continuously in the marrow of certain bones, and transport oxygen from the lungs to body tissues and carbon dioxide from the tissues to the lungs. The protein hemoglobin, the primary constituent of red blood cells, combines with oxygen to allow the red blood cells to carry out their work. Hemoglobin turns bright red when it is combined with oxygen, which gives red blood cells (and blood) their characteristic color.

White blood cells, which are manufactured in the lymph system and in the bone marrow, protect the body from infection. The blood of an individual with an injury or infection has a high count of white blood cells. These cells are needed to combat the infection. In the event of a localized infection, such as a cut or scrape, white blood cells surround the infection zone to keep the infection from spreading.

The platelets play a vital role in the process of blood clotting. When blood flows from a cut, the platelets release a substance that combines with plasma to form fibrin. When fibrin combines with red and white blood cells and platelets, a clot forms to stop bleeding from blood vessels. This is why bleeding from superficial cuts usually stops by itself.

### The Pump

The principal organ of the circulatory system is the heart, a muscular, pear-shaped organ about the size of a fist (Figure 2.24). It is convenient to

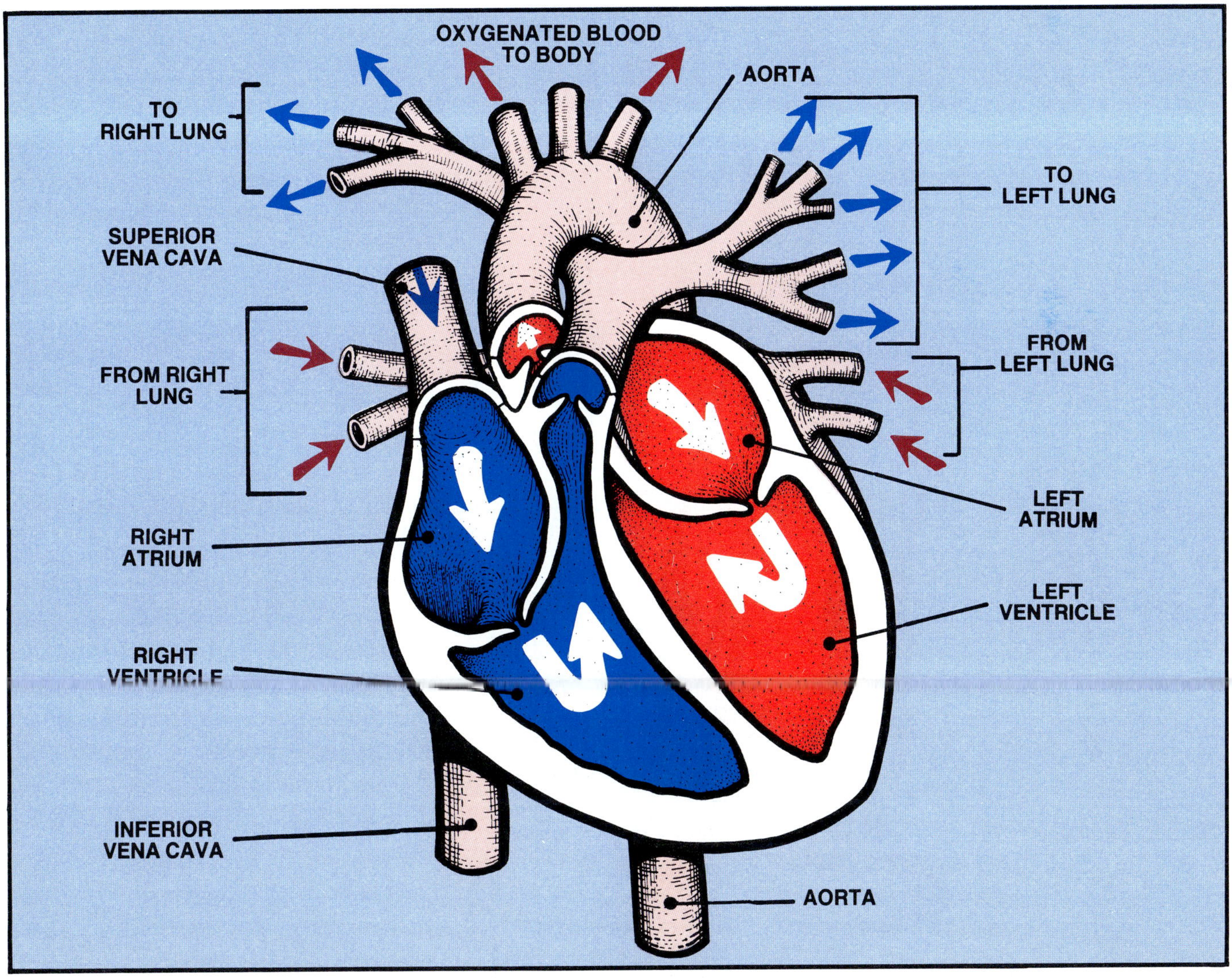


**Figure 2.24** The principal organ of the circulatory system is the heart, a muscular, two-sided pump.

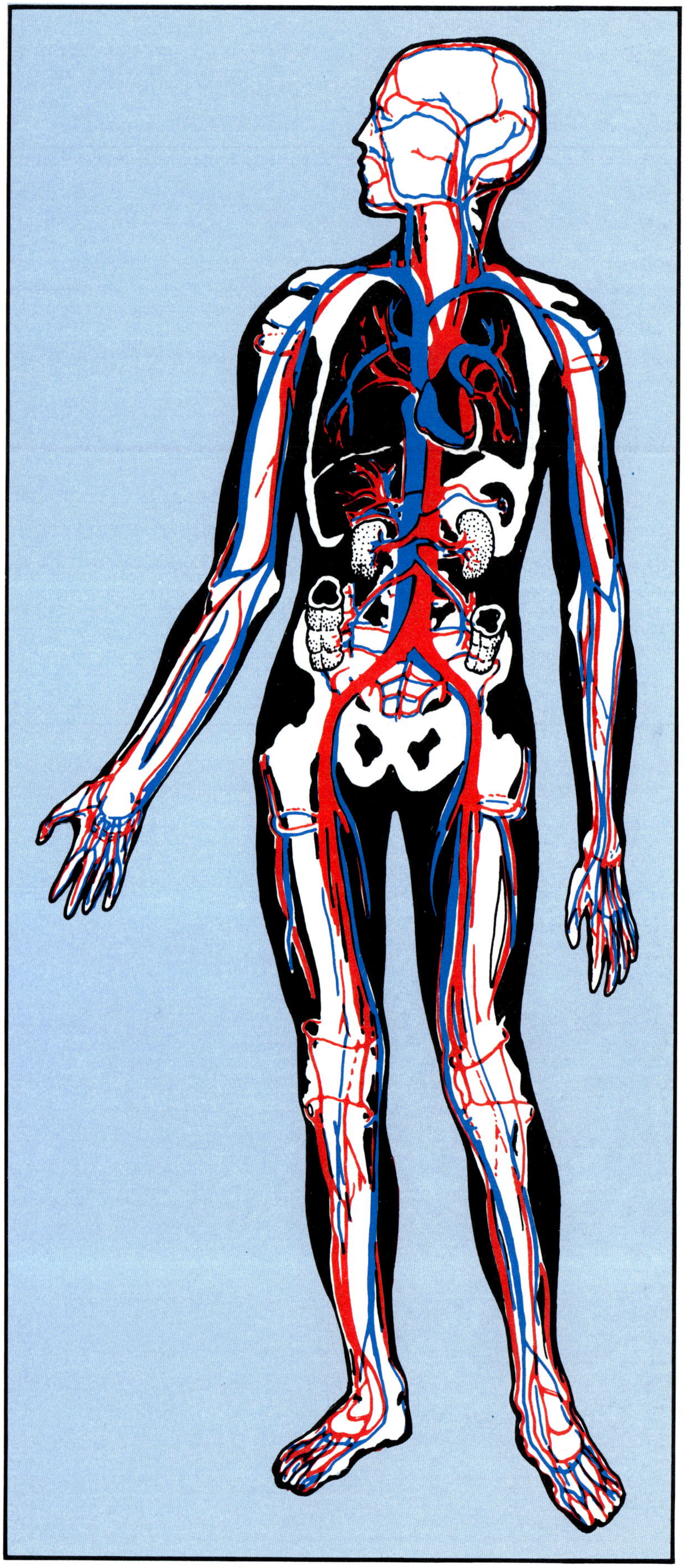

think of the heart as a pump; actually, it is two pumps, the left heart and the right heart. Each side is divided into a receiving chamber (atrium) and a pumping chamber (ventricle). The two sides of the heart are separated by a thin wall called the septum.

### The Network of Tubes

Arteries are vessels that carry blood *away* from the heart, while the veins carry blood *toward* the heart. The largest artery is the aorta, which rises from the left atrium and delivers blood to all parts of the body. The aorta branches into arteries, which become progressively smaller as arterioles, and finally, tiny capillaries, which are only one cell wall thick. Capillaries combine into slightly larger vessels called venules, which in turn join to form veins. The veins finally come together at the right atrium to form the body's largest vein, the vena cava (Figure 2.25).

### Circulation

Oxygen-poor blood from the vena cava empties into the right atrium. From there it passes into the right ventricle, which contracts and pumps blood out through the pulmonary artery into the lung capillaries. There the blood deposits the carbon dioxide it has gathered from other body tissues and absorbs oxygen from the lungs (Figure 2.26).

From the lungs the blood, now oxygen-rich, travels through the pulmonary vein to the left atrium, then to the left ventricle. The left chamber pumps the blood into the aorta, which carries blood to the smaller arteries and finally to the capillaries in the body tissues. There the blood deposits the oxygen and nutrients it has carried from the lungs, and the circulatory cycle begins again (Figure 2.27).

**Figure 2.25** Arteries and veins branch throughout the body to deliver oxygenated blood to the body's cells and to transport deoxygenated blood back to the lungs.

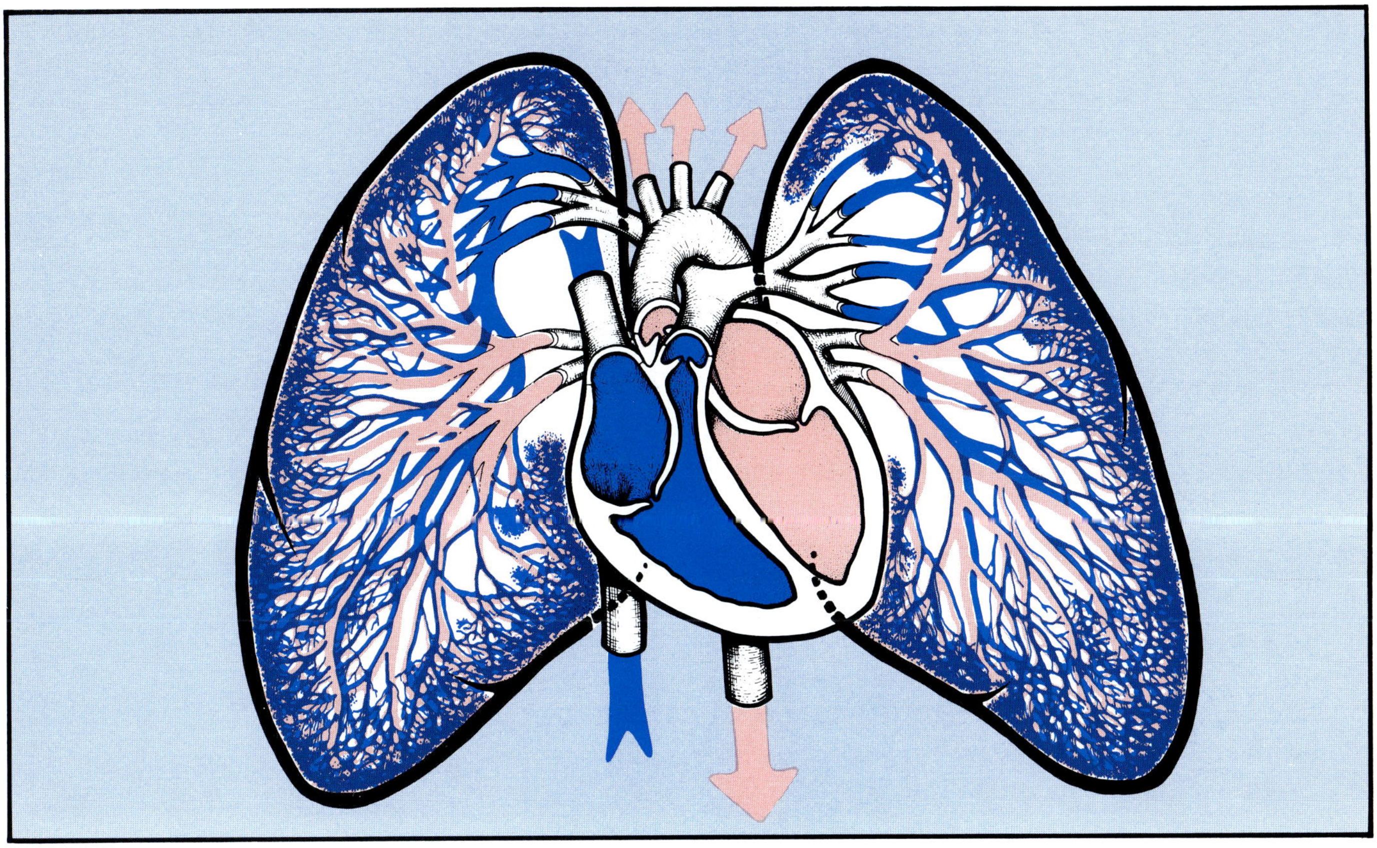

**Figure 2.26** Oxygen-poor blood is pumped from the right ventricle to the lungs.

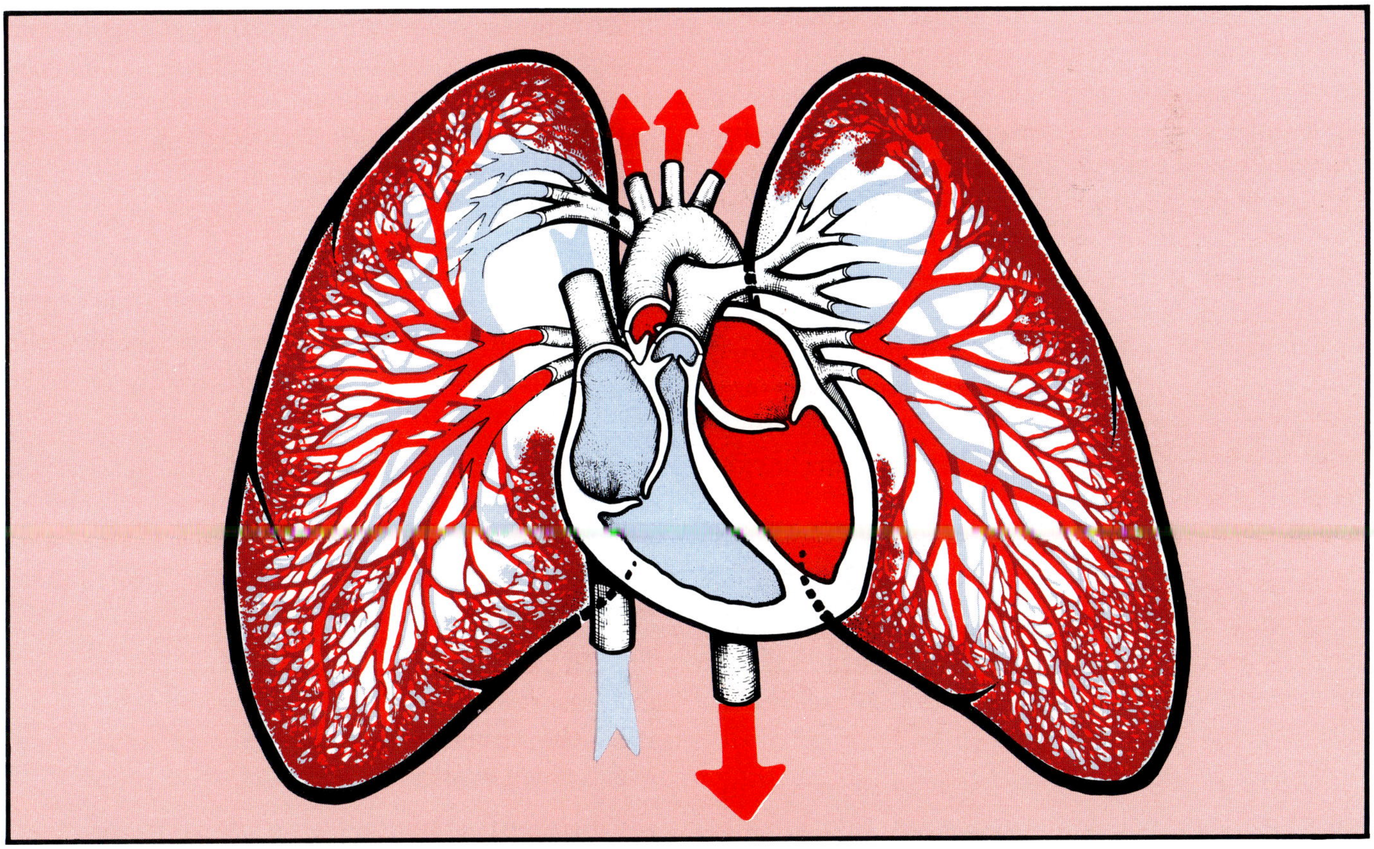

**Figure 2.27** Oxygen-rich blood travels back to the heart, where it is pumped out to the body through the aorta.

## THE DIGESTIVE SYSTEM

The digestive system converts food and liquid into chemical forms that the body can use. Although the process of digestion begins in the mouth, most of the organs of digestion lie in the abdominal cavity. The abdominal cavity extends almost to the nipple line: the diaphragm forms the upper boundary of the abdominal cavity and the pelvic bones form the lower boundary. The back boundary of the abdominal cavity consists of the lumbar spine, the sacrum, and the coccyx. The abdomen contains the organs of digestion and excretion, including the liver, gallbladder, spleen, pancreas, kidneys, stomach, intestines, urinary bladder, and rectum. The entire abdominal cavity is lined by a smooth, thin tissue called the peritoneum.

The digestive organs are of two types: solid and hollow. The solid organs are solid masses of tissue, while the hollow organs are tube- or sac-like organs that transport material to other parts of the digestive system.

### The Solid Organs

The solid organs of the digestive system are the liver, spleen, and pancreas (Figure 2.28). The liver is the largest organ in the abdominal cavity; it lies just below the diaphragm and is partially protected by the rib cage. This protection is important because the liver has many large and small blood vessels and if it is ruptured or lacerated (cut) in an accident, hemorrhage can be severe. The liver performs a number of vital functions, such as producing bile, (a fluid needed to digest fats), storing vitamins and minerals, and breaking down fats and proteins into usable forms. The liver can also render certain dangerous drugs and poisons harmless to the body.

The spleen, located in the upper left-hand part of the abdominal cavity, retires old red blood cells and produces new ones. Because the liver and bone marrow can assume this function if the spleen must be removed, the spleen is not considered a vital organ.

The pancreas is a firm, flat organ just within the upper right part of the abdominal cavity. This digestive organ performs two vital functions: it releases chemical enzymes needed for digestion and it releases insulin into the bloodstream. The pancreatic enzymes break down food substances in the small intestine, while insulin regulates the amount of sugar in the blood.

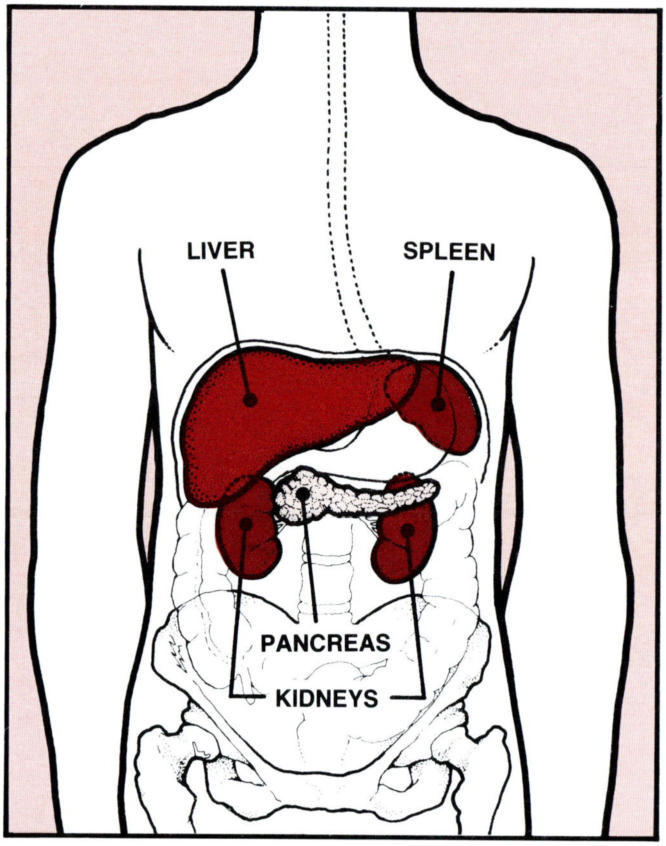


**Figure 2.28** The solid organs of the digestive system are the liver, spleen, pancreas, and kidneys.

### The Hollow Organs

The hollow organs pass material or fluids through the digestive system. They include the gallbladder, stomach, and small and large intestines (Figure 2.29).

The gallbladder is a small sac located just under the liver. It stores and concentrates the bile produced by the liver until the bile is needed during digestion. Then, the gallbladder allows bile to enter the small intestine.

The stomach's primary purpose is to act as a food reservoir. Digestive enzymes and acids, along with the churning action of the stomach, help break down food early in the digestive process.

From the stomach food passes into the small intestine, where bile and enzymes from the pancreas act vigorously upon it. Nearly all absorption of the nutrients from food takes place in the small intestine.

When food enters the large intestine from the small intestine, it is almost completely digested. The large intestine, which is six to seven feet (1.8 m to 2.1 m) long, serves as a reservoir for digested food, absorbs water, and excretes waste materials through the rectum and anus.

The appendix is attached to the large intestine but serves no known function; however, it is important to emergency care personnel because it can become inflamed (appendicitis) and must be removed by emergency surgery.

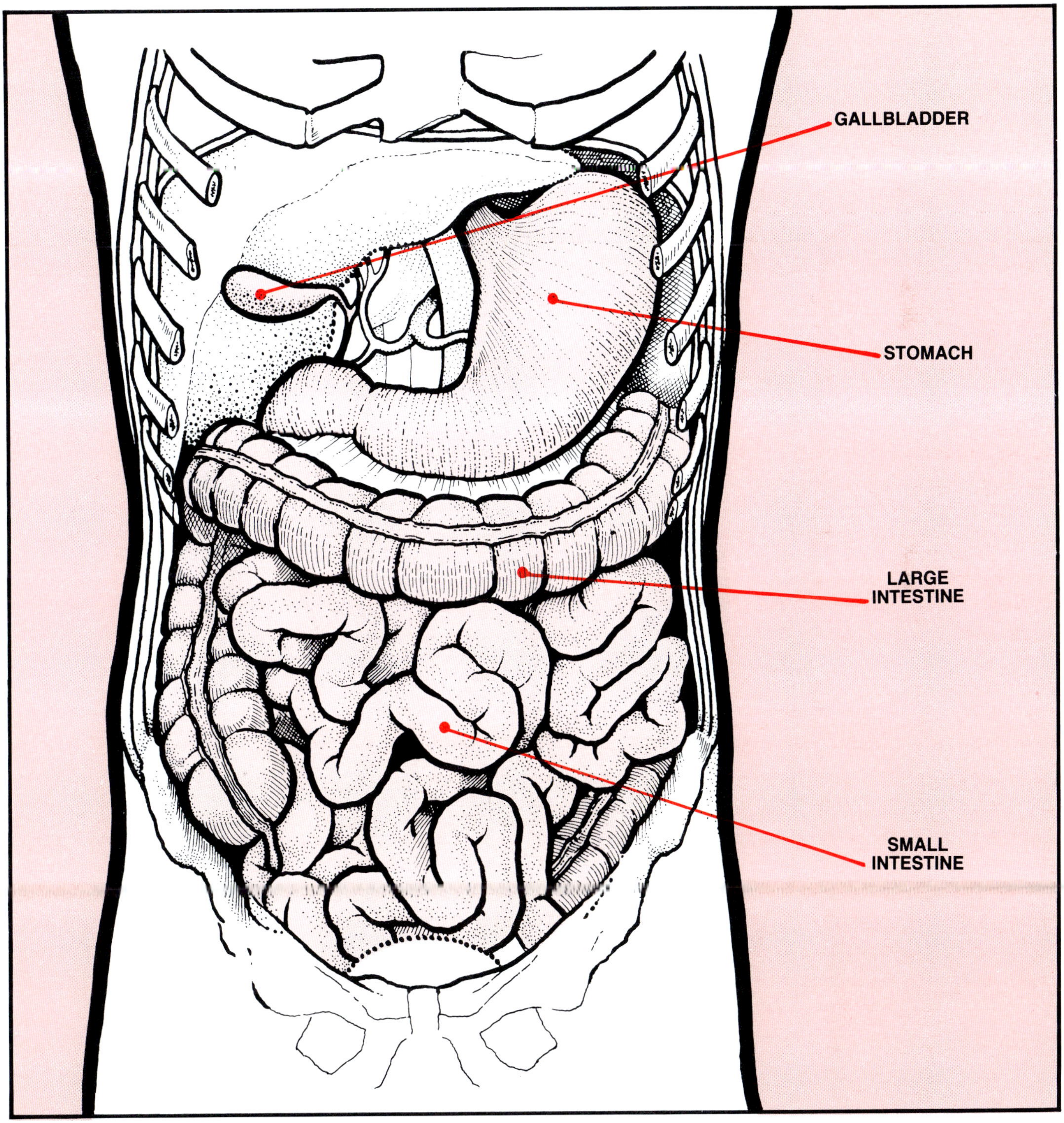


**Figure 2.29** The hollow organs pass material or fluids through the digestive system.

## THE URINARY SYSTEM

The function of the urinary system is to remove liquid waste products from the body. The major organs of this system are the kidneys, urinary bladder, ureters, and urethra (Figure 2.30). The kidneys are two solid organs that lie on the back wall of the abdomen. Their job is to filter impurities and excess water from the blood and to eliminate these materials in the form of urine. The urine then passes to the bladder through two small tubes called ureters. The urinary bladder, just below the kidneys and behind the pubic bone, stores urine until it is almost full; then sensory nerves notify the brain that the bladder is ready to be emptied. Urine leaves the body through a passage called the urethra. In males, the urethra is longer and discharges urine through the penis; in females, the urethra is shorter and discharges urine just in front of the vagina.

## THE GENITAL (REPRODUCTIVE) SYSTEM

The genital, or reproductive system, consists of the male and female genitalia and in males, the urethra. The function of the genitalia is to allow for sexual intercourse and reproduction.

The female reproductive organs are almost entirely internal. They include the ovaries, fallopian tubes, uterus, cervix, and vagina (Figure 2.31). The ovaries produce female hormones and ova

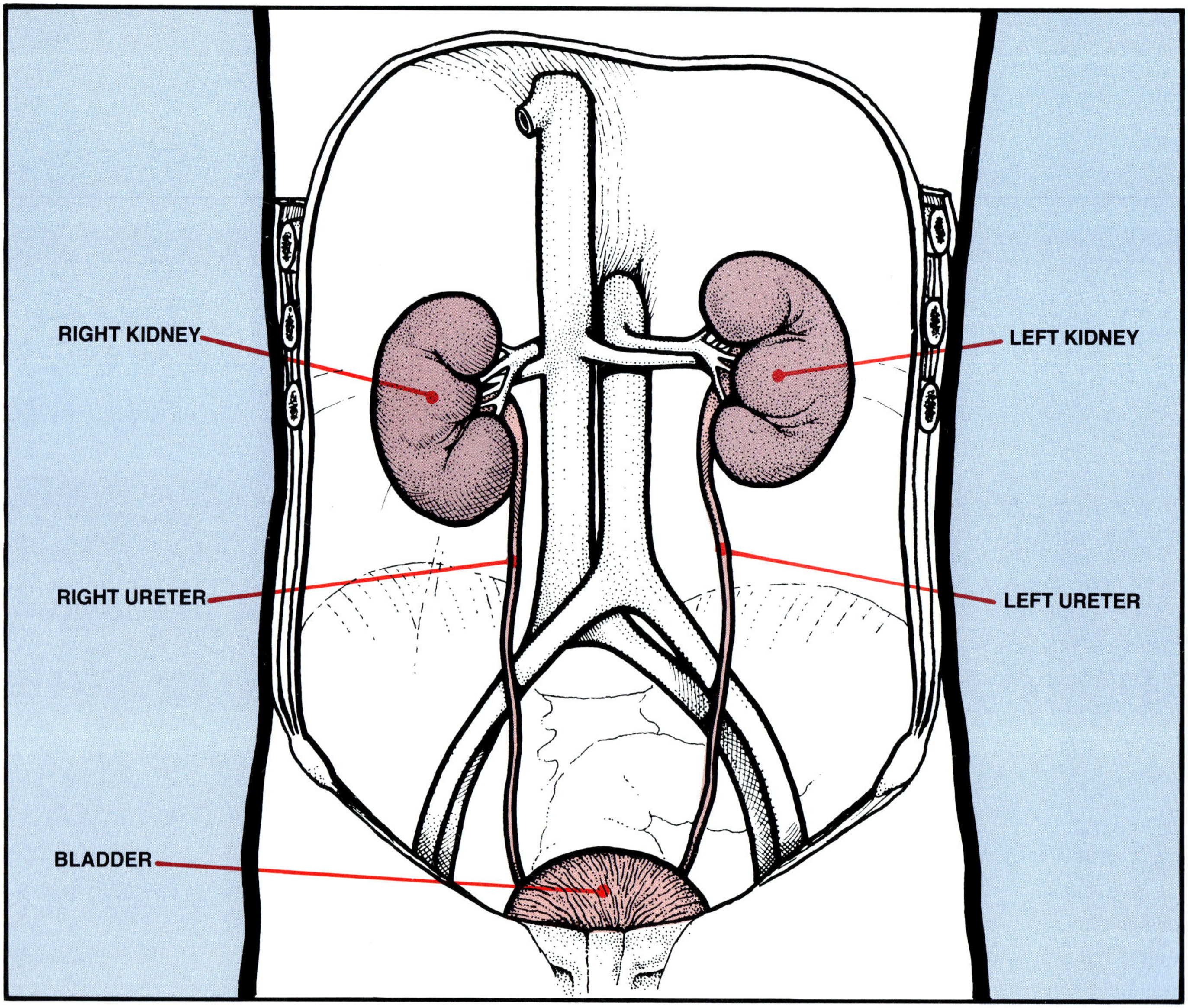


**Figure 2.30** The urinary system removes liquid waste products from the body.

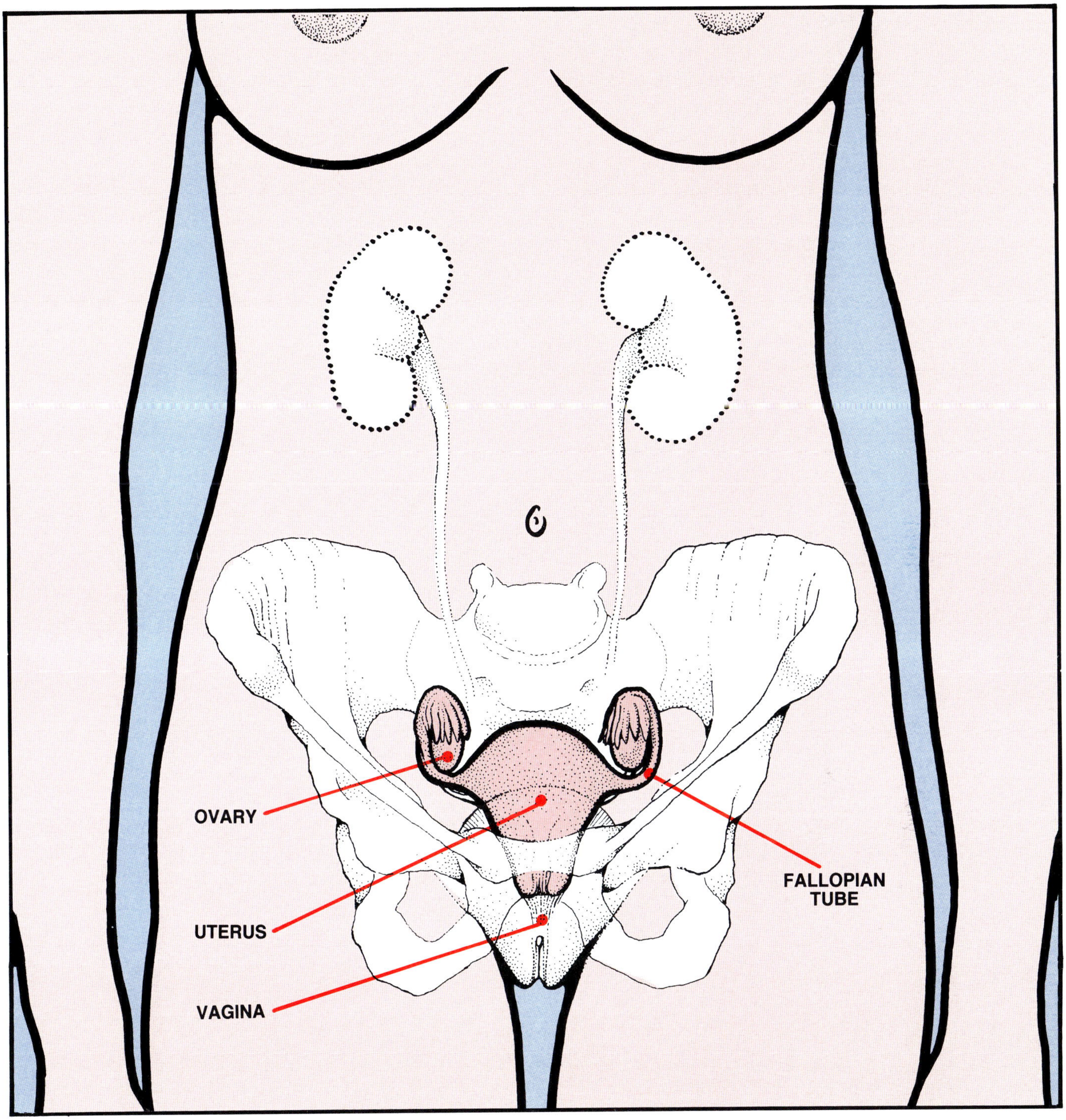


**Figure 2.31** The organs of the female reproductive system are pictured above. Notice that they are almost entirely internal

(eggs). About every 28 days the ovaries release an egg, which travels to the uterus through the fallopian tubes. The uterus is a muscular, pear-shaped organ designed to nourish and protect the fertilized egg until it has developed into an infant. If the egg has been fertilized by a male sperm, it implants in the thickened lining of the uterus and begins to grow. Otherwise, the egg and lining are shed during menstruation.

The cervix is a narrow opening from the uterus to the vagina. It permits male sperm cells to pass into the uterus and allows menstrual flow to pass through the vagina. The vagina opens to the external female genitalia, the vulva.

The male reproductive organs are primarily external. They include the testicles, seminal vesicles, vas deferens, urethra, and penis (Figure 2.32). The main sexual glands are the testicles, which occupy a sac called the scrotum. The testicles manufacture male hormones and sperm cells. The hormones are absorbed by the bloodstream for use in the body, while the sperm cells and semen are stored in the seminal vesicles. During sexual arousal, the penis becomes erect and ejaculates sperm through the urethra. Because these organs are quite vascular (contain many blood vessels) and have many nerve endings, injuries to the male (and female) genitalia are very painful.

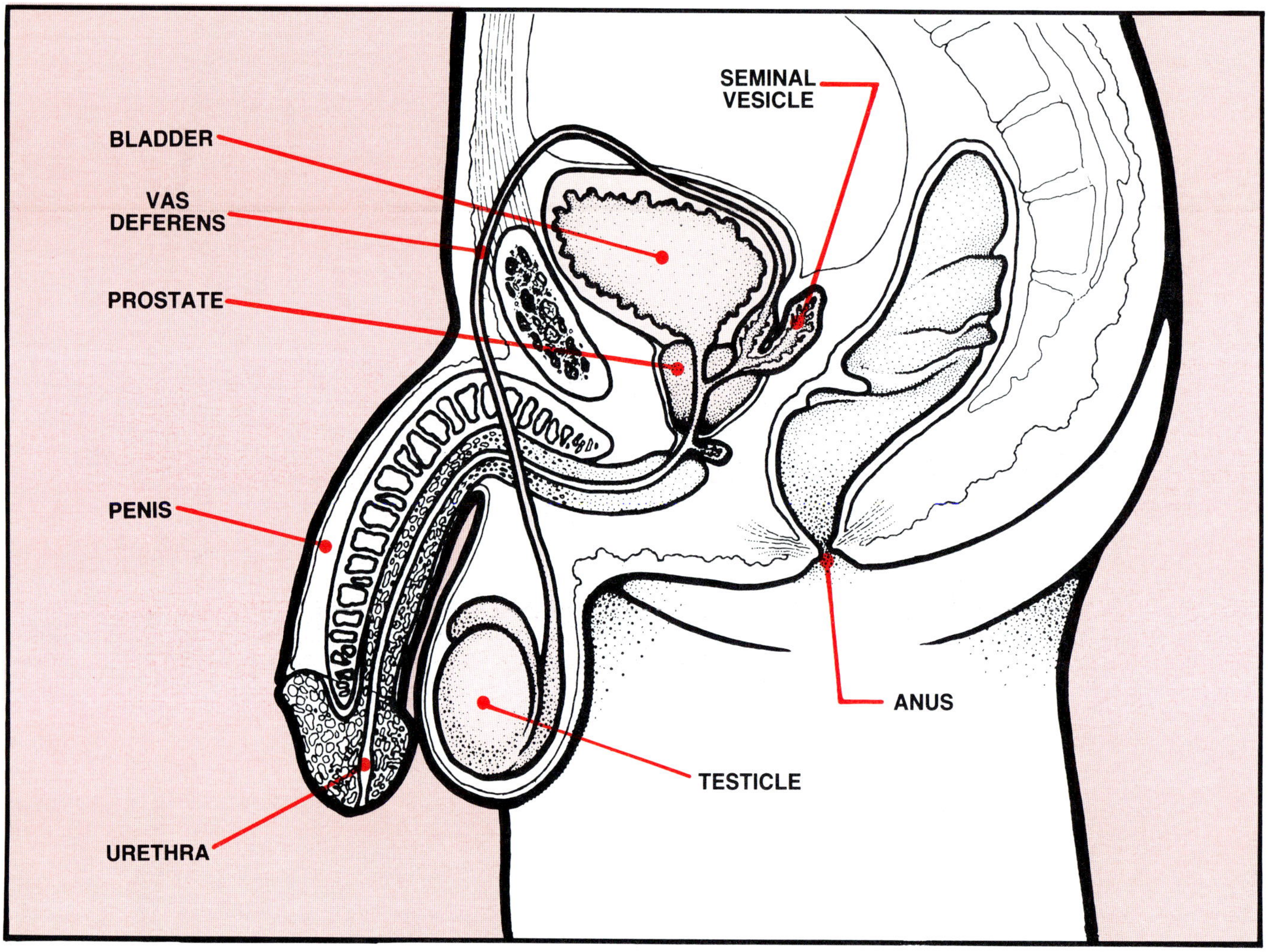


**Figure 2.32** The male reproductive organs are almost entirely external.

# 3

# Scene Assessment and Safety

# Chapter 3
# Scene Assessment and Safety

The primary duty of the first responder is to assist those who are injured or suddenly taken ill until other emergency medical care personnel arrive. Before attending to the physical needs of the patient, however, the first responder must carefully size up each scene and continue size-up throughout the call. Size-up means using one's senses to get the "big picture," then having extra personnel and equipment dispatched as soon as possible. Scene safety is also a prerequisite to good patient care; first responders must look to their own welfare as well as that of the patient. **In fact, identifying the special circumstances at the scene and calling for assistance is one of the most valuable services the first responder can perform, both in terms of scene safety and patient care.**

Many emergency scenes are either too large or too complicated to handle alone. Hazards at the scene, such as spilled chemicals or fire, require additional engine companies or specialized teams. Motor vehicle accidents often require a larger emergency medical response and specialized power tools to free trapped passengers.

Not only can the physical surroundings themselves present a challenge, so can the people at the scene. People are naturally under a great deal of stress when a loved one is suddenly taken ill; an already stressful situation compounded by alcohol, drugs, weapons, or crowds can become dangerous for both the first responder and the patient. Unstable scenes that carry the threat of violence require police assistance. Under these circumstances, first responders must ensure their own safety lest they become patients themselves.

Scene assessment and control depend on a well-functioning communications system, so this chapter begins with a brief overview of communications systems and the roles they play in emergency care. Following are descriptions of different types of scenes, including special considerations for size-up and safety for each scene. The scenes described are as follows:

- Residential scene
- Industrial/business scene
- Motor vehicle accidents
- Unstable or violent scenes that require police assistance
- Scenes complicated by hazardous substances — hazardous materials, radiation, or utility emergencies

The chapter concludes with a discussion of a hazard present at many emergency scenes, but one that EMS personnel tend to overlook: infectious diseases. Guarding against infection while still providing needed patient care requires strict attention to sanitary practices and keeping inoculations up-to-date.

## COMMUNICATIONS

A well-functioning communications system is vital to an EMS system. All components — notification, dispatch, transmissions to hospital or other emergency personnel — must work smoothly if first responders are to provide timely, quality care to the patient. Communications involves more than hardware; it also requires face-to-face exchange of information with the patient, other emergency care providers such as EMTs and paramedics, and hospital personnel.

Good communications are even more important at the emergency scene — to manage resources at hand, request additional aid, and prepare other emergency personnel to continue to treat the patient.

The complexity of an EMS communications system varies, depending on the size of the area, the number and type of emergency calls handled, or the number and type of medical facilities in the area. However, certain elements are common:

- Base station — Dispatch and coordination area
- Mobile transmitter/receiver — hand-held radios used by EMS personnel or physicians not working in a hospital
- Repeaters — Extend range of telemetry or voice communications; may be in vehicle or in fixed location
- Remote center — Usually in the emergency room of a hospital; receives voice and telemetric transmissions from the field
- Telemetry — used to transmit patient data; used by paramedics and certain EMTs (Figure 3.1)

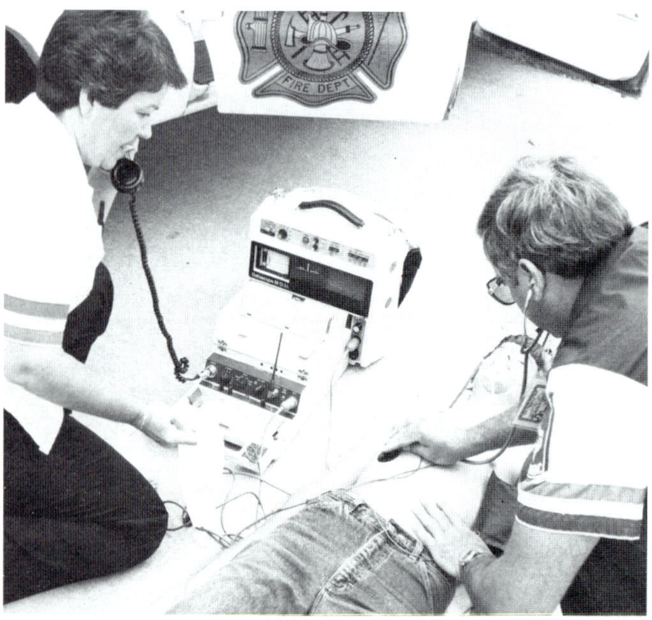


**Figure 3.1** Telemetry equipment uses radio waves to transmit a patient's heart signals to a physician in a hospital. *Courtesy of Colbert, Oklahoma Fire Department.*

- Backup communications system — such as landlines (telephones) to be used if the main system fails or in the event of a disaster or other emergency that overloads or disables the system

Linking so many different components requires careful coordination and strict attention to protocols. Communication failures, whether mechanical or human, waste precious minutes needed for patient care and can make the difference between life or death. Misdirected emergency vehicles, unreported patient signs and symptoms, and failed radio transmissions can cause a department to be sued, and cost it vitally needed public support.

## RECEIPT OF ALARM

Most calls for emergency assistance are received by telephone, although they may be received by radio, microwave, or intercom. As soon as the alarm is received, it is the dispatcher's job to obtain as much information about the emergency as possible and to dispatch the appropriate vehicles. After determining the nature of the emergency, the dispatcher fills out an emergency alarm report form, recording the caller's telephone number, name, address, and cross streets (Figure 3.2). The following information should be obtained for every call:

- The exact location of the patient. This includes the street address, direction, apartment number, and cross streets. In rural areas, it may be necessary to establish landmarks such as nearby businesses, water towers, mile markers, or cross roads to point the way for the emergency responders.
- The telephone number of the caller. This is necessary in case the connection is broken or the caller has to be redialed.
- The caller's perception of the patient's problem. Through careful questioning the dispatcher can quickly learn specifics about the patient (unconscious, bleeding severely, not breathing). This information helps the dispatcher determine which units to send or any extra equipment that may be needed.

## STILLWATER FIRE DEPARTMENT EMERGENCY MEDICAL SERVICE REPORT

| 1 DATE | 2 RUN NO | 3 UNIT NO | 4 ROAD CONDITION | FOLIO# |
|---|---|---|---|---|

| 5 NAME | SEX | AGE/DOB |
|---|---|---|

| ADDRESS | CITY | STATE | ZIP | PHONE |
|---|---|---|---|---|

| PATIENT LOCATION | PATIENT DESTINATION |
|---|---|

| GUARANTOR'S NAME | PHYSICIAN |
|---|---|

| ADDRESS | CITY | STATE | ZIP | PHONE |
|---|---|---|---|---|

| 6 | TYPE OF RUN | 7 | SKIN | 8 | SYMPTOMS/COMPLAINTS | 9 | LEVEL OF CONSCIOUSNESS |
|---|---|---|---|---|---|---|---|
| A | MEDICAL EMERGENCY | A | COOL | A | CONSCIOUS | EYE OPEN | SPONTANEOUSLY |
| B | TRANSFER | B | CLAMY | B | UNCONSCIOUS | | TO SPEECH |
| | | C | DRY | C | NUMBNESS | | TO PAIN |
| 10 | PUPILS | D | HOT | D | LOSS OF MOTION | | NONE |
| A | CONSTRICTED | E | RED | E | VISION DISTURBANCE LOSS | VERBAL | ORIENTED |
| B | DILATED | F | PALE | F | BREATHING DIFFICULTY | | CONFUSED |
| C | NON REACTIVE | G | ASHEN | G | DIZZINESS FAINT WEAK | | INAPPROP. WORDS |
| D | NORMAL/EQUAL | H | CYANOTIC | H | CHEST PAIN | | INCOMPREHENSIVE |
| E | SLUGGISH | I | NORMAL | I | VOMITING NAUSEA | | WORDS |
| F | UNEQUAL | | | | | | NONE |
| G | FIXED | | | | | MOTOR | OBEY COMMANDS |
| 11 | VITAL SIGNS | | | | | | LOCALIZED PAIN |
| | | | | | | | FLEXION TO PAIN |
| | | | | | | | EXTENTION TO PAIN |
| | | | | | | | NONE |

| TIME | B/P | PULSE | RESPIRATION |
|---|---|---|---|
| | | | |
| | | | |
| | | | |
| | | | |

EQUIP. LEFT AT HOSP.

12 COMMENTS/HISTORY/TREATMENT AT SCENE

| 13 DISPATCH | | 14 EQUIPMENT USED |
|---|---|---|
| | CALL RECEIVED | |
| | DISPATCHED | |
| | ARRIVE SCENE | 15 OTHER ASSISTANCE |
| | DEPART SCENE | 16 HOSPITAL NOTIFIED |
| | ARRIVE HOSPITAL | 17 DISPOSITION OF VALUABLES |
| | BACK IN SERVICE | |
| | BACK IN QUARTERS | 18 RECEIVED-HOSPITAL |
| | TOTAL TIME | 19 CREW SIGNATURES |
| 20 MILEAGE IN | | |
| OUT | | |
| TOTAL | | |

ORIGINAL COPY/AMBULANCE CANARY COPY/DATA PROCESSING PINK COPY/HOSPITAL

**Figure 3.2** The emergency alarm report form is used to record critical information about an emergency. *Courtesy of Stillwater, Oklahoma Fire Department.*

- If the call concerns an accident with possible multiple casualties, such as an automobile or industrial accident, the dispatcher should try to determine the
  - — Number and type of vehicles involved (cars, trucks, buses). If trucks are involved it is useful to know what type of load they are carrying.
  - — Number of persons involved and whether or not they appear to be trapped or seriously injured.
  - — Hazards at the scene, such as spilled or leaking chemicals, downed electrical lines, or fire.
  - — Location of vehicles — on or off the road, number of lanes blocked, direction of travel (such as eastbound or westbound lanes).
  - — The caller's location and the time elapsed since he or she left the scene.

By asking a series of ordered questions the dispatcher can control the conversation and obtain critical information about the patient's condition and circumstances at the scene. This additional information can be relayed to give responding units a better idea of the situation while they are en route. The dispatcher may also keep the caller on the line and give first aid instructions or advise what actions to avoid. This coaching helps to reduce the caller's anxiety and may help save the patient's life.

When a call comes in, listen carefully to the dispatcher. Get the correct address (write it down if possible) and note the nature of the call. Certain calls, such as shooting or fight victims, domestic violence, psychological disturbance, or attempted suicide, should immediately alert you to ask for police assistance. Other calls, such as accidents with multiple victims or hazards at the scene, will also require a larger response and specialized equipment. If the call is of an unknown nature, ask the dispatcher to obtain more information and relay it to you.

Before leaving, know exactly how to get to the address. Take into account the time of day, weather, and traffic. Everyone in the emergency vehicle should wear seat belts when driving to or from every emergency call.

## SIZE-UP AND SCENE CONTROL

Size-up begins on the way to the emergency scene and continues throughout the entire call. En route to the scene, begin to form a mental picture of what to expect based on the nature of the call. Review treatment procedures and remember to assess the ABC's first. This mental planning is the first step in size-up.

Shut off the siren several blocks away from the destination to avoid broadcasting your arrival. As you arrive at the scene, use your eyes and ears to get the "big picture." Particularly at night, it is easy to focus on only one aspect of the scene. For example, a person may be injured and lying on the ground; if all your attention is immediately directed toward that one person, you may miss the fact that there is another victim lying nearby. If it is necessary, provide lighting as soon as possible after arriving on the scene.

If the emergency scene involves multiple casualties and additional ambulances are needed, use the following rule of thumb when determining how many ambulances will be needed:

- One patient requiring advanced life support (ALS) per ambulance. ALS includes persons needing IV therapy, those in shock, patients with shortness of breath, chest pain, severe head or chest injuries, or multiple trauma.
- Two patients requiring basic life support (BLS) per ambulance.

Additional time is needed for extra personnel and equipment to reach the scene, so the sooner they are dispatched, the better.

First of all, remember that your own safety is of prime importance, because if you are disabled you cannot provide help to anyone else. Different types of calls require different approaches to ensure safety for yourself and the patient. Carry a portable radio at all times so that you can communicate with the dispatcher.

### Residential Scene

A residential call requires coordination between first responders and other incoming EMS vehicles. Many times the ambulance will want to back into the driveway to make it easier to load the patient. If requested to do so, work out a system for marking the house or apartment. Shining a spotlight or parking in front of the house can save time for incoming units. Be sure to take a first aid kit, the keys, and lock the vehicle.

As you walk toward the house or apartment, keep your eyes and ears open for any threatening situations. Stand to the side of the door, knock, and loudly announce who you are. Then wait for someone to open the door.

Family members can be both a help and a hindrance. Usually, relatives are very concerned about the patient and are eager to help. However, it is a frightening experience to have to call for emergency medical help; anxiety levels are high, and family members who are terrified that a loved one will die may themselves collapse. Try to reduce anxiety levels by keeping family members informed of your actions. If possible, give them a simple task, such as holding equipment or going outside to flag down incoming vehicles. By keeping busy, family members can reduce their own anxiety about the patient. If necessary, have your partner interview family members while you interview the patient separately. Then you can compare notes.

When a child is the patient, remember that the parents are the ones who make the decisions; therefore, they must be completely informed. Do not attempt to separate very young children from their parents. This action only increases anxiety in both parents and child; besides, parents often will have to do the talking for the children.

**THE INJURY OR ILLNESS OF A LOVED ONE CAUSES SEVERE ANXIETY IN FAMILY MEMBERS. REDUCE THIS ANXIETY BY DISPLAYING A CALM, PROFESSIONAL MANNER AND BY KEEPING FAMILY MEMBERS INFORMED OF YOUR ACTIONS.**

### Business/Industrial Scene

Because of the increased hazards encountered at a business or industrial site, it is very important to have complete information from the dispatcher. This information should include pre-incident plans that detail the type of business, entrances, chemicals stored on the premises, and any other special hazards. Some plant entrances are only open at certain times. If the emergency is at a large industrial complex, you may have to go to a guard shack and get further directions to the site of the accident. If the accident involves a chemical, take in the scene before getting out of the vehicle. If people are lying on the ground for no apparent reason, be very careful. Many chemicals are colorless, odorless, and attack the sense of smell.

If the plant is a large one, you may be directed to a first aid station staffed by a nurse. If the patient is somewhere in the plant, ask a supervisor or someone who knows the plant to accompany you and provide technical assistance. Ask how the injury occurred and if it is safe to work around the machinery. If there are multiple injuries, begin triage as soon as possible. Remember that an ambulance can handle one patient requiring advanced life support and two patients requiring basic life support.

### Motor Vehicle Accident

When arriving on the scene of a motor vehicle accident, park your vehicle so as to provide safety and to allow access for other EMS vehicles. Park so that a motorist who is watching the accident rather than the road will not strike your vehicle, you, or the patient. Note quickly whether gasoline or chemicals have been spilled; if so, call for another engine immediately. Any sign of smoke or fire also requires a call for assistance. If it looks like power tools will be needed for extrication, have them dispatched.

If a truck is involved, try to determine what the truck is carrying. Look for a placard on the truck indicating a hazardous material or check the manifest in the cab. Keep in mind that *any* vehicle, not just a truck, can be carrying hazardous materials; automobiles sometimes carry radioactive materials or disease specimens. Remember that materials weighing less than 1,000 lbs. (454 kg) are not required to carry placards. (For further discussion of hazardous materials, see the Hazardous Materials section later in this chapter.)

If the accident involves more than one person, begin triage as soon as possible. Remember that people who are bleeding or yelling are not necessarily the most seriously injured; a very quiet patient may be in much more serious trouble. When calling for more ambulances, remember the formula for patients — patient needing advanced life support, two patients needing basic life support, per ambulance. Be ready to spot incoming EMS vehicles.

## Unstable Scenes

Unstable scenes are scenes that carry the threat of violence, either from the patients themselves or from people at the scene. Often police assistance is required to restrain violent people or to keep others from the patient or rescue workers. Each department has its own procedures for dealing with violent or potentially violent situations; follow these procedures rigorously. **Remember that your own safety comes first; you cannot assist others if you are injured.** Finally, remember that all calls require careful size-up; just because a call is to a neat, well-kept residence does not mean that someone inside may not be armed or violent.

### CRIME SCENE

If a scene is already known to be unstable (called in as a person assaulted, stabbed, or shot), wait until the police have secured the scene before entering. Note the position of the patient, and move the patient only if necessary to provide treatment. Do not touch anything inside unless absolutely necessary, and place equipment carefully so as not to destroy evidence. Do not handle weapons unless they must be moved off or away from the patient. Assume that any gun is cocked and ready to fire. If you must move a gun, keep the barrel pointed away and pick it up very carefully by the end of the grip (Figure 3.3). NEVER push a pencil or similar object down the barrel of a gun; to do so may rescore the barrel, making any ballistics tests useless. When a knife is the weapon, use several gauze pads to protect your fingers, then pick up the knife by the tip of the blade. Lastly, when cutting away clothing to view a wound, cut clothing around the wound rather than through the point of entry. Cutting clothing in this manner helps to preserve evidence.

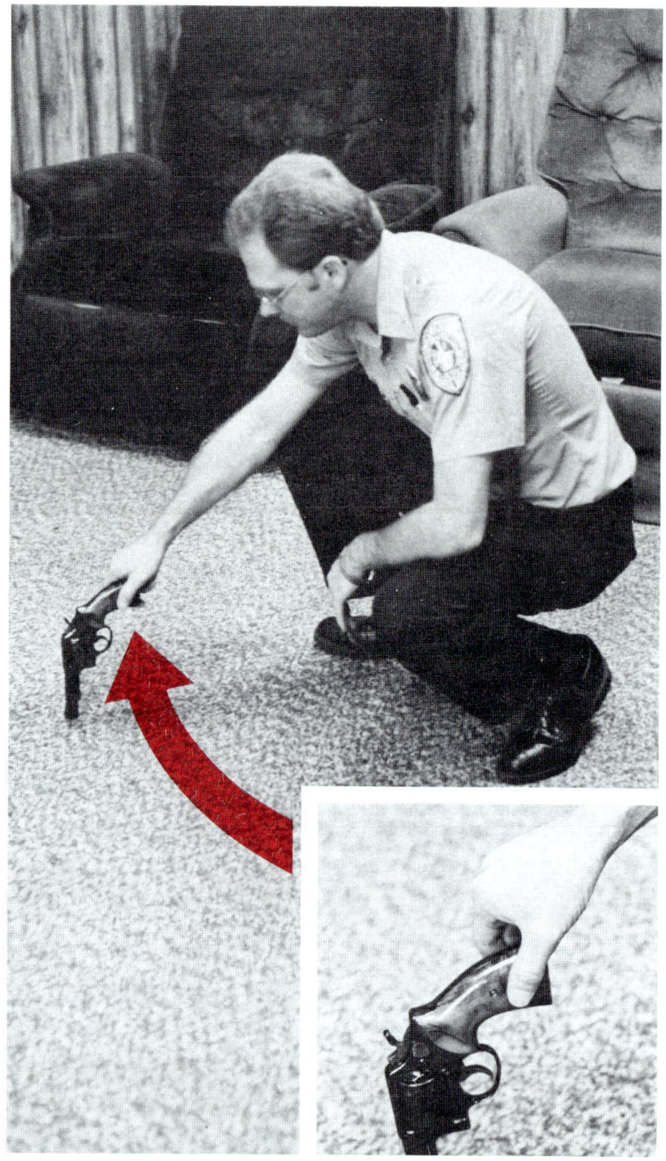

**Figure 3.3** If you must handle a gun, pick it up very carefully by the end of the grip.

### DOMESTIC VIOLENCE

Police officers are more likely to be assaulted at a domestic violence scene than at any other, so first responders should exercise extra caution. Call for police to secure the scene first; they can also subdue someone who becomes violent. If it does become necessary to enter a residence without police backup, take extra precautions because people behave unpredictably. Stand to the side of the door and announce yourself loudly, then wait for someone to answer the door (Figure 3.4). Do not walk in alone even if requested to do so.

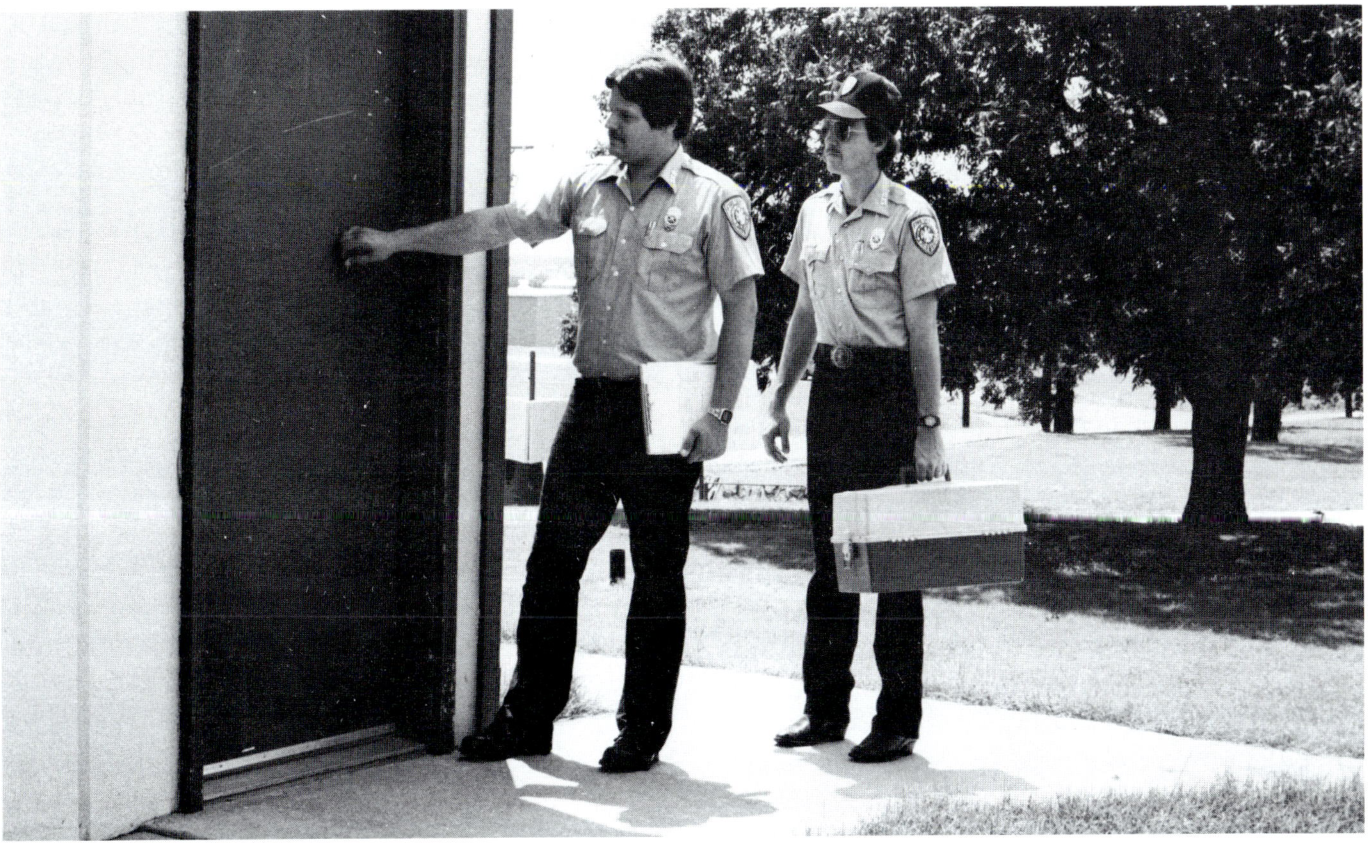

**Figure 3.4** Take extra caution when responding to calls that may involve violence. Stand to the side of the door and announce yourself loudly, then wait for someone to open the door.

## AID TO PERSON IN MOTOR VEHICLE

Safety is the first consideration when approaching an automobile that does not seem to have been involved in an accident; someone slumped over the wheel of a car may well be ill, but may also be intoxicated or armed. Position the rescue vehicle a safe distance behind the car and turn the wheels slightly to the left; if it becomes necessary to back up rapidly, the vehicle will not go deeper into the shoulder of the road. If it is dark, use your headlights to illuminate the interior of the car. Make sure the trunk of the car is locked. Stand to the driver's rear and try to see if the driver is holding any weapons. Have another rescuer approach from the passenger side and open that door first if possible. Watch the patient's hands at all times. If the patient does become violent, retreat quickly and call for police assistance.

## CROWD CONTROL

One thing all EMS scenes have in common is the ability to draw a crowd. Some people want to help; others just want to watch. Bystanders range from the merely curious to sidewalk "doctors," who are eager to tell you exactly what to do. If possible, find something for these people to do: holding supplies, flagging down incoming vehicles, or keeping other bystanders clear. A task will help focus their energy and keep them out of your way. If anyone claims to be a physician, nurse, or EMS specialist and wants to assist, request identification. Remind that person that he or she must stay until the ambulance arrives and, if necessary, ride with the patient to the medical facility.

Crowds can degenerate into angry crowds, particularly if several people feel that care is not being rendered fast enough. Maintain a professional demeanor at all times; getting mad and yelling at people will not help the situation. Merely ignoring abuse is not always wise, however; if people become threatening, call for police assistance.

## BARKING OR VICIOUS DOGS

Dogs can become very agitated at the sight of strangers entering the home, particularly when the scene inside may already be chaotic. At best they can be distracting, upsetting the patient and making it more difficult to conduct an examination, and at worst they can be dangerous. Have someone who can handle the dog lock it in another room. A dog outside in a yard can make it difficult to get to the house. Some departments use a booster line or a $CO_2$ extinguisher to make the dog retreat.

## ENVIRONMENTAL HAZARDS

Environmental hazards may involve the release of hazardous materials, gas leaks, or downed electrical lines. Emergency scenes that are complicated by hazards such as these demand the intervention of persons or teams trained in dealing with the specific hazard. As with scenes that require police intervention, it is vitally important that you act to protect yourself first. Rushing into an unsafe environment without proper protective equipment may only create additional patients; if this happens, the first responder is not only unable to provide assistance, but also complicates matters by presenting other emergency care personnel with even more victims. Again, **recognizing the special circumstances at the emergency scene and then calling for expert assistance is one of the most valuable services the first responder can perform, both in terms of scene safety and patient care.**

### Electric and Gas Hazards

Utility hazards require the assistance of trained personnel. For electrical hazards, such as downed lines, park at least one span away (Figure 3.5). Watch for falling poles; a pole may take other poles with it. Do not touch any wires, power lines, or other electrical sources until they have been deactivated by a power company employee. Assume that all downed wires are live wires until informed otherwise by a power company employee. It is not just the wires themselves that are hazardous: any metal that they touch also becomes energized. Fences that become energized are energized for their entire length as long as they are unbroken. Of course, be careful around running or standing water since it is an excellent conductor of electricity.

Both natural gas and liquefied petroleum gas (LPG) are nontoxic but are classified as asphyxiants because they displace breathing air. In

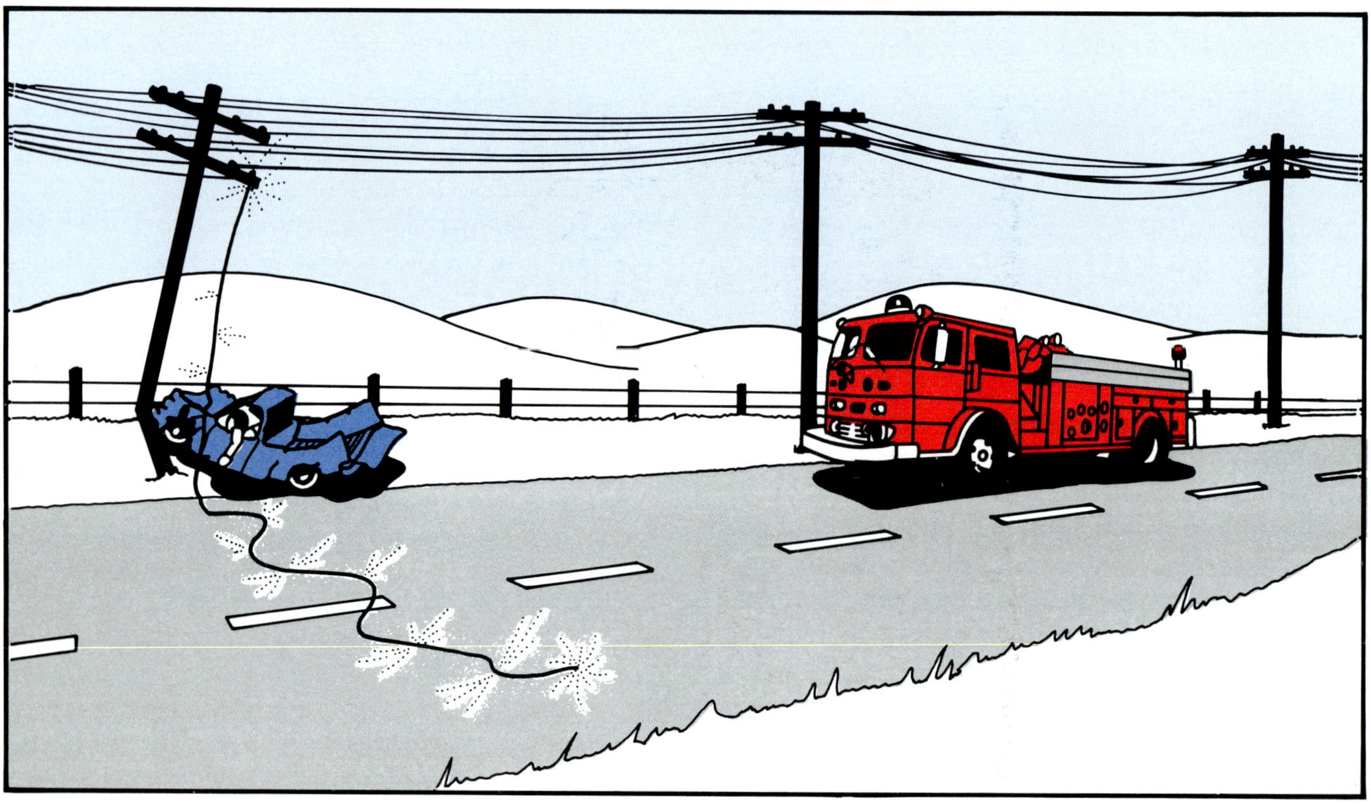

**Figure 3.5** Park the rescue vehicle at least one span away from downed lines.

addition, both types of gas are explosive. If an emergency involves leaking gas, call the gas company immediately. Allowing power company employees to turn off power sources ensures that the job is done properly and that power is not disrupted to more sources than is necessary. If a patient has been overcome by leaking gas, wear positive-pressure self-contained breathing apparatus immediately. Remove the patient from the atmosphere before beginning treatment.

### Hazardous Materials

The manufacture and transport of hazardous materials has made every area the potential site of a hazardous materials incident. Hazardous materials are routinely transported by truck, rail, water, air, and car. Some examples of materials commonly transported are trucks shuttling 55 gallon (208.2 L) drums of chemicals between plants; trucks carrying compressed gases used for welding; gasoline tankers; and cars transporting radioactive materials to hospitals. As a first responder it is imperative that you be aware of the risks posed by hazardous materials and act accordingly. In many cases, it is just as important to know what *not* to do as what *to* do.

What is a hazardous material? The U.S. Department of Transportation defines a hazardous material as "any substance or form which may pose an unreasonable risk to health and safety of property when transported in commerce." Hazardous materials range from chemicals in liquid or gas form to radioactive materials to etiologic (disease-causing) agents. Moreover, hazardous materials pose risks to health and safety in many ways. They may be flammable, explosive, toxic, corrosive, radioactive, unstable, or reactive.

Some large population centers route hazardous materials through less-congested areas, while other large areas allow bulk loads to pass through them. Most transportation of hazardous materials is routed around large population centers; however, smaller shipments are frequently involved in accidents. The two most common types of hazardous materials incidents likely to be encountered by the first responder are motor vehicle accidents and industrial accidents.

Ideally, initial size-up should include information obtained during pre-incident planning. Information about stored hazardous materials, transportation routes, terrain, and evacuation procedures should be available. Sometimes a particular address by itself will alert you to the possibility of hazardous materials at the scene. As outlined at the beginning of this chapter, the dispatcher should ask for additional information upon receipt of the alarm and transmit it to responding units. Weather conditions and wind direction and velocity are also important to note and remember.

Trying to determine whether an accident is complicated by the release of hazardous materials requires caution and careful approach. The natural response of a first responder is to approach any patient and begin assessment and treatment immediately. However, in the case of hazardous materials, this approach is neither feasible nor wise. First responders who follow their natural instincts and rush into the scene without first sizing up the situation may only complicate the incident by creating more patients. If first responders are disabled, treatment for the original victims is delayed and more personnel and equipment are required to remove and treat the increased number of victims.

### Motor Vehicle Accident

If the alarm has not already been dispatched as a known hazardous materials incident, look for signs of possible hazardous materials involvement when approaching the scene. Such signs include container failure, placards, vapor clouds, smoke, or any unusual odors. If any of these signs are present, stay **UPWIND** of the accident scene and evaluate it before approaching. Remember the saying: "Attack with binoculars." In an open area, stay 1,000 feet (304.8 m) away, in residential or light commercial areas, stay one block away, and in large complexes or when the incident is hidden by a building, maintain a distance of at least 500 feet (152.4 m). If you detect any unusual odors, put on positive-pressure self-contained breathing apparatus immediately. Call for additional help immediately: more engine companies, ambulances, and a hazardous materials team detailing their response route. Notify the police department so that they can establish an isolation zone of 2,500 feet

(762 m) in all directions. Keep any additional responding vehicles from entering the area until it has been evaluated.

Look to see if the vehicle has a placard on it (Figure 3.6 on next two pages). On the placard there may be a four-digit identification number. This identification number can usually be looked up in the U.S. Department of Transportation *Emergency Response Guidebook* to determine both the name of the chemical involved and instructions for handling the initial scene. Be aware that a vehicle carrying a bulk load of mixed materials may necessitate more than one placard. Sometimes a mixed load is placarded as dangerous. **CAUTION:** Do not assume that a vehicle without a placard has no hazardous materials. Truck regulations do not require placards for many hazardous material loads of less than 1,000 pounds (454 kg).

Try to identify the material involved. Consult pre-incident plans, note warning signs, container color and shape, or try to obtain shipping papers. Again, identification may require the use of binoculars. If several people must make a closer approach to identify the hazardous material, they should do so **ONLY** after donning protective clothing, including positive-pressure self-contained breathing apparatus. The wrists, ankles, and waist should be secured.

After the material is identified, call CHEMTREC (1-800-424-9300) for further information on dealing with the situation. CHEMTREC is staffed 24 hours a day in order to provide assistance with hazardous materials.

## Industrial Accident

At the scene of an industrial accident, pre-incident planning is vital for obtaining rapid information about the chemical involved. Information should already be available about chemicals stored at the plant. In addition, safety personnel at the plant can supply additional information in the form of a Material Safety Data Sheet (MSDS) that gives information about the chemical. The information most important for the first responder is the first aid section, which describes specific treatment for exposure to a chemical. If you cannot obtain adequate information about the chemical, call CHEMTREC.

**Figure 3.6** The identification number on a placard can be looked up to determine the name of the chemical and how to handle it. *Courtesy of Office of Hazardous Materials, (DHM-51), Materials Transportation Bureau, Research and Programs Administration, U.S. Department of Transportation.*

The NFPA 704 system gives quick information about the hazards of a particular chemical. This system is used on fixed facilities only, such as buildings or tanks. The 704 label looks similar to a placard but gives different information (Figure 3.7). The 704 sign gives the firefighter/first responder information about the severity of a chemical without stating the name of the chemical. The diamond is divided into four different colored sections. Three sections have a number from 0 to 4; 4 is the most hazardous and 0 is the least hazardous. The bottom section contains special information, such as radiation hazard or instructions not to use water.

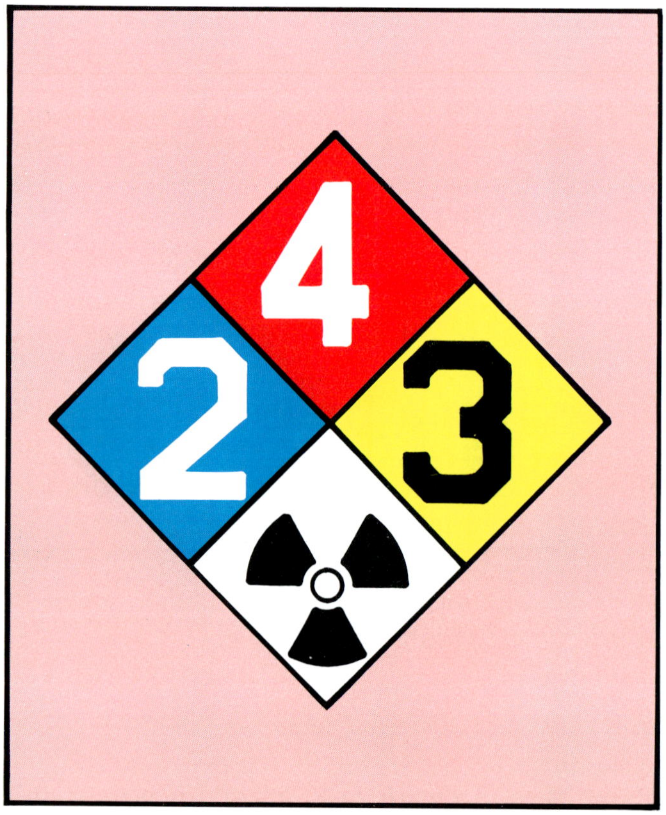


**Figure 3.7** The NFPA 704 system gives vital information about chemicals stored in fixed facilities. *Reprinted with permission from NFPA 704-1985, Standard System for the Identification of Fire Hazards of Materials, Copyright 1985, National Fire Protection Association, Quincy, MA 02269. This warning system is intended to be interpreted and applied only by properly trained individuals to identify fire, health and reactivity hazards of chemicals. The user is referred to a certain limited number of chemicals with recommended classifications in NFPA 49 and NFPA 325.*

# Hazardous Materials Warning Placards

## DOMESTIC PLACARDING

Illustration numbers in each square (1 through 18) refer to TABLES 1 and 2 below.

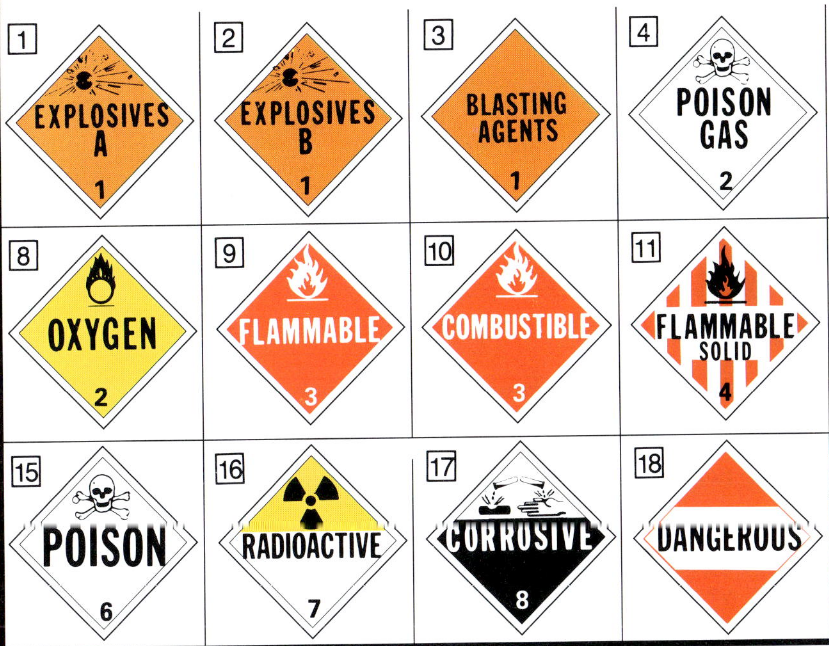


**(WHITE) SQUARE BACKGROUND FOR PLACARD**

**HIGHWAY**

- Used for "HIGHWAY ROUTE CONTROLLED QUANTITY OF RADIOACTIVE MATERIALS". (Sec. 172.507)

**RAIL**

- Used for RAIL SHIPMENTS-"EXPLOSIVE A." "POISON GAS" and "POISON GAS-RESIDUE" placards. (Sec. 172.510(a))

## TABLE 1

| HAZARD CLASSES | *NO. |
|---|---|
| Class A explosives | 1 |
| Class B explosives | 2 |
| Poison A | 4 |
| Flammable solid (DANGEROUS WHEN WET label only) | 12 |
| Radioactive material (YELLOW III label) | 16 |
| Radioactive material: | |
| Uranium hexafluoride fissile (containing more than 1.0% $U^{235}$) | 16 & 17 |
| Uranium hexafluoride, low-specific activity (containing 1.0% or less $U^{235}$ | 16 & 17 |

NOTE: For details on the use of Tables 1 and 2, see Sec. 172.504 (See footnotes at bottom of tables.)

## Guidelines

**(CFR, Title 49, Transportation, Parts 100-177)**

- Placard *motor vehicles, freight containers,* and *rail cars* containing *any quantity* of hazardous materials listed in TABLE 1.
- Placard *motor vehicles, freight containers* and *rail cars* containing 1,000 pounds or more gross weight of hazardous materials classes listed in TABLE 2.
- Placard *freight containers* 640 cubic feet or more containing *any quantity* of hazardous material classes listed in TABLES 1 and/or 2 when offered for transportation by air or water. Under 640 cubic feet see Sec. 172.512(b).

CAUTION

*CHECK EACH SHIPMENT FOR COMPLIANCE WITH THE APPROPRIATE HAZARDOUS MATERIALS REGULATIONS:

Proper Classification, Marking, Placarding, Packaging, Labeling, Documentation

PRIOR TO OFFERING FOR SHIPMENT

## TABLE 2

| HAZARD CLASSES | *NO. |
|---|---|
| Class C explosives | 18 |
| Blasting agent | 3 |
| Nonflammable gas | 6 |
| Nonflammable gas (Chlorine) | 7 |
| Nonflammable gas (Fluorine) | 15 |
| Nonflammable gas (Oxygen, cryogenic liquid) | 8 |
| Flammable gas | 5 |
| Combustible liquid | 10 |
| Flammable liquid | 9 |
| Flammable solid | 11 |
| Oxidizer | 13 |
| Organic peroxide | 14 |
| Poison B | 15 |
| Corrosive material | 17 |
| Irritating material | 18 |

## INTERNATIONAL PLACARDING

- Most International placards are similar (color and pictorial symbol(s) to the Domestic placards illustrated above.
- International placards are enlarged ICAO or IMO labels (See International Labeling—Otherside).
- Placard MUST correspond to *hazard class* of material.
- Placard *ANY QUANTITY* of hazardous materials when loaded in FREIGHT CONTAINERS, PORTABLE TANKS, RAIL CARS and HIGHWAY VEHICLES.
- International placards *may* be used *in addition* to DOT placards for international shipments.

When required, *Subsidiary Risk placards* must be displayed in the same manner as *Primary Risk placards.* Class numbers are *not shown* on Subsidiary Risk placards.

- COMPATIBILITY GROUP DESIGNATORS *must* be displayed on EXPLOSIVES PLACARDS.
- UN CLASS NUMBERS and DIVISION NUMBERS *MUST* be displayed on hazard class placards when required.

## UN and NA Identification Numbers

- The four digit UN or NA numbers must be displayed on all hazardous materials packages for which identification numbers are assigned. Example: ACETONE UN 1090.
- UN (United Nations) or NA (North American) numbers are found in the Hazardous Materials Tables, Sec. 172.101 and 172.102 (CFR, Title 49, Parts 100-199)
- Identification numbers may not be displayed on "POISON GAS," "RADIOACTIVE" or "EXPLOSIVE" placards. (Sec. 172.334)
- UN numbers are displayed in the same manner for both Domestic and International shipments.
- NA numbers are used only in the USA and Canada.

When hazardous materials are transported in Tank Cars, Cargo Tanks and Portable Tanks, UN or NA numbers *must* be displayed on:

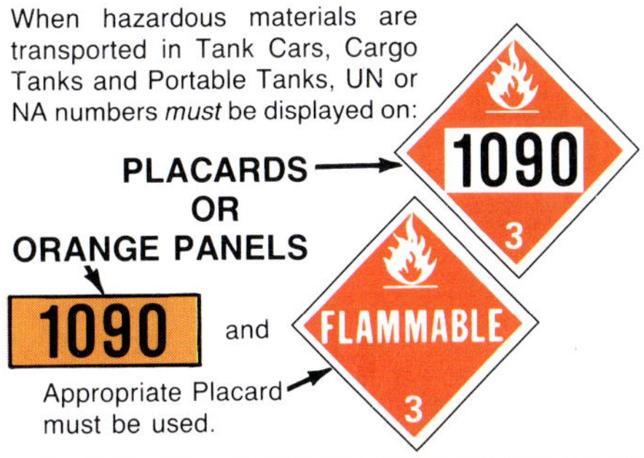

PLACARDS
OR
ORANGE PANELS
1090
3
1090
and
FLAMMABLE
3
Appropriate Placard must be used.


EUROPEAN NUMBERING SYSTEM—

**Top Number**—Hazard Index (Identification of Danger, 2 or 3 figures) Example: 33 = highly inflammable liquid.

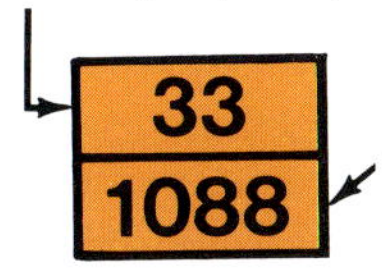

33
1088


**Bottom Number**—UN Number of substance Example: 1088 ACETAL

For more complete details on identification Numbers see Sec. 172.300 through 172.338.

For sale by the Superintendent of Documents, U.S. Government Printing Office, Washington, D.C. 20402

# Hazardous Materials Warning Labels

## DOMESTIC LABELING

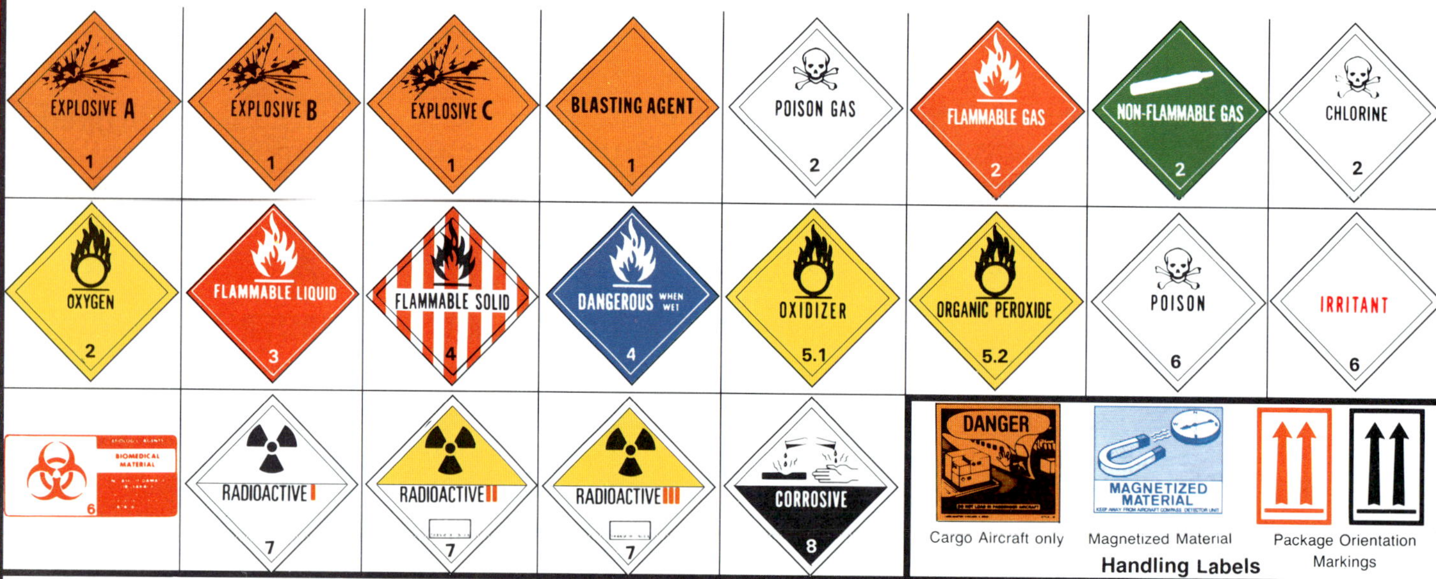


## General Guidelines on Use of Labels

**(CFR, Title 49, Transportation, Parts 100-177)**

- Labels illustrated above are normally for *domestic shipments*. However, some air carriers *may* require the use of International Civil Aviation Organization (ICAO) labels.
- Domestic Warning Labels *may* display UN Class Number, Division Number (and Compatibility Group for Explosives only.) Sec. 172.407(g).
- Any person who offers a hazardous material for transportation MUST label the package, if required. [Sec. 172.400(a)].
- The Hazardous Materials Tables, Sec. 172.101 and 172.102, identify the proper label(s) for the hazardous materials listed.
- Label(s), when required, must be printed on or affixed to the surface of the package near the proper shipping name. [Sec. 172.406(a)].
- When two or more different labels are required, display them next to each other. [Sec. 172.406(c)].
- Labels may be affixed to packages (even when not required by regulations) provided each label represents a hazard of the material in the package. [Sec. 172-401].

Check the Appropriate Regulations

Domestic or International Shipment

## UN Class Numbers

Class 1—Explosives

Class 2—Gases (compressed, liquified or dissolved under pressure)

Class 3—Flammable liquids

Class 4—Flammable solids or substances

Class 5—Oxidizing substances
Division 5.1-Oxidizing substances or agents.
Division 5.2-Organic peroxides.

Class 6—Poisonous and infectious substances

Class 7—Radioactive substances

Class 8—Corrosives

Class 9—Miscellaneous dangerous substances

## INTERNATIONAL LABELING

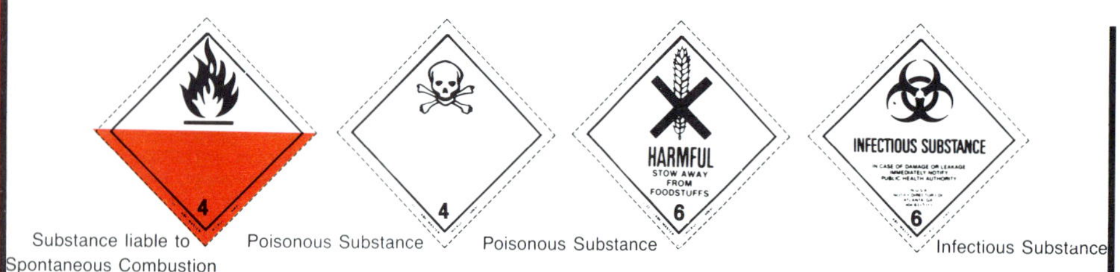


### EXAMPLES OF INTERNATIONAL LABELS

- These are examples of International Labels not presently used for domestic shipments.
- Text, when used Internationally *may* be in the language of the country of origin.
- **Most of the domestic labels ( illustrated above) *may* be used Internationally.**

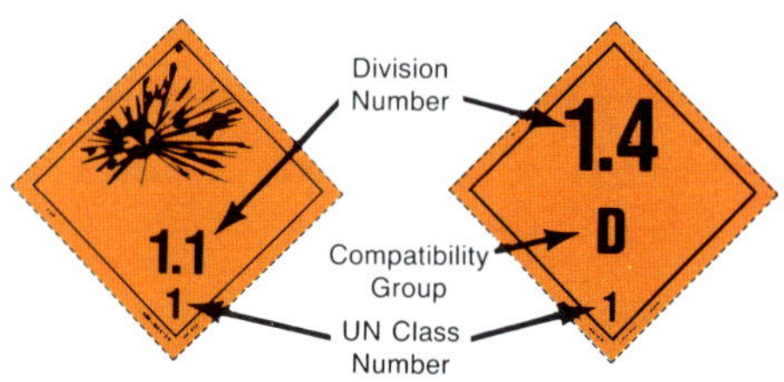


### EXAMPLES OF EXPLOSIVE LABELS

- The NUMERICAL DESIGNATION represents the CLASS or DIVISION.
- ALPHABETICAL DESIGNATION represents the COMPATIBILITY GROUP (for Explosives Only)
- DIVISION NUMBERS and COMPATIBILITY GROUP combinations can result in over 30 different "Explosives" labels (see IMDG Code/ICAO).

For complete details, refer to one or more of the following:

- Code of Federal Regulations, Title 49, Transportation. Parts 100-199. [All Modes]
- International Civil Aviation Organization (ICAO) Technical Instructions for the Safe Transport of Dangerous Goods by air. [Air]
- International Maritime Organization (IMO) Dangerous Goods Code. [Water]
- "Transportation of Dangerous Goods Regulations" of Transport Canada. [All Modes]


U.S. Department of Transportation

**Research and Special Programs Administration**

Washington, D.C. 20590

CHART 8
REV. FEBRUARY 1986

The left section, which is blue, gives information about the health effects of the chemical. The top section is red: it gives information about the flammability of the chemical. For example, a chemical with a rating of 0 will not burn and one rated 4 burns readily, needing only an ignition source. Be sure that the ignition source does not come from your vehicle's engine or the spark created when keying up a radio transmitter. The third section is yellow and gives information about the stability of the chemical. Chemicals with a rating of 4 are readily capable of detonating; chemicals with a rating of 0 are normally stable.

In summary, **DO NOT** rush into a known or suspected hazardous materials scene without first performing a careful size-up. If at all possible, let hazardous materials experts handle the situation. **NEVER** enter a dangerous atmosphere without first donning full protective clothing and positive-pressure self-contained breathing apparatus.

## Radiation Hazards

The thought of radiation is frightening to many people, and indeed exposure to radiation can be lethal. However, it is safe to treat people who have been exposed to radiation. People who absorb radiation may become ill but they are not dangerous to others. Radiation hazards, like the release of hazardous materials, are most likely to be encountered at industrial and motor vehicle accidents.

A radioactive substance is unstable and emits particles to become stable. Particle emission is known as ionizing radiation. Some substances are naturally radioactive, while other substances can be made unstable. There are three types of ionizing radiation: alpha, beta, and gamma rays.

Alpha particles are the largest and slowest radioactive particles. Alpha particles do not travel very far in the air and can be stopped by a piece of paper, clothing, or even the skin. If alpha particles do enter the body through inhalation or ingestion, however, they can do significant damage.

Beta particles are smaller and faster than alpha particles. Beta particles can be stopped by heavy clothing or a thin sheet of metal. Like alpha particles, beta particles can enter the body through inhalation or ingestion.

Gamma rays are the most penetrating and the most dangerous of the ionizing rays. Gamma rays easily penetrate the entire body, and can only be stopped by heavy lead shielding or very thick concrete. Gamma rays are basically x-rays. When used for medical diagnosis, gamma rays are rendered safe by using very brief exposure times.

Radiation is colorless, odorless, and cannot be felt. It can only be detected with special instruments, such as a Geiger counter or dosimeter. Remember that as a first responder you do not have the tools or expertise to handle a radiation incident alone. If an incident involves release of radioactive materials, immediately call for additional help from any local organizations that have expertise in handling radioactive materials: Civil Defense, university laboratories, or private businesses. If the incident is a motor vehicle accident and you see the universal radiation symbol, immediately request help (Figure 3.8).

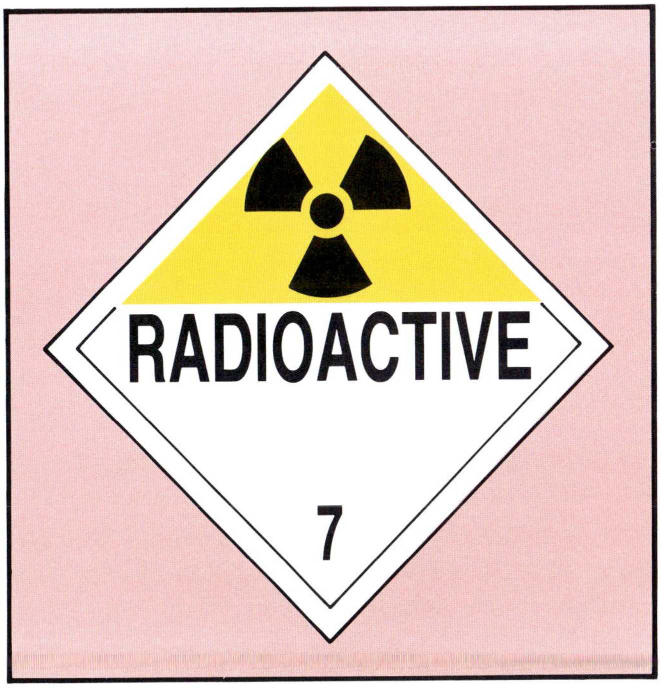


**Figure 3.8** If you see the universal radiation symbol on a vehicle involved in an accident, call for additional help immediately.

Park **UPWIND** of the accident scene; in addition, park upwind of any liquid spills or leaks. Wear full protective clothing and positive-pressure self-contained breathing apparatus. The clothing does not protect against gamma rays, but wearing breathing apparatus prevents inhalation of radioactive particles. Reduce your exposure by using **TIME, DISTANCE, AND SHIELDING.** Spend as little time in the "hot" zone (the area closest to the incident) as possible to reduce total exposure. If necessary, work in relays. Increase your distance from the source of radiation as much as possible. Radiation follows the inverse square law: as distance is increased, the amount of radiation decreases as the square of the distance. For example, doubling your distance from a radioactive source gives you one-fourth the exposure. Remove the patient from the area of heaviest contamination as rapidly as possible and assess the patient's ABC's.

An "intermediate zone" may be established for decontamination of any patients and rescue workers. It is in this area that everyone's clothing must be washed and removed. Then each person must be checked for contamination before being allowed to leave. By following these procedures, contamination that clings to boots, clothing, and personal articles is not spread elsewhere. If everyone is not decontaminated at the scene, they may have to be decontaminated in the hospital, in a separate area away from the Emergency Room.

## INFECTION CONTROL: GUARDING AGAINST COMMUNICABLE DISEASES

**NOTE:** Much of the information that follows was adapted with permission from *Emergency Concepts: Infection Control* by Katherine H. West, R.N., B.S.N., copyright 1984.

Because of the many elements associated with scene assessment and patient care, it is easy for the first responder to forget to take personal precautions against communicable diseases. These precautions must not be overlooked because lack of attention to infection control can have serious consequences for anyone involved in health care. The fact is, sick people have germs, and many of these germs are communicable, that is, they can be spread from one person to another. Anyone who cares for sick people must learn basic techniques of infection control, and practice these techniques on every call. Infections are spread in four basic ways:

1. Direct contact — such as a handshake or kiss with an infected person
2. Indirect contact — coming in contact with an object that has been handled by an infected person
3. Droplet infection — inhaling droplets that are discharged when an infected person coughs or sneezes
4. Sexual contact — transmission through close sexual contact

Although anyone may be harboring a communicable disease, be especially careful around the patient who

- Has a fever of unknown origin
- Has diarrhea
- Has draining wounds
- Is bleeding
- Has jaundice
- Is receiving dialysis
- Has a rash
- Is known to have communicable disease

Figure 3.9 lists some communicable diseases and the way they are transmitted.

### AIDS

Acquired Immune Deficiency Syndrome (AIDS) deserves special mention because it is a communicable disease and it is deadly. AIDS is a very serious disorder in which the body loses its ability to fight off infection. More than 16,000 cases of AIDS have been diagnosed in the United States since 1981, and half of those afflicted have died. It is estimated that up to 1 million people will develop AIDS. At this writing, AIDS is a fatal disease and there is no known cure.

Naturally, AIDS has caused a great deal of concern in the general public and in health care providers. This concern can be alleviated somewhat by knowing which groups are at high risk of contracting AIDS, and by taking precautions to guard against infection.

First, although AIDS is a communicable disease, **it is not transmitted through casual contact.** It is not transmitted through airborne spread, direct casual contact with AIDS patients, or contact with body fluids. AIDS is transmitted through intimate sexual contact or through blood-to-blood

| COMMON COMMUNICABLE DISEASES | | | |
|---|---|---|---|
| **DISEASE** | **SOURCE AND MODE OF TRANSMISSION** | **PERIOD OF COMMUNICABILITY** | **CARE OF PERSONNEL** |
| Chicken Pox | Respiratory tract secretions; droplet contact | One day before skin lesions appear to six days afterwards | Wash hands, shower, change clothes |
| Diphtheria | Discharge from nose and throat; direct or indirect contact | | Immunization; wear mask if not immunized |
| German Measles (Rubella) | Discharge from nose and throat; direct and indirect contact with droplets | One week before rash appears to four days after | Wash hands |
| Gonorrhea | Discharge from mucous membranes; sexual intercourse | Months to years | Wash hands |
| Hepatitis A (viral or infectious hepatitis) | Direct contact with blood or feces | Unknown | Wash hands |
| Hepatitis B (serum hepatitis) | Sexual contact, blood, or mucous membranes; contaminated needles, blood transfusions; indirect contact with dishes, clothing, or bed linens | Unknown | Wash hands |
| Meningitis | Secretions from nose and throat; direct contact; droplet contact | Varies | Contact physician if direct contact occurs |
| Mononucleosis | Respiratory tract secretions; direct contact | Unknown | Wash hands |
| Pneumonia/Flu/Cold | Respiratory tract secretions; direct or indirect contact | Varies | Wash hands |
| Syphilis | Saliva, semen, blood, vaginal discharge during infectious period; direct contact through mucous membranes or open wound | Variable | Wash hands; contact physician if scratched or skin is broken |
| Tuberculosis | Respiratory secretions; occasionally milk; direct or indirect contact | Variable | Wash hands; contact physician |

**Figure 3.9** Infectious diseases are common and can be spread in a variety of ways.

contact, such as occurs among abusers of intravenous drugs who share needles. The groups of people most at risk for contracting AIDS are

- Homosexual or bisexual men with multiple sex partners (73 percent of reported cases)
- Abusers of intravenous drugs who share needles (17 percent of reported cases)
- Hemophiliacs and other people who have required transfusions of blood or blood products (2 percent of reported cases)

At present, there are no cases of EMS personnel having contracted the AIDS virus while providing emergency medical care, even in the procedures of greatest concern: mouth-to-mouth resuscitation, suctioning, and accidental needle sticks. However, because concern about AIDS is understandably high, the following procedures are recommended to minimize the chances of infection. These infection control procedures are useful for other infectious diseases as well:

- Use an airway and pocket mask when administering mouth-to-mouth resuscitation or CPR (Figure 3.10).

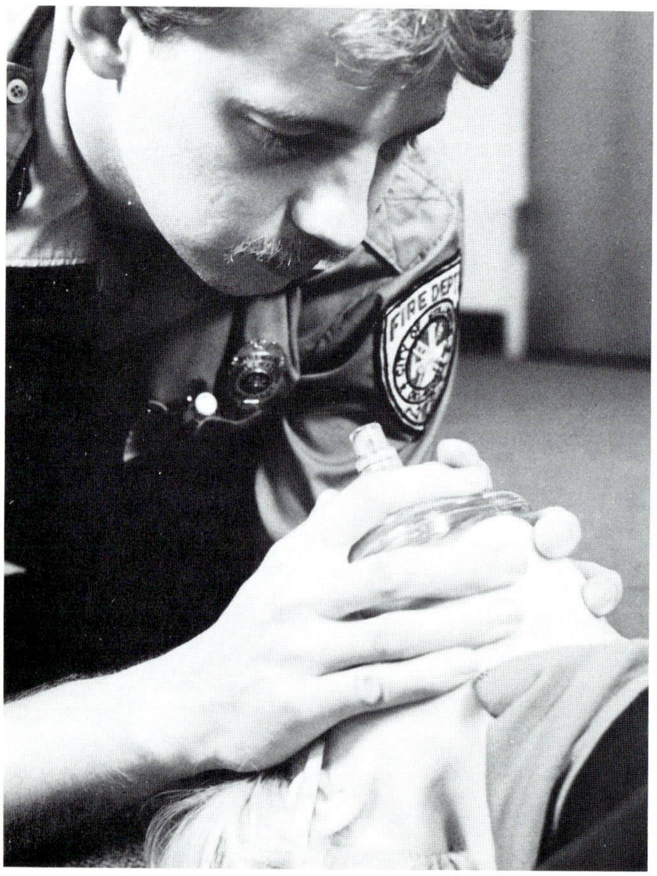

**Figure 3.10** Using a pocket mask when performing rescue breathing or CPR is a good way to guard against infectious diseases.

- If possible, wear rubber surgical gloves when handling blood or body fluids.
- If you handle needles, take extra care to avoid needle sticks.
- Avoid direct skin and mucous membrane contact with blood and body fluids of an AIDS patient. If exposure does occur, wash thoroughly with soap and water as soon as possible.
- Clean blood spills on equipment with a solution of chlorine bleach and water. Use one-fourth cup (57 mL) of bleach per gallon (3.78 L) of water.
- Place clothes or linens soiled by blood or body fluids in a plastic bag marked "blood contaminated." Launder the items using one-half cup (114 mL) of bleach per load.

While it is impossible to completely avoid exposure to communicable diseases, there are several basic procedures that form the foundation of infection control: keeping your hands and equipment clean and keeping inoculations up-to-date.

Your hands are what you use to examine a patient and they are an excellent means for transmitting germs; to avoid this, keep them as clean as possible. **FIRST OF ALL, KEEP YOUR HANDS AWAY FROM YOUR FACE IN ORDER TO AVOID THE INTRODUCTION OF GERMS THROUGH THE MUCOUS MEMBRANES** (Figure 3.11). Avoid touching open skin lesions or

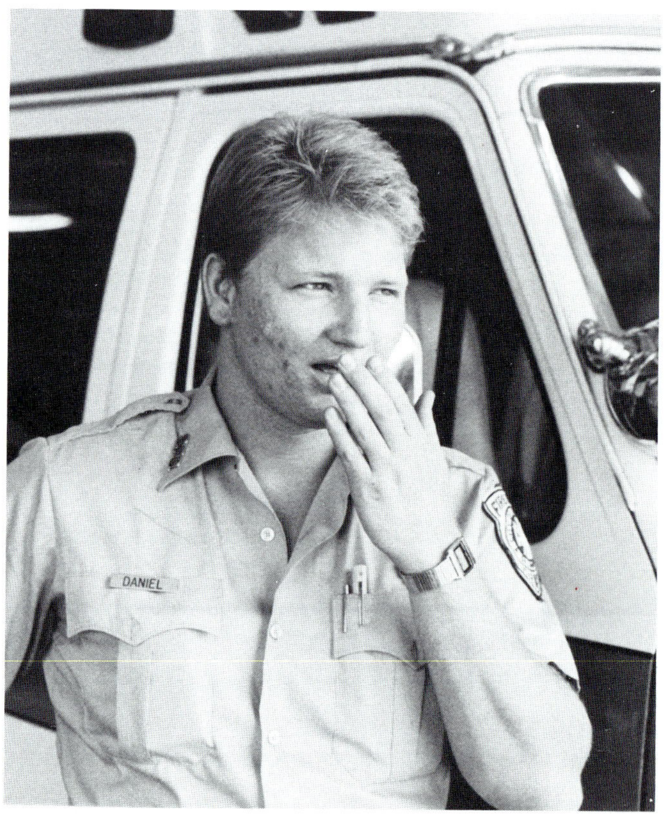


**Figure 3.11** Learn to keep your hands away from your face to lessen the spread of germs.

any draining wounds. Use disposable rubber gloves when necessary to provide an added measure of protection. Wash hands thoroughly with soap after each patient contact; be sure to clean under the fingernails. If you do not have access to soap, use a foam hand cleaner.

Several other methods can be used to make patient contact safer. Wear a disposable mask around a patient known to have a communicable disease. Use an airway and pocket mask when administering CPR.

Be sure that all equipment and supplies are cleaned or disposed of after each use. Of particular importance are airway adjuncts and suction equipment. Linens that are soiled should be placed in plastic bags for disposal or sterilization. Disposable items should be bagged for disposal.

### Inoculations

Avoiding unnecessary exposure to communicable disease while on the job is one way to guard against the spread of infection; another way to guard against disease is to keep inoculations up-to-date. The following inoculations are recommended:

- Dpt (Tetanus-Diptheria). A booster required every ten years. Tetanus is combined with diptheria because the population has not kept up immunization against diptheria. Since this is primarily a disease that affects children, people who are involved in their care should maintain their level of immunity.
- Influenza. Flu vaccine, required yearly. This should be offered on a voluntary basis. Participation should be encouraged as it will reduce provider illness and reduce patient exposure.
- Mumps vaccine. One-time dose. EMS personnel who have never had the mumps may wish to receive this vaccine. This may be an important consideration for males since 25 percent of males who acquire the disease in adulthood develop inflammation of the testes.
- Rubella vaccine. (German measles). One-time dose. This is recommended for women in EMS who have not had German measles. It is especially important for those of childbearing age. There is an effort being made to eradicate rubella worldwide. In keeping with this effort, all persons susceptible to rubella should be immunized.
- Hepatitis B vaccine. One-time dose, though there is a possible need for a booster after five years. Vaccine against hepatitis B is recommended for providers susceptible to the acquisition of hepatitis B. Recent studies have shown that persons with frequent blood contact are most at risk and should be immunized.

# 4

# Patient Assessment and Triage

## NFPA STANDARD 1001
## EMERGENCY MEDICAL CARE
### Fire Fighter I

**3-4.1** The fire fighter shall identify a primary survey for life-threatening injuries.

### FIRE FIGHTER II

**4-4.1** The fire fighter shall identify four sources from which information might be gathered pertaining to the nature of an accident victim's injuries.

**4-4.2** The fire fighter, given specific situations shall identify what injuries might be suspected from observation of the injury-producing mechanisms in addition to those injuries that are obvious.

**4-4.3** The fire fighter, given a victim, shall conduct a secondary survey for other than life-threatening injuries.



## U.S. DEPARTMENT OF TRANSPORTATION
### First Responder Training Course

**Objectives:**

- Given each vital sign, describe its normal and abnormal states and how you would check for the sign.
- Identify the medical identification symbol.
- Given a "patient," perform a complete head-to-toe primary and secondary patient assessment.
- Given descriptions of patients, identify priority for triage purposes.
- Given "patients," perform complete assessments for illnesses and injuries and describe appropriate emergency care procedures.

# Chapter 4
# Patient Assessment and Triage

A first responder is the first person arriving at the scene of an emergency who is trained to mitigate the emergency. Mitigating the emergency means identifying a patient's problem(s) and providing emergency care in the field for life-threatening problems. It means alleviating the anxiety that accompanies emergency situations. And, it means obtaining critical information about patients in the field and transmitting that information to medical personnel. Mitigating the emergency, in a very fundamental sense, means communicating effectively.

## COMMUNICATING WITH PATIENTS

Communication may be either verbal or nonverbal. From the moment you arrive at the scene of an emergency, whether you realize it or not, you begin to send important messages to the patient, family members, and bystanders. For example, your physical and personal appearance make a strong impression on the public and on patients. The attitude you display, both verbally and nonverbally, when working with patients is a crucial factor in establishing a productive, trusting atmosphere in emergency situations.

Maintaining a professional and positive attitude is not always easy for emergency care providers since they deal, almost without exception, with people who are at their worst: sick, injured, frightened, angry, intoxicated, or any combination of these things. Patients and their family members are much more likely to communicate in a helpful way and to view you as an ally if your attitude is kind and assuring. If you have a hostile, sarcastic, or indifferent attitude, patients are likely to respond in the same way. Similarly, swearing, joking, or making disparaging remarks is highly unprofessional and will only increase tension at the scene. On the subject of remarks, **never assume that a patient cannot hear or understand you, even if he or she appears to be unconscious.**

When you arrive at the scene of an emergency, first introduce yourself to the patient and explain why you are there. Learn the patient's name and use it during the examination. Thoughtfulness in the simple matter of introductions is an important aspect of establishing trust and opening communications with the patient. For example, if the patient is your age or younger, you will probably instinctively use only his or her first name as you conduct the examination, while you may hesitate to address an older patient so informally. This is a sound instinct, and the best way to know how to address the patient is to ask, "What would you like for me to call you?"

Situations in which the first responder and the patient speak different languages can be highly complex. Try to find an interpreter at the scene. It often happens that the best interpreter available is a child, so remember to keep the level of your language appropriate for the circumstances. Ask only one question at a time and try not to hurry the interpreter. The interpretation process takes time.

The physical and emotional distress patients experience in emergency situations is often heightened by a feeling of a loss of control. Whether the chief complaint is a traumatic injury or a behavioral emergency, the patient is thrust into a situation in which he or she essentially feels helpless. The effective use of some standard communications techniques can restore, at least in part, some sense of control for the patient.

One technique involves maintaining *eye contact* with the patient. This practice communicates a certain sincerity to the patient: it indicates not only that you are *listening* to what the patient has to say, but also that you feel that the patient's responses are *important*. Maintaining good eye contact requires that you stay at the patient's *eye level*. Whether the patient is standing up, sitting, or lying down, adjust your position accordingly (Figure 4.1).

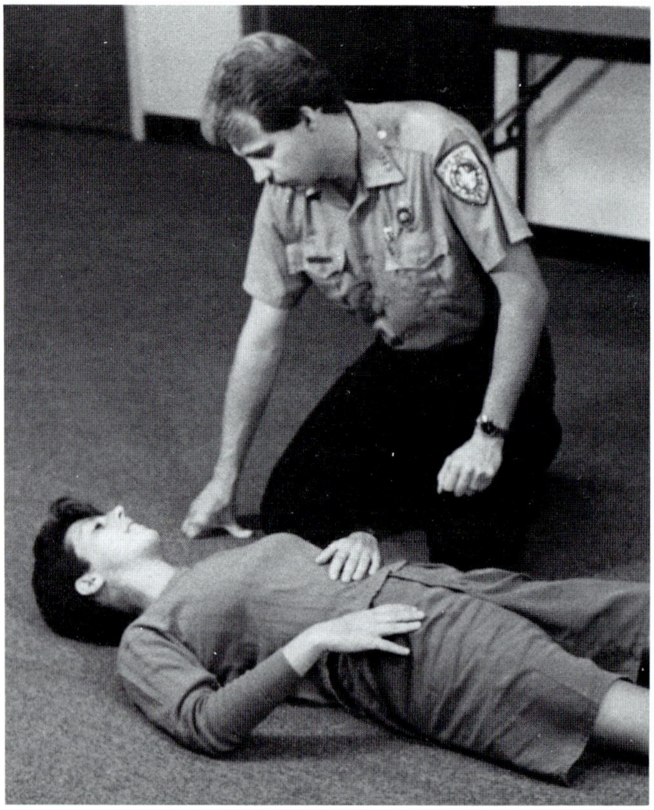

**Figure 4.1** Help to put the patient at ease by placing yourself at same eye level as the patient.

Another important aspect of nonverbal communication, particularly in emergency situations, is *physical contact* with the patient. Unfortunately, this physical contact may be interpreted as invasive or even offensive. This type of touching is not intended to be comforting: it is necessary in order to gather information about a patient's condition. However, it is possible to ease the patient's anxiety about the prodding of the examination by being discreet and professional and by dispersing onlookers. In addition, you can communicate a genuine sense of caring to patients through touching that is not associated with the physical examination. A simple touch on the shoulder or hand may ease the patient's emotional distress significantly.

Keep your *voice* low and calm as you speak with the patient. This is especially important with elderly patients, who tend to be particularly anxious in emergency situations because of a heightened awareness of their own mortality. Some of these patients are disagreeable while some are apologetic for being an inconvenience. Make every effort to be kind and patient. Many elderly patients also suffer some hearing loss. Avoid shouting questions at these patients: simply move closer to them and speak distinctly, at the same time raising the volume of your voice slightly.

Speak softly with children also, since they are easily frightened. If possible, have a parent or someone who knows the child hold him or her during the examination. Children are naturally curious, so if the situation permits, let the child "help" with the examination. If the child must be put on a stretcher, have a familiar face nearby. Also, remember that children often cry loudly, so do not take it personally. The sight of an injured child is unnerving, even terrifying, to most emergency medical care providers, thus it is doubly important to control your own anxiety and go about the examination calmly and methodically (Figure 4.2).

## PATIENT ASSESSMENT

One of the first responder's most important jobs is to carefully but quickly assess a patient's overall condition. A complete patient assessment has two parts: a *primary survey* to identify life-threatening conditions, and a *secondary survey* to identify important but non-life-threatening conditions. The information that is gathered during the primary and secondary surveys is recorded and transmitted as a *patient history* to arriving EMTs and paramedics. In the field, history-taking and patient assessment serve three purposes:

- To win the patient's confidence and thereby relieve some of his or her anxiety
- To identify the patient's problem(s) and to establish which problem(s) require immediate care in the field
- To obtain information about the patient that may not be readily available later at

## GENERAL POINTS IN DEALING WITH CHILDREN:

How you approach little people can have everything to do with whether you can even get close enough to examine — much less treat — their little maladies. Some pointers which seem to be of universal value include but probably aren't limited to:

1. Don't have your hands full of instruments; have your hands as empty as possible. Make the child look at your face and not at your tools.
2. Get down on the patient's level. You are less intimidating that way. In fact, it may be a good idea to sit *next* to a child, on the floor, say, or possibly with the child sitting on its mother's lap rather than to sit *facing* the child initially. This has the advantage of "telling" the patient that the encounter they face is not necessarily a confrontation.
3. Talk in a calm, quiet voice, and feel free to use baby talk if the child's age warrants it.
4. Take the time to develop and maintain eye contact. In asking questions of the parents, you might face the child and act as though you are asking the child your questions. Talk to the child, not just to the parents.
5. In using equipment, let the child handle your equipment. For instance, you could let a child listen to your heartbeat in exchange for your listening to his or hers; use terminology that your patient can relate to. A stethoscope can be a telephone; a blood pressure cuff can be a choo-choo.
6. Tell the truth. (Yes, it's probably going to sting a little bit, but it will make you better.)
7. Don't degrade your patient, as he's at a disadvantage already. (For instance, don't say "I have a child of three who acts better than you do." Instead, you might say "You're only six? I thought you were ten!")
8. Don't cheat your pediatric patients out of the advantages of field treatment when they need it, simply because they're kids. But don't forget the advantages of the controlled environment which a hospital setting can offer, either.

**Figure 4.2** Dick, Thom and Glenda Jenkins. "Looking at Little People," *JEMS* Vol. 6, No. 7, (July 1981). Reproduced with permission.

the hospital (for example, observations about the environment in which the patient was found)

The amount and depth of information you gather through history-taking and patient assessment depends upon the skill with which you perform these procedures. Patient assessment must be unhurried and systematic; a hasty, haphazard approach only leads to the omission of important information. Thus, it is critical that you learn to take a history and perform the primary and secondary surveys systematically.

In the sections that follow, the method for performing the primary survey is presented first, followed by methods for obtaining a history and performing the secondary survey.

Circumstances will dictate which aspects of the secondary survey — history of the present illness or the head-to-toe examination — are most relevant and merit more emphasis. The physical exam will be influenced by whether the patient is suffering from a medical problem or is the victim of trauma, whether the patient is conscious or unconscious, and whether life-threatening conditions are present.

## THE PRIMARY SURVEY: ABC'S

The primary survey is the first step in assessing the patient and **ALWAYS** takes precedence over all other aspects of history-taking and physical examination.

The purpose of the primary survey is to find and correct life-threatening conditions. It does no good to carefully and competently splint a broken leg if the patient cannot breathe because of a blocked airway. Since our lives depend upon a constant supply of oxygen, anything that threatens the respiratory system (which takes oxygen into the lungs) or the circulatory system (which delivers the oxygen to the body's cells) is a life-threatening condition. For these reasons, the primary survey **ALWAYS** requires that you check and correct the ABC's — **AIRWAY, BREATHING, CIRCULATION, AND SEVERE BLEEDING** — before doing anything else. The only tools needed are your senses of sight, hearing, touch, and smell. You also need a watch with a sweep hand and, if it is dark, a flashlight.

These skills are interdependent and must be performed in ABC order. The patient must have an open **AIRWAY** in order to breathe. If the patient is breathless, begin rescue **BREATHING** before taking the pulse and assessing **CIRCULATION.** Finally, assess the patient's **CIRCULATION** before attempting to control **SEVERE BLEEDING** (Figure 4.3).

Many times the primary survey can be completed in short order: when, for example, you encounter the alert, communicative patient with medical problems. On the other hand, close examination will be required to accomplish the primary survey if the patient is unconscious or the victim of major trauma. If the patient is not alert and communicative, you will have to establish responsiveness by shaking and shouting.

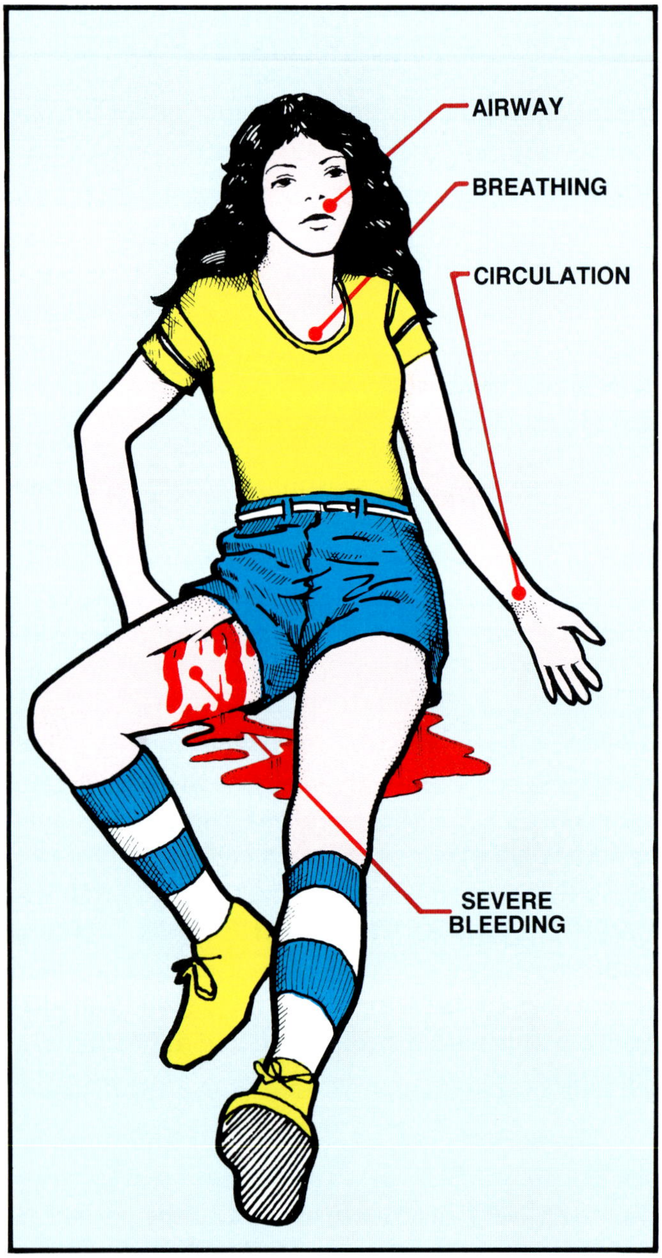


**Figure 4.3** The primary survey is always the first step in patient examination. Assess the patient's airway, breathing, circulation, then look for signs of severe bleeding.

**CAUTION:** You must assume that anyone who is unconscious has a spinal cord injury. **DO NOT** move the patient's neck. If the patient does not respond, assume that he or she is unconscious.

**1. AIRWAY** — In order to breathe, the patient must first have an open airway. A blocked airway is a true medical emergency and will cause death in minutes if not corrected. The most common airway obstruction is the tongue, which tends to relax and fall back into the throat in unconscious individuals. If this is the problem, repositioning the patient's head or jaw will reopen the airway. Food or foreign objects caught in the throat must be removed as quickly as possible (see Chapter 5, Basic Life Support: The ABC's).

**CAUTION:** Use only the Modified Jaw Thrust maneuver to open and maintain the airway of a trauma victim.

**2. BREATHING** — Once the airway is open, determine whether or not the patient is breathing. Inhaling oxygenates the blood and exhaling removes waste products. To determine whether the patient is breathing, lean over the patient's head and place your ear within an inch (3 mm) of the patient's mouth and nose. Listen and feel for sounds and movement of air coming from the patient's nose and mouth and watch the patient's chest for movement (Figure 4.4). If the patient is not breathing, begin artificial respiration immediately (see Chapter 5, Basic Life Support: The ABC's).

Look now for any severe open chest wounds, such as a sucking chest wound. A wound of this type needs to be covered as soon as possible with an occlusive dressing to prevent more air from entering the wound. If you have no dressing, use your hand. Be aware that covering a sucking chest wound can cause complications later. (See Chapter 8, Injuries to the Skull, Spine, and Chest.)

**3. CIRCULATION** — When blood receives oxygen from the lungs, the heart must pump it to all parts of the body (especially the brain, which is damaged in minutes without oxygen). Check circulation by carefully taking the patient's pulse. The most reliable pulse site is the carotid (neck) pulse

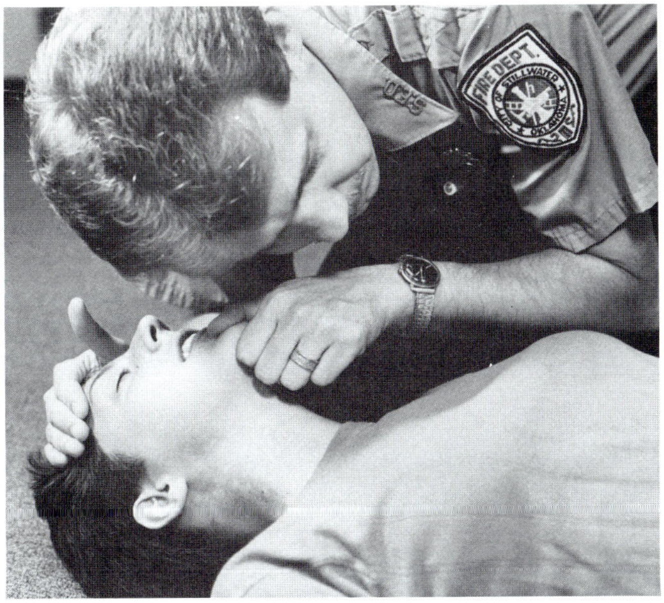

**Figure 4.4** To determine if the patient is breathing, look for the rise and fall of the chest, listen for sounds of air moving from the patient's nose and mouth, and feel for movement of air on your cheek or ear.

since it can be felt when other pulses are too weak to detect. Check the patient's pulse for at least five seconds and as much as ten seconds if necessary. **NEVER** begin chest compressions on someone whose heart is still beating, even if the pulse is very weak. If you cannot find a pulse, begin chest compressions at once (see Chapter 5, Basic Life Support: The ABC's).

A patient who is alert and able to answer questions obviously has an open airway, is breathing, and has a heartbeat, so the ABC check is especially important for a semiconscious or unconscious patient who is unable to respond to questions or to describe symptoms.

**4. SEVERE BLEEDING** — Bleeding from a major wound or a large artery or vein can cause shock and death within minutes if it is not stopped (see Chapter 6, Shock). However, controlling bleeding does no good if the patient is not breathing, so assess and correct the patient's **AIRWAY, BREATHING,** and **CIRCULATION** first.

## Taking a History

During the primary and secondary survey, the first responder's job is to gather and record as much information as possible about the patient's illness or injury. This *patient history* — information about the patient's chief complaint — comes from a variety of sources. History-taking may involve the patient, the patient's family, and bystanders. In general, if the patient is able to communicate, it is best to question him or her rather than the others. The patient is thus reassured that he or she is the center of medical interest and still retains some control over the situation. If it is necessary to question others, do so one at a time; it is difficult to determine what is happening from a chorus of voices. On some occasions, it is advisable to have a partner question a family member in another room while you interview the patient, especially if there are conflicting reports from the two sources.

Information received from the patient, of course, can be helpful, but your observations of the patient's environment and the probable mechanism(s) of injury, along with the information you gather during the primary and secondary survey are critical to the patient history. Record patient information on a patient survey form (Figure 4.5). The report on the patient should include, at the very least, the following:

- Patient's name, age, and gender
- Signs and symptoms of the injury or illness presented by the patient
- Description and cause of the patient's injury or illness
- Medications used by the patient and any known allergies

To gather this information, you must carefully phrase and ask a series of questions. The questions, naturally, depend upon the circumstances of the emergency, but the first question to ask (*after* you have introduced yourself and asked the patient his or her name) is always the same, that is, "What happened here?" or, "Why did you call for help?" If the patient is conscious and communicative or if there are bystanders at the scene, you may get an approximate idea of what has happened. On the other hand, circumstances may be such that you actually ask yourself the question, and arrive at an answer through your observations of the scene and of the patient.

In general, the questions you ask the patient should be open-ended questions, that is, they should be questions that require the patient to des-

**FRONT**

SCENE ______ PT.NO. ____ AGE ____ M F
INJURY ____________________
____________________
____________________
HIST. OF ILL. ____________________
____________________
B/P ____ P ____ R ____ TIME ____
____ ____ ____ ____
ST. CON. ________ AIRWAY ________
PUPILS ________ SKIN ________
MEDS. ____________________
PAST MED. HIST. ____________________
____________________
____________________
ASSMT. ____________________
____________________
____________________
EKG: ____________________
ACTION ____________________
____________________
____________________
HOSP. ________ ETA ________
DOCTOR ____________________
NAME ____________________

**BACK**

CHIEF COMPLAINT OF PAIN
1) QUALITY OF THE PAIN
____________________
____________________
2) DURATION
____________________
3) INCITING EVENT
____________________
____________________
4) NAUSEA OR VOMITING?
____________________
5) DIAPHORESIS?
____________________
6) S.O.B.?
____________________
7) RADIATION OF THE PAIN
____________________
____________________
____________________
8) RELIEVING EVENT
____________________
____________________
____________________
____________________
____________________

**Figure 4.5** The information recorded on a patient survey form gives valuable assistance to other emergency care personnel.

cribe symptoms rather than give a simple "yes" or "no" answer.

Be aware that some patients, for whatever reason, may conceal or even lie about certain aspects of the injury or illness. If you cannot obtain a history from the patient, you can question bystanders or family members, but family members and friends, depending upon the situation, may also be evasive or even dishonest in responses to your questions. Patients, for a number of reasons, may also fake semiconsciousness or unconsciousness.

## THE SECONDARY SURVEY

Once the primary survey is complete, the next step is to proceed to the secondary survey. The purpose of the secondary survey is to form an impression of the patient's overall condition and to locate any non-life-threatening but significant medical conditions. The secondary survey consists of the following:

FOR ALL PATIENTS

- An assessment of the patient's level of consciousness and overall appearance
- Patient history
- Vital Signs

FOR MEDICAL PATIENTS

- Descriptions of the chief complaint
- History of present illness
- Description of any additional medical problems
- Modified head-to-toe examination

FOR UNCONSCIOUS PATIENTS OR VICTIMS OF MAJOR TRAUMA

- Events leading up to the accident
- Mechanism of injury
- Description of the chief complaint, if possible
- Head-to-toe examination

All patients need to be evaluated for general overall appearance, level of consciousness, and vital signs. The rest of the secondary survey, however, must be carried out according to the patient's needs. For the medical patient, emphasis is placed on a history of the present illness and relevant past medical history. A patient who is unconscious or the victim of major trauma is unable to describe symptoms, so you must perform a head-to-toe examination in an attempt to discover additional medical problems. In this situation, relatives or bystanders must be relied upon to provide a patient history.

In many cases, it is best to take the history as you perform the physical examination — the practice, aside from being efficient, also lessens the possibility of any lapse in communication with the patient during the exam. With two first responders, one can interview the patient while the other takes vital signs and performs a quick head-to-toe survey. This system allows the interviewer to talk with the patient to obtain a history while the examiner counts pulse, respirations, and so on without interruption.

In the sections that follow, methods for performing an overall patient assessment and taking vital signs are described first, since they apply to all patients. The Medical Survey that follows contains detailed questions for eliciting information about the patient whose chief complaint is illness. Finally, the Trauma Survey presents methods for performing a head-to-toe examination when the patient is unconscious or seriously injured.

## General Assessment and Vital Signs

The secondary survey, like the primary survey, is a hands-on skill. Since you work with very few tools, you must look, listen, and feel while examining the patient. When examining a patient, it is important that you be aware of the significance of certain diagnostic signs and symptoms. The distinction between *signs* and *symptoms* is important: signs can be seen, felt, or heard by the examiner, while symptoms cannot. Examples of signs include labored breathing, flushed skin, or dilated pupils. Symptoms are reported verbally by the patient. Pain, dizziness, and shortness of breath are examples of symptoms. Symptoms, then, cannot be directly observed by the examiner, and signs can only be gathered by direct observation.

The general assessment, which is needed for all patients, consists of an evaluation of the following:

- General appearance of patient
- Level of consciousness
- Skin color and condition
- Vital signs: Temperature<br>Pulse<br>Respiration<br>Blood pressure (if this skill is taught in your jurisdiction)
- Pupil reaction
- Medical identification tags

## General Appearance of Patient

Your impression of the *general appearance* of the patient begins as soon as you see the patient.

Before asking a single question, take a quick look at the patient's environment. If the patient is at home, what is its appearance? Is it clean and well maintained? Are there bottles of medication nearby that might give a clue to the patient's illness? Do empty bottles or glasses give evidence of alcohol consumption? If the patient is a victim of trauma, in what position is the patient found? Does the placement of the patient and any objects at the scene give a clue to the mechanisms of injury? Take note of certain characteristics of the patient — posture, dress, facial expression, and attitude. Does the patient seem to be in pain or discomfort? Does the patient seem frightened?

### Level of Consciousness

An assessment of *level of consciousness* (LOC) reveals vital information about the gravity of any patient's condition. Because injuries and illnesses often affect the level of consciousness, it is important to begin assessing the patient's level of consciousness as soon as possible after you arrive at the scene. The traditional terms for different states of consciousness are not precise: confused, disoriented, stuporous, and comatose may mean different things to different people. Thus, it is best to record the patient's exact responses to various stimuli, whether the responses are verbal or nonverbal. Any *change* in level of consciousness, positive or negative, is important and should be noted.

With a conscious patient, level of consciousness is best determined by conversation. An alert patient will be able to answer questions and will be oriented to person, place, and time. Start by asking several questions:

- What is your name? (person)
- Do you know where you are? Where do you live? (place)
- What day is this? Can you tell me the date? The year? (time)

The patient who can answer each of these questions appropriately is said to be "oriented," or "alert and oriented times three" (oriented to person, place, and time). If, on the other hand, the patient knows his or her name and the date, but cannot answer your other questions, the patient is said to be "confused — oriented to person and time, but not to place." Time is first to go.

There are further aspects of the patient's verbal response that need to be noted and reported: Does the patient respond appropriately to questions? Is the patient's speech normal, garbled, incomprehensible, or absent? Slurred or garbled speech can be a sign of drug reaction or stroke.

The patient who is semiconscious or unconscious may only respond to shouts or physical stimuli. Physical stimuli include such actions as squeezing the upper arm, rubbing the sternum, or pinching the skin between the shoulder and the neck (Figure 4.6). Observe whether the patient grimaces, groans, or tries to move away from the pain. Record exactly what stimuli are applied and how the patient reacts.

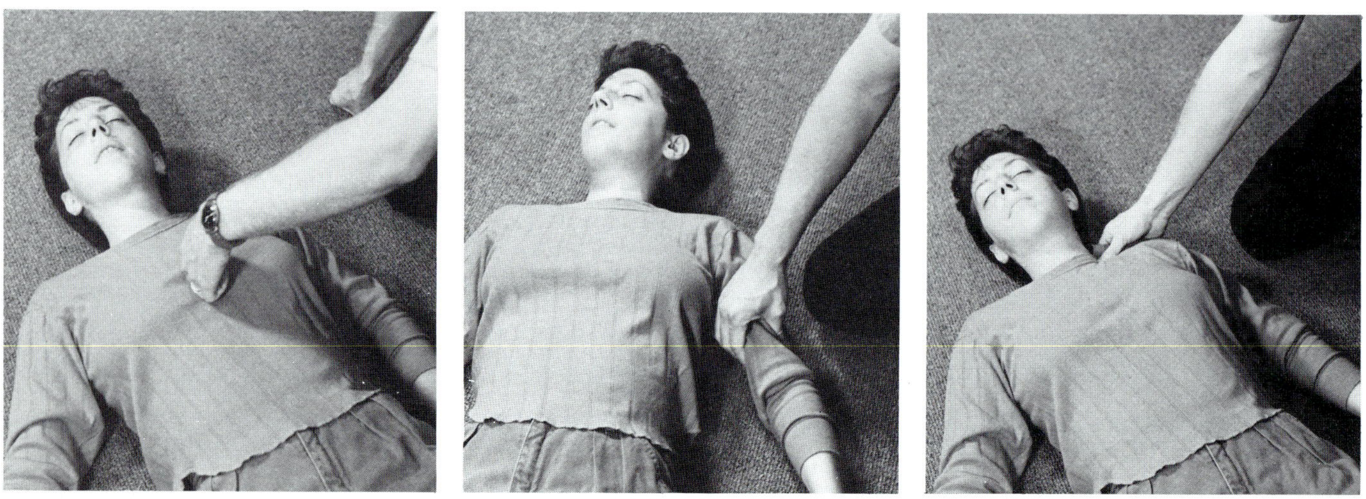

**Figure 4.6** If the patient is not responsive, rub the sternum, pinch the upper arm, or pinch the skin between the neck and shoulder and note the patient's reaction.

**CAUTION:** You *must* assume that anyone who is unconscious has a spinal cord injury. **DO NOT** move the patient any more than necessary for examination (see Chapter 8, Injuries to the Skull, Spine, and Chest).

### Skin Color and Appearance

Every patient assessment must include an examination of the skin, irrespective of the patient's problem or chief complaint, since the appearance of the skin gives important clues to the patient's condition (Figure 4.7). Skin *color* is an indication of how effectively the blood is circulating and of the oxygen levels within the blood.

| SKIN COLOR | | |
|---|---|---|
| **FLUSHED** | **PALE** | **CYANOTIC** |
| Heat Stroke | Insufficient Circulation | Heart Failure |
| Heart Attack | Fright | Poisoning |
| High Blood Pressure | Heart Attack | Airway Obstruction |
| CO Poisoning | Shock | Cold |
| Fever | Cold | |

**Figure 4.7** Skin color and appearance give important clues to a patient's condition.

During a fever or an allergic reaction blood vessels dilate and move toward the surface of the skin to help the body dissipate (give off) excess heat. Consequently, the skin becomes warm and pink or reddish. This reddening also occurs in the early stages of carbon monoxide poisoning.

Excessive blood loss, fright, or anemia may cause the blood vessels to constrict and retreat from the skin surface, thus the skin becomes cool, moist, and pale. The constriction of the blood vessels reduces circulation to the extremities and allows for an increased blood flow to the vital organs. The reduced blood supply to the surface of the skin causes *pallor*, or lack of color. Pallor also causes the lips to appear more prominent and circles to show under the eyes in light-skinned patients.

Decreased oxygen levels in the blood cause the skin to become bluish or grayish (cyanotic). Patients in shock or those who have been exposed to extreme cold are often cyanotic. Some types of shock cause the skin to appear blotchy or mottled (uneven in color).

It is easier to note variations in skin color in light-skinned patients; however, dark-skinned patients who are in shock may appear grayish. You can detect pallor in a dark-skinned patient by examining the mucous membranes of the eyes and mouth (inside the lower lip) and by checking the fingernail beds to see whether they appear unusually pale. Cyanosis in dark-skinned patients can be detected in the same way: check the mucous membranes of the eyes and mouth and the fingernail beds for a bluish or grayish color.

Some patients may also have abnormal skin color due to disease. For example, disease of the liver or gallbladder may cause the skin to turn yellow, a condition known as *jaundice*. You can detect jaundice in dark-skinned patients by examining the whites of the eyes for yellow discoloration. Some diseases of the circulatory system can give skin a purple or blue cast.

When examining the patient's skin, note whether the skin color and appearance are consistent with conditions at the scene. For example, you would not expect to find a patient with cool, clammy skin on a hot summer day. Such a sign might indicate a heat-stress condition.

If the patient's condition and mechanism of injury suggest internal injury with shock, check skin perfusion (oxygenation of tissues) by performing a capillary refill test. To do this, pinch the patient's fingernails until the nailbeds are white. Then let go. If color returns within two seconds (the amount of time it takes to say "capillary refill"), the tissues are adequately perfused. If color returns later than two seconds or not at all, assume that the patient is in shock.

### Vital Signs

The vital signs are *temperature, pulse, respiration,* and *blood pressure*. Assessing each of these body functions reveals important clues to the patient's condition. Take vital signs every 5 to 10 minutes. Their importance for proper body functioning is discussed on the following pages.

### TEMPERATURE

Normal body temperature is 98.6°F (37°C). The skin is largely responsible for temperature regulation since it radiates heat and evaporates water from the skin. Thus, skin may be hot and wet, hot and dry, cold and wet (clammy), or cold and dry. During emergency work, estimate temperature by feeling the patient's forehead with the back of your hand and judge whether it is hot or cold compared with your own skin.

### PULSE

The pulse is the rhythmic throbbing of the arteries as the heart pumps blood throughout the body. A pulse can be measured at any point on the body where an artery can be compressed against a bone. The principal locations for taking the pulse during emergency work are the neck (carotid pulse), the wrist (radial pulse), and the groin (femoral pulse) (Figure 4.8). If the patient is an infant (less than one year old), the upper arm (brachial pulse) is the preferred location for taking the pulse. If you have a stethoscope, you can place it on the infant's chest and listen to the heartbeat (apical pulse). The pedal pulse, located at the top of the foot, is used to check for circulation when there has been an injury to the leg.

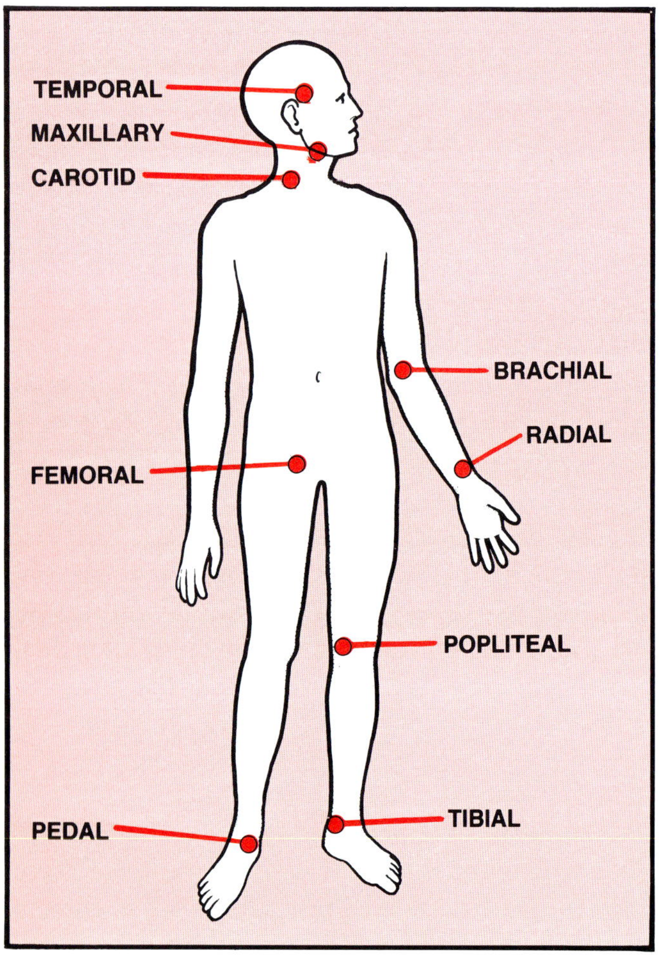


**Figure 4.8** The principal pulse sites are shown. The radial and carotid pulses are used most often for adults. The brachial pulse is preferred for infants.

The pulse is measured for its *rate, rhythm,* and *strength.* The normal resting pulse rate for an adult is about 60-80 beats per minute. The rate for a male is usually about 8-10 beats slower per minute than that for a female. A child's heart rate (that is, someone between one and eight years old) is faster, about 80-100 beats per minute. An infant's heart rate is faster still, about 100-200 beats per minute.

A very slow or very fast pulse is usually an indication of illness, although a well-conditioned person may have a very slow resting heart rate (below 50 beats per minute) and a person who is very anxious or upset may have a pulse as fast as 150 beats per minute. A very slow pulse can indicate heart damage or drug overdose. An individual's pulse rate typically accelerates during a fever or shock. If the patient's pulse rate consistently increases, assume that shock is imminent and treat the patient accordingly (see Chapter 6, Shock).

The *rhythm* is the regularity of the intervals between heartbeats. Note and record whether the beats are regular or irregular. A patient who has had a pacemaker implanted will have a regular, steady heart rate that does not change.

The *strength* of the pulse is assessed by determining whether it is full, bounding, or thready. A regular pulse is said to be *full,* a very strong pulse is called *bounding,* and a weak pulse is termed *thready.*

Take the pulse using your index and middle fingers. Do not use your thumb because it has its own pulse, which may cause you to confuse it with the patient's. To take the carotid pulse, first locate the patient's Adam's apple with your fingertips, then slide your fingers back toward you into the groove beside the Adam's apple. Do not reach across the throat. Press lightly to feel the pulse with the most sensitive part of your fingertips (Figure 4.9). If the patient is alert and sitting up, it will be more comfortable for the patient if you take a radial wrist pulse.

It may be difficult to find the pulse if it is very weak or irregular. Remember to take your time: take at least 5 seconds, and, if necessary, as much as 10 seconds to locate the pulse. Count the pulse for 30 seconds and multiply by 2, or count for 15 seconds and multiply by 4, to estimate the rate per minute. If the pulse seems irregular or abnormal, count it for a full 60 seconds. Report the pulse by describing its rate, rhythm, and strength, for example: "The patient's pulse is 70, regular, and full."

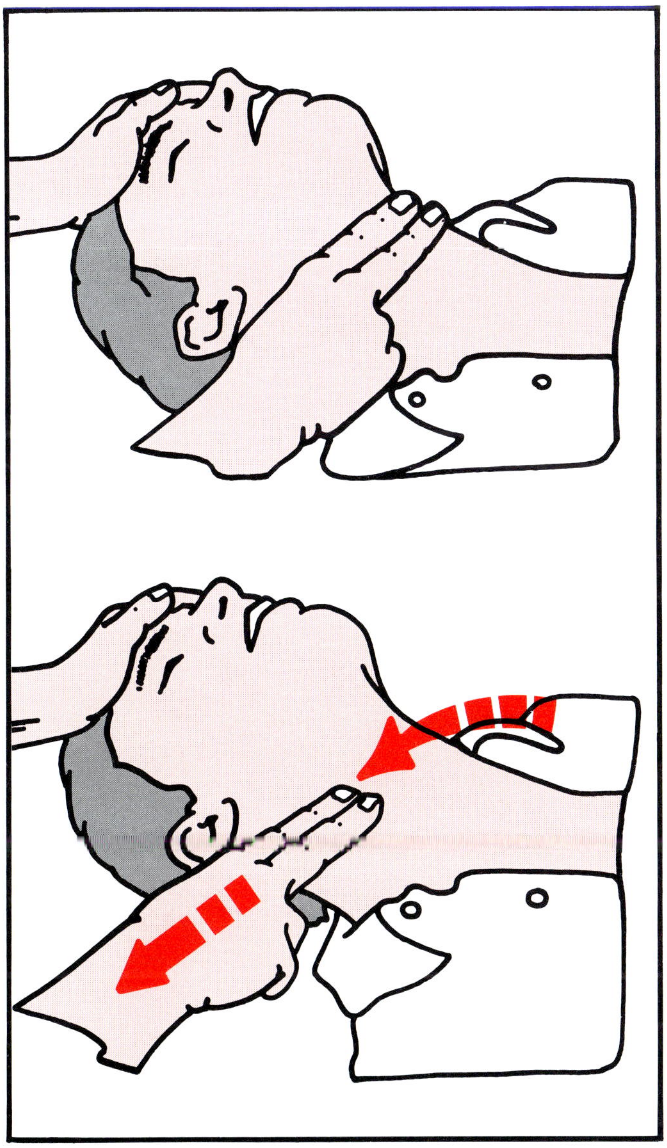

**Figure 4.9** Take the carotid pulse by sliding your fingertips into the groove beside the patient's Adam's apple.

## RESPIRATION

Respiration is the act of breathing in air, exchanging oxygen for the waste gases within body tissues, and breathing out the waste gases. Breathing is assessed for its *rate* and *quality*. Normal breathing is automatic, regular, and quiet.

*Rate* of breathing is calculated by determining the number of breaths taken over a given period of time, usually one minute. The average adult breathes (an inspiration and expiration counts as one breath) 12-20 times per minute. Children breathe somewhat faster, about 20-32 times per minute, and infants breathe about 30-40 times per minute.

Very slow breathing (less than 12 respirations per minute) or very fast breathing (more than 25 respirations per minute for an adult) is often caused by illness or injury and should be noted. Very slow breathing may be caused by a stroke, an injury to the nervous system, or a drug reaction or overdose. Very rapid breathing is usually seen in patients suffering from lung disorder, shock, or extreme anxiety.

A good time to count respirations is right after taking the patient's pulse. Without moving your fingers from the pulse site, quietly shift your gaze to the patient's chest or abdomen and observe it rising and falling. It is best to measure respirations without the patient being aware of it since people's breathing rates often change when they know that they are being watched. Count respirations for 30 seconds and multiply by 2 to determine the rate per minute.

Breathing is also assessed for its *quality*. Quality is determined by listening for how deeply the patient is breathing and for any unusual noises. Note whether breathing is shallow or deep, noisy, labored, or gasping. Report any unusual odors, such as alcohol or the fruity smell noted in diabetic acidosis (see Chapter 10, Medical Emergencies). If the patient is not breathing, respirations are termed absent.

## BLOOD PRESSURE

Blood pressure is the pressure that exists in the large arteries at the height of the pulse wave. This pressure is highest during *systole*, or that part of the heart cycle during which the heart contracts and forces blood to surge through the aorta and the pulmonary artery. Blood pressure is lowest during *diastole*, or the period of the heart cycle in which the heart relaxes, dilates, and fills with blood.

Blood pressure varies according to age, sex, altitude, muscular development, and according to states of worry and fatigue. It is usually lower in women than in men, low in children, and high in elderly patients. Blood pressure falls during sleep or relaxation and rises during activity or excitement.

If measuring blood pressure is a skill practiced by first responders in your jurisdiction, you have ready access to the tools for measuring blood pressure: a stethoscope and a blood pressure cuff (sphygmomanometer). Blood pressure cuffs are available in sizes for adults, infants, and children. Special femoral cuffs that measure blood pressure in the upper leg are also available. While the cuffs vary according to size and make, all consist basically of three parts: an inflatable cuff, a pressure gauge, and a rubber bulb (Figure 4.10).

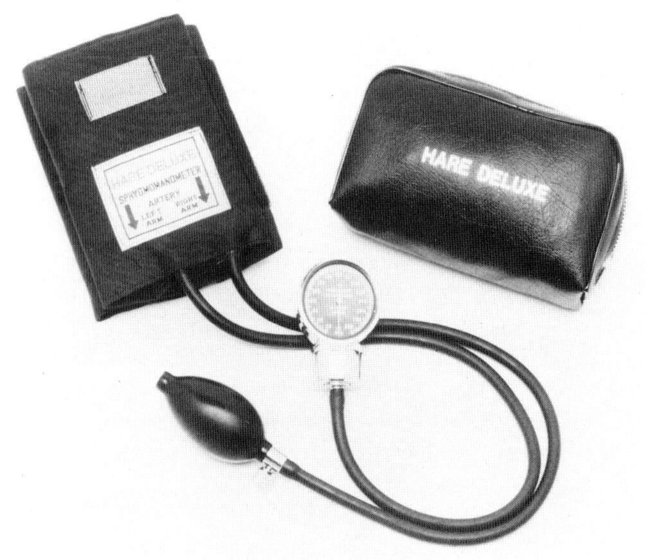


**Figure 4.10** A blood pressure cuff (sphygmomanometer) and stethoscope are used to measure blood pressure.

Unless both of the patient's arms are seriously injured, measure the blood pressure at one of the brachial arteries. Most medical personnel measure blood pressure from the patient's right arm. In any case, when monitoring a patient's blood pressure over time, take the measurement from the same arm each time.

First, see that the patient is either sitting or lying down, and that the arm from which you take the blood pressure is level with the patient's heart (Figure 4.11). Position the arrow on the blood pressure cuff over the patient's brachial artery. Locate the pulse, which is on the little finger side of the patient's arm (Figure 4.12). This is where you will place the stethoscope. Place the earpieces of the stethoscope in your ears and lightly tap the diaphragm of the stethoscope.

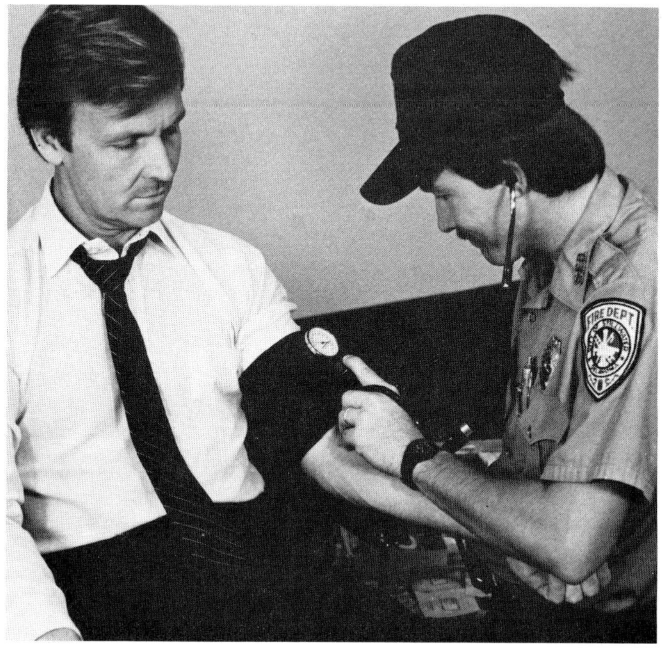

**Figure 4.11** The arm from which you take the blood pressure should be level with the patient's heart.

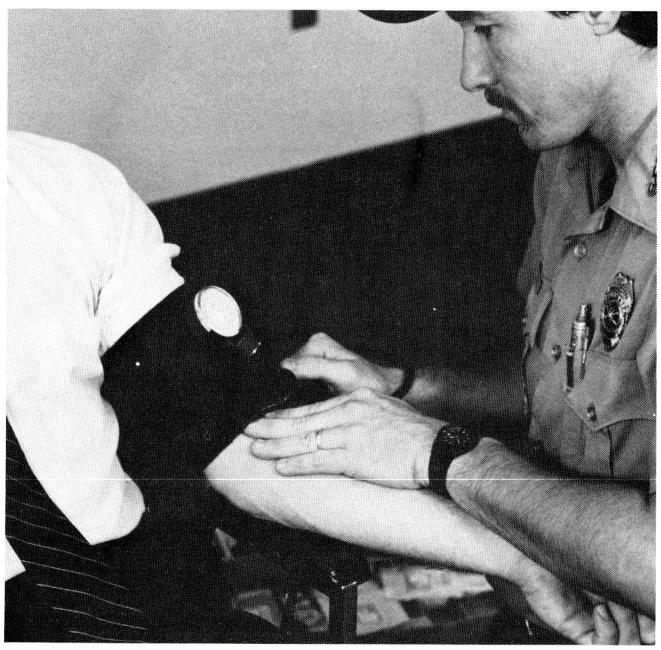

**Figure 4.12** Locate the pulse on the little finger side of the patient's arm.

**NOTE:** Dual-head stethoscopes have a bell-type head for listening to heart tones and a diaphragm side for listening to breath sounds and blood pressures (Figure 4.13). If you do not hear any sounds when you tap the stethoscope, turn the head and tap it again.

Place the diaphragm over the brachial pulse. Do not press the diaphragm too hard against the skin or you will get a false reading. Inflate the cuff by squeezing the rubber bulb until the needle on the gauge reads over 200.

Begin to let air out of the cuff SLOWLY by turning the pressure control valve. The first pulse sound you hear after you begin to deflate the cuff is the high or *systolic pressure*. Note the gauge reading when you hear the first sound. Continue to deflate the cuff slowly and watch the gauge. The point at which sounds are no longer heard is the low or diastolic pressure. Note the gauge reading when the pulse sounds disappear. If you miss one or both of the pulse sounds, deflate the cuff completely and take the blood pressure again. If you reinflate the cuff after it has been only partially deflated, you will get an inaccurate blood pressure reading.

**NOTE:** Sounds heard over the brachial artery change in quality at some point prior to the point the sounds disappear altogether, and some consider this the diastolic pressure.

For convenience, blood pressure is recorded as two figures separated by a slant. For example, 110/70 indicates systolic pressure of 110 and diastolic pressure of 70. Each time you measure blood pressure, record the figures and the time of measurement immediately. See Table 4.1 for normal blood pressure values in resting infants, children, and adults.

**TABLE 4.1**
**RANGES OF BLOOD PRESSURES**

| | |
|---|---|
| Adults | 100/65—150/90 |
| Children | 90/60—105/65 |
| Infants | 74/40—85/60 |

### Taking Blood Pressure by Palpation

If there is too much noise to hear pulse sounds, you may have to take the blood pressure by palpation. To palpate the blood pressure, first find the radial pulse. Place the blood pressure cuff over the patient's brachial artery as before and pump the cuff up until the needle or gauge reads over 200. You should not be able to feel the radial pulse. SLOWLY let the pressure control valve go and, keeping your fingers on the radial pulse, note the reading on the gauge when you do feel a pulse. This

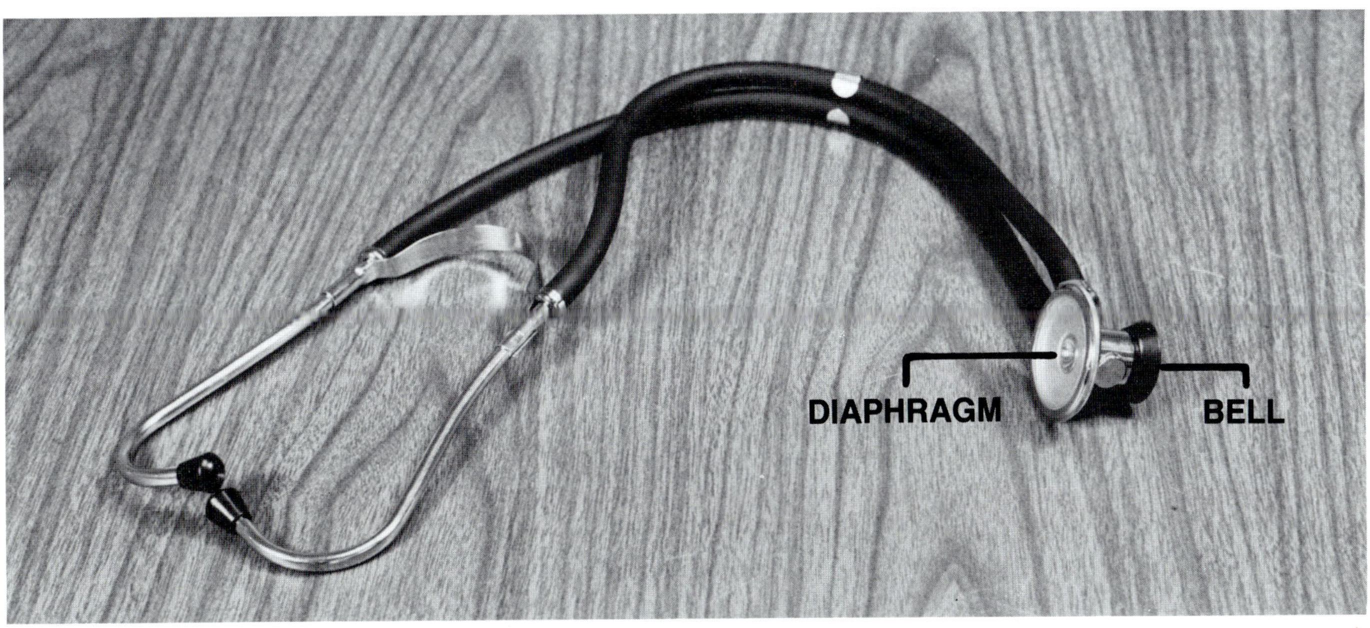


**Figure 4.13** Use the diaphragm side of a dual-head stethoscope for measuring blood pressures.

method of taking blood pressure gives only a systolic reading, so it would be reported, for example, "The patient's blood pressure was 140 by palpation." If you cannot find a radial pulse at all, assume that the patient's arm is injured or that the blood pressure is less than 90, which indicates shock. Try the other arm; if no pulse is felt, check the carotid pulse.

### Pupils

Check both pupils to see if they are the same size and react to light. Although two to four percent of the population naturally have pupils of unequal sizes, pupils that are different sizes are often an indication of head injury (Figure 4.14). If you are in a brightly-lit area, check reaction to light by covering the patient's eyes for 30 seconds and then taking your hand away. The pupils should contract in about one second. Note whether pupil reaction is normal, slow, or absent. If pupil reaction is very slow it may be evidence of injury to the central nervous system. Pupils that remain dilated when exposed to light may indicate heart attack, brain injury, or the presence of drugs such as amphetamines or hallucinogens. Pupils that remain constricted can be a sign of narcotic drugs, such as heroin, morphine, or codeine, or a central nervous system disorder. Of course, if you are in dim light you will need a penlight or flashlight to check the pupils. To make the check, hold the flashlight about 12 inches (305 mm) from the patient's face and, with a sweeping motion, briefly shine the light into one eye and then move it immediately toward the side of the patient's face away from the eye (Figure 4.15). This entire motion should take about one second. Note the pupil reaction to the light and to the absence of light. If the patient is conscious, ask if he or she notices blurred vision, spots, or halos.

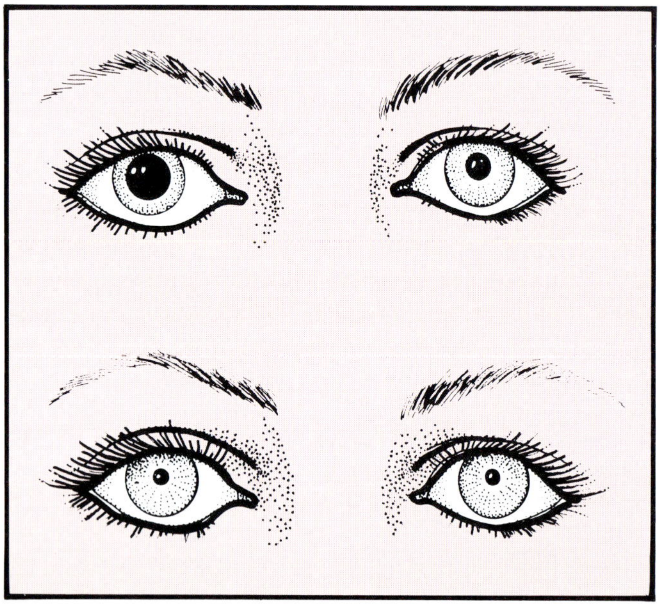

**Figure 4.14** Pupils that are different sizes are often a sign of head injury.

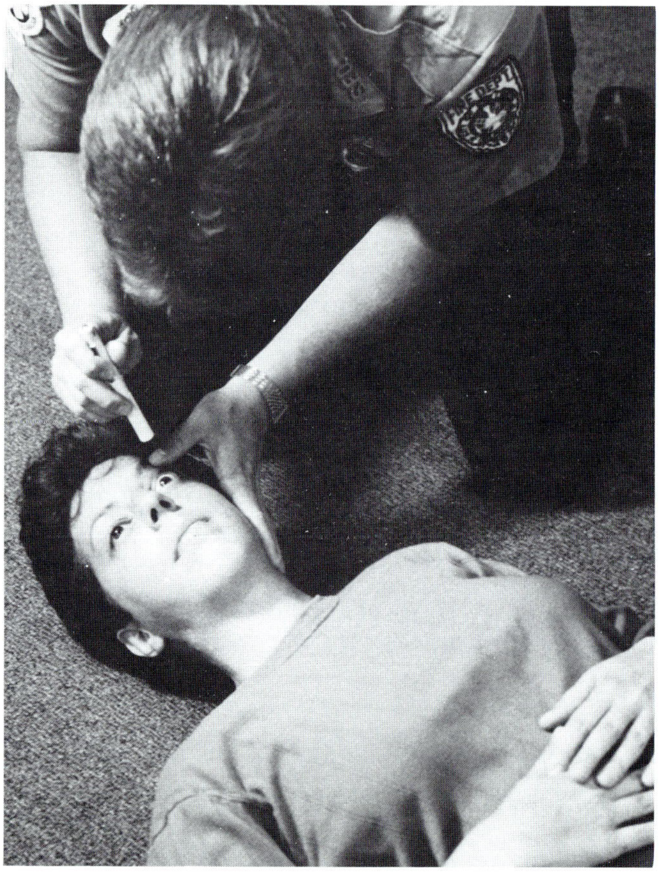

**Figure 4.15** To check pupil reaction to light, briefly shine a penlight into the patient's eye, then move it immediately toward the side of the patient's face.

### Medical Survey

For a patient who is conscious and whose chief complaint is a medical problem, such as pain in the chest, the rest of the secondary survey should concentrate on evaluating the patient's overall appearance, obtaining a history of the present illness, and learning of any additional medical problems that might complicate treatment. (For information on different types of medical emergencies, see Chapter 10, Medical Emergencies.)

First of all, notice the patient's *appearance*. In what position is the patient? Does the patient seem to be in pain? What is the appearance of the skin? Is it flushed, pale, mottled? Is the patient sweating heavily? Does the patient appear frightened?

Talk with the patient to determine the patient's *level of consciousness*. Level of consciousness is a particularly important sign because changes in the state of consciousness are often the first clues to an alteration in the patient's condition. Is the patient oriented to person, place, and time (time of day, day of week, and date)? An alert and oriented patient will be able to pay attention and to answer questions. Note the patient's speech. Progressive slurring of words or vagueness when answering questions, especially if the patient's normal speech is clear and coherent, indicates a decreased level of consciousness. If the patient cannot speak, determine whether the patient can understand by giving a simple command, such as: "Squeeze my hand." Estimate the alertness of young children and infants by noting their interest in their surroundings and by observing their voluntary movements.

Determine the patient's *chief complaint* by asking: "Why did you call for help?" Most chief complaints are characterized by pain, abnormal function, some change from a normal state, or an observation made by the patient. Obtain a *history of the present illness* by asking a series of questions designed to provide more information about the chief complaint. The information that makes up the history of the present illness should include answers to the following:

- PAIN. Is there pain? Where is it?
- QUALITY. What does the pain feel like? Dull? Sharp? Cutting? Throbbing? Crushing? Does the pain cause difficulty in breathing? How?
- RADIATION. Does the pain radiate (spread to another part of the body)? Where? Under what circumstances?
- SEVERITY. How bad is the pain? The patient's response will be a mixture of the actual severity of the pain and the patient's reaction to that pain. Therefore, you will have to form a quick impression of the patient's temperament to interpret the description of pain.
- TIME. When did the pain begin? How long has it lasted? What was the patient doing when symptoms began?
- ALLEVIATION. Does anything make the symptoms better or worse?
- MODIFICATION OF SYMPTOMS. Has the patient taken any medications or made any other attempts to alleviate symptoms?
- ASSOCIATED COMPLAINTS. Are there any other problems, such as shortness of breath, nausea, or dizziness?

Avoid asking questions that can be answered with a yes or no; instead, ask open-ended questions that allow the patient to explain in his or her own words what happened. Do not suggest answers to the patient; allow the patient to answer in his or her own words. Thus, it is better to ask "When does the pain come on?" and not "Does the pain come on after exertion?" It may be helpful to provide the patient with alternatives, for example: "Does the pain stay in one place or does it move around?"

After completing questions about the present illness, ask about the patient's *past medical history*. Focus on those aspects of the patient's past medical history that relate to the current problem, either because they are directly related to the present problem, or because they could complicate care and treatment of the problem. For example, it would be important to learn that a patient whose chief complaint was chest pain also had emphysema, because the presence of emphysema complicates oxygen administration. To complete the past medical history, obtain information about the following:

- MAJOR UNDERLYING MEDICAL PROBLEMS. Does the patient have any major underlying medical problems, such as heart disease, lung disease, diabetes, or epilepsy? Is the patient currently under a doctor's care for any medical condition?
- MEDICATIONS. Does the patient take any medications regularly? If so, what are they?

Has the patient taken his or her prescribed medications today? When? Were any other drugs or alcohol taken during the past several hours? If so, when? How much?

- ALLERGIES. Does the patient have known allergies? Although people often volunteer information about food allergies, concentrate specifically on allergies to medications.
- DOCTOR. Does the patient regularly see a particular doctor? At a particular hospital? In an area where there are several hospitals close together, it is preferable to take the patient to the hospital where his or her medical records are on file. Record this information and pass it on to other members of the EMS team.
- VITAL SIGNS. Take and record vital signs.

Vital signs are often taken while obtaining the past medical history. It may be more efficient if one first responder interviews the patient and another first responder takes the patient's vital signs. In that way, the examiner taking vital signs can concentrate on one task and the interviewer can concentrate on another. First, explain to the patient what you both are going to do. It is important that you ask questions about a given body area or organ system before examining it. If you examine an area first and then ask questions, the patient may conclude that something is wrong, which will only increase the patient's anxiety.

After obtaining as much information as possible about the patient's chief complaint, conduct a modified head-to-toe examination. Just because a patient's chief complaint is medical in nature does not mean that he or she cannot have signs and symptoms of other illness or even evidence of trauma. Ask the patient to smile. Note whether one side of the patient's face droops. Look for signs of difficulty in breathing: tracheal tugging (the trachea pulls up on inspiration) and tracheal deviation (the trachea pulls to one side during inspiration). Examine the patient's chest: notice whether both sides of the chest move evenly during respiration; notice also whether the patient makes use of muscles in the chest and neck to breathe. Listen for abnormal breathing sounds, such as wheezing or gurgling. Ask the patient to squeeze your hands and to push against your hands with his or her feet; note if one side is markedly weaker than the other. Check pulses on both sides of the body. Notice if the patient's face, hands, or ankles seem swollen. If the patient's chief complaint is abdominal pain, note the patient's position: is he or she guarding the abdominal area? Do not poke at the patient's abdomen; touch the abdomen only to see if it is rigid. A rigid abdomen indicates possible internal bleeding or inflammation.

### Trauma Survey: The Head-To-Toe Examination

The patient who is unconscious or the victim of trauma is unable to report symptoms or to give a history of the present illness. For this type of patient, the secondary survey consists of a general assessment of the patient's appearance and level of consciousness, followed by a head-to-toe physical examination. Of course, you must assess and correct the patient's ABC's before proceeding to the head-to-toe examination.

It is often difficult to assess patients who have suffered trauma. Because their mental functioning is often impaired, they may be unable to give a patient history or to cooperate in physical examinations. In such cases, you must obtain information from careful observation, not only of the patient, but also of the scene of the accident.

Answers to the following questions are particularly important:

- *What* happened?
- *When* did the accident occur?
- *How* did it occur? What were the mechanisms of injury? Was the spine flexed, extended, or twisted?
- Was the patient unconscious at any time? For how long? Did unconsciousness occur immediately after the accident, or later?
- If the patient is able to communicate, what is the chief complaint? Does the patient experience any pain, numbness, tingling, or paralysis? Have the symptoms changed since the accident?

- Did the patient vomit? Children frequently vomit after head injury, but vomiting in adults may indicate serious brain injury.
- What symptoms does the patient have now? Headache? Dizziness? Nausea? Weakness? Can the patient move all extremities? Does the patient have numbness or a tingling sensation?
- Are there possible complicating factors such as significant underlying medical problems? Do not assume that just because a patient has suffered trauma that he or she may not also suffer from a medical problem, such as heart disease, lung disease, or diabetes. If the patient is unconscious, look in his or her wallet for a Medic Alert card (do this in the presence of witnesses).

As with a medical patient, notice the patient's *general appearance*. In what position is the patient lying? If the patient is the victim of an accident, where is the patient in relation to the site of the accident? If there is a major neurological injury, the patient may exhibit stereotyped postures known as *decorticate* and *decerebrate*. In decorticate posturing, the arms are flexed but the legs remain extended (Figure 4.16). In decerebrate posturing, both arms and legs are extended. Patients may either exhibit these postures in response to a painful stimulus, or may assume and maintain them indefinitely. Note the color and appearance of the patient's skin. Is the patient pale, cyanotic, or sweating heavily?

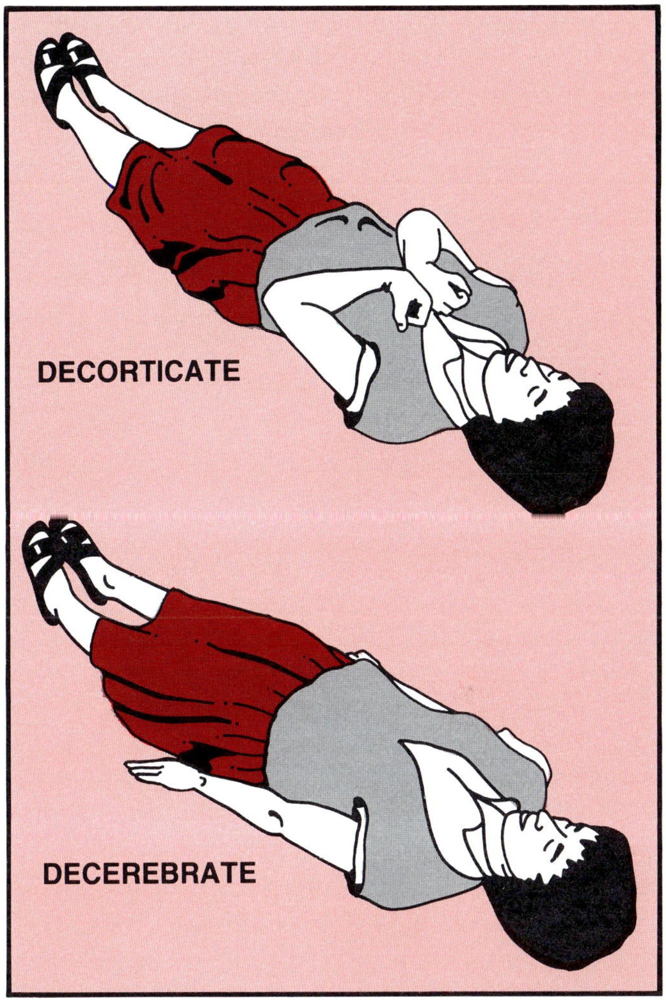


**Figure 4.16** These postures are a sign of major neurological injury. In decorticate posturing, the arms are flexed; in decerebrate posturing, the arms are extended.

After taking the patient's vital signs, try to determine the *mechanism of injury*, that is, the way in which the patient was injured. First, try to determine whether the injuries sustained by the patient were blunt or penetrating.

Blunt injuries transfer energy to the body in general without penetrating the skin. The amount of energy transferred determines the amount of injury. A punch thrown into the region of the stomach may transfer 100 to 150 pounds (45.5 kg to 68 kg) of energy. In an automobile accident, the body continues to travel at the impact speed after the automobile stops. Because the laws of physics dictate that energy can be neither created nor destroyed, the energy generated by the impact, which can be as much as 5,000 pounds (2 268 kg) must be absorbed. Energy is absorbed in the bending, tearing, and deformation of body tissues. When confronted with blunt trauma then, it is important to indentify the type of instrument that produced the injury and, if possible, to assess the amount of energy involved in the blow or at least the speed of impact.

Penetrating trauma transfers energy to the body in the form of lacerated or torn tissues. Gunshot wounds and stabbings are two of the most common causes of penetrating trauma. In the thoracic (chest) region, hemorrhage and air leaks to either the inside or the outside of the body are likely. In the abdomen, blood loss leading to shock is the prime danger. In the head, neurological damage may be of major importance. Look for an exit wound (perforating wound) as well as an entry wound, particularly in the case of a shooting victim (Figure 4.17). For more information on management of soft-tissue injuries, see Chapter 7, Bleeding Control and Soft-Tissue Injuries.

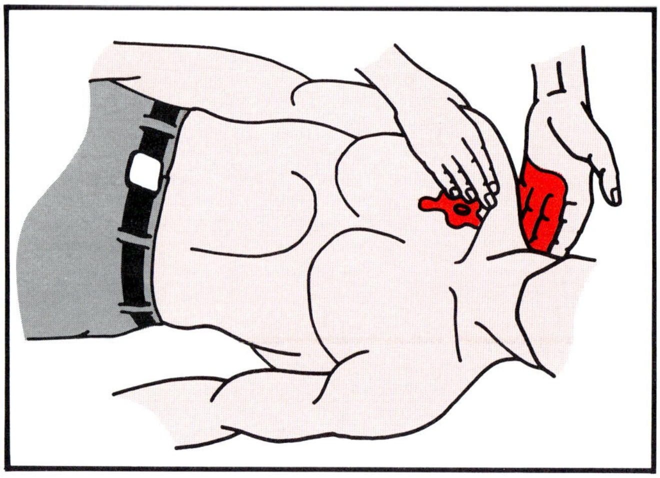

**Figure 4.17** If a patient has been shot, look for an exit wound as well as an entry wound.

Mechanism of injury as it relates to motor vehicle accidents deserves special attention because these accidents are such a common cause of traumatic injury. If the patient has been in a motor vehicle accident, try to determine the direction of impact (frontal, side, rear, rotational, or rollover) in order to reconstruct, in your mind, the pathway traveled by the occupant(s) of the vehicle. The parts of the body that strike the interior compartment of the automobile are most likely to have been injured. In this manner, you can anticipate the most likely severe injuries (Figure 4.18).

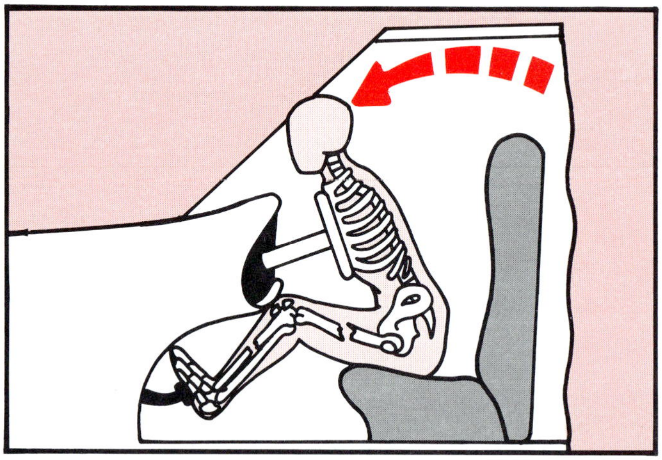

**Figure 4.18** For the victim of an automobile accident, multiple injuries are common, particularly if the patient did not wear a seat belt.

For example, a frontal collision could result in fractured ribs, pneumothorax, or cardiac injuries resulting from chest compression. Laceration and hemorrhage of abdominal organs, facial injuries, and cervical spine fractures are also possible. A posterior fracture of the hip, a common injury, occurs when the knee strikes the dash.

A side impact collision could cause flail injuries to the lateral part of the chest and a pneumothorax. A fractured clavicle (collarbone) is also common when the arm is driven inward.

Rear impact collisions are doubly complicated because the initial impact forces the head back over the seat. As the car comes to a stop, the body moves forward and strikes the dash or the steering column, resulting in injuries similar to those in a frontal collision (Figure 4.19).

Because of the many directions that an unrestrained occupant can travel in a rollover collision, the injury pattern is difficult to predict.

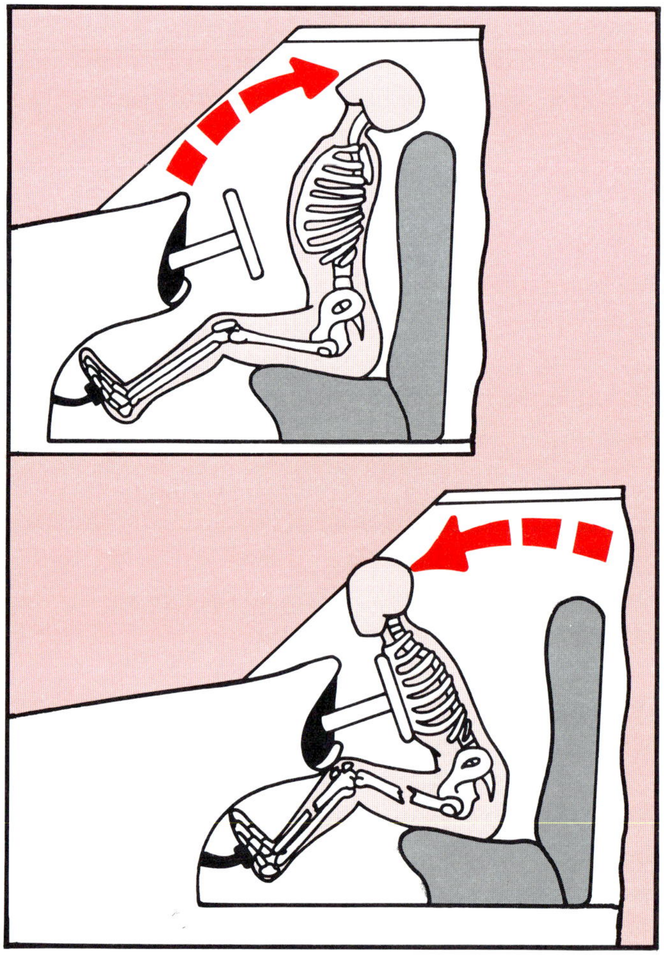

**Figure 4.19** In a rear-impact collision, the head and neck are forced back, then forward, as the car comes to a stop.

In addition to possible patterns of injury, other information that is important to obtain in the case of a motor vehicle accident includes the following:

- Were any passengers wearing seat belts? Did the patient suffer a direct blow to the head or spine? Was there a rapid deceleration?
- Was the patient unconscious at any time? For how long? Did unconsciousness occur immediately after the accident, or later?
- If the patient is able to communicate, what is the chief complaint? Does the patient experience any pain, numbness, tingling, or paralysis? Have the symptoms changed since the accident?
- Has the patient been moved before emergency help arrived? If so, document the fact that the patient has been moved.
- In what condition is the steering wheel? Is it bent up or down?
- What cracks or holes are in the windshield? Does the windshield have a star pattern of cracks, indicating that the driver or passengers struck the windshield?

**Glasgow Coma Scale**

| | | | Total Glasgow Coma Scale Points |
|---|---|---|---|
| **Eye Opening** | Spontaneous | 4 | |
| | To Voice | 3 | |
| | To Pain | 2 | 14-15=5 |
| | None | 1 | 11-13=4 |
| **Verbal Response** | Oriented | 5 | 8-10=3 |
| | Confused | 4 | 5- 7=2 |
| | Inappropriate Words | 3 | 3- 4=1 |
| | Incomprehensible Words | 2 | |
| | None | 1 | |
| **Motor Response** | Obeys Command | 6 | |
| | Localizes Pain | 5 | |
| | Withdraw (pain) | 4 | |
| | Flexion (pain) | 3 | |
| | Extension (pain) | 2 | |
| | None | 1 | |
| **Total Trauma Score** | | 1-16 | |

**Figure 4.20** The Glasgow Coma Scale is used to assess a patient's verbal, motor, and eye-opening responses. *Courtesy of Dr. Howard Champion.*

## LEVEL OF CONSCIOUSNESS

With the unconscious or severely injured patient, it is not possible to assess the patient's level of consciousness through conversation. For this type of patient, the Glasgow Coma Scale is often used to determine the severity of unconsciousness or to note any changes in the level of consciousness (Figure 4.20). This coma scale was developed to allow emergency personnel to assess a patient's verbal, motor, and eye-opening responses. The total from the three categories of assessment is the patient's "score." The highest score on the Glasgow Coma scale is 16, and the lowest score is 1.

To check the patient's eye-opening response, note whether the patient opens his or her eyes spontaneously, in response to the sound of your voice, in response to a painful stimulus, or not at all. The standard painful stimulus consists of pressing your knuckles into the patient's sternum with varying degrees of pressure.

The patient's motor response to painful stimuli is also an important indicator of mental functioning. If the patient attempts to push your arm away, movements are purposeful, and he or she is said to "localize" pain. If the patient moves away from a painful stimulus, then on the Glasgow scale he or she is said to "withdraw" in response to pain. If the patient has suffered a spinal cord injury, he or she may respond to painful stimulus with decorticate or decerebrate posturing.

In order to keep from overlooking any main areas of the body, always conduct the head-to-toe examination in the same order — starting at the head and working toward the feet. There is one exception to this rule: when examining a child, it may be easier to conduct the examination from feet-to-head. Many children are wary of strangers, and they may feel less threatened if you begin the examination at their feet and work gradually toward the more sensitive areas.

Begin by examining the head. Again, if you have any reason to suspect a spinal cord injury, **DO NOT** move the patient's head or neck during the examination. Look for blood from cuts or abrasions, and feel carefully through the hair for any unusual lumps or depressions. Touch depressions very carefully to avoid pushing any pieces of broken glass into the soft tissue of the brain.

Examine the ears and nose for signs of injury, such as cuts, swelling, or deformity. Blood or clear fluid coming from the ears or nose may indicate skull fracture and leakage of cerebrospinal fluid. **DO NOT** attempt to stop the flow, since such action may cause pressure to build up inside the skull. Note ecchymoses (bruises) behind the ears, which are known as Battle's sign (Figure 4.21). Battle's sign is an indication of basal skull fracture.

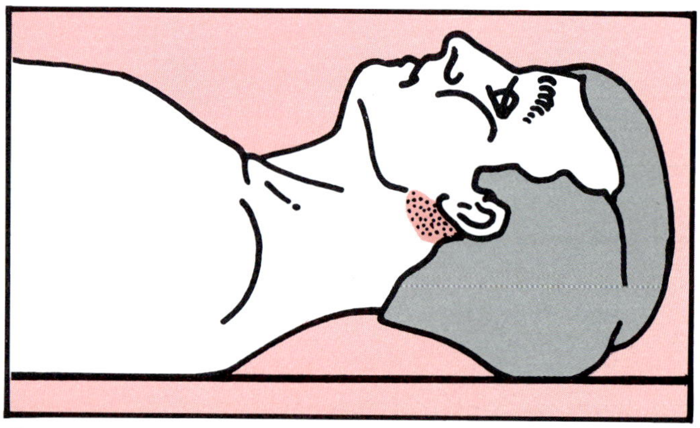

**Figure 4.21** Bruises behind the ears, known as Battle's sign, are a sign of skull fracture.

Examine the eyes for swelling, bruises, or other signs of injury. Two black eyes are known as "coon's eyes" and indicate possible skull fracture.

Observe the motion of the eyes. Normally, the eyes move together (conjugately). In head injury or direct trauma to the eyes, the eyes may turn in different directions or may not move together. This is known as dysconjugate gaze. If the patient is conscious, ask him or her to follow your finger as you move it 180 degrees up, down, and to the left and right (Figure 4.22). Note whether the gaze is paralyzed in any direction. Patients with fractures of the orbit often have a paralyzed upward gaze, while patients with stroke may have paralyzed gaze to the right or left. Note the reaction of the pupils in response to light. Pupils that react sluggishly may be an indication of head injury.

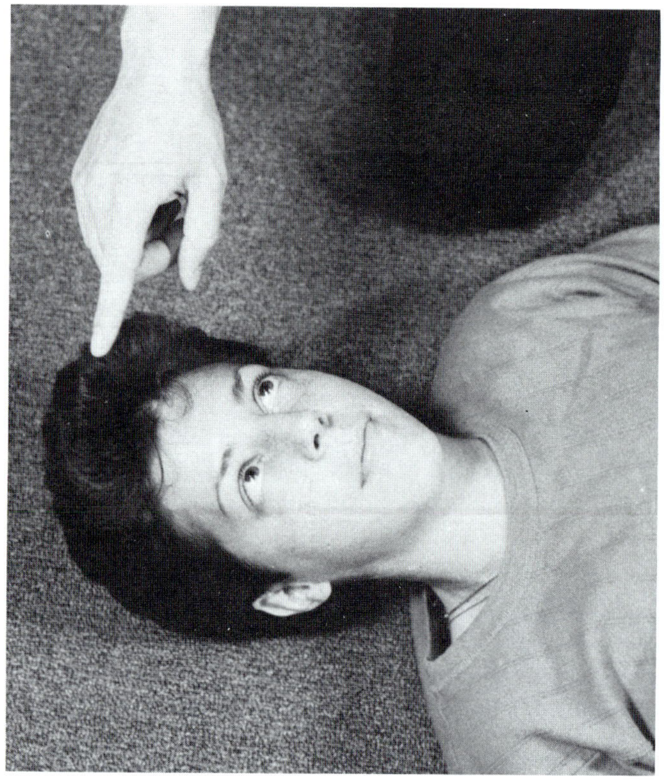

**Figure 4.22** Check to see if both eyes move together by asking the patient to follow your finger as you move it up, down, and to the left and right.

The mouth should now be inspected more carefully for foreign objects, food, loose teeth, or blood. Clear the mouth with a clean, soft cloth to ensure an open airway and to keep the patient from choking. If you have mechanical suction equipment and are trained to use it, suction the mouth and airway to clear it of foreign matter (see Chapter 5, Basic Life Support: The ABC's).

Examine the patient's neck by placing one hand on each side of the neck and feeling gently and carefully for alignment of the neck structures. Check for open wounds or obvious deformities. Note whether gentle pressure on the neck or vertebrae seems painful to the patient. Note if jugular veins are distended, which can be an indication of chest trauma. Grasp the patient's trachea and notice whether the trachea deviates (pulls to one side) during inspiration (Figure 4.23). Tracheal deviation is another sign of chest trauma. Loosen the patient's collar and look for a stoma (opening) at the front of the neck. The presence of a stoma indicates that the patient has had surgery and breathes either partially or completely through the neck opening. Look for a Medic Alert tag around the pa-

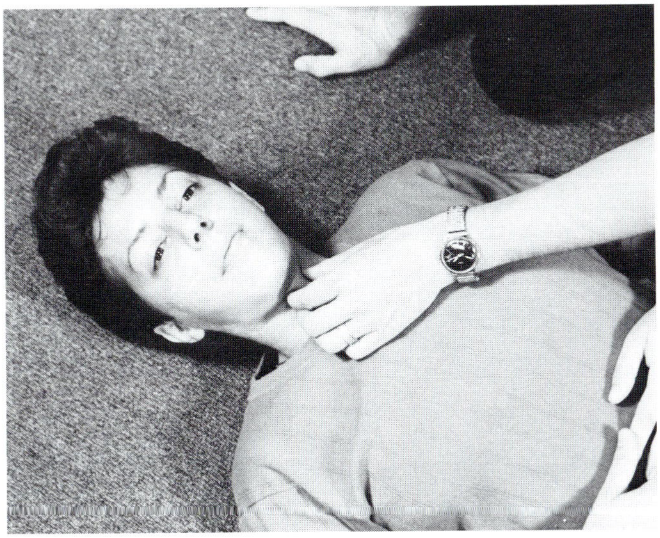

**Figure 4.23** Grasp the patient's trachea and note whether it pulls to one side as the patient inhales.

tient's neck. The Medic Alert tag lists medical conditions or allergies that are important in the event that the patient is ill or injured. These tags also contain patient identification numbers that should be recorded and relayed to other emergency care personnel. Medical alert tags may be worn around the neck, wrist, or ankle (Figure 4.24). Stabilize

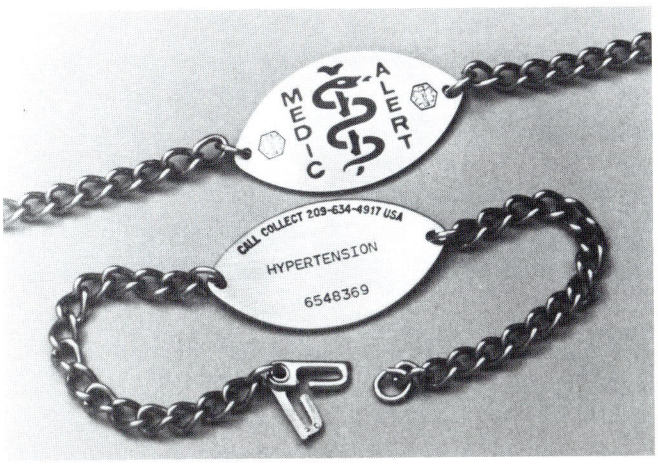


**Figure 4.24** The Medic Alert tag contains valuable information about underlying medical conditions. These tags are worn around the neck, wrist, or ankle. *Courtesy of Medic Alert Foundation.*

the patient's neck with a cervical collar. Do not allow the patient to sit up or move around. Watch, too, for signs of nausea: if the patient begins to vomit, he or she will have to be turned as a unit in order to avoid further injury to the cervical spine.

Move the patient as little as possible, but slide one hand under the patient's shoulder blades and use your other hand to check the patient's back, feeling for tenderness, deformities, or possible bleeding wounds (Figure 4.25).

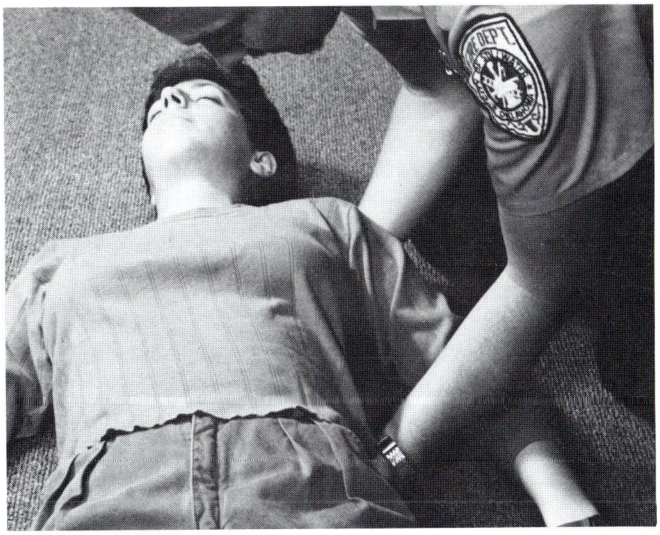

**Figure 4.25** Carefully slide one hand under the patient's shoulder blades and use your other hand to check for abnormalities.

Move toward the patient's chest. Feel along the collarbone and down the sternum for fractures, which are indicated by deformities or tenderness. Place both hands on the upper chest and press down firmly but gently; then place your hands on the sides of the chest and squeeze the chest inward. If the patient is conscious, ask if the examination or breathing is painful. Listen for labored or abnormal breathing. Note whether both sides of the chest expand and contract evenly during respiration (Figure 4.26). If they do not, the patient is probably suffering from a chest injury and is un-

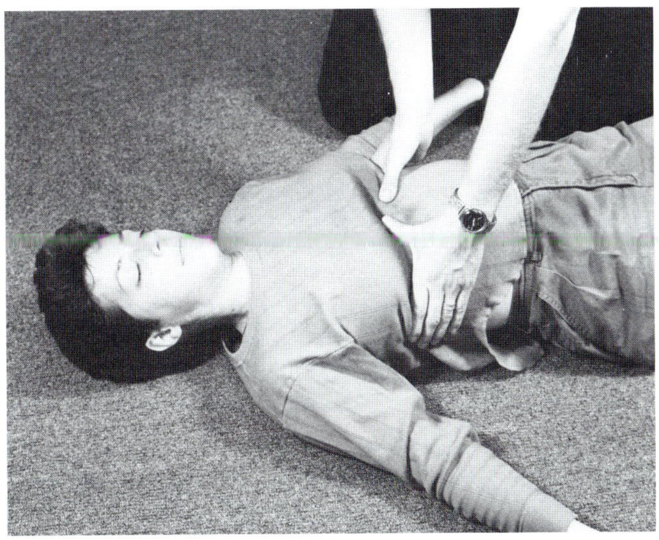

**Figure 4.26** Place your hands on both sides of the patient's chest; note whether both sides of the chest expand evenly during respiration.

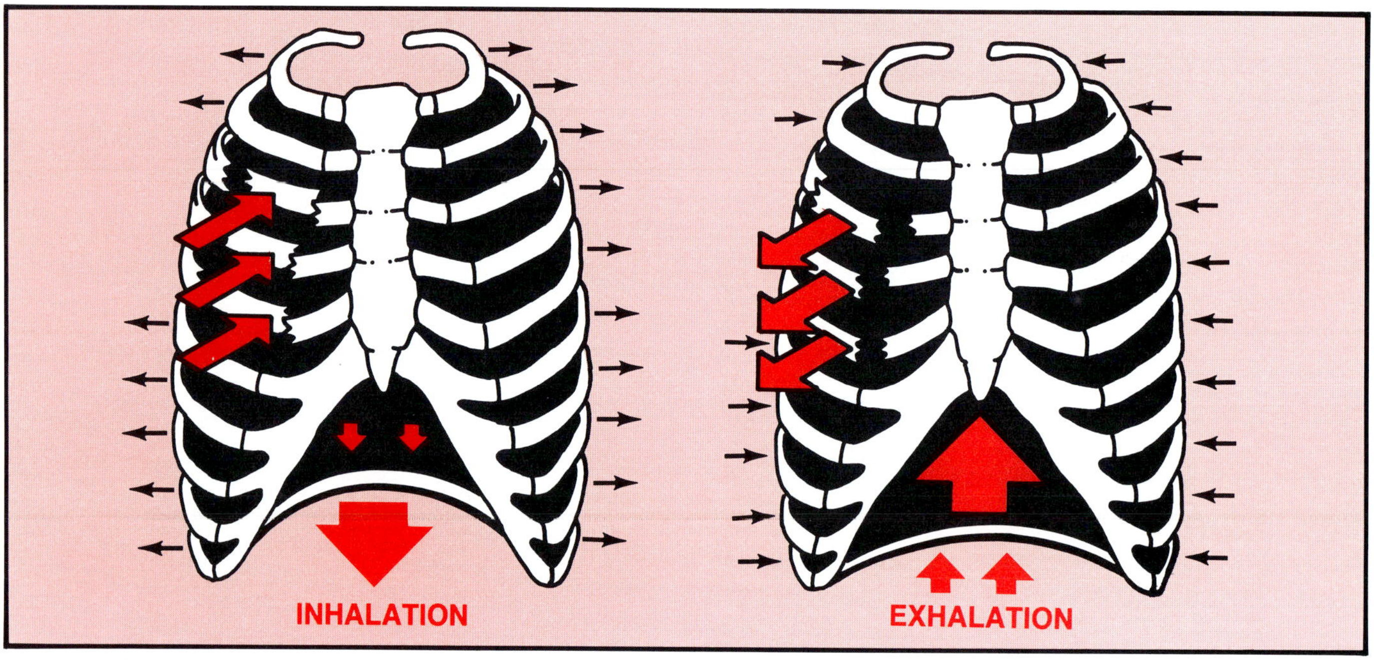


**Figure 4.27** During paradoxical chest movement, a portion of the chest expands while the rest of the chest contracts.

able to breathe properly. Look also for paradoxical chest movement, another sign of chest injury. During paradoxical chest movement, a portion of the chest, say a flail segment caused by broken ribs, expands while the rest of the chest contracts (Figure 4.27). Place a sandbag on the flail segment to stabilize it temporarily. Look for bleeding, wounds (entry and exit points), and bruises. For more information on evaluating injuries to the chest, see Chapter 8, Injuries to the Skull, Spine, and Chest.

Check the abdomen for wounds, tenderness, and rigidity. Ask a conscious patient to relax the stomach muscles and observe whether the abdominal area stays rigid. Rigidity indicates possible internal bleeding, which can lead to shock. Abdominal swelling is also a sign of internal injury.

Next, check the pelvis for tenderness and bruises. Remove any of the patient's clothing that interferes with the examination and shield the patient from the sight of onlookers. Place your hands on the patient's pelvic bones (hip bones) and press straight down (Figure 4.28). Then squeeze the pelvic bones together, if possible one at a time. If the patient has a fractured or dislocated pelvis, this action will cause discomfort. Note whether the patient's genitals are bruised, swollen, or bleeding.

Begin to examine the lower extremities, one leg at a time. Encircle the leg with both hands and palpate (feel) the entire length of the leg. Pay special attention to any deformities or unusual positions, which indicate a possible fracture or dislocation. If either leg seems injured, remove clothing from the legs, cutting it off if necessary to avoid jarring the patient. Note if one leg seems rotated or

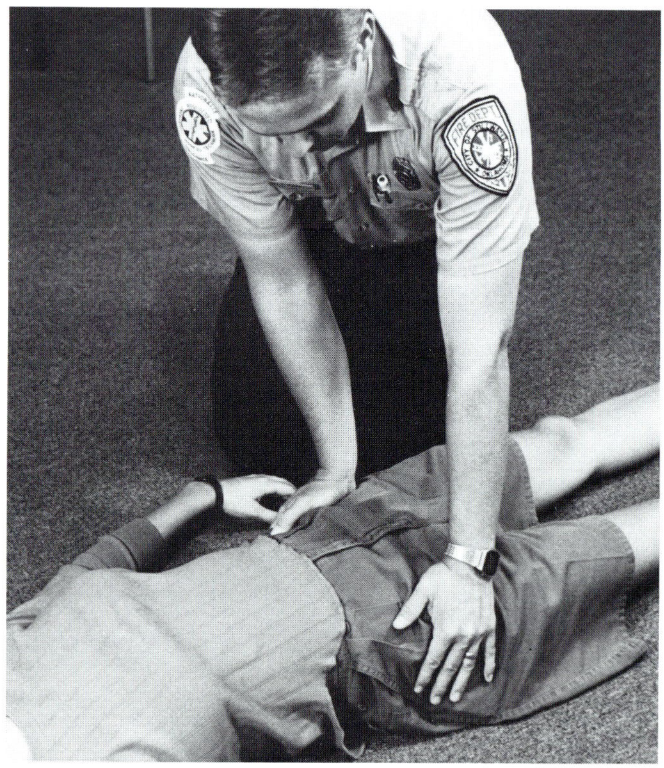

**Figure 4.28** Check for pelvic injuries by pressing the patient's pelvic bones straight down, then squeezing them together.

shortened, a sign of a fractured hip (Figure 4.29). Examine each leg carefully for tenderness, bruises, or cuts. Check pulses in both feet; absence of a pulse indicates a loss of circulation. Check perfusion of tissues by performing a capillary refill test. Press a nailbed enough to make the skin blanch; it should return to full color within one to two seconds. Ask the patient if he or she can feel your touch as you conduct the examination. Then ask the patient to flex and extend each foot. If the patient has no feeling in the leg, reports numbness or tingling, or cannot move on command, it is an indication of possible spinal cord injury and should be noted.

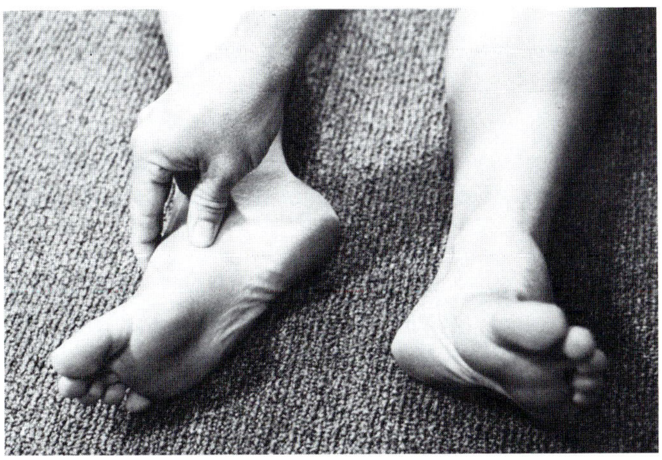

**Figure 4.29** If one leg is rotated or shortened, the patient probably has a fractured hip.

Examine both arms: feel the entire arm and note tenderness or any unusual positions. If the arm seems to be injured, remove any clothing that inhibits the examination and examine it carefully for bruises, cuts, dislocations, and fractures. Listen for crepitus, a scraping sound made when the ends of a broken bone rub together. **NOTE:** Some first responders examine the arms after examining the neck; others move directly to the chest and abdomen after examining the neck. The reason for proceeding directly to the chest and abdomen is that this area is much more likely to reveal life-threatening problems. Whatever method you use, follow the same order each time so that no body areas go unexamined.

Check radial pulses in both arms and ask the patient whether he or she has sensation in the arm or feels numbness or tingling. Ask the patient to squeeze your hands; note whether one side seems markedly weaker than the other. As with legs, lack of sensation, inability to move the arm, and numbness or tingling are indications of possible spinal cord injury. Check perfusion of tissues by performing a capillary refill test. Finally, be sure to note the presence of a Medic Alert tag around the patient's wrist.

Various trauma scales may be used to evaluate the severity of trauma. They are similar to the Glasgow Coma Scale in that they assign numerical values to different body functions. The Trauma Score is composed of the Glasgow Coma Scale and measurements of cardiorespiratory function (Figure 4.30). The patient is evaluated for re-

**Trauma Score**

The Trauma Score is a numerical grading system for estimating the severity of injury. The score is composed of the Glasgow Coma Scale (reduced to approximately one third total value) and measurements of cardiopulmonary function. Each parameter is given a number (high for normal and low for impaired function). Severity of injury is estimated by summing the numbers. The lowest score is 1, and the highest score is 16.

| | | |
|---|---|---|
| **Respiratory Rate** | 10-24/min | 4 |
| | 24-35/min | 3 |
| | 36/min or greater | 2 |
| | 1-9/min | 1 |
| | None | 0 |
| **Respiratory Expansion** | Normal | 1 |
| | Retractive | 0 |
| **Systolic Blood Pressure** | 90 mm Hg or greater | 4 |
| | 70-89 mm Hg | 3 |
| | 50-69 mm Hg | 2 |
| | 0-49 mm Hg | 1 |
| | No Pulse | 0 |
| **Capillary Refill** | Normal | 2 |
| | Delayed | 1 |
| | None | 0 |

**Glasgow Coma Scale**

| | | | **Total Glasgow Coma Scale Points** |
|---|---|---|---|
| **Eye Opening** | Spontaneous | 4 | |
| | To Voice | 3 | |
| | To Pain | 2 | 14-15=5 |
| | None | 1 | 11-13=4 |
| **Verbal Response** | Oriented | 5 | 8-10=3 |
| | Confused | 4 | 5- 7=2 |
| | Inappropriate Words | 3 | 3- 4=1 |
| | Incomprehensible Words | 2 | |
| | None | 1 | |
| **Motor Response** | Obeys Command | 6 | |
| | Localizes Pain | 5 | |
| | Withdraw (pain) | 4 | |
| | Flexion (pain) | 3 | |
| | Extension (pain) | 2 | |
| | None | 1 | |
| **Total Trauma Score** | | | 1-16 |

**Figure 4.30** The Trauma Score is composed of the Glasgow Coma Scale and measurements of the patient's respiration and circulation.

spiratory rate, respiratory expansion, systolic blood pressure, and adequacy of capillary refill; each category is given a score from 0 to 4. These scores are then added to the Glasgow Coma Scale (which is reduced to one-third) to arrive at the patient's total trauma score. The lowest score is 1, and the highest score is 16.

### Reporting Information Concerning the Patient's Condition

The examination and gathering of information are conducted in a systematic manner so that arriving EMTs and other emergency care personnel can be advised of the patient's condition quickly and completely. This allows EMTs to continue with any further treatment without having to ask a lot of questions. The following is a sample of an oral report that a first responder may give to an EMT:

> "We have a 63-year-old male found about 30 minutes ago after an apparent fall from a ladder. Upon report he was unable to move his right arm and leg. Upon arrival the patient was alert times three. The patient's vital signs are pulse 120, respirations 28, blood pressure 130/90, pupils normal, skin warm and dry with normal color. We have the patient lying flat and covered with a blanket to maintain body temperature."

## TRIAGE

Patient assessment is usually performed on one patient at a time; however, a problem arises when several or even many persons are injured at the same time: who should be treated first? Why? In emergency services, multiple casualties are rapidly assessed and categorized in a process known as *triage*.

Triage is a French word meaning "to sort." The purpose of triage is to ensure that patients with life-threatening injuries receive immediate treatment and transportation to a medical facility. Patients with injuries that are not life-threatening can be treated and transported after the patients with more urgent injuries are treated. Patients who are already dead or who are injured so severely that death seems imminent must be passed over in favor of patients who are salvageable. The goal of triage is to perform the greatest good for the greatest number of people, so one victim who *may* be saved by an all-out effort of several rescuers may have to be bypassed in favor of several victims who can be stabilized through simple procedures.

Although many people associate triage with a mass casualty incident (MCI), triage is necessary any time an incident results in more patients than there are emergency personnel and resources to care for them. An automobile accident involving five injured people is an example of a common occurrence that is likely to require triage.

As the first-arriving emergency personnel on the scene of an accident, be sure to park the rescue vehicle off the road so that it does not create a traffic hazard. Conduct a rapid size-up: park UPWIND of any spilled chemicals, away from any downed power lines, and make sure that the scene is safe before you begin assessing patients (see Chapter 3, Scene Assessment and Safety). Immediately call for extrication equipment, wreckers, and ambulances.

Begin triaging the patients. At a smaller incident, such as a motor vehicle accident, patients are usually triaged in place unless a hazard at the scene requires that they be moved first. At a mass casualty incident, patients will be moved to a triage area for evaluation.

One first responder should act as triage officer until more highly trained personnel arrive. The triage officer identifies those patients most urgently in need of medical attention. Other first responders begin stabilization and treatment of the most critically injured patients. It is vitally important that the triage officer get to each patient as rapidly as possible, conducting a primary survey of each patient. The triage officer does not stop during the survey, except to make rapid corrections of the ABC's. The number of patients and the severity of their injuries will dictate whether or not it is possible to make a rapid secondary survey. The secondary survey may have to wait until other emergency personnel arrive.

There are two methods of triage, and both are presented here. The first, and more traditional method, categorizes patients according to injury classification. Based on the assessment of the rescuer, patients are classified as first priority, second priority, delayed priority, or dead/nonsalvageable, and tagged appropriately. The second method of triage, known as the START plan (Simple Triage and Rapid Treatment), calls for rescuers to assess breathing, perfusion (adequacy of circulation), and mental status, and to tag patients as high or low priority based on the results of those tests.

Both triage systems make use of a triage tag to rapidly categorize and identify patients. The Mettag is one of the most commonly used triage tags (Figure 4.31). The colored strips on the tag are used to indicate the patient's status:

- GREEN indicates walking wounded. This patient does not need to be hospitalized at all; his or her injuries can be managed by first aid.

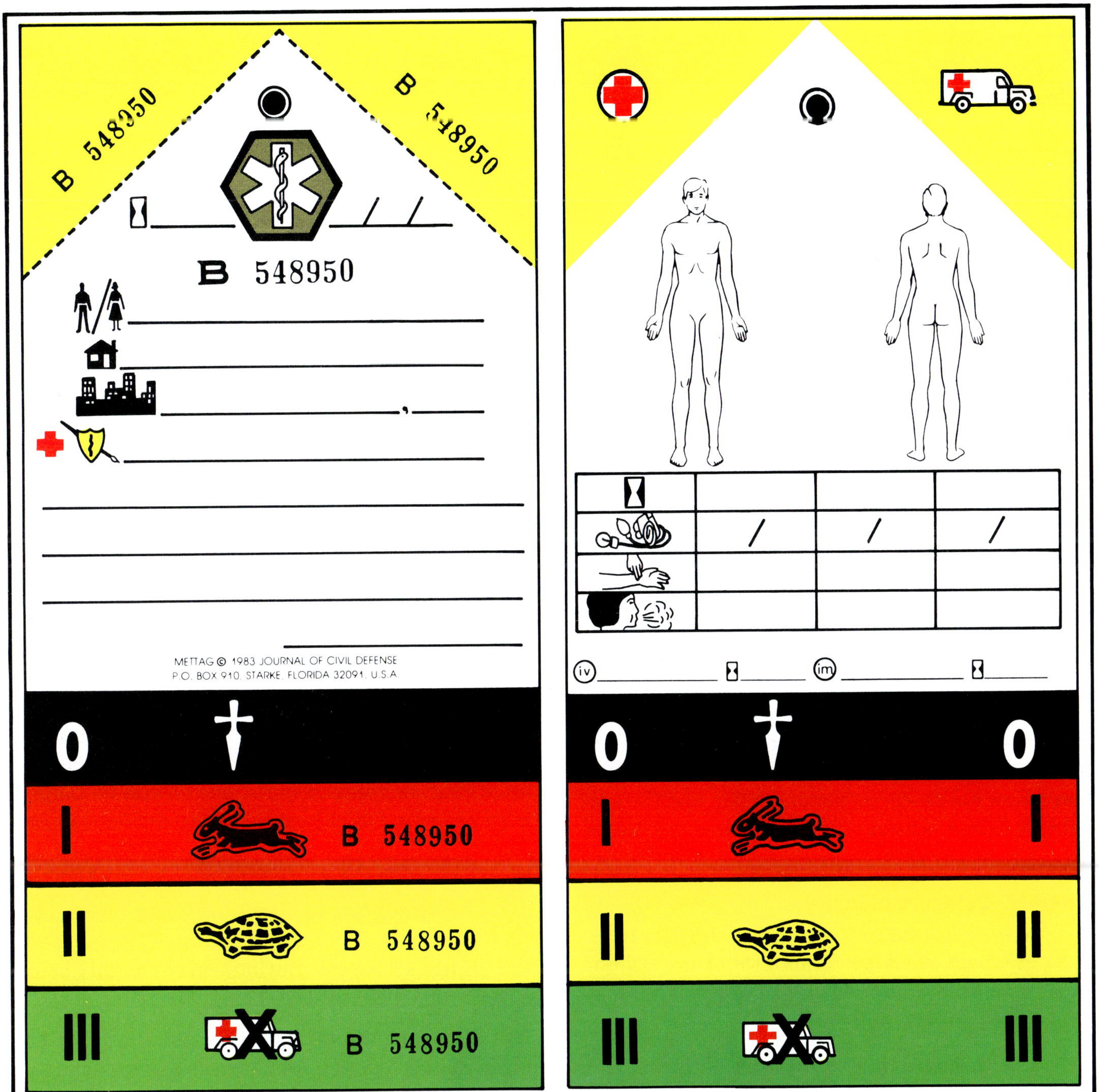


**Figure 4.31** A four-color triage tag, such as the Mettag shown above, is used to rapidly categorize and identify patients. *Courtesy of Journal of Civil Defense, Starke, Florida.*

- YELLOW indicates a need for hospital care, but delayed transportation will be sufficient.
- RED indicates that immediate care and transportation are necessary. Patients in this category should receive attention before all others.
- BLACK indicates a patient who is dead or nonsalvageable. Patients in this category receive no care.

To use the Mettag, the rescuer tears off the strips that do not apply to the patient, leaving the bottom strip to identify the patient's need for treatment. For example, a rescuer with a patient needing immediate care would tear off the green and yellow strips, leaving the red strip to alert other rescuers who actually begin stabilization and treatment. The rescuer performing triage can also mark, on the triage tag, the area of the patient's body that requires immediate attention. The rescuer then places the triage tag around the patient's neck or wrist so that it is easily visible to other rescuers.

The numbers on the triage tag are used to keep track of patients at a mass casualty incident. When the rescuer tears strips from the bottom of the triage tag, he or she keeps the strips; then, the triage officer can identify which patients were triaged by which rescuer. The identical numbers at the upper corners of the triage tag are used when the patient is transported to a medical facility. At a mass casualty incident, a transportation officer keeps track of the number of ambulances (and patients) going to various hospitals. The transportation officer keeps one corner of the tag, and the ambulance driver, who may be a first responder, keeps the other corner of the tag.

### Triage by Category of Injury

To perform triage by category of injury, the rescuer or triage officer performs a rapid assessment and tags the patient based on his or her determination of the patient's injuries.

As with any patient care, threats to the airway, breathing, and circulation receive the highest priority. However, the priority of treatment may change, depending on the number and severity of people injured and the number of rescuers present to give emergency care. A patient who requires intense resuscitative efforts, such as a person in cardiac arrest, may have to be classified as a delayed priority if there are more persons with life-threatening injuries than there are emergency personnel available to care for them. It may be necessary not to commit one or two rescuers to such a patient in order that a greater number of other people may be saved.

Begin triage by conducting a rapid primary survey of each patient. It is critically important that every patient receive an ABC assessment.

**A BLOCKED AIRWAY WILL CAUSE DEATH IN MINUTES IF NOT CORRECTED. THE ABC'S ARE CRITICAL!**

First, determine if the patient's airway is open or if the patient is bleeding into the airway. Quickly clear the patient's mouth of blood, debris, or loose teeth. If a simple correction can be made, such as repositioning the patient's head or turning the patient onto his or her side, do so. If possible, insert an oral airway. In a mass casualty incident, the usual cervical spine precautions may have to be ignored when opening the airway due to the large number of victims and the necessity for reaching everyone as rapidly as possible. Saving a patient's life takes precedence over everything else.

Once the patient's airway is open, determine if he or she is breathing. Difficulty breathing, pain on breathing, or rapid respirations should be tagged high priority. Quickly observe the patient's chest: seal sucking chest wounds with an occlusive dressing and tag the patient high priority (red). Flail chest is serious but can wait until other, more urgent injuries are taken care of. If the patient is not breathing, assist ventilations mechanically or by mouth-to-mouth resuscitation.

Take the patient's pulse to assess circulation. If the pulse is rapid or weak, assume shock and tag the patient high priority. Check perfusion by performing a capillary refill test. Pinch the patient's lip or a nailbed hard enough to make the skin blanch. Normal color should return within two seconds; if it does not, assume that the patient is in shock. If the patient has no pulse, available resources will dictate whether it is possible to begin cardiac compressions. If there are a sufficient number of rescuers, begin cardiac compressions at once. If there are many patients and few rescuers, the patient in cardiac arrest may have to be bypassed in order that other patients with better chances of survival can be reached.

The patient who is bleeding heavily requires a high-priority (red) tag. Very quickly attempt to control severe bleeding with bulky dressings and roller bandages. If the patient is conscious, ask him or her to hold the dressing in place. If there are many casualties, it may be necessary to apply a tourniquet to control bleeding. Remember, salvage of life takes precedence over salvage of limb. (See Chapter 7, Bleeding Control and Soft-Tissue Injuries for instructions on applying a tourniquet.)

**PERFORM A RAPID SECONDARY SURVEY ONLY AFTER ASSESSING EVERY PATIENT'S ABC'S!**

If time and resources permit, perform a rapid secondary survey to identify injuries that require medical attention or that may cause the patient's condition to deteriorate. As with a single trauma patient, perform a rapid head-to-toe examination. Examine the head for evidence of skull fracture, noting Battle's sign or coon's eyes. Look for facial fractures that could cause bleeding into the airway. The neck is an especially important and vulnerable part of the body: examine it for open wounds, tracheal deviation (the trachea pulls to one side during inspiration), damage to the trachea, subcutaneous emphysema (air trapped beneath the skin due to air leaking from the trachea), or distended jugular veins. Any of these signs indicates that the patient's ability to breathe has been seriously compromised; tag these patients high priority. Examine the chest for even expansion of the lungs, bruises, or fractured ribs. Examine the abdomen for open wounds, evisceration, rigidity, and pain. Rigidity is a particularly important sign because it may indicate internal bleeding, which leads rapidly to hypovolemic shock. Check the pelvis by first pushing straight down on the pelvic bones, then pressing them together. If these actions cause pain, assume injury to the pelvic area. Quickly examine all extremities for deformities and pulses. If the patient is conscious, ask if he or she can feel your touch. Conversation is also the best way to assess the patient's mental status: a patient who is unable to answer questions must be assumed to have injuries serious enough to require medical attention.

Based on this rapid patient assessment, tag the patient as first priority, second priority, delayed priority, or no treatment (dead). The following is a list of emergency priorities commonly used:

FIRST-PRIORITY INJURIES (RED TAG)

- Airway and breathing difficulties
- Cardiac arrest
- Uncontrolled or suspected severe bleeding
- Shock
- Open chest or abdominal wounds
- Burns covering 20 percent or more of body surface
- Severe head injuries

SECOND-PRIORITY INJURIES (YELLOW TAG)

- Burns covering less than 20 percent of body surface
- Major multiple fractures
- Back injuries with or without spinal cord damage
- Moderate bleeding
- Head injuries with decreasing level of consciousness

DELAYED-PRIORITY INJURIES (GREEN TAG)

- Fractures or other injuries of a minor nature

NO TREATMENT (BLACK TAG)

- Injuries that are so severe that death appears certain
- Obvious death

## The START System of Triage

**NOTE:** (The following information on the START system of triage was adapted with permission from *START: A Triage Training Module,* written by Victoria Cleary, R.N., Mary Hewett, R.N.; and Alan Schmehl, EMT-P. Copyright 1983, Hoag Memorial Hospital, Newport Beach, CA).

The START plan (Simple Triage and Rapid Treatment Plan) was developed to allow first responders to triage victims in 60 seconds or less based on only 3 observations: breathing, perfusion (adequacy of circulation), and mental status. This plan is based on the observation that trauma victims die during the first hour after injury because they cannot breathe, they bleed to death, or because they have central nervous system injuries so severe that regulation of breathing and perfusion by the brain is lost. The START plan calls for rescuers to rapidly correct the two main threats to life: a blocked airway and severe bleeding. As with triage by injury classification, patients are tagged with four-color triage tags as immediate, delayed, dead/nonsalvageable, or no hospital care needed (Figure 4.32).

The first step of the START plan is to ask all who can walk to move to a designated area. Victims who can walk rarely have life-threatening injuries; in fact, some of them may be able to assist with patients who are more seriously injured.

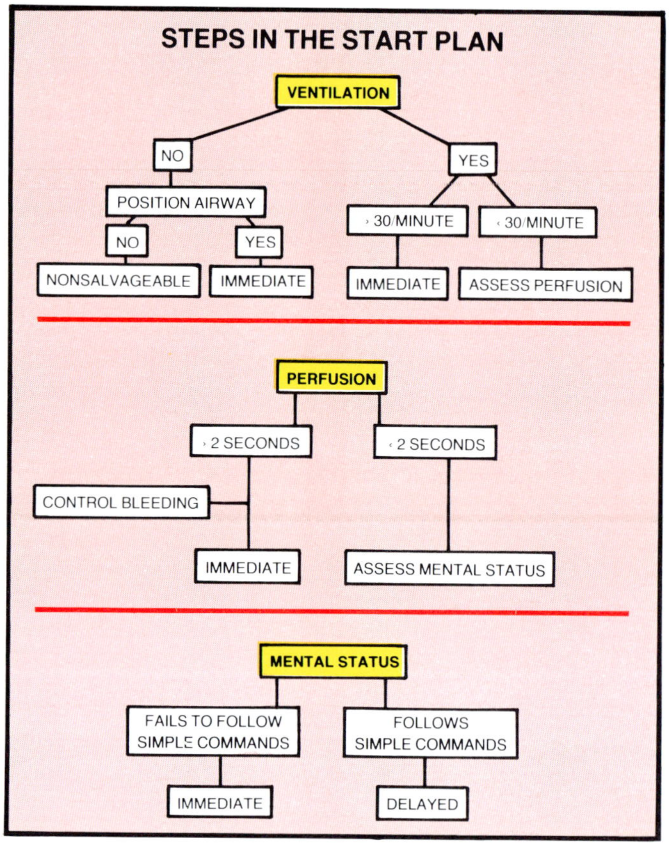


**Figure 4.32** Shown above are the steps in the START system of triage. Reproduced with permission from *START: A Triage Training Module,* by Victoria Cleary, R.N., Mary Hewett, R.N., and Alan Schmehl, EMT-P. Copyright 1984, Hoag Memorial Hospital Presbyterian, Newport Beach, California.

### VENTILATION (BREATHING)

Every patient is quickly assessed for adequacy of ventilation. If the patient is not breathing, the rescuer quickly removes dentures or foreign matter from the mouth or repositions the patient's head by hyperextending the cervical spine. The usual cervical spine precautions may have to be ignored; it is better to open the airway, prop the victim in a new position, and move on to other victims. If possible, the walking wounded may be enlisted to help maintain the airway of the unconscious victim. Any victim who needs help in maintaining an open airway is tagged immediate (red).

If the victim does not breathe after attempts are made to open the airway, he or she is tagged dead/nonsalvageable (black). Victims with respirations greater than 30 a minute are tagged immediate (red). Victims with respirations less than 30 a minute are not tagged at this time.

Of course, 30 respirations a minute is an arbitrary cutoff point. Rescuers do not have time to count respirations; however, they should be able to quickly recognize very rapid respirations.

### PERFUSION

The most rapid method for assessing perfusion (adequacy of oxygenation) is by performing the capillary refill test. The rescuer places pressure on the victim's lip or nailbed and then releases it. The area should regain its normal color within two seconds. If it does not, the victim has signs of inadequate perfusion and should be tagged immediate (red). If color does return within two seconds, perfusion is adequate and the victim is not tagged until his or her mental status is evaluated.

The radial (wrist) pulse can also be used as a test of adequate perfusion. In most people, the radial pulse cannot be felt when the systolic blood pressure falls below 80. Therefore, a victim without a readily detectable radial pulse is assumed to have inadequate perfusion and is triaged into the immediate group.

Rescuers can employ two rapid stabilization methods for victims with inadequate perfusion. First, the patient or one of the walking wounded may apply pressure to bleeding areas. Second, rescuers should elevate the victim's legs to maximize perfusion of the victim's heart, lungs, and brain. (For more information on perfusion, see Chapter 6, Shock).

### MENTAL STATUS

The final test, mental status, is used for patients whose respirations are adequate and whose tissues are adequately perfused. To test a victim's mental status, rescuers ask the victim to follow a simple command, such as opening and closing the eyes or squeezing the rescuer's hand. If the victim is able to follow commands, he or she is triaged into the delayed (yellow) category. If the victim is unable to follow simple commands, triage into the immediate (red) category is indicated.

The START plan is a primary triaging system. It is designed to enable rescuers to *rapidly* identify patients most in need of critical care. It is expected that as more personnel and resources arrive on the emergency scene, patients will be retriaged. People who have been injured do not always remain in the same condition, and some patients who were initially triaged as delayed may have developed problems that require immediate attention.

## Triage at a Mass Casualty Incident (MCI)

At a mass casualty incident (MCI), patients may have to be moved to a triage area first, so that they and their rescuers are safe from any hazards, such as fire or spilled chemicals. At a large incident, triage is conducted in rounds, with the first round of triage concentrating only on identifying those patients with high-priority injuries. First responders begin conducting the first round of triage, and physicians, nurses, and other medical personnel conduct additional rounds in designated treatment areas. Separate treatment areas will be set up for first priority, second priority, and delayed priority patients (red, yellow, and green tags). As patients are brought to the treatment areas (remember, patients with red tags are moved first), they are rapidly triaged again and stabilized.

Repeat patient assessments are important because injured people do not always remain in a stable condition. A person who was first triaged as a second-priority injury may develop complications and slip into a state of high-priority injury. After patients are stabilized, they are moved to a separate staging area, which contains waiting ambulances, and transported to a medical facility.

The duties of a first responder at a mass casualty incident are many: upon arrival, immediately call for more assistance and begin triage. As soon as physicians, nurses, and EMTs arrive, they will take over triage duties. You may be asked to perform any of the following:

- Serve as litter bearer, helping to move patients to treatment areas.
- Stay in a treatment area and assist with patient care, for example, taking vital signs.
- Procure supplies for other emergency personnel.
- Help move stabilized patients to a staging area so that they can be transported.
- Drive the ambulance or rescue vehicle.

If you are asked to serve as litter bearer, remember to SEARCH FOR AND MOVE THE PATIENTS WITH THE RED TAGS FIRST. These patients are in the most urgent need of help. Resist the temptation to move the first patient you see, who may have a yellow or green tag. When all patients with red tags have been moved to a treatment area, search for and move all the patients with yellow tags to the appropriate treatment area. Only when all the red-and yellow-tagged patients have been moved should the patients with green tags be moved. After all the living patients have been accounted for, the dead should be moved to a separate area and covered.

# 5

# Basic Life Support: The ABC's

## NFPA STANDARD 1001
### Emergency Medical Care
### Fire Fighter I

**3-4.2** The fire fighter shall identify procedures for determining whether or not a victim has an open airway.

**3-4.3** The fire fighter shall identify procedures for establishing an open airway in a nonbreathing person.

**3-4.4** The fire fighter shall demonstrate mouth-to-mouth and mouth-to-nose resuscitation.

**3-4.5** The fire fighter shall demonstrate oronasal ventilation.

**3-4.6** The fire fighter shall identify the three signs of cardiac arrest.

**3-4.7** The fire fighter shall demonstrate cardiopulmonary resuscitation.

### Fire Fighter II

**4-4.13** The fire fighter shall identify the heart-lung-brain relationship as it affects life and shall define what occurs when an airway obstruction is not corrected.

**4-4.14** The fire fighter shall demonstrate cardiopulmonary resuscitation employing the two-person technique.

**4-4.16** The fire fighter shall demonstrate the use of breathing aid equipment.



## U.S. DEPARTMENT OF TRANSPORTATION
### First Responder Training Course

**Objectives:**

- Describe the signs of adequate and inadequate breathing.
- Given an adult manikin, perform the five techniques for maintaining an open airway.
- Given an adult manikin, perform mouth-to-mouth and mouth-to-nose pulmonary resuscitation.
- Given an infant manikin, perform pulmonary resuscitation.
- Given an adult manikin, perform procedures for removing an obstruction from the airway for conscious and unconscious patients and for standing, seated, and supine patients using both abdominal and chest thrusts.
- Given an infant manikin, perform procedures for removing an obstruction from the airway.
- Describe variations in design of the respiratory system for partial and total laryngectomees.
- Describe airway care and resuscitation procedures for the laryngectomee.
- Given a diagram of the heart and its related organs, identify these organs and complications if CPR is performed incorrectly.
- List the signs of cardiac arrest.
- Given an adult manikin, perform one-man cardiopulmonary resuscitation.
- Given an infant manikin, perform cardiopulmonary resuscitation.
- Given an adult manikin and a partner, perform two-man cardiopulmonary resuscitation, including changing positions.
- List the signs of effective CPR.

## Chapter 5

# Basic Life Support: The ABC's

### INTRODUCTION

All living cells in the human body require oxygen for survival, but for the cells of the brain and nervous system, oxygen is particularly important: without it, these cells die within four to six minutes. When brain cells begin to die, irreversible brain damage and death soon follow.

**NOTE:** Under certain circumstances, especially drowning or prolonged exposure to very cold temperatures, brain cells may survive intact for much longer.

Respiratory arrest (cessation of breathing) is a critical medical emergency that interrupts the functioning of the brain and heart as well as that of the lungs. The lungs supply the heart and circulatory system with oxygen to nourish the body tissues, including brain tissue. Because the brain regulates the activities of the heart and lungs, an interruption in the air supply to the lungs ultimately interferes with the brain's regulatory activity. If breathing is not restored, the heart stops in a matter of minutes, and death follows rapidly. Cardiac arrest (cessation of the heartbeat) is an equally critical emergency that may occur either as the cause or the effect of respiratory arrest. When the heart stops, breathing also stops within seconds.

In cases of respiratory or cardiac arrest, *immediate* action is essential. The oxygen in the lungs and bloodstream is usually adequate to sustain life for up to six minutes. When breathing stops, the heart continues to pump blood for several minutes, carrying the oxygen remaining in the victim's lungs to the brain, heart, and other vital organs. When this oxygen is depleted, the heart itself stops and brain cells begin to die. Prompt emergency intervention can reverse this deadly process.

As you remember from the previous chapter, the primary survey - an assessment of the patient's Airway, Breathing, and Circulation - is ALWAYS the first step in patient assessment. Since our lives depend upon a constant supply of oxygen, anything that threatens the respiratory system (which takes oxygen into the lungs) or the circulatory system (which delivers the oxygen to the body's cells) is a life-threatening emergency.

Opening the airway, removing an airway obstruction, recognizing the signs of adequate and inadequate breathing, resuscitating a nonbreathing patient, and administering cardiopulmonary resuscitation are critical skills for every first responder. The efficient, proper execution of these skills (basic life support) may mean the difference between life and death to patients in respiratory and cardiac arrest.

This chapter is divided into three sections. Taken together, these sections describe the skills of basic life support. Section 1, AIRWAY CARE, describes methods for opening a nonresponsive patient's airway and for removing a foreign body obstruction from the airway. Section 2, RESCUE BREATHING AND OXYGEN ADMINISTRATION, describes rescue breathing techniques and includes a discussion of supplemental oxygen administration for both conscious and unconscious patients. Section 3, CARDIOPULMONARY RESUSCITATION (CPR), builds on the skills learned in the first two sections and adds another: external cardiac compressions. This section begins with an overview of CPR that includes the major causes of cardiac arrest and legal considerations associated with CPR. After a brief review of the ABC's of CPR, the techniques of CPR are discussed, including step-by-step instructions for one- and two-rescuer CPR, and CPR for infants and children. The section concludes with a discussion of two special situations that involve CPR: near-drowning and electric shock. These situations warrant special treatment because these victims must be rescued before rescuers can make any attempts at resuscitation.

## SECTION 1: AIRWAY CARE

In order to breathe, the patient must have an open airway. Naturally, a conscious, talking patient has an open airway, but a seemingly unconscious patient must be examined more closely to determine whether he or she is in fact unconscious, and whether the airway is open. If the patient's tongue is blocking the airway, you must use one of the standard maneuvers to open the airway. Likewise, if the patient's airway is blocked by a foreign object, such as a piece of food, you must take steps to remove it.

Once the patient's airway is open, it must be kept open or the patient will not be able to breathe. Maintaining an open airway by repositioning the patient's head or body, inserting an oral airway, and suctioning vomitus or secretions from the patient's mouth are all essential elements of airway care.

### Establishing Unresponsiveness

When you come upon a patient who seems to be unconscious, you must establish that the patient is unresponsive and not merely asleep. Do this by kneeling beside the patient, tapping the patient on the shoulder, and shouting, "Are you all right?" Other methods of establishing unresponsiveness include squeezing the upper arm, rubbing the sternum, or pinching the skin between the shoulder and the neck. If the patient is an infant or small child, you may also establish unresponsiveness by flicking your fingers against the soles of the feet.

If the patient does not respond, contact the dispatcher and make sure that additional medical help is on the way. Then take immediate steps to open the patient's airway.

### Opening the Airway

In unconscious individuals, the most common airway obstruction is the tongue, which tends to relax and fall back into the throat, thereby blocking the airway. If this is the case, tilting the patient's head back, which moves the jaw forward, will reopen the airway (Figure 5.1). Since the tongue is attached to the lower jaw, forward movement of the jaw lifts the tongue away from the back of the throat.

Two methods are commonly used to open an airway:

- Modified jaw-thrust maneuver
- Head-tilt chin-lift maneuver

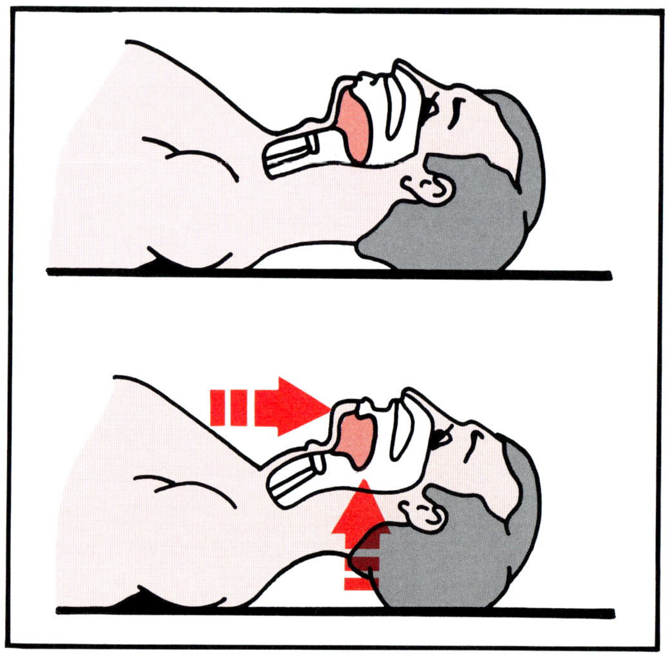

**Figure 5.1** Forward movement of the jaw lifts the tongue away from the back of the throat.

#### MODIFIED JAW-THRUST MANEUVER

The modified jaw-thrust maneuver allows you to open a patient's airway without repositioning the head. If the patient is an accident victim, you *must* suspect a spinal injury. To avoid aggravating (worsening) an actual or suspected spinal injury, DO NOT move the patient's head or neck. The patient must be lying face up for this maneuver (see Chapter 8, Injuries to the Skull, Spine, and Chest for the principles and procedures for handling patients with spinal injuries). To perform the modified jaw-thrust maneuver,

Step 1: Kneel at the patient's head.

Step 2: Place your hands on both sides of the patient's head and hold the head in such a way that the neck remains in a fixed, neutral position without being extended (Figure 5.2).

Step 3: Place your fingers behind the angle of the lower jaw on each side of the patient's head (Figure 5.3).

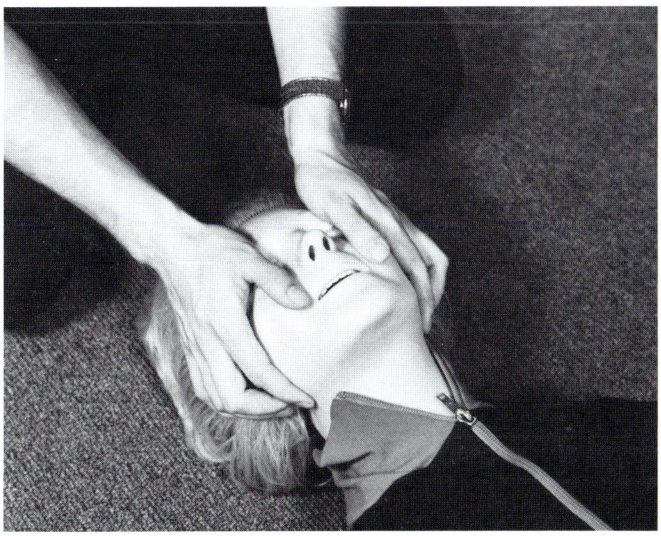

**Figure 5.2** Place your hands on both sides of the patient's head, holding the head and neck in a fixed, neutral position.

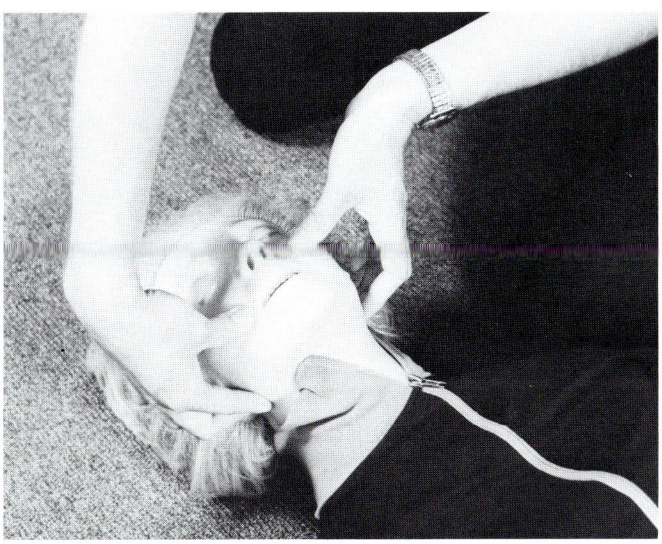

**Figure 5.3** Place your fingers behind the angle of the lower jaw on each side of the patient's head.

Step 4: Move the jaw forward with your fingers, taking care not to tilt the head back or to move it to either side (Figure 5.4).

Naturally, the modified jaw-thrust maneuver may also be used on patients in whom there is no reason to suspect a spinal injury.

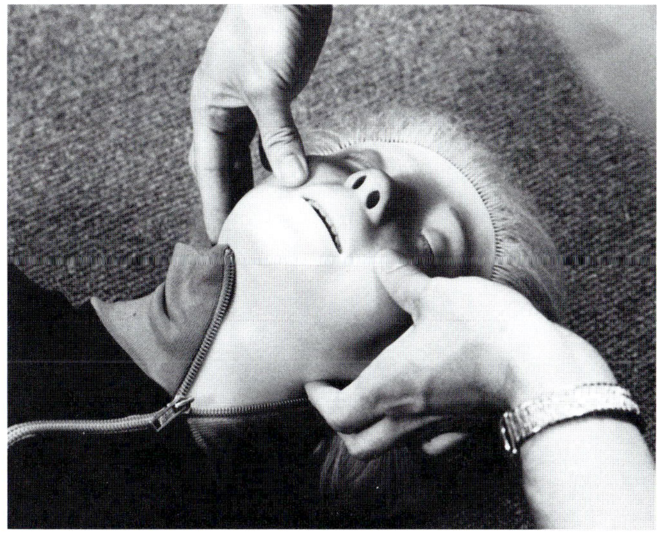

**Figure 5.4** Carefully move the jaw forward with your fingers, taking care not to move the head.

### HEAD-TILT CHIN-LIFT MANEUVER

DO NOT use this maneuver on a patient with a suspected spinal injury. The patient must be lying face up for this maneuver.

Step 1: Kneel beside the patient's head.

Step 2: Place one hand on the patient's forehead and press back firmly with your palm. This action tilts the head back and moves the tongue away from the back of the throat (Figure 5.5).

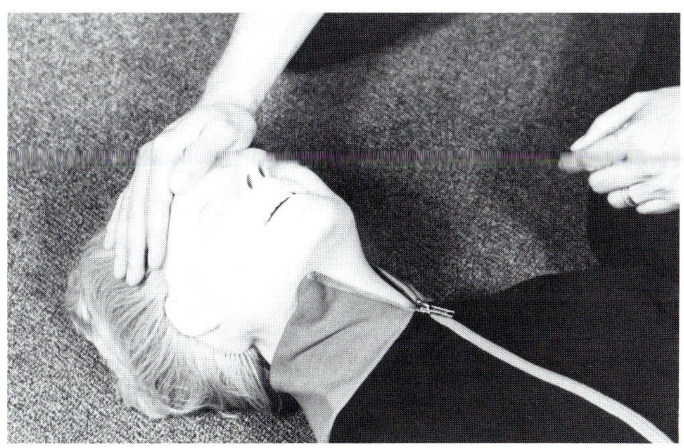

**Figure 5.5** To begin the head-tilt chin-lift maneuver, place your hand on the patient's forehead and press back with your palm.

Step 3: Grasp the patient's chin with the fingertips of your other hand and lift up and forward until the teeth are nearly closed (Figure 5.6). Be sure to grasp just below the bony part of the chin; do not press into the soft tissues under the chin or you may obstruct the airway.

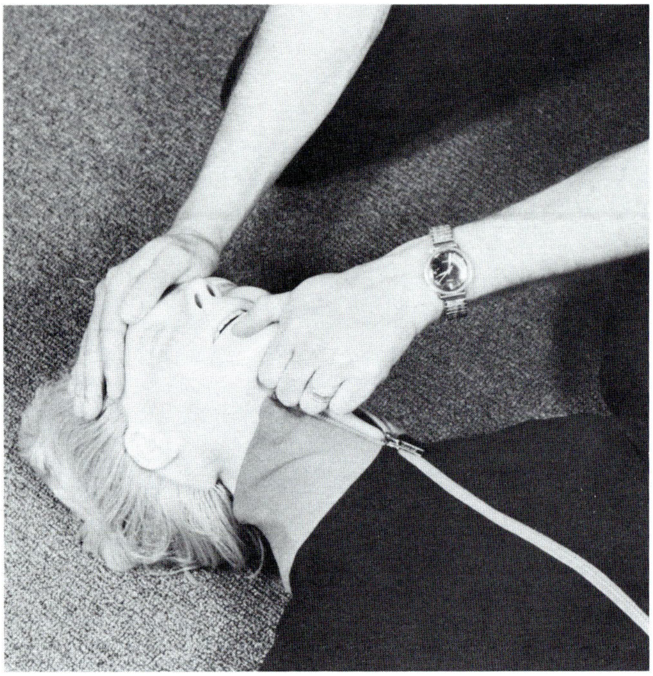

**Figure 5.6** Grasp the patient's chin with the fingertips of your other hand and lift up and forward until the teeth are nearly closed.

Step 4: If necessary, insert your thumb between the patient's teeth to ensure that the patient's mouth remains slightly open.

Three other maneuvers may be used to open a patient's airway:

- Head-tilt neck-lift maneuver
- Face-down maneuver
- Jaw-thrust maneuver

None of these maneuvers is recommended for the patient with an actual or suspected spinal cord injury.

### HEAD-TILT NECK-LIFT MANEUVER

This maneuver allows you to open a patient's airway by repositioning the head. DO NOT use this maneuver on a patient with a suspected spinal injury. The patient must be lying face up for this maneuver.

Step 1: Kneel beside the patient's head.

Step 2: Place one hand on the patient's forehead and the other under the neck (Figure 5.7).

Step 3: Push down firmly with the hand that is on the forehead as you *gently* pull upward with the hand that is under the neck (Figure 5.8).

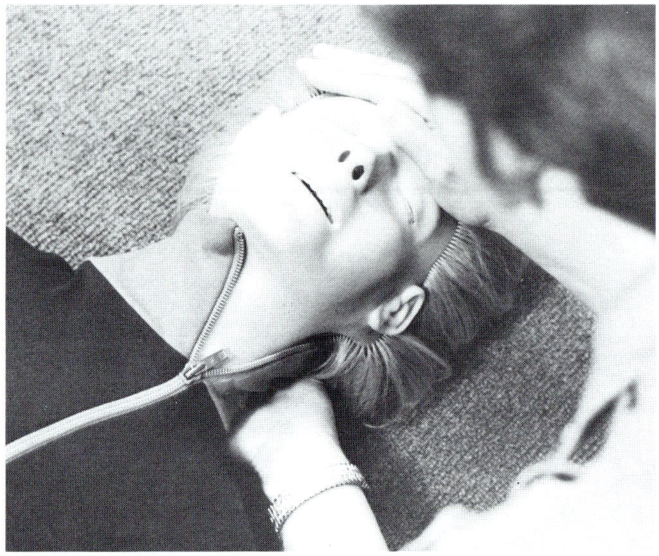

**Figure 5.7** Place one hand on the patient's forehead and the other under the neck.

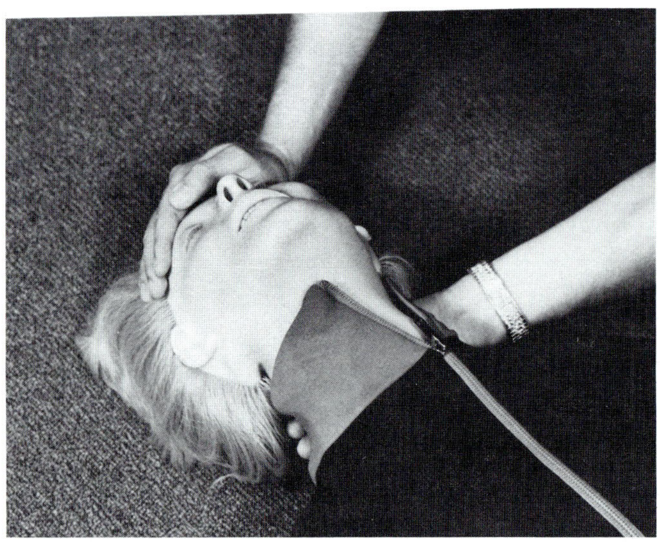

**Figure 5.8** Push down firmly on the forehead as you *gently* pull the neck upward.

### JAW-THRUST MANEUVER

Use this maneuver if neither of the Head-Tilt maneuvers is effective. DO NOT use this maneuver on a patient with a suspected spinal injury. The patient must be lying face up for this maneuver.

Step 1: Kneel above the patient's head.

Step 2: Place your hands on both sides of the patient's head with your fingers behind the angles of the lower jaw and your thumbs on either side of the lower lip (Figure 5.9).

Step 3: Push the jaw forward as you tilt the head backward. Open the lower lips with your thumbs (Figure 5.10).

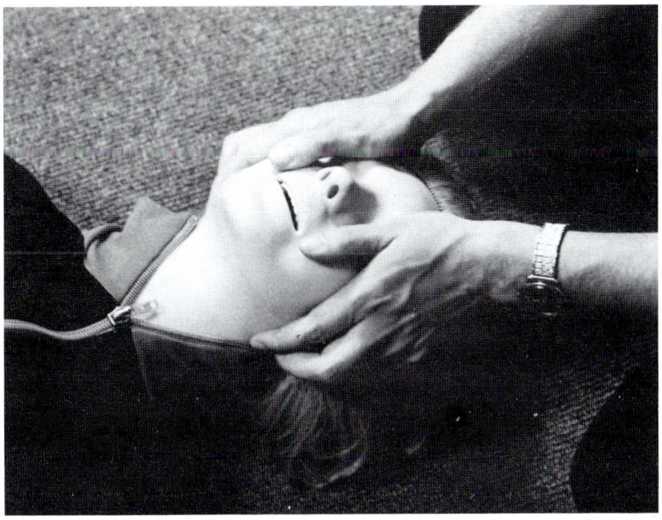

**Figure 5.9** Place your hands on both sides of the patient's head with your fingers behind the angles of the lower jaw and your thumbs on either side of the lower lip.

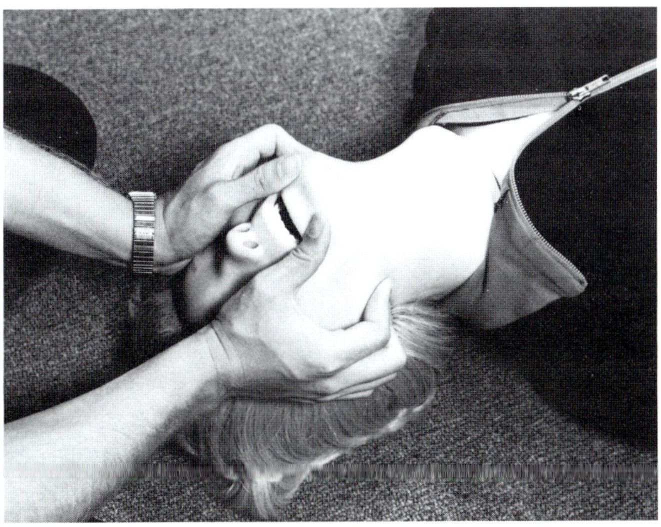

**Figure 5.10** Push the jaw forward as you tilt the head backward; open the lower lips with your thumbs.

## FACE-DOWN MANEUVER

This maneuver lets the tongue fall forward, away from the back of the throat. It also permits saliva, mucus, and blood to drain from the mouth. DO NOT use this maneuver on a patient with a suspected spinal injury unless the patient is immobilized on a long backboard. In this situation, the backboard can be tipped on its side to help keep the patient's airway open. The patient must be lying face up when you begin this maneuver.

Step 1: Kneel at the patient's side.

Step 2: Grasp the patient's farthest shoulder with one hand and the farthest hip with the other (Figure 5.11).

Step 3: Roll the patient gently toward you until he or she is resting on the side nearest you. The patient's tongue should fall forward, thereby opening the airway (Figure 5.12).

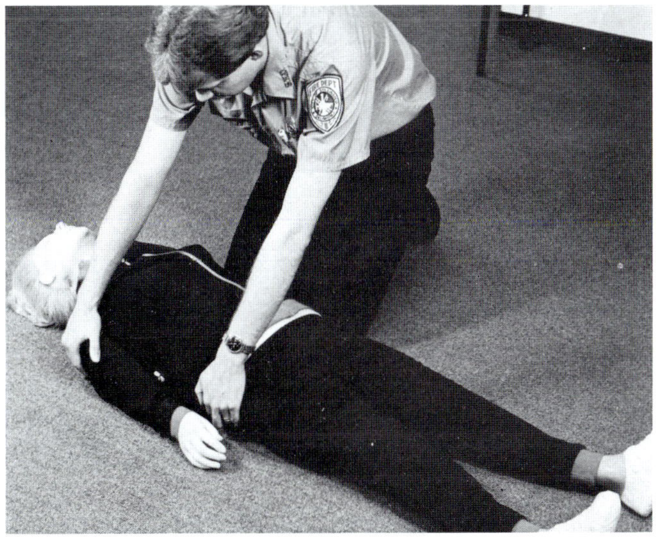

**Figure 5.11** Grasp the patient's farthest shoulder and hip with your hands.

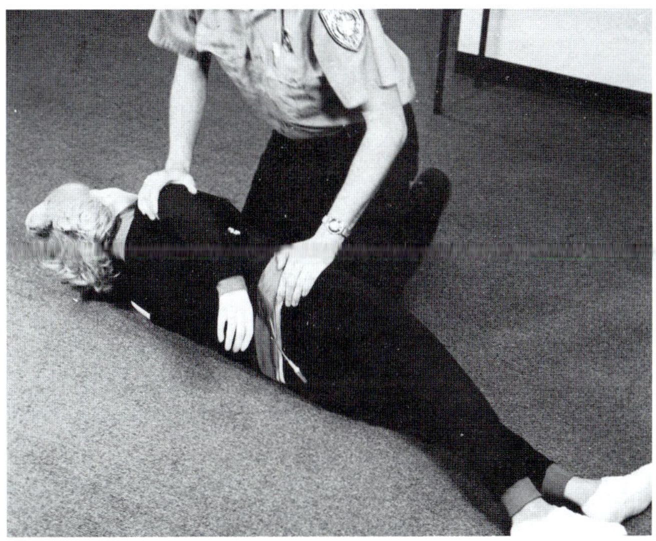

**Figure 5.12** Roll the patient gently toward you until he or she is resting on the side nearest you.

## DISLODGING A FOREIGN OBJECT FROM THE AIRWAY

### (Conscious Patients)

Deaths due to asphyxia (a condition that results from insufficient oxygen) caused by airway obstructions number almost 2,000 in the United States annually. The most common airway obstruction is the human tongue, which often relaxes in unconscious patients and lodges against the back of the throat. Foreign objects, too, such as food, toys, or dentures, may lodge in any other part of the airway to obstruct the flow of air into the lungs. Similarly, the aspiration of water in drowning victims causes a laryngeal spasm that ultimately closes the airway and causes the victim to suffocate. Finally, the accumulation of fluids such as vomitus, blood, or mucus in the back of the throat may obstruct the airway.

Foreign body obstruction of the airway usually occurs during a meal, with meat the most common cause of choking. Other factors that contribute to choking incidents are

- Drinking excessive amounts of alcohol before and during a meal
- Trying to eat large pieces of food, particularly if the individual wears dentures
- Talking and laughing with the mouth full

Because the signs of choking often resemble those of a heart attack, deaths due to airway obstruction by food have come to be known as "cafe coronaries." (Remember that a patient who has collapsed in a restaurant or seems to be a choking victim may actually be suffering a heart attack. Under these circumstances, quickly try to find out what the patient was doing before he or she collapsed.)

An airway obstruction may be either complete or partial. A conscious patient with a *complete* obstruction usually displays the universal distress signal (Figure 5.13). A patient suffering a *partial* obstruction of the airway may be coughing, choking, wheezing, turning blue (cyanosis), or exhibiting a combination of these symptoms, as well as displaying the universal distress signal.

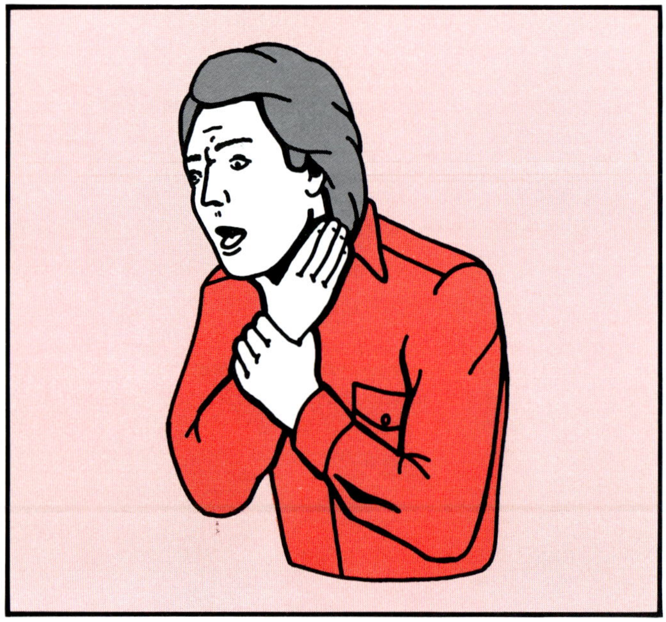

**Figure 5.13** Most choking victims display the universal distress signal.

If the patient is conscious and seems to be choking on a foreign object, first ask, "Are you choking?" If the patient can speak or is coughing, stand back and allow the patient to continue to cough and try to dislodge the obstruction. If the patient cannot speak or cough, perform the Heimlich maneuver to dislodge the object.

Step 1: Stand behind a standing or sitting patient and wrap your arms around the patient's waist.

Step 2: Make a fist with one hand and place the thumbside of your fist against the patient's abdomen, slightly above the navel and well below the xiphoid process (Figure 5.14). Correct hand position is very important: compressing the xiphoid process can cause laceration of internal organs.

Step 3: Grasp the fist with your other hand and press the fist into the patient's abdomen 6 to 10 times with quick, inward and upward thrusts (Figure 5.15). Each thrust should be distinct and delivered with the intent of relieving the airway obstruction.

The resulting compression of the abdomen and diaphragm forces the lungs to expel the air that they hold, thereby driving the foreign object from the patient's throat. If the choking patient is a child, you will need to lessen the force of the thrusts.

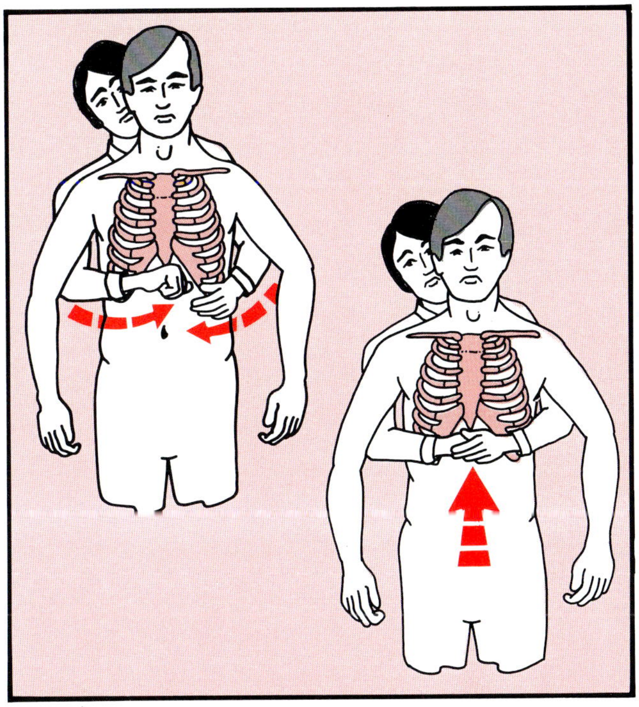

**Figure 5.14** Make a fist with one hand and place the thumbside of your fist against the patient's abdomen, slightly above the navel and well below the xiphoid process.

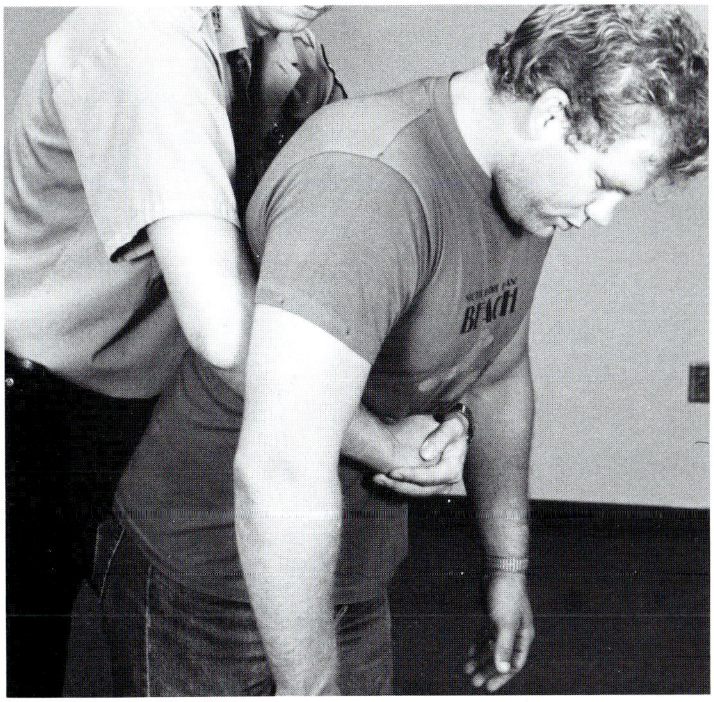


**Figure 5.15** Press your fist into the patient's abdomen and give 6 to 10 sharp, upward thrusts.

## DISLODGING A FOREIGN OBJECT FROM THE AIRWAY

### (Unconscious Patients)

If the choking patient lapses into unconsciousness, perform the Heimlich maneuver with the patient lying on his or her back. To do this,

Step 1: Either kneel at the patient's side or straddle the patient's body so that you are facing his or her head, then place the heel of one of your hands on the patient's abdomen, slightly above the navel and well below the xiphoid process. With your other hand, press the heel of that hand into the patient's abdomen with 6 to 10 sharp, forward thrusts (Figure 5.16).

Step 2: Move back to the patient's head, hook your thumb over the patient's teeth and pull the jaw up. Look into the patient's mouth. If you see the foreign object, carefully pull it out. Do not jam your fingers blindly into the patient's throat or you may push the object back down the throat (Figure 5.17).

Step 3: Open the patient's airway using the head-tilt chin-lift method. Pinch the patient's

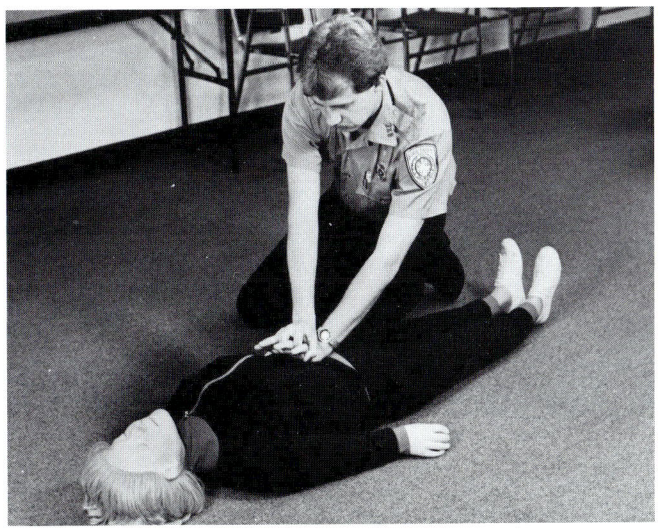

**Figure 5.16** Place the heels of your hands on the patient's abdomen, below the xiphoid process, and give 6 to 10 sharp, forward thrusts.

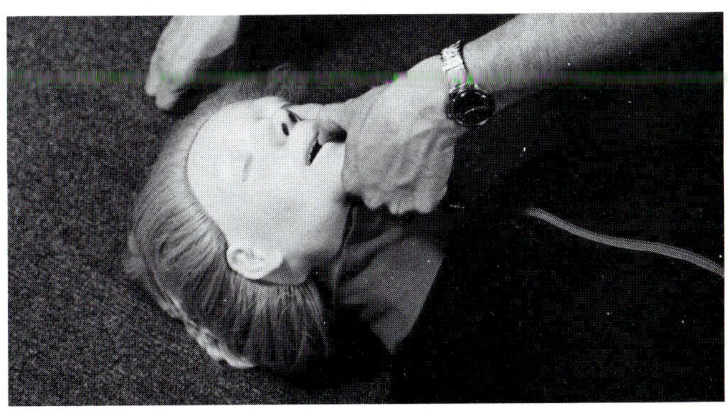

**Figure 5.17** Pull the patient's jaw up and look into the mouth. If you see the foreign object, carefully pull it out.

nose closed with the thumb and index finger of the hand that is on the forehead as you maintain pressure on the forehead with the heel of that same hand (Figure 5.18).

Step 4: Open your mouth widely, take a deep breath, and enclose the patient's mouth with your own, making a tight seal. Blow into the patient's lungs with *two* full breaths. Each breath should last 1 to 1½ seconds.

Step 5: Lift your mouth from the patient's by turning your head toward the patient's chest. Watch for the rise and fall of the chest.

Step 6: If you are unable to ventilate the patient's lungs, reposition the head and try again.

Step 7: Repeat steps 1 through 6 if necessary. If you cannot completely dislodge the foreign object, you may be able to move it enough to permit ventilation of the lungs.

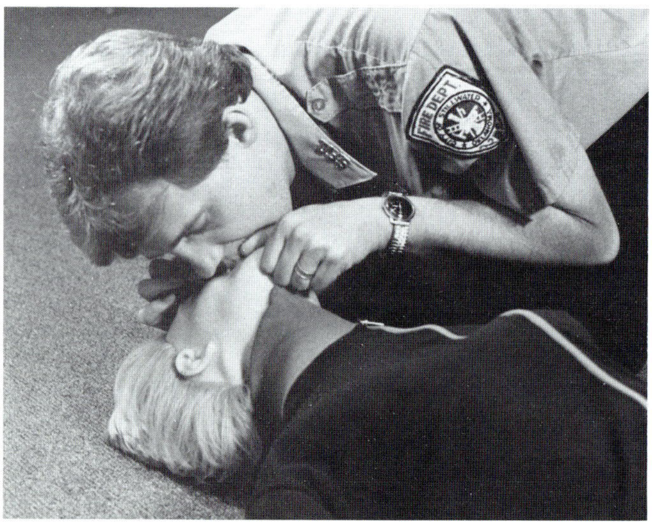

**Figure 5.18** Attempt to ventilate the patient's lungs.

### Chest Thrusts

Chest thrusts performed to relieve a foreign body airway obstruction should be used *only* when the choking victim is in an advanced stage of pregnancy or when the victim is markedly obese. These instances are rare, but if it is impossible to compress the patient's diaphragm, chest thrusts are an alternative method for dislodging a foreign object.

If the choking victim is standing or sitting, administer chest thrusts in the following manner:

Step 1: Stand behind the patient and encircle the patient's chest with your arms. Make a fist with one hand and place the thumbside of your fist against the middle of the patient's sternum (breastbone). Take care to avoid the xiphoid process.

Step 2: Grasp the fist with your other hand and press backward 6 to 10 times. Each thrust should be administered with the intent of relieving the obstruction.

If the choking victim becomes unconscious, administer chest thrusts in the following manner:

Step 1: Place the victim on his or her back and kneel close to the side of the patient's body.

Step 2: Place your hands on the patient's chest in the same manner as you would to deliver external cardiac compressions (see Section 3 of this chapter).

Step 3: Press straight down 6 to 10 times. Each thrust should be delivered slowly, distinctly, and with the intent of relieving the obstruction.

Step 4: Move back to the patient's head, hook your thumb over the patient's teeth and pull the jaw up. Look into the patient's mouth. If you see the foreign object, carefully pull it out. Do not jam your fingers blindly into the patient's throat or you may push the object back down the throat.

## DISLODGING A FOREIGN OBJECT FROM THE AIRWAY OF AN INFANT

If the choking victim is an infant, hold the infant face down so that he or she straddles your forearm. Hold the head lower than the rest of the body and support it by holding the jaw (Figure 5.19). Rest your arm on your thigh and deliver four sharp back blows (about one blow per second) between the infant's shoulder blades with the heel of your hand. After you have delivered the four back blows, place your free arm along the victim's back so that his or her head and body are sandwiched between your hands and arms (Figure 5.20). Care-

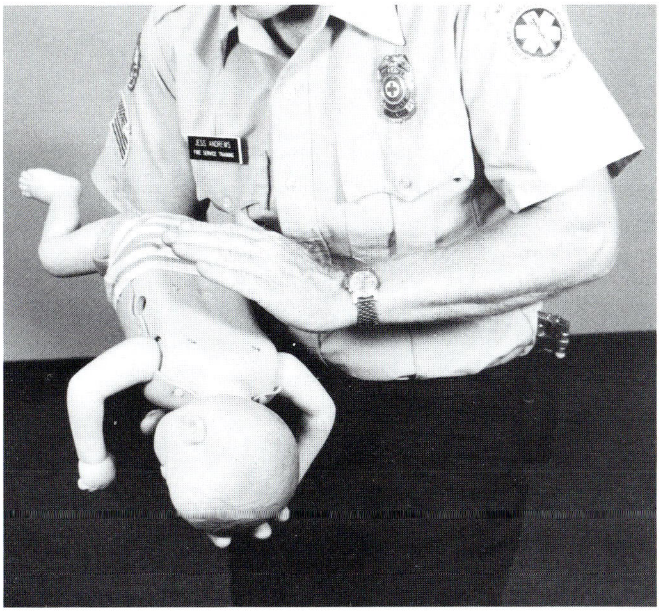

**Figure 5.19** Hold the infant face down on your forearm, supporting the head by holding the jaw.

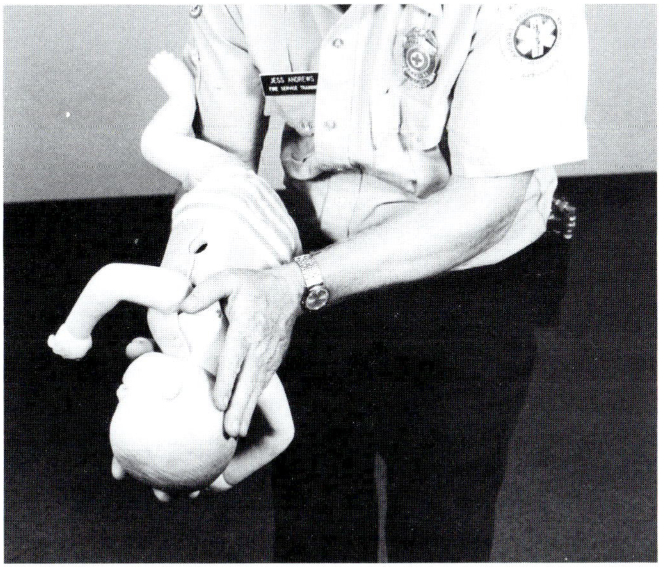

**Figure 5.20** Place your free arm along the infant's back so that the head and body are sandwiched between your hands and arms.

fully turn the infant over and position him or her on your thighs so that the head is lower than the rest of the body. Now, imagine a line across the infant's chest that intersects both nipples (the nipple line). Place three fingers of one hand just below this line where it intersects the sternum. Lift the finger closest to the nipple line and use the remaining two fingers to administer four chest thrusts — again, about one thrust per second (Figure 5.21). Look into the baby's mouth for the foreign obstruction. If you cannot see it, repeat the sequence of back blows and chest thrusts until you are successful.

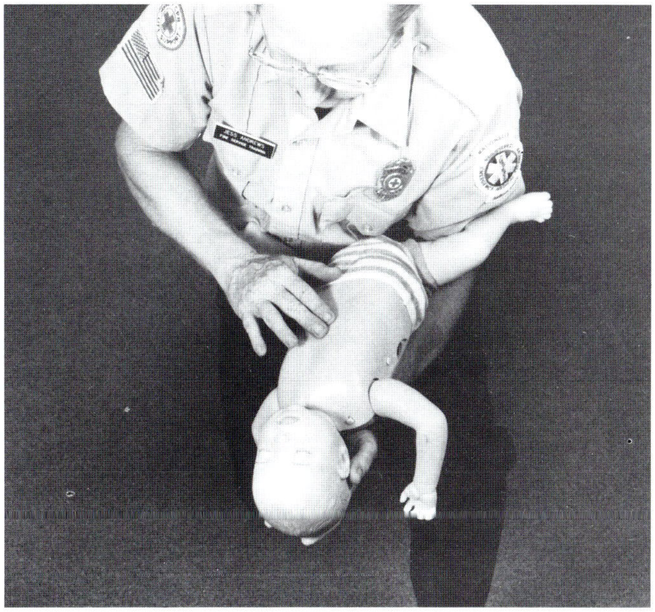

**Figure 5.21** The proper compression area on an infant is one finger's width below the nipple line, over the midsternum.

## SECTION 2: RESCUE BREATHING AND OXYGEN ADMINISTRATION

This section focuses on the second step of the ABC's: Breathing. The steps for determining whether or not a patient is breathing are described first, followed by rescue breathing techniques for adults, infants, and children. Gastric distention, a condition that may interfere with rescue breathing, is discussed next, followed by a discussion of adjunctive equipment for maintaining the airway and assisting with rescue breathing.

The second part of this section, Assisting the Breathing Patient: Supplemental Oxygen, concentrates on the patient who requires supplemental oxygen. A number of injuries and illnesses can interfere with an individual's ability to take in enough oxygen and/or to deliver sufficient oxygenated blood to adequately nourish body tissues. Also discussed are oxygen equipment and methods of administering oxygen, including the nasal cannula, various oxygen masks, and the demand valve.

## RESCUE BREATHING: RESUSCITATING THE NONBREATHING PATIENT

Once you have opened the patient's airway using one of the methods described in the previous section, you must determine whether or not the patient is breathing. To do this, lean over the patient's head and face the chest (Figure 5.22). Place your ear within an inch (25.4 mm) of the victim's mouth and nose, and

*Look* to see whether the patient's chest and abdomen rise and fall.

*Listen* for air movement at the nose and mouth.

*Feel* for air movement on your cheek or ear.

The critical indications of breathing are feeling and hearing breathing at the patient's mouth and nose. If an individual is moving air into and out of the lungs, the air passes through the mouth and/or nose.

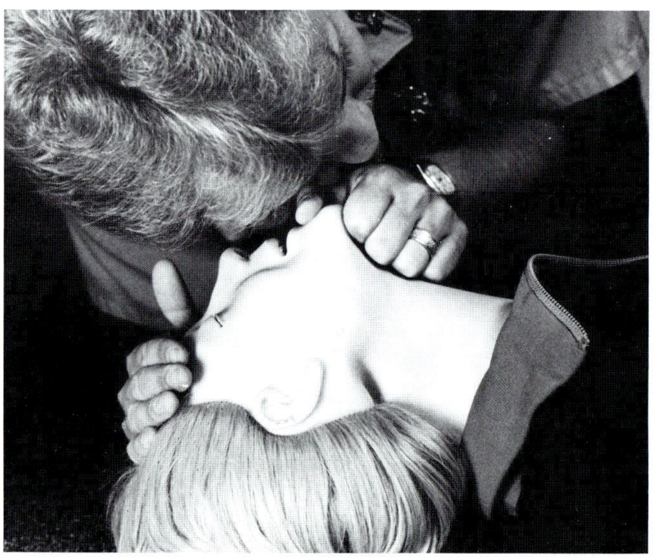

**Figure 5.22** Look, listen, and feel for the movement of air from the patient's mouth and nose.

If the patient *is* breathing, continue to maintain the airway in an open position. This may be done manually or with an oral airway. Monitor the patient's pulse and vital signs and arrange for rapid transport to a medical facility. It may be advisable to administer supplemental oxygen as well (see Oxygen Administration later in this section).

If the patient is *not* breathing, begin rescue breathing immediately. Rescue breathing is the movement of air into and out of the lungs of a person whose breathing has stopped. You may use either your own lungs or mechanical means to force air into a nonbreathing patient's lungs.

The air that we inhale from the atmosphere contains about 21 percent oxygen, while the air that we exhale is about 16 percent oxygen. Thus, our bodies use only about one-fourth of the oxygen we inhale. Clearly, the remaining three-fourths of the oxygen that we exhale is adequate to sustain life in another human being. In the absence of mechanical oxygenation equipment, the air you exhale is the best air you can give a nonbreathing patient.

Depending upon the size and physical condition of the patient, you may choose one of the following rescue breathing techniques:

- Mouth-to-mouth ventilation (adults)
- Mouth-to-mouth ventilation (infants and small children)
- Mouth-to-nose ventilation
- Mouth-to-stoma ventilation
- Mouth-to-mask ventilation

Remember that the patient's head must still be in the correct position so that the airway is open, otherwise ventilation efforts will be ineffective. A foreign body lodged in the airway will also make rescue breathing impossible. Do *not* take the time to look for foreign objects lodged in the airway unless their presence is known or strongly suspected. Your efforts to ventilate the patient's lungs will reveal whether or not a foreign object is present.

### Mouth-To-Mouth Technique

Step 1: Kneel beside the patient.

Step 2: Open the patient's airway using the head-tilt chin-lift maneuver (use the modified jaw-thrust maneuver if you have reason to suspect a spinal injury).

Step 3: Pinch the patient's nose closed with the thumb and index finger of the hand that is on the forehead as you maintain pressure on the forehead with the palm of that same hand (Figure 5.23). If you have used the modified jaw-thrust maneuver to open the patient's airway, use the side of your cheek to close the patient's nostrils (Figure 5.24).

Step 4: Open your mouth widely, take a deep breath, and enclose the patient's mouth with your own, making a tight seal (Figure 5.25). If the patient has dentures, try to keep them in place — it is easier to ensure a good seal around the patient's mouth if the dentures are in place. If the dentures slip or interfere with ventilation efforts, simply remove them.

Step 5: Blow into the patient's lungs with *two* full breaths and watch for the patient's chest to rise. Each breath should last 1 to 1½ seconds. Allow the patient's chest to deflate between breaths. This technique is now recommended to lessen the possibility of gastric distention (see Gastric Distention later in this section.)

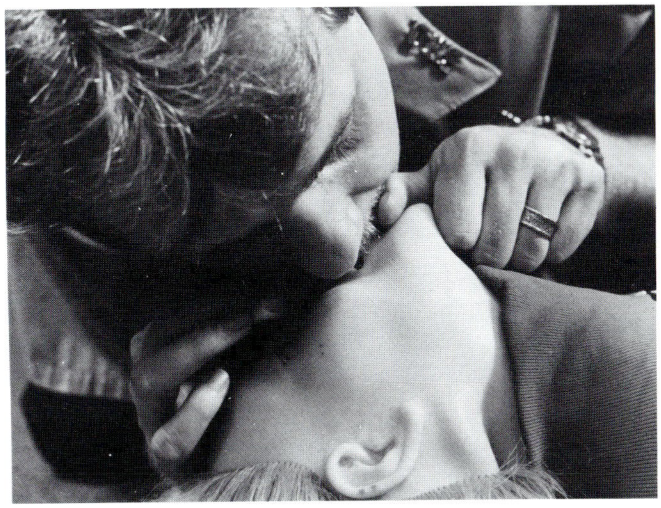

**Figure 5.25** Open your mouth widely, take a deep breath, and enclose the patient's mouth with your own, making a tight seal.

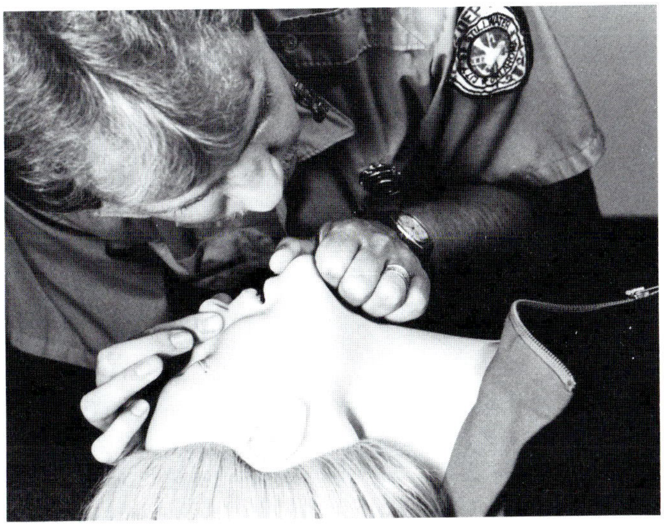

**Figure 5.23** Pinch the patient's nose closed with the thumb and index finger of the hand that is on the forehead as you maintain pressure on the forehead with the heel of that same hand.

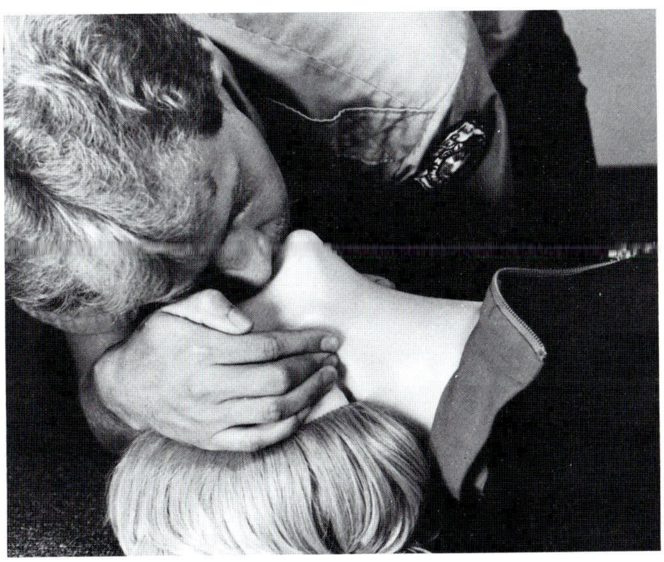

**Figure 5.24** If you use the modified jaw-thrust maneuver to open the patient's airway, use the side of your cheek to close the patient's nostrils.

Step 6: Remove your mouth from the patient's to allow air to escape from the airway. Do this by just lifting your mouth and turning your head toward the patient's chest (Figure 5.26). You will know that ventilation is adequate if you can

- *Feel* the patient's lungs yield to your respirations.
- *See* the patient's chest rise and fall.
- *Hear* and feel air escaping from the patient's lungs after each ventilation.

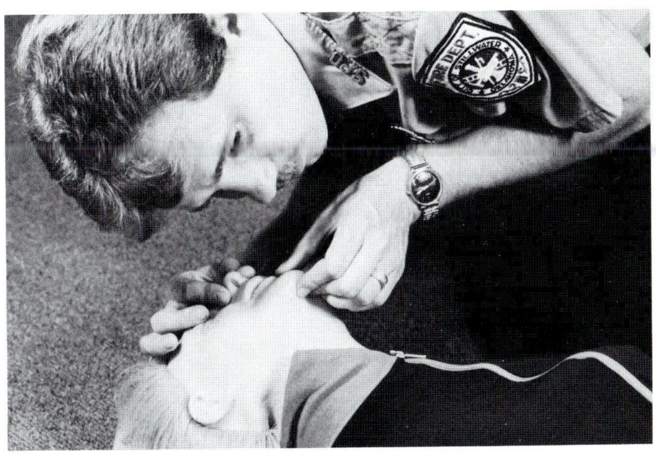

**Figure 5.26** Lift your mouth away from the patient's mouth and turn your head toward his or her chest.

Step 7: If you do not see the chest rise and fall, reposition the head and try again, watching for the rise and fall of the chest. If repositioning the head is not effective, you must suspect a foreign body obstruction and perform the Heimlich maneuver to dislodge the obstruction.

Step 8: If the patient's chest *does* rise and fall, take the patient's pulse at the carotid artery. Maintain the airway by continuing the downward pressure of your hand on the forehead. Use the hand that is holding the patient's chin up to feel for the pulse. Slide your fingers down from the chin and find the Adam's apple with your fingertips, about halfway between the patient's chin and collarbone. Draw your fingers back toward you into the groove beside the Adam's apple (Figure 5.27). Press *lightly* to feel the pulse with the most sensitive part of your fingertips. Remember not to use your thumb because it has its own pulse. Feel very carefully to find a pulse: take at least 5 seconds and up to 10 seconds if necessary. If there is no pulse, begin external cardiac compressions (see Section 3, Cardiopulmonary Resuscitation).

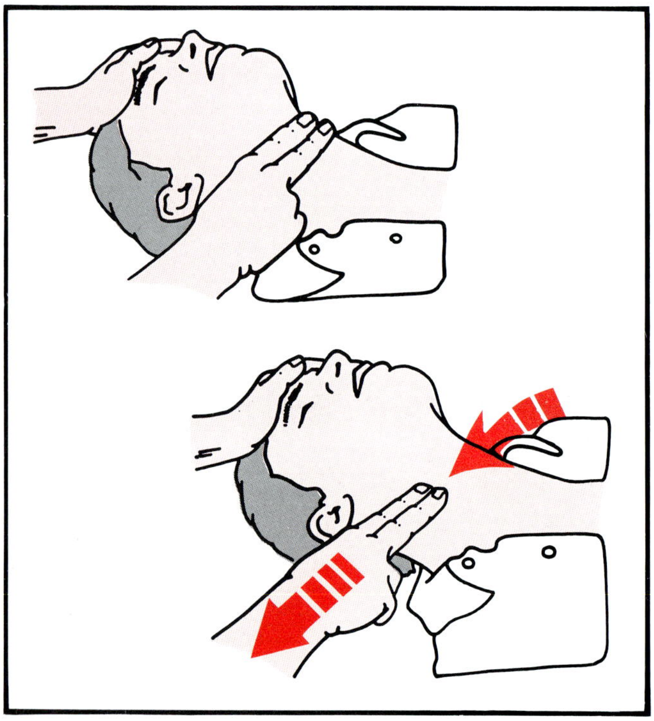

**Figure 5.27** Draw your fingers back toward you into the groove beside the Adam's apple.

**CAUTION: NEVER** begin chest compressions on someone whose heart is still beating, even if the pulse is weak or irregular. Performing compressions on a person whose heart is functioning causes the heart to stop.

Step 9: If the patient has a pulse, continue rescue breathing at a rate of once every 5 seconds, or 12 times per minute. Lift your mouth away after each inflation, turn your head, and watch the patient's chest fall as you allow time for the lungs to empty after each breath.

Step 10: Check the pulse once a minute (after every 12 breaths) to be sure that the heart is still circulating blood even though breathing has stopped. Continue to breathe for the patient as long as the breathing inadequacy continues or until additional help arrives.

If the unconscious victim begins to breathe voluntarily while you are doing rescue breathing, discontinue rescue breathing but maintain the airway. If vomiting occurs at this point, turn the patient to one side as you continue to monitor breathing. Let the stomach contents drain from the mouth and wipe the mouth clean.

Always arrange to transport anyone who has required rescue breathing to the nearest medical facility. Even if the patient regains consciousness and claims to be fine, he or she must be evaluated by a physician to avoid any possible complications of the respiratory emergency.

## Mouth-To-Mouth Technique for Infants and Children

The techniques for administering rescue breathing to infants and children are very similar to those for adults, but with some important differences. For the purposes of basic life support, an infant is less than one year old, and a child is one to eight years old. The recommended treatment for children eight years old and older is the same as that for adults.

### MOUTH-TO-MOUTH TECHNIQUE FOR CHILDREN

The recommended techniques for performing mouth-to-mouth rescue breathing for children are essentially the same as those for adults. To perform mouth-to-mouth rescue breathing for a child,

Step 1: Kneel beside the patient.

Step 2: Open the airway by gently positioning the head using the head-tilt chin-lift method.

Step 3: Make a seal with your mouth around either the child's mouth or mouth *and* nose, depending upon the size of the child.

Step 4: Give *two* breaths, using only enough force to cause a normal chest rise. Use a little more force than you would for an infant, but less than you would for an adult. Allow 1 to 1½ seconds for each breath, and allow the chest to deflate after each breath.

Step 5: If you do not see the chest rise, reposition the head and try again, watching for the rise and fall of the chest. If repositioning the head is not effective, you must suspect a foreign body obstruction and take steps to dislodge it using the techniques described in Section 1 of this chapter.

Step 6: If the chest rises, check the child's pulse at the carotid artery. If the child has a pulse, continue rescue breathing at a rate of once every 4 seconds, or 15 times per minute. If there is no pulse, begin cardiac compressions (see Section 3, Cardiopulmonary Resuscitation).

### MOUTH-TO-MOUTH TECHNIQUE FOR INFANTS

The recommended rescue breathing techniques for infants differ in several important ways from recommended techniques for adults. When you perform mouth-to-mouth rescue breathing for an infant,

- Make a tight seal with your mouth over the infant's nose *and* mouth.
- Use a much smaller volume of air to inflate the lungs; puffs of air from your cheeks are usually sufficient.
- Check the pulse at the brachial rather than the carotid artery.

To perform mouth-to-mouth rescue breathing for infants,

Step 1: Position the infant. There are two methods for doing this (Figure 5.28). One is to support the infant on your forearm, supporting the head in the palm of one hand. The other method is to place the infant lying face up on a firm surface, such as a table.

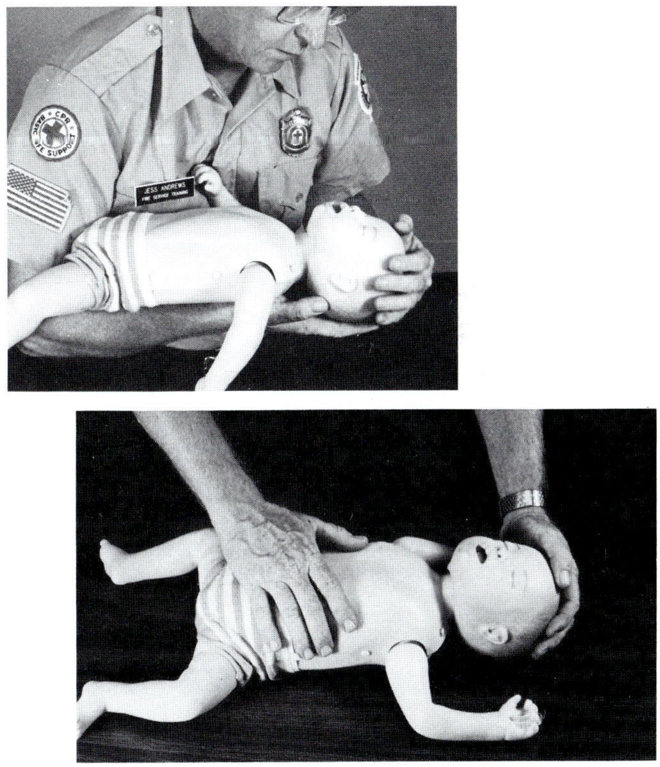

**Figure 5.28** Position an infant either on your forearm, supporting the head in the palm of one hand, or lying face up on a firm surface.

Step 2: Open the airway (Figure 5.29). If you are holding the infant, tip the head back slightly so that the infant looks as though

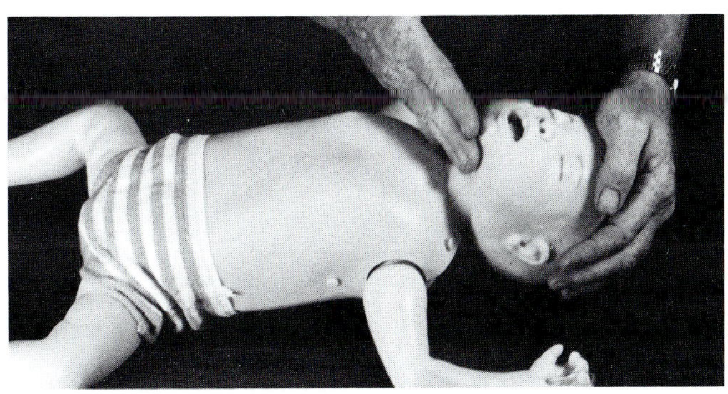

**Figure 5.29** Open the infant's airway by gently positioning the head using the head-tilt chin-lift method, tilting the head only to the sniffing position.

he or she is sniffing (see Figure 5.28). If the infant is lying on a firm surface, gently position the head using the head-tilt chin-lift method, again tilting the head only to the sniffing position (Figure 5.29). If tilting the head lifts the shoulders, slip your hand under the infant's shoulders and neck. This action maintains the infant's airway in an open position and provides a firm surface beneath the infant in the event that chest compressions are necessary.

Step 3: Make a seal with your mouth around the infant's mouth *and* nose, and use a small volume of air to inflate the lungs. In general, puffs of air from your cheeks provide sufficient ventilation for infants, but remember that the correct volume of air is the volume that causes the chest to rise and fall (Figure 5.30).

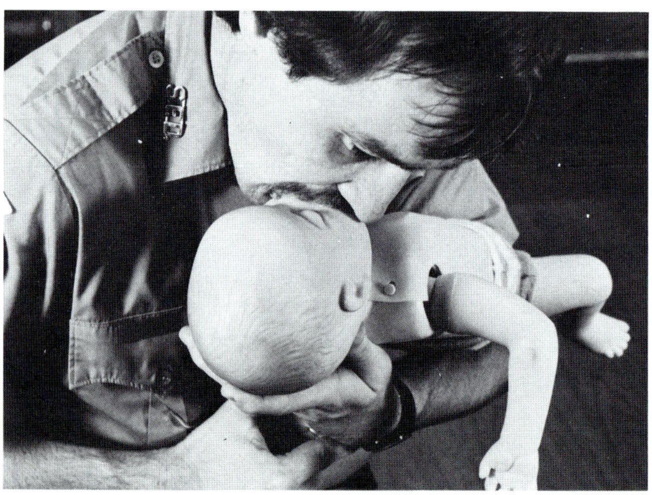

**Figure 5.30** Puffs of air from your cheeks provide sufficient ventilation for infants.

Step 4: Give *two* breaths, using only enough force to cause a normal chest rise. Allow 1 to 1½ seconds for each breath, and allow the chest to deflate after each breath.

Step 5: If you do not see the chest rise, reposition the head and try again, watching for the rise and fall of the chest. If repositioning the head is not effective, you must suspect a foreign body obstruction and try to dislodge it using the techniques described in Section 1 of this chapter.

Step 6: If the chest rises, check the infant's pulse. The carotid pulse is very difficult to find on an infant's short, fat neck. The brachial artery in the upper arm is easier to find; therefore, it is the recommended pulse site for infants and small children. To find the brachial artery, gently move the infant's arm away from the body and turn it palm up. Place your thumb on the outside of the arm between the shoulder and elbow and your first two fingers on the inside of the arm. Press gently into the humerus (upper arm bone) to feel the pulse (Figure 5.31). The brachial artery lies in the groove between the two muscles on the side of the upper arm that touches the body.

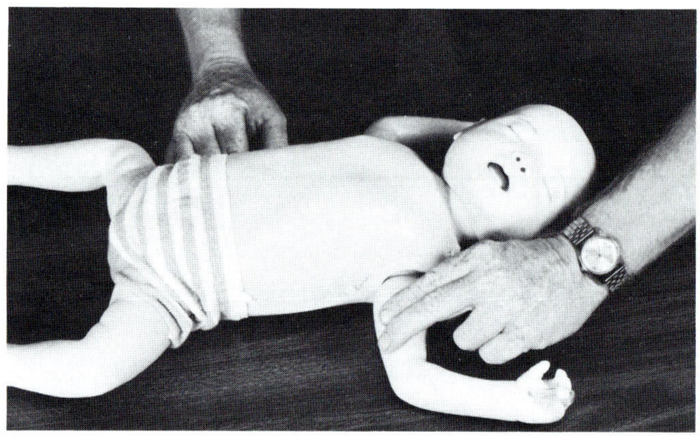

**Figure 5.31** Check an infant's pulse at the brachial artery.

Step 7: If the infant has a pulse, continue rescue breathing at a rate of once every 3 seconds, or 20 times per minute. If there is no pulse, begin cardiac compressions (see Section 3, Cardiopulmonary Resuscitation).

If a child is very small, say only one or two years old, he or she may require essentially the same rescue breathing techniques as an infant. Use a little more force to inflate the lungs than you would use for an infant. Again, exhale only enough to cause a normal chest rise.

## Mouth-To-Nose Technique

If the nonbreathing patient has a severe injury to the face or mouth, or if the patient's mouth is extremely large, it may be difficult or even impossible to use the mouth-to-mouth technique. You may be required to treat a patient who has very large teeth or no teeth at all. In each of these instances, the difficulty with the mouth-to-mouth technique is that it may be impossible to make a tight seal over the patient's mouth with your own. An alternative method is the mouth-to-nose technique. To perform the mouth-to-nose technique,

Step 1: Kneel beside the patient's head.

Step 2: Open the patient's airway using the head-tilt chin-lift maneuver or the modified jaw-thrust maneuver. Use your fingertips to lift the lower jaw and close the patient's lips.

Step 3: Take a deep breath, seal your lips around the patient's nose, and give *two* full breaths, taking 1 to 1½ seconds for each breath (Figure 5.32). Allow the chest to deflate between each breath. Watch the patient's chest to be sure that the quantity of air you exhale is sufficient but not excessive.

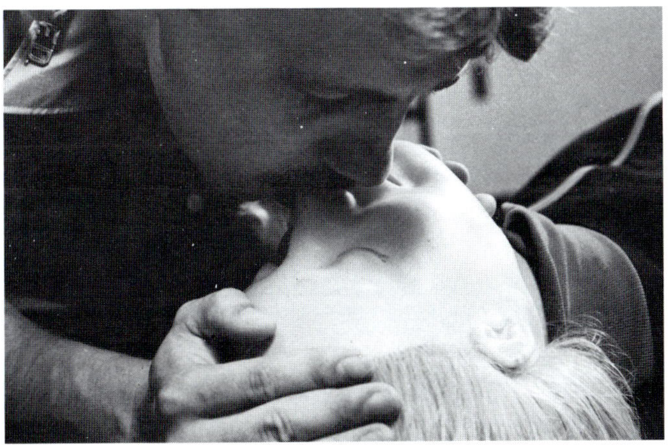

**Figure 5.32** Lift the lower jaw and close the patient's lips, then make a seal over the patient's nose with your mouth. Give two full breaths, with each breath lasting 1 to 1½ seconds.

Step 4: Remove your mouth from the patient's nose to allow air to escape. Open the patient's mouth, if necessary, to make exhalation easier.

Step 5: If the chest rises, check the patient's pulse at the carotid artery. If the patient has a pulse, continue rescue breathing at a rate of once every 5 seconds, or 12 times per minute.

## Mouth-To-Stoma Technique

You may encounter patients in respiratory distress who breathe through a surgical opening (stoma) in the front of the neck. The stoma is an artificial airway that joins the trachea with the surface of the neck. This artificial airway allows the patient to breathe directly through the opening rather than through the nose and mouth. The opening may be either temporary or permanent, depending upon the surgical procedure involved.

A tracheotomy is the operation of cutting directly into the trachea through the front of the neck, usually for the insertion of a breathing tube (Figure 5.33). The opening is usually temporary, maintained only until the obstruction that necessitated the surgery can be eliminated. A plastic or silver tube may protrude from the opening, and the patient may cover the opening with a light cloth pad.

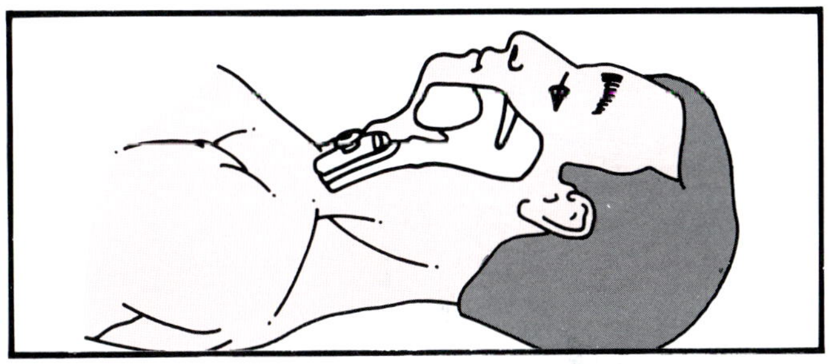

**Figure 5.33** A tracheotomy is the operation of cutting directly into the trachea through the front of the neck, usually for the insertion of a breathing tube.

In cases involving severe illness or injury to the upper airway, a laryngectomy may be performed to create a permanent opening in the front of the neck. This operation involves the removal of some or all of the patient's larynx (voice box). The trachea is then sewn to the skin of the neck to allow the patient to breathe (Figure 5.34). Patients who

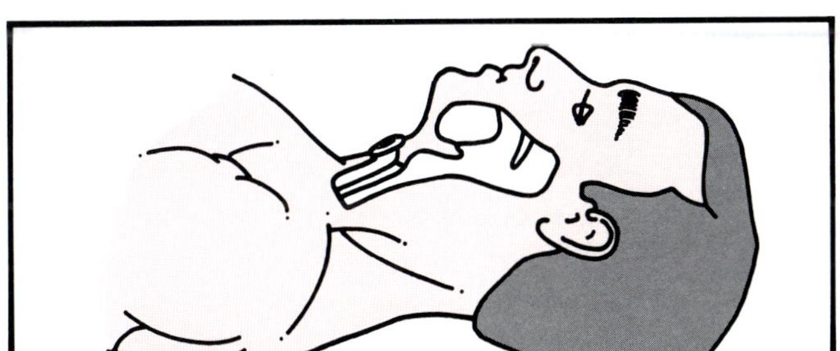

**Figure 5.34** A laryngectomy is the operation of removing some or all of the patient's larynx and sewing the trachea to the skin of the neck to allow the patient to breathe.

have had the entire larynx removed breathe only through the opening in the neck, while those whose larynx has been only partially removed breathe both through the neck and the nose and mouth. Partial neck breathers have a tube graft that connects the stoma with the base of the tongue, providing a so-called speaking tube.

Laryngectomees (those who have had a laryngectomy) are rare, but it is important to be aware of the condition and to know how to ventilate these patients. Always check the neck of a nonbreathing patient for a stoma. To perform rescue breathing for a patient who has a stoma,

Step 1: Kneel beside the patient.

Step 2: Remove all coverings (scarves, ties, necklaces, protective coverings) from the stoma area, baring the entire neck down to the breastbone.

Step 3: Clear the stoma of all foreign matter.

Step 4: Take a deep breath and make a seal with your mouth over the stoma (Figure 5.35).

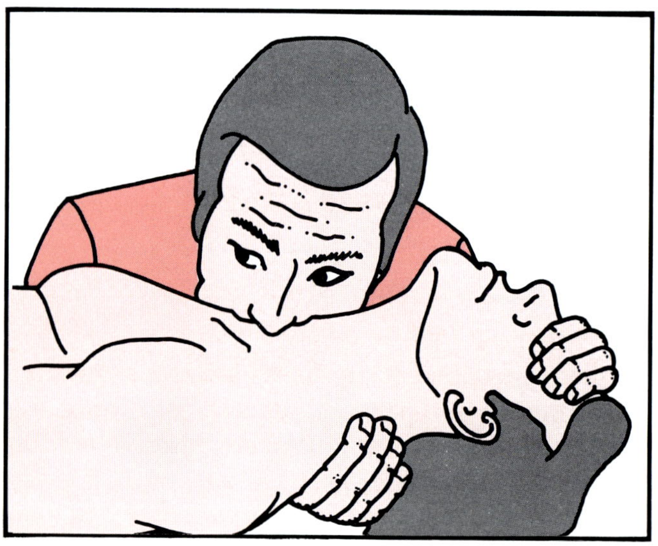

**Figure 5.35** Take a deep breath and make a seal with your mouth over the stoma.

Step 5: Blow into the stoma with two full breaths. If the chest does not rise, the patient may be a partial neck breather. Seal the patient's nose and mouth with one hand and try again to ventilate the lungs. To seal the nose and mouth, pinch the patient's nose closed with your third and fourth fingers and seal the lips with the palm of your hand. Place the thumb of that same hand under the patient's chin and press upward and backward on the jaw (Figure 5.36).

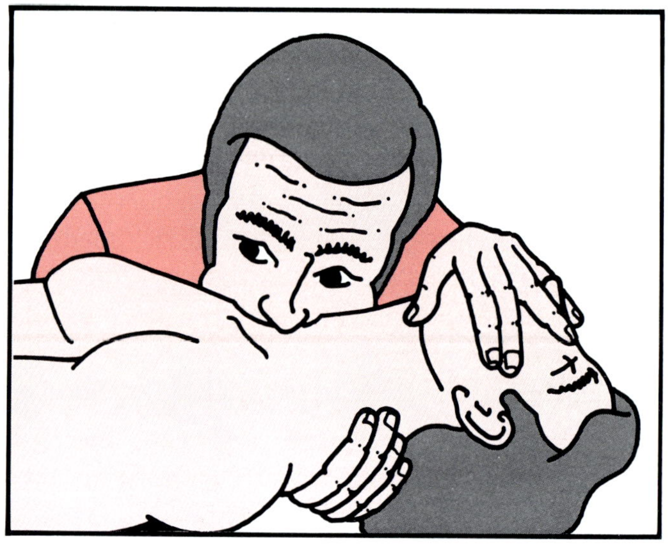

**Figure 5.36** Place your thumb under the patient's chin and press upward and backward on the jaw.

Step 6: Give *two* full breaths, allowing 1 to 1½ seconds for each breath. Remove your mouth from the stoma to allow air to escape. Watch for the rise and fall of the patient's chest between each breath.

Mouth-to-stoma ventilation is simple and safe. You need not be concerned about obstructions of the nose, mouth, tongue, or larynx since they are bypassed through the opening in the neck. Filling the lungs of these patients requires less effort and may be less objectionable than using the mouth-to-mouth or mouth-to-nose methods.

## Gastric Distention

Gastric distention, or inflation of the stomach, can occur as a complication of rescue breathing. Gastric distention may be caused by an incompletely open airway or by an excessive volume of air blown into the patient's lungs. If it is severe, gastric distention can cause the patient to vomit, resulting in airway problems and the possibility of the patient aspirating stomach contents into the airway or lungs. Foreign material in the lungs can cause aspiration pneumonia, which may be fatal.

If the victim has an open airway, air moves more easily into the lungs than into the stomach. If the airway is not completely open, the pressure of your breath in the narrow passageway may cause air to enter the stomach as well as the lungs. Even if the airway is properly opened, an excessively large breath can overwhelm the capacity of the lungs and pass into the stomach.

Gastric distention is most common in children but can also occur in adults. It may be dangerous if it is severe, since it exerts upward pressure on the diaphragm. This pressure on the diaphragm reduces the capacity of the lungs and increases the danger of vomiting.

The best way to deal with gastric distention is to try to prevent it. Avoid excessive pressure when you breathe and watch the patient's chest and stomach to be sure that you exhale only enough to get a good chest rise.

If the stomach does become inflated, you will notice obvious bulging in the patient's stomach area. To relieve the distention, roll the patient to one side, then press briefly on the patient's stomach with your hand to force the air from the stomach. Because this action may also cause the patient to vomit, be prepared to clear vomitus from the throat. Reposition the airway and continue rescue breathing.

**CAUTION:** Attempting to relieve gastric distention can have dangerous consequences. **DO NOT** try to relieve gastric distention unless the patient's abdomen becomes so rigid that ventilation is impossible. You should have suction equipment at hand and be prepared to use it.

## ADJUNCTIVE EQUIPMENT

### Airway Adjuncts

If the patient's airway cannot easily be maintained by positioning the head and jaw, especially in an unconscious patient, adjunctive equipment may be useful. The airway adjuncts most commonly used by first responders are oral airways, S-tubes, and suctioning equipment. Remember that even with adjunctive equipment, proper placement of the patient's head must be maintained in order to allow ventilation of the lungs.

#### ORAL (OROPHARYNGEAL) AIRWAY

The oropharyngeal airway is a curved device that fits over the back of the tongue and holds it away from the back wall of the throat. NEVER use an oral airway on a patient with functioning gag reflexes because it can stimulate gagging and vomiting. Oral airways come in different sizes and must be measured for proper fit. To select the proper size, place the airway on the side of the patient's face; it should extend from the angle of the jaw to the corner of the mouth (Figure 5.37).

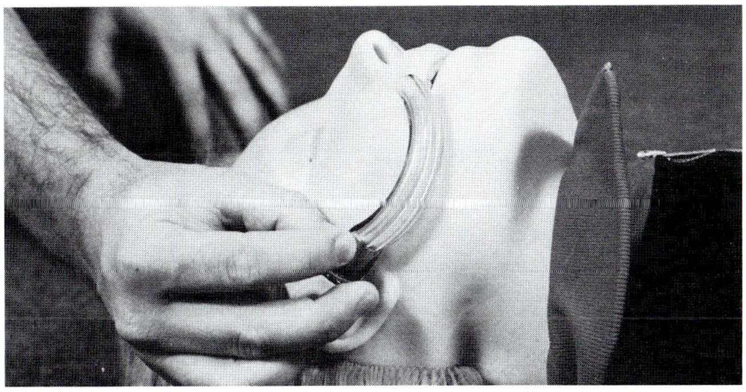

**Figure 5.37** The oral airway should extend from the angle of the jaw to the corner of the mouth.

There are two methods for inserting an oral airway. One method consists of inserting the airway upside down (tip upward) into the mouth and then rotating it as the tip reaches the back of the throat (Figure 5.38). Be especially careful not to

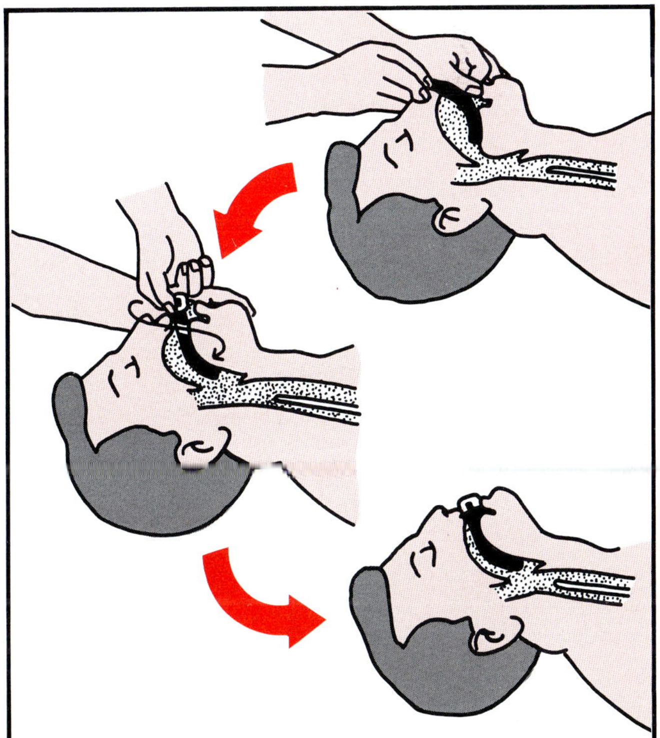

**Figure 5.38** Insert the oral airway upside down into the mouth and rotate it as the tip reaches the back of the throat.

push the tongue backward into the patient's throat as you insert the oral airway. The other way to insert an oral airway is to hook your thumb over the patient's lower teeth and pull the jaw up. Then insert the airway, tip down, following the contour of the mouth (Figure 5.39).

If a patient begins to gag while you are inserting an oral airway, remove it immediately.

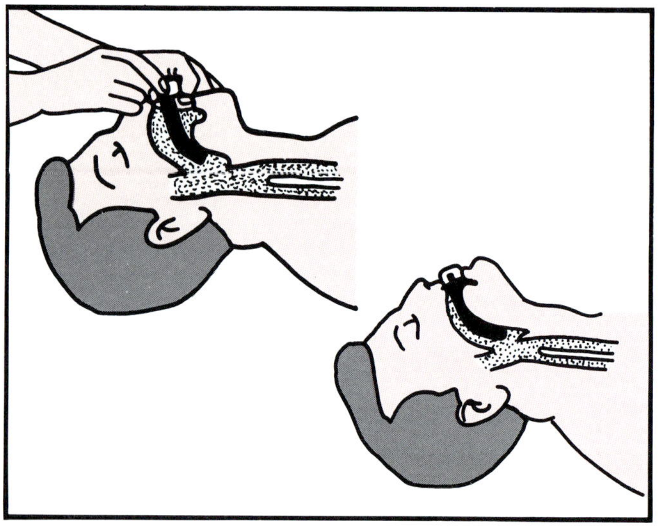

**Figure 5.39** Lift the patient's lower jaw and insert the oral airway, tip down, following the contour of the mouth.

### S-TUBE

An S-tube is made of flexible plastic and is used much like an oral airway. The S-tube is particularly useful for rescue breathing. After insertion, another S-tube can be attached to the first one with a flange. This arrangement allows the rescuer to ventilate the patient without direct mouth-to-mouth contact (Figure 5.40).

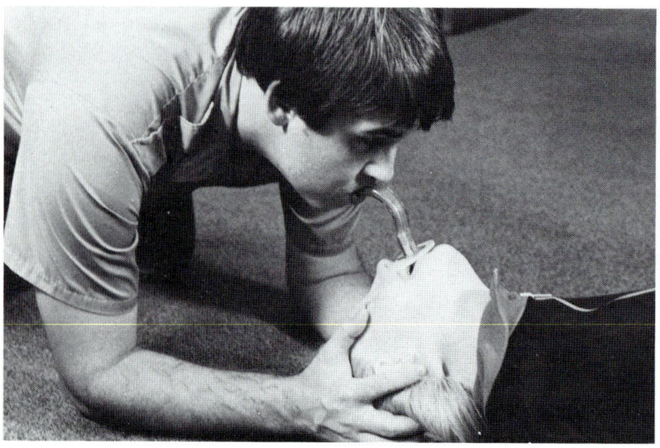

**Figure 5.40** Attaching one S-tube to another allows the rescuer to ventilate the patient without direct mouth-to-mouth contact.

S-tubes, like oral airways, must be sized for each patient. Measure the S-tube for proper fit and insert it as you would an oral airway.

### SUCTIONING EQUIPMENT

Suctioning equipment is particularly useful for clearing secretions such as blood, mucus, or vomitus from the airway. Suctioning the mouth and throat is most easily performed with a rigid tonsil tip catheter, a device that can be quickly directed to the desired location. Make sure you can see where you are directing the tonsil tip catheter. Direct it into the mouth carefully; do not jam it blindly into the patient's mouth or throat (Figure 5.41). Suction only the back part of the mouth; do not push the tip into the throat or you will stimulate the patient's gag reflex. Between suctioning attempts, clear the catheter in sterile water or saline and oxygenate the patient.

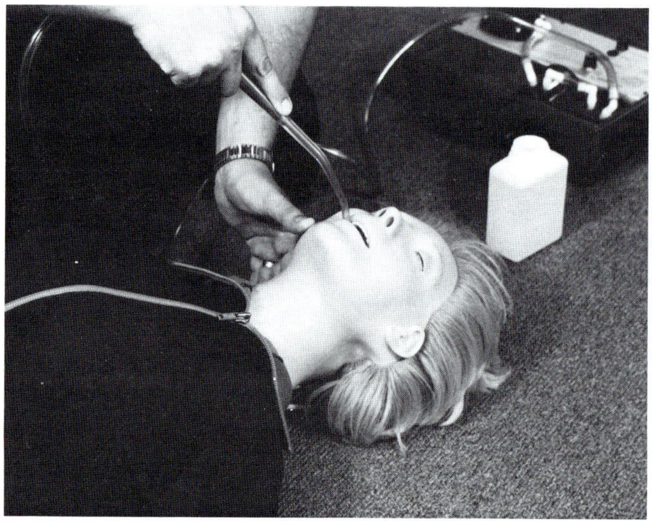

**Figure 5.41** Direct the tonsil-tip catheter carefully into the patient's mouth — never jam it blindly into the patient's mouth or throat.

If a patient begins to vomit, turn him or her to one side to allow secretions to drain from the mouth (if the patient has a suspected spinal injury, he or she must be turned as a unit — see Chapter 8, Injuries to the Skull, Spine, and Chest). Then direct the tonsil tip catheter into the mouth and begin suctioning. Do not suction for more than 15 seconds at a time.

If possible, preoxygenate the patient before applying suction. Preoxygenation is especially beneficial for the patient who is not breathing or who is not breathing adequately.

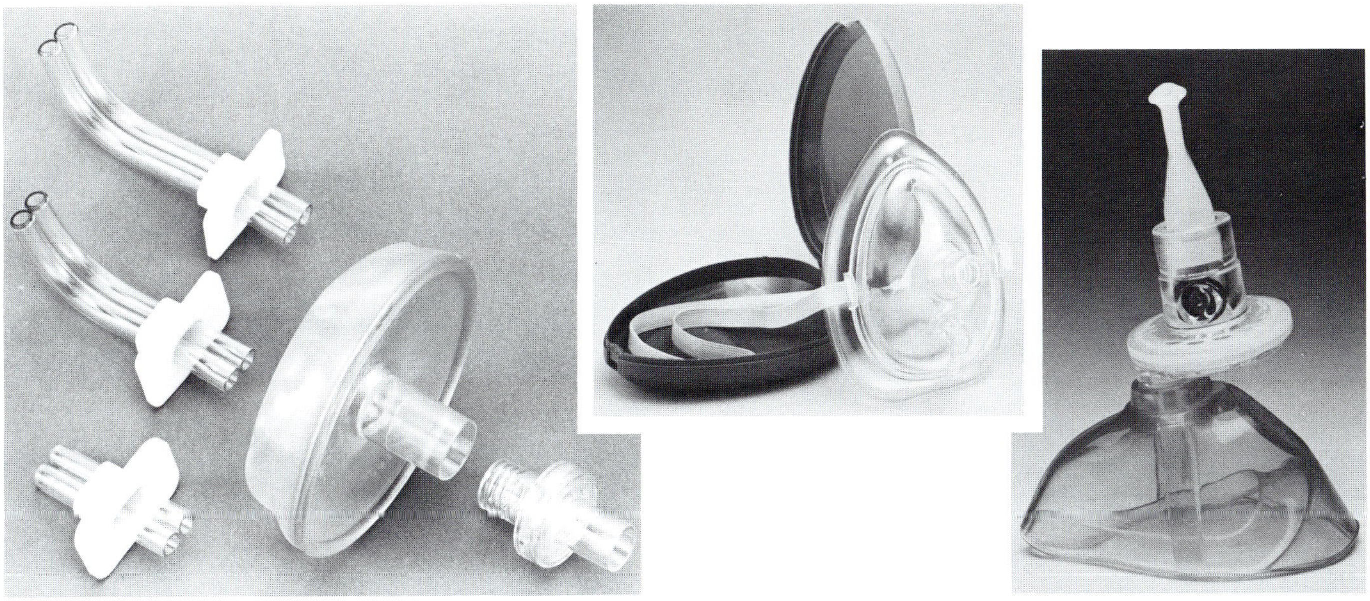

**Figure 5.42** Pocket masks are used to administer rescue breathing without direct mouth-to-mouth contact. *Photos courtesy of Armstrong Industries Inc., Northbrook, IL and Dyna Med.*

To preoxygenate the patient, give several full breaths using the mouth-to-mouth or mouth-to-mask techniques, or by using a bag-valve mask (see Breathing Adjuncts below). If you use a bag-valve mask, give two or three ventilations, then begin suctioning. Do not suction for more than 15 seconds at a time. Remember that the patient will not be receiving any oxygen during suctioning.

## Breathing Adjuncts

Two ventilation devices are commonly used by first responders to treat patients who need rescue breathing: the pocket mask and the bag-valve mask.

### POCKET MASK

The pocket mask with an oxygen inlet valve allows a rescuer to perform rescue breathing without having to make direct contact with the patient's nose and mouth (Figure 5.42). An oxygen source connected to the mask's inlet valve permits mouth-to-mask ventilation with up to 50 percent oxygen at a flow rate of 10 L/min. A pocket mask may also be used with an oral airway or S-tube. Because you can use both hands to maintain an open airway with a pocket mask, masks of this type are easier to use than bag-valve masks.

The steps for using a pocket mask are described as follows:

*Method 1: For the patient with actual or suspected spinal injury*

Step 1: Open the victim's airway using the modified jaw-thrust maneuver or an oral airway to maintain the open airway.

Step 2: Place the rim of the pocket mask between the patient's lower lip and chin. With one hand, retract the lower lip and hold the mouth open (Figure 5.43).

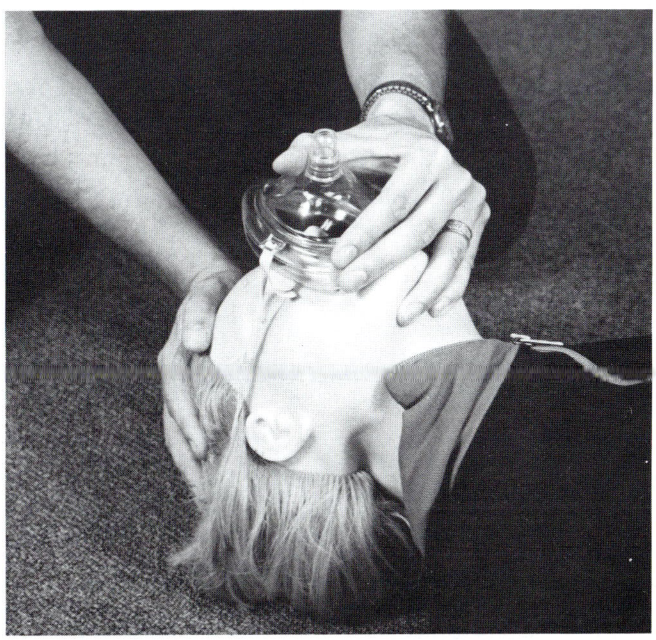

**Figure 5.43** Place the rim of the pocket mask between the patient's lower lip and chin, and with one hand, retract the lower lip and hold the mouth open.

Step 3: Place both thumbs along the side of the mask and press the remainder of the mask to the face. Grasp the jaw just beneath the angles with your fingers to maintain the forward thrust of the jaw (Figure 5.44).

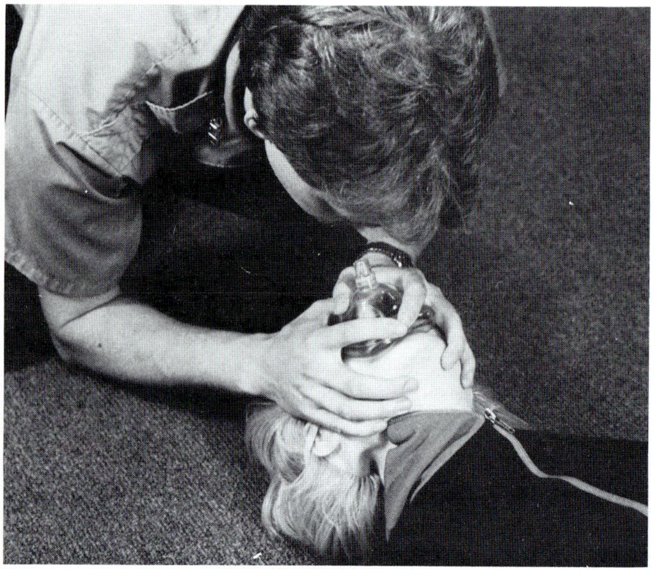

**Figure 5.44** Grasp the jaw just beneath the angles with your fingers to maintain the forward thrust of the jaw.

Step 4: Exhale into the mask, forcing your breath, which is enriched with oxygen, into the patient's lungs.

*Method 2: For the patient without suspected spinal injury*

Step 1: Position yourself behind the patient's head or at the side of the head. Open the victim's airway using the head-tilt chin-lift method. (Remember that an oral airway may also be used.)

Step 2: Clamp the mask between the patient's lower lip and chin. Use your thumbs and forefingers to seal the mask over the patient's nose and chin. The rest of your fingers should hook over the lower jaw. Apply pressure with these fingers to help keep the patient's mouth open. If necessary, press your knees against the patient's forehead to help maintain the backward tilt of the head.

Step 3: Exhale into the mask, forcing your breath into the patient's lungs (Figure 5.45). As with any other means of rescue breathing, watch for the rise and fall of the patient's chest, which indicates adequate ventilation.

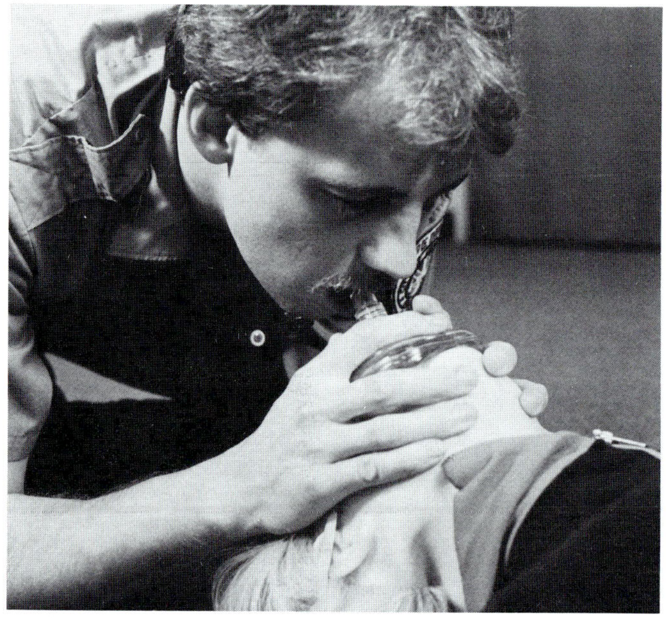

**Figure 5.45** Exhale into the mask to ventilate the patient's lungs.

Step 4: Additional oxygen may be connected to the mask's inlet valve using oxygen connecting tubing. If the oxygen flow rate is high enough (15 L/min), periodically close off the opening of the mask with your tongue and allow the oxygen flow to ventilate the patient. This technique will produce an inspired oxygen concentration higher than 50 percent. Again, make sure that the patient's chest rises normally but not excessively.

**NOTE:** To use a pocket mask on an infant, turn the mask over so that the narrower part fits over the infant's chin and the wider part fits over the infant's nose and mouth. Remember to use small puffs of air from your cheeks. Again, exhale only enough to cause a normal chest rise.

### BAG-VALVE MASK

Like the pocket mask, the bag-valve mask permits rescue breathing without direct contact with the patient's nose and mouth. A bag-valve mask consists of a mask, system of valves, self-inflating bag, and an oxygen tube connector (Figure 5.46). The mask is designed to form an airtight seal around a patient's mouth and nose. The bag reinflates itself after it has been squeezed and released. Through a system of valves, air enters the patient's lungs when the bag is squeezed, but air returning from the lungs leaves the mask through an exhaust valve. Bag-valve masks are available in different sizes for infants, children, and adults (Figure 5.47).

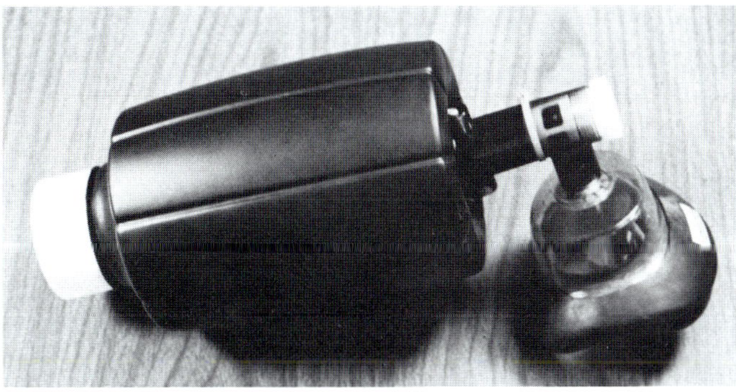

**Figure 5.46** A bag-valve mask consists of a mask, system of valves, self-inflating bag, and an oxygen tube connector.

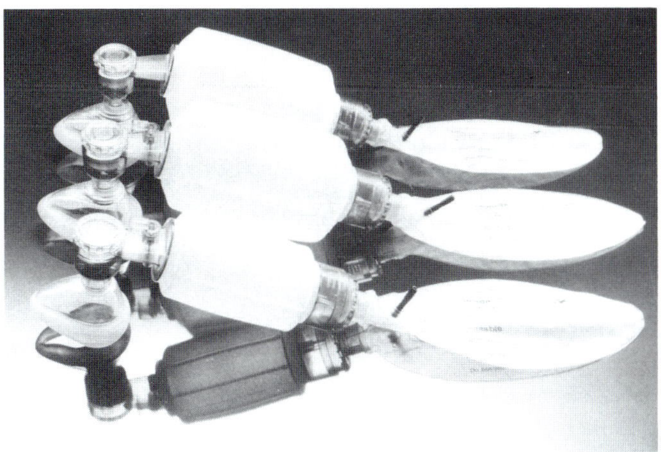

**Figure 5.47** Bag-valve masks are available in different sizes for infants, children, and adults. *Photo courtesy of Dyna Med.*

The bag-valve mask delivers a more enriched oxygen mixture than mouth-to-mouth or mouth-to-mask ventilation. Keep in mind, however, that the bag-valve mask does not provide as much volume for ventilation as is possible with mouth-to-mouth or mouth-to-mask ventilation. When used without supplemental oxygen, bag-valve masks deliver room air (21 percent oxygen) to the patient. If an oxygen source with a flow rate of 12 L/min is attached to the bag-valve mask, the delivered oxygen concentration can be increased to 40 percent. Adding an oxygen reservoir to the bag can further increase the inspired oxygen concentration to about 90 percent.

The mask used with a bag-valve device should be transparent so that vomitus or secretions around the patient's mouth can be seen. To correctly employ the bag-valve mask,

Step 1: Insert an oral airway and position yourself at the top of the patient's head. Tip the patient's head back.

**CAUTION:** If you suspect a spinal injury, use the modified jaw-thrust method to open the airway. Then insert the oral airway.

Step 2: Apply the mask so that it fits snugly beneath the patient's lower lip and over the bridge of the patient's nose (Figure 5.48).

Step 3: Place your thumb and index finger on the mask with your thumb above the patient's nose and below the valve connection. Use the other fingers to grip the patient's lower jaw and form a tight seal (Figure 5.49). Be careful not to push the patient's head forward.

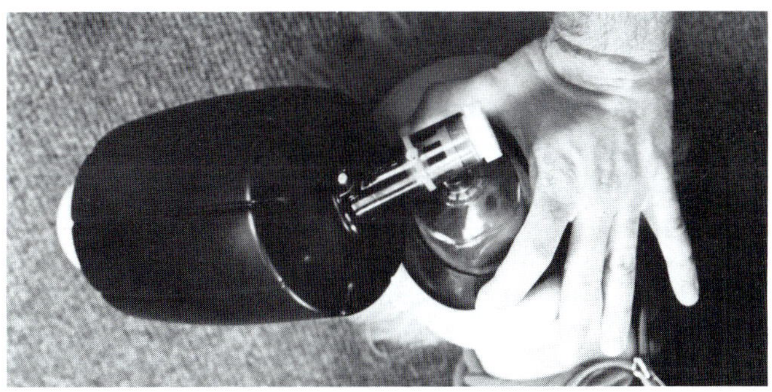

**Figure 5.48** Apply the mask so that it fits snugly beneath the patient's lower lip and over the bridge of the patient's nose.

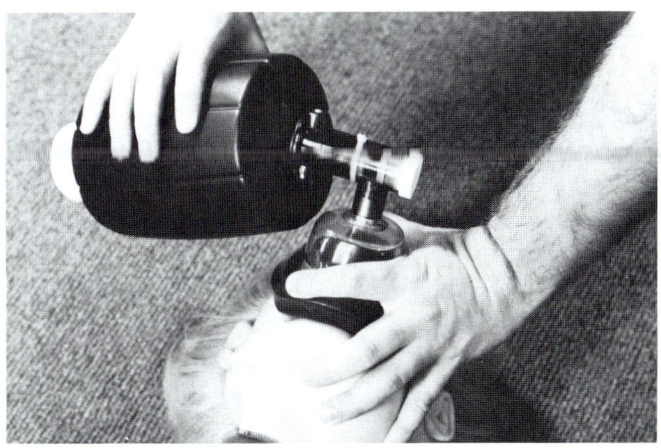

**Figure 5.49** Use your fingers to grip the patient's lower jaw and form a tight seal.

Step 4: Maintain a tight seal between the mask and the patient's face with one hand while you squeeze the bag rhythmically with the other hand (Figure 5.50). Do not remove the mask from the patient's face for exhalation because exhaled air passes through the exhalation valve.

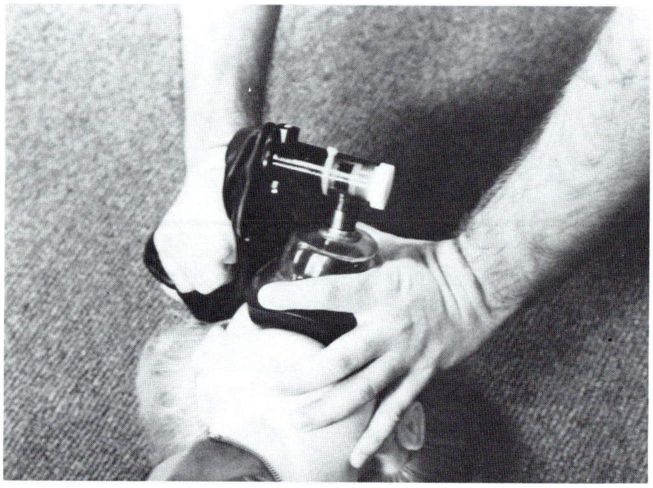

**Figure 5.50** Maintain a tight seal between the mask and the patient's face with one hand while you squeeze the bag rhythmically with the other hand.

Step 5: Watch for the rise and fall of the chest to be certain that ventilation is occurring. Continue to ventilate the adult patient with 12 breaths per minute, the child with 15 breaths per minute, and the infant with at least 20 breaths per minute.

Bag-valve masks with oxygen supplementation may also be used to assist a spontaneously breathing patient. Apply the mask to the patient's face in the manner described above, and gently squeeze the bag as the patient takes a breath.

## ASSISTING THE BREATHING PATIENT: SUPPLEMENTAL OXYGEN

A patient may be breathing and conscious, yet require additional oxygen. A wide number of illnesses and injuries interfere with an individual's ability to take in enough oxygen to supply the body's tissues. If this is the case, early administration of oxygen can save a patient's life, particularly in cases of heart attack or difficulty breathing. Supplemental oxygen enables the blood to carry more oxygen, thereby decreasing the amount of work the heart must perform to keep the vital organs supplied with oxygen. In particular, give oxygen to any patient who suffers from the following:

- Cyanosis, which indicates lack of oxygen in body tissues
- Chest pain
- Shock
- Difficulty breathing
- Trauma to the chest
- Suspected stroke
- Exposure to products of fire or toxic gases
- Seizure
- Near-drowning
- Obvious signs of respiratory distress, for any reason, including
  — Nasal flaring: the nostrils open wide on inspiration
  — Tracheal tugging: the Adam's apple pulls upward as the patient inhales
  — Retraction of the intercostal muscles (the muscles between the ribs) during inhalation
  — Use of the diaphragm and neck muscles during breathing

The amount of oxygen administered differs according to the patient's condition and the amount of difficulty he or she has breathing. In general, for the patient who is suffering from illness, such as a heart attack, administer oxygen in moderate amounts. Oxygen delivered at 4 to 6 L/min by nasal cannula is usually sufficient for these patients. If the patient also suffers from Chronic Obstructive Pulmonary Disease (COPD), administer oxygen at 2 to 4 L/min by nasal cannula. Before administering oxygen, always ask a patient if he or she suffers from COPD. (See Chapter 10, Medical Emergencies for more information about COPD).

The patient who has suffered trauma to the chest or is in shock requires greater amounts of oxygen. Administer oxygen to these patients at 10 to 12 L/min by mask. Do not try to administer oxygen by nasal cannula at amounts greater than 6 L/min. Do not administer oxygen by mask at amounts less than 6 to 8 L/min.

When you are administering supplemental oxygen, particularly to the patient in respiratory distress, observe the patient carefully for signs that the patient is receiving enough oxygen. In particular, look for an improvement in color and easing of the patient's respiratory efforts. If the patient is not improving, he or she needs more oxygen.

**NOTE:** These are only very general guidelines. Follow your local guidelines for the amount of oxygen to be administered.

## Oxygen Equipment

There are several methods for supplying oxygen to the patient who is breathing on his or her own but who requires supplemental oxygen. Since first responders do not arrive in an ambulance, they will have portable oxygen equipment (Figure 5.51).

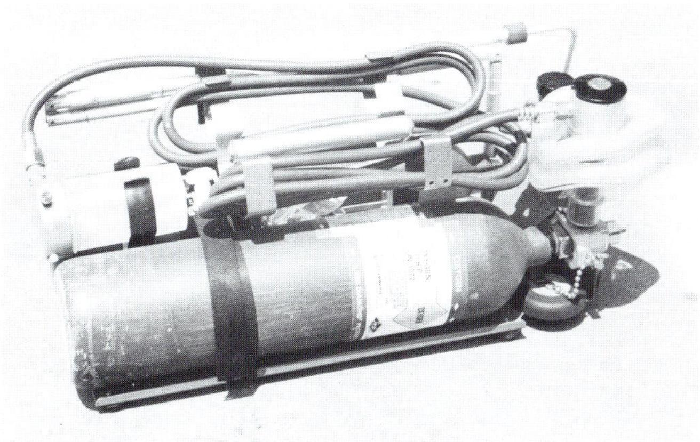

**Figure 5.51** Since first responders do not arrive in an ambulance, they carry portable oxygen equipment. *Courtesy of Geneva, IL Fire Department.*

Oxygen is a colorless, odorless gas, normally present in the atmosphere in approximately a 21 percent concentration. Pure or 100 percent oxygen is obtained commercially by fractional distillation, a process in which air is liquefied and the gases other than oxygen (primarily nitrogen) are boiled off. The resulting liquid oxygen is then converted under high pressure to a gas and stored in steel cylinders. These cylinders, under pressure of about 2,000 pounds per square inch (psi) (13 790 kPa) are given letter designations according to size. For example, an "E" cylinder is about 4.5 inches (114 mm) in diameter and 30 inches (762 mm) tall; a "G" cylinder, about 8.5 inches (215 mm) in diameter and 55 inches (1 397 mm) tall.

Gas flow from an oxygen cylinder is controlled by a regulator that reduces the cylinder's high gas pressure to a safe range (around 50 psi [345 kPa]) and controls the flow from 1 to 15 L/min. The regulators are attached to the cylinder by a yoke, which is designed so that its pins will fit only one type of gas cylinder (Figure 5.52). All gas cylinders

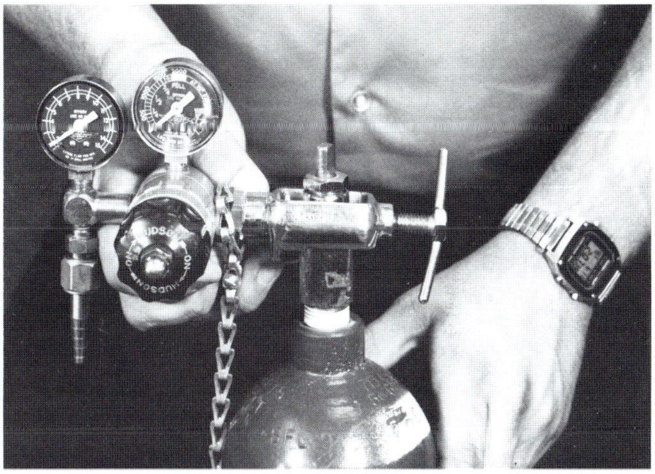

**Figure 5.52** The yoke is designed so that its pins fit only one type of gas cylinder.

are color coded by contents; in the United States, oxygen cylinders are always green. When you handle oxygen cylinders,

- Keep combustible materials, such as oil or grease, away from the cylinders and the cylinder regulators, fittings, valves, and hoses.
- Do not smoke in any area where oxygen cylinders are in use or are being stored.
- Do not subject oxygen cylinders to temperatures above 120°F (49°C).
- Do not use oxygen cylinders without safe, properly fitted regulator valves. Never modify regulator valves for a specific gas for use with another gas.
- Close all valves when oxygen cylinders are not in use, even if they are empty.
- Secure the oxygen cylinders to prevent them from toppling over. In transit, keep them in a proper carrier or rack or strap them onto the stretcher with the patient.

- When you work with an oxygen cylinder, always stay to one side of the cylinder. Never place any part of your body over the cylinder valves. A loosely fitting regulator can be launched off a cylinder with enough force to demolish any object in its path.

With these safety precautions in mind, administer oxygen following these steps:

Step 1: Secure the cylinder in an upright position and move to one side of the cylinder.

Step 2: "Crack" the tank valve with the appropriate wrench and slowly open, then quickly close the cylinder to flush out debris.

Step 3: Inspect the regulator valve to be certain that it is the right type for an oxygen cylinder and that its washer is intact.

Step 4: Apply and tighten the regulator valve.

Step 5: Open the main cylinder valve slowly to about one-half of a turn beyond the point where the regulator valve becomes pressurized.

Step 6: Open the control valve to the desired flow rate.

After the ambulance arrives on the emergency scene and you have exchanged information about the patient, it will be necessary to switch the patient to the oxygen equipment carried on the ambulance. Disconnect your equipment, assist with transferring the patient to another source of oxygen, then turn off your oxygen equipment:

Step 1: Shut off the control valve, which returns the flow rate to zero.

Step 2: Shut off the main cylinder valve.

Step 3: "Bleed" the valves by opening the control valve until the needle or ball indicator moves to indicate zero (zed) flow.

Step 4: Close the control valve.

Check cylinders frequently and replace them when pressure is low. If possible, carry a backup cylinder in the emergency vehicle. You do not want to come to the aid of a gasping patient with flashing lights and sirens only to discover that the oxygen cylinder is empty.

## OXYGEN ADMINISTRATION

Oxygen is delivered to the patient by one of several types of masks or by nasal cannula. The nasal cannula is the most easily tolerated method of delivering oxygen, and is preferred for the patient who is breathing spontaneously and who needs moderate amounts of oxygen. Plastic face masks are capable of delivering oxygen at higher concentrations. Some patients, however, can barely tolerate the masks and complain of feelings of suffocation. No matter what device you choose, explain to the patient its function and why it is needed. If you are using a mask, let the patient know that the mask may feel confining but that it actually provides more air than unaided breathing. Such an explanation may help the patient accept the mask without anxiety. If the patient becomes very anxious, it may be better to administer oxygen through a nasal cannula.

### NASAL CANNULA

A nasal cannula is a plastic tube with two short extensions that fit into a patient's nostrils (Figure 5.53). The cannula can deliver 25 to 40 percent oxygen at a flow rate of 4 to 6 L/min. A cannula is the most comfortable device for delivering oxygen to the patient but should not be used when high-flow, high-concentrations of oxygen are needed.

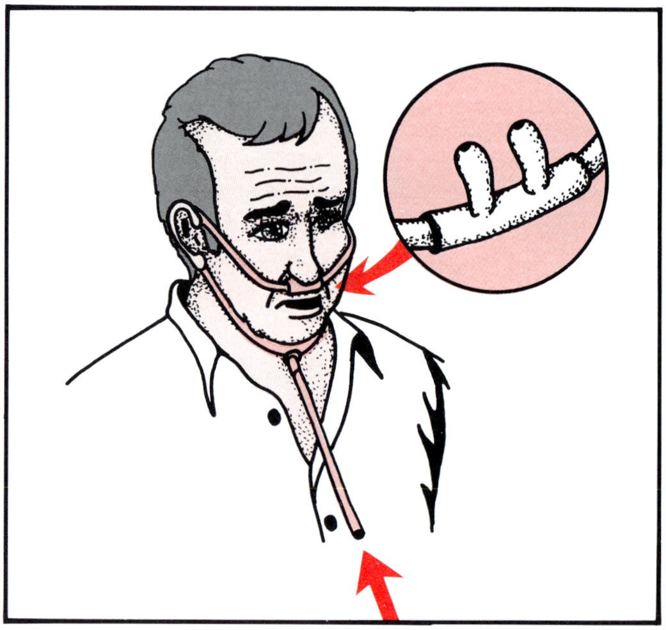

**Figure 5.53** A nasal cannula has two short extensions that fit into the patient's nostrils.

### SIMPLE FACE MASK

A simple face mask is made of clear, molded plastic and is designed to fit over the patient's nose and mouth (Figure 5.54). Although the face mask is not as well tolerated as a nasal cannula, it can deliver 40 to 60 percent oxygen at a flow rate of 10 L/min.

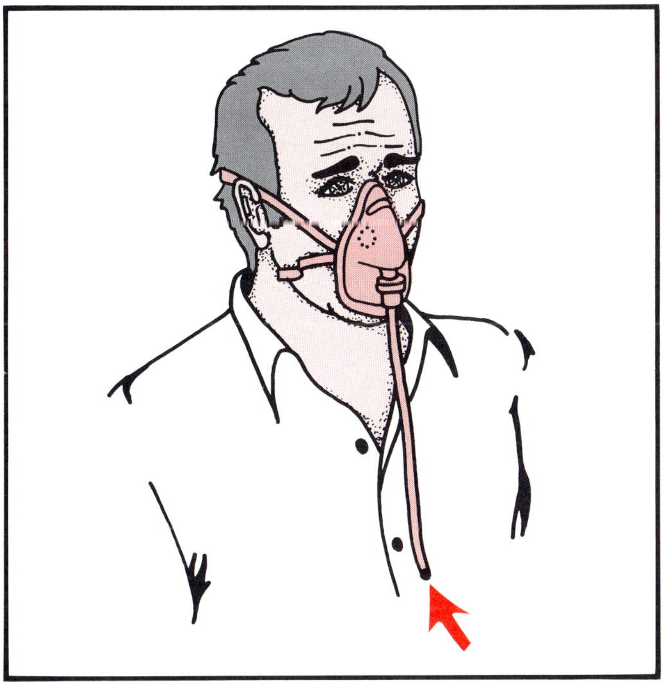

**Figure 5.54** A simple face mask is designed to fit over the patient's nose and mouth.

### PARTIAL REBREATHING MASKS

Partial rebreathing masks look like plastic face masks but they have reservoir bags that allow the patient to rebreathe about one-third of the air he or she exhales (Figure 5.55). This air comes principally from areas of the patient's respiratory tract where gas exchange does not take place. Therefore, the mask contains mostly oxygen inspired during the previous cycle. At flow rates of 6 to 10 L/min, partial rebreathing masks can provide oxygen concentrations of 35 to 60 percent.

### NONREBREATHING MASKS

Nonrebreathing masks are similar to partial rebreathing masks in that they have reservoir bags, but they are also equipped with a one-way valve that enables the patient to inhale oxygen from the reservoir bag but keeps exhaled air from entering the reservoir bag (Figure 5.56). The oxygen flow rate, usually about 10 to 12 L/min, is ad-

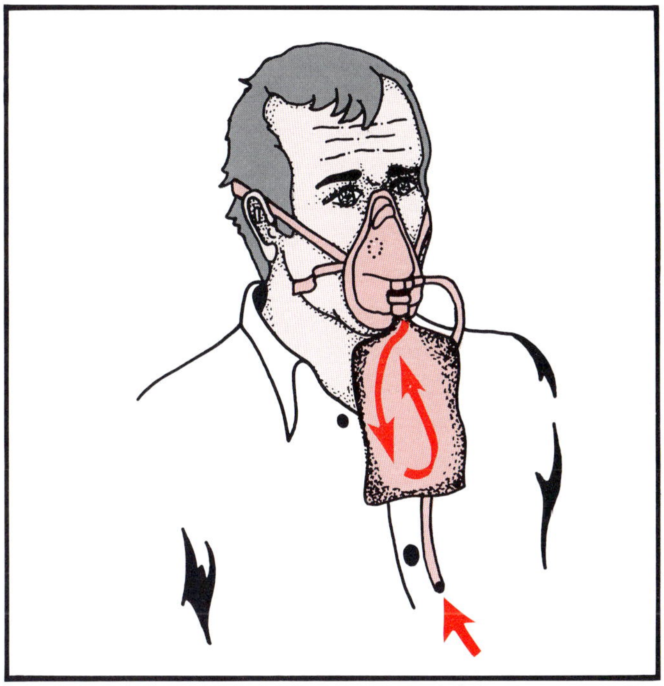

**Figure 5.55** A partial rebreathing mask has a reservoir bag that allows the patient to rebreathe about ⅓ of the air he or she exhales.

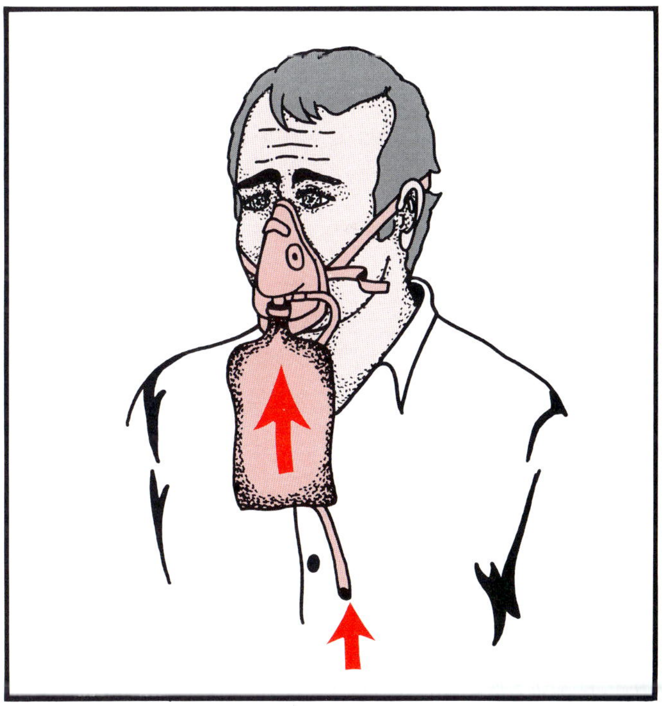

**Figure 5.56** A nonrebreathing mask has a one-way valve that permits the patient to inhale oxygen from the reservoir bag but keeps exhaled air from entering the reservoir bag.

justed to prevent collapse of the bag as the patient inhales. If the mask is fitted tightly to the face, it can deliver oxygen concentrations approaching 100 percent. Therefore, a nonrebreathing mask is well suited to situations in which the patient needs as much oxygen as possible.

### PORTABLE RESUSCITATOR (DEMAND VALVE)

Portable resuscitators are used in many ambulances and rescue vehicles. Many first responders favor these devices because they are easier to use than bag-valve masks. Moreover, they can be used for a number of purposes because they include suction equipment, manually triggered ventilation devices (demand valves), and flowmeters for providing oxygen by mask or cannula (Figure 5.57). Portable resuscitators can also be connected to an endotracheal tube, esophageal obturator airway (both inserted by EMTs or paramedics), or a mask. Portable resuscitators are best used to assist the spontaneously breathing patient.

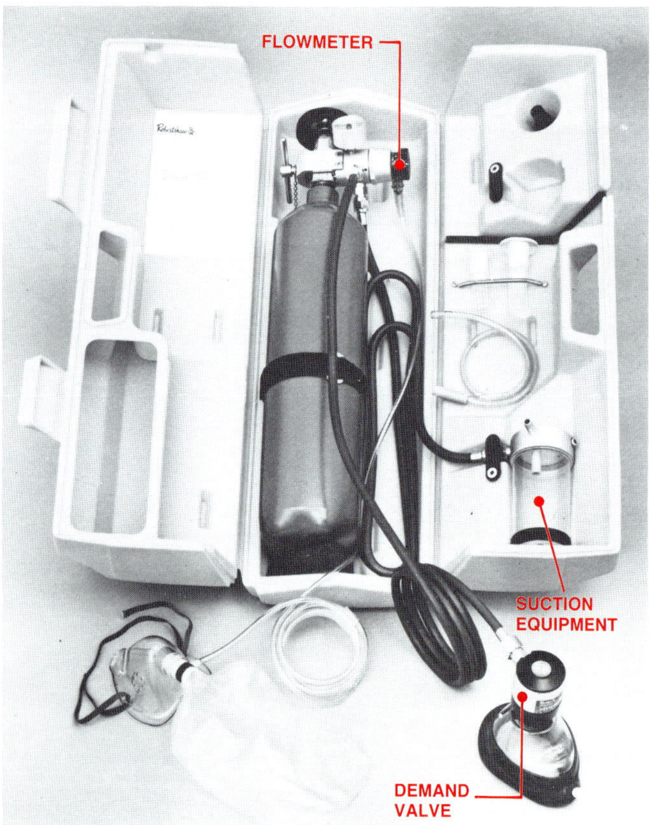


**Figure 5.57** Portable resuscitators include suction equipment, manually triggered ventilation devices (demand valves), and flowmeters for administering oxygen by mask or cannula. *Photo courtesy of Armstrong Industries Inc., Northbrook, IL.*

The demand valve can be used to administer oxygen to the breathing or nonbreathing patient. For the breathing patient, oxygen flow is triggered by a slight negative pressure produced when the patient inhales. When the patient stops inhaling, the negative pressure ceases and exhaled gases leave through a nonbreathing valve. Using the demand valve in this way is not the most effective way to administer supplemental oxygen because the patient has to work to trigger the oxygen flow. A more efficient way to assist the breathing patient is to set the flowmeter to the desired rate and deliver oxygen at a steady flow by mask or cannula.

To use the demand valve on a nonbreathing patient, use both hands to seal the mask on the patient's face. Press the demand button with your thumb or use your chin to trigger the oxygen flow (Figure 5.58). Release the button when the patient's chest rises. Continue to rhythmically force air into the patient's lungs and release the flow until additional help arrives.

TAKE CARE WHEN USING A DEMAND VALVE NOT TO OVERINFLATE THE PATIENT'S LUNGS. Monitor the patient carefully for signs of gastric distention. Do not use the demand valve at all on patients under 12 years old.

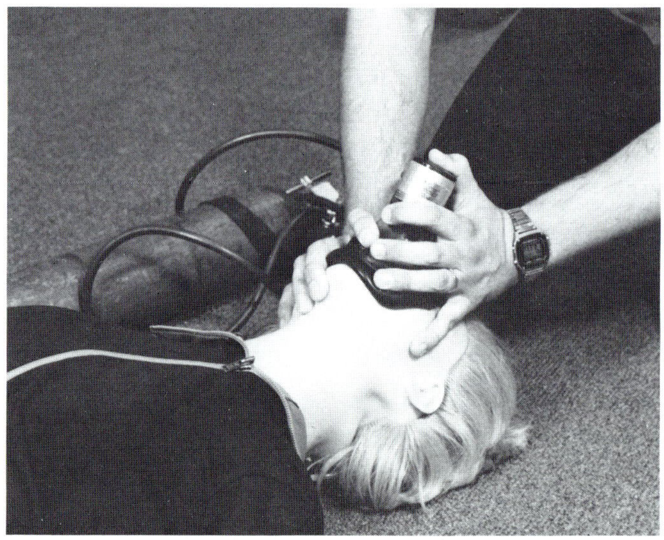

**Figure 5.58** To use the demand valve on a nonbreathing patient, use both hands to seal the mask on the patient's face. Press the demand button with your thumb and use your chin to trigger the oxygen flow.

## SECTION 3: CARDIOPULMONARY RESUSCITATION

The first two sections of this chapter dealt with the Airway and Breathing aspects of the ABC's. This section deals with the third aspect: Circulation. As you can see, these body processes are interdependent. Breathing is not possible without an open airway, and circulation is not possible unless an individual is breathing. If the heart is not beating, an open airway and adequate breathing are useless.

This section begins with a discussion of the causes of cardiac and respiratory arrest, general considerations for CPR, and legal issues concerning CPR. Step-by-step procedures for CPR are given, beginning with establishing unresponsiveness, opening the airway, assessing breathing, removing an airway obstruction, performing rescue breathing, and administering external cardiac compressions. The techniques for opening the airway, removing an airway obstruction, and performing rescue breathing have already been discussed in Sections 1 and 2 of this chapter, so special emphasis is placed on techniques for administering external cardiac compressions and assessing the effectiveness of CPR.

The principles for administering CPR to small children and infants are the same as those for adults, but the techniques differ, so these are discussed after adult CPR. The chapter concludes with two special situations requiring resuscitation: near-drowning and electric shock. These situations are special because the victims must be rescued before resuscitation efforts can begin.

## CAUSES OF RESPIRATORY AND CARDIAC ARREST

There are many causes of sudden respiratory or cardiac arrest, including heart attack, drowning, smoke inhalation, electric shock, drug overdose, and anaphylaxis (severe allergic reaction). By far the most common cause of sudden arrest is heart attack, which claims more than 500,000 lives each year. More than half of these deaths occur outside a hospital, within two hours of the onset of symptoms. **NOTE:** Heart disease and heart attacks are discussed in more detail in Chapter 10, Medical Emergencies.

## GENERAL CONSIDERATIONS FOR CPR

Once breathing and circulation stop, the victim is clinically dead. Clinical death means that the heartbeat and breathing have stopped. This death may be reversible through CPR and advanced life support provided by paramedics, nurses, and doctors. Biological death is permanent death due to lack of oxygen. This type of death is not reversible. Since permanent damage for lack of oxygen occurs first in the brain, speed is essential if the patient is to have any chance of meaningful recovery.

To be effective, CPR *must* be performed on a firm, flat surface, such as a floor or backboard (Figure 5.59). In addition, the patient's head must not be higher than the heart. If it is necessary to pull a patient from a car or from a bed to the floor, do so as quickly as possible; any spinal or internal injuries the patient may have suffered are secondary to basic life support.

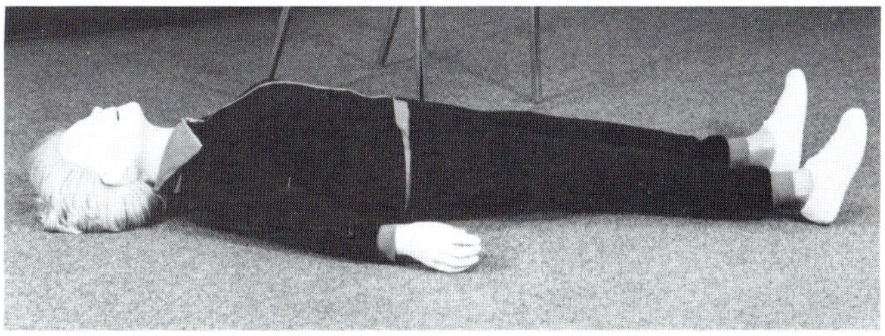

**Figure 5.59** To be effective CPR *must* be performed on a firm, flat surface, such as a floor or backboard.

### Legal Considerations

Calls involving cardiopulmonary resuscitation do not always run smoothly. First of all, family members or bystanders may have already begun CPR and might want to assist you. Since lay people are taught only one-rescuer CPR techniques, it is not a good idea to try to "train" someone to assist you on the spot. It is best to have these individuals assist by flagging down EMS vehicles, holding equipment, and so on.

Another complication of CPR is dealing with a terminally ill patient. Such a patient may be part of a hospice program in which he or she has made plans to die peacefully at home, with no heroic measures instituted to sustain life. In spite of such plans, however, family members may panic and call for emergency assistance when a loved one's condition suddenly deteriorates. Follow the guidelines in your local area for dealing with such cases. When in doubt, begin CPR and continue until additional emergency personnel arrive.

Once you have begun CPR, you are obligated to continue until

- The patient's heart resumes normal beating.
- A physician or other properly trained person responsible for emergency medical services assumes responsibility for the patient.
- You are exhausted and unable to continue.

## THE ABC'S OF CPR

Cardiopulmonary resuscitation involves three basic rescue skills: Airway, Breathing, and Circulation. These skills are interdependent and must be performed in ABC order.

First, the patient must have an open AIRWAY before he or she can breathe. Remember that the tongue is the most common cause of airway obstruction in the unconscious victim. Since the tongue is attached to the lower jaw, moving the lower jaw forward lifts the tongue from the back of the throat and opens the airway.

Once the airway is open, the patient must be BREATHING. Inhaling oxygenates the blood and exhaling removes waste products. If the victim is not breathing, perform rescue breathing until the victim begins to breathe again or until other EMS personnel arrive and take over. The quickest and most effective way to perform rescue breathing is through mouth-to-mouth resuscitation.

The victim must have adequate CIRCULATION. If the victim's heart is not beating, you must perform chest compressions in addition to rescue breathing. Chest compressions provide artificial circulation to keep the brain, lungs, and other vital organs adequately oxygenated.

## TECHNIQUES OF CPR

The steps of CPR must be performed *in sequence*: first assess the airway, then perform rescue breathing, then administer cardiac compressions plus rescue breathing. If you discover that the victim's airway is obstructed by a foreign body, the obstruction must be dislodged or the patient cannot be ventilated. Learning to perform CPR correctly and efficiently requires practice on manikins under the guidance of a certified instructor.

**CAUTION:** PRACTICE CPR SKILLS ONLY ON MANIKINS. DO NOT, UNDER ANY CIRCUMSTANCES, PRACTICE THESE SKILLS ON OTHER PEOPLE.

The steps of CPR are as follows:

Step 1: AIRWAY
- Determine unresponsiveness
- Call for help
- Position the patient
- Open the airway

Step 2: BREATHING
- Assess breathing; determine breathlessness
- Perform rescue breathing
- Dislodge a foreign object from the airway

Step 3: CIRCULATION
- Assess circulation; determine pulselessness
- Activate EMS system
- Begin chest compressions

Step 4: ASSESS EFFECTIVENESS OF CPR
- Look for chest rise and improvement in color
- Determine pulselessness

Step 5: CONTINUE CPR

### Determine Unresponsiveness

The first step to take when you encounter a patient who seems to be unconscious is to establish unresponsiveness. Do this by gently tapping the patient's shoulder or face and shouting, "Are you all right?" (Figure 5.60). IF YOU HAVE ANY REASON TO SUSPECT A SPINAL INJURY, DO NOT MOVE THE PATIENT'S HEAD OR NECK. If the patient does not respond, take immediate steps to open the airway.

### Call for Help

As a first responder, you should make sure that EMTs or paramedics are on their way. If you are in a home or do not have access to a radio, enlist the help of relatives or bystanders to telephone for additional help.

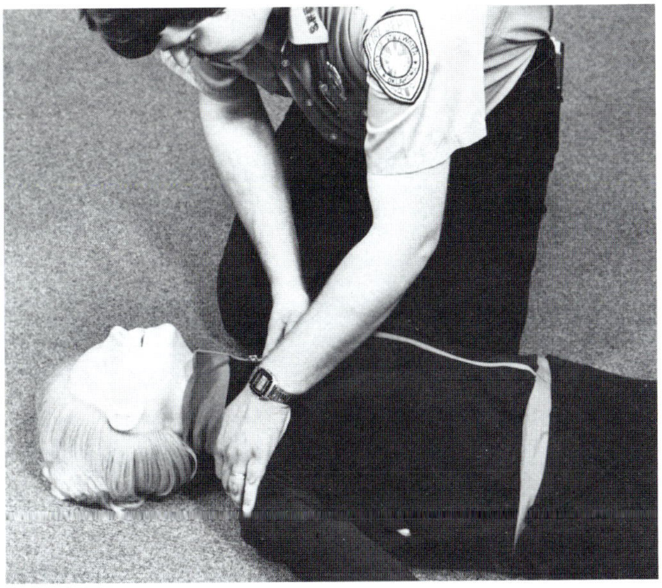

**Figure 5.60** Determine unresponsiveness by tapping the patient on the shoulder and shouting, "Are you all right?"

## Position the Patient

If the patient is found crumpled and lying face down, turn the patient over. The patient must be turned as a unit so that the head, shoulders, and torso move at the same time. To do this,

Step 1: Kneel beside the patient and straighten the patient's arms above the head. Slide your hand under the near arm close to the shoulder and place the palm of your hand over the back of the victim's head near the neck. Be sure that your hand is in a position to support the weight of the head as you roll the patient (Figure 5.61).

Step 2: Place your other hand on the victim's hip. Roll the patient away from you, being careful not to twist the body. Follow the patient on your knees as he or she rolls to help keep your balance and to provide support for the patient's head and neck. Keep your hands in their original positions until the patient is flat on the floor (Figure 5.62). If there are two rescuers, one rescuer can remain at the patient's head and provide axial traction during the move (Figure 5.63). (See Chapter 8, Injuries to the Skull, Spine, and Chest, for the principles and procedures for handling patients with suspected spinal injuries.)

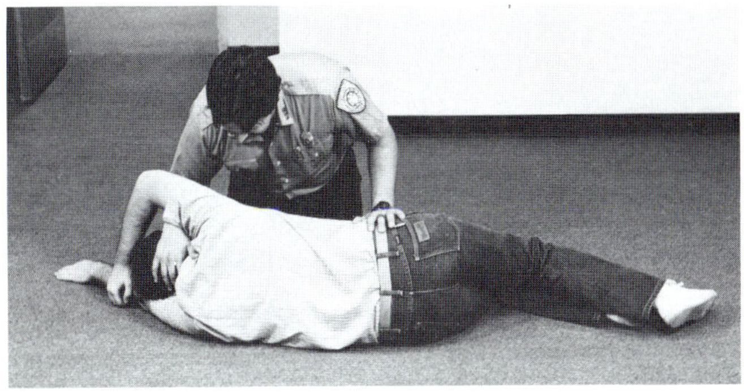

**Figure 5.61** Be sure that your hand is in a position to support the weight of the head as you roll the patient.

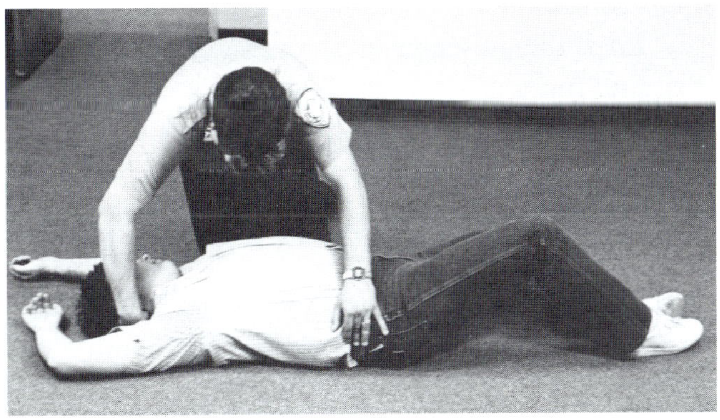

**Figure 5.62** Keep your hands in their original positions until the patient is flat on the floor.

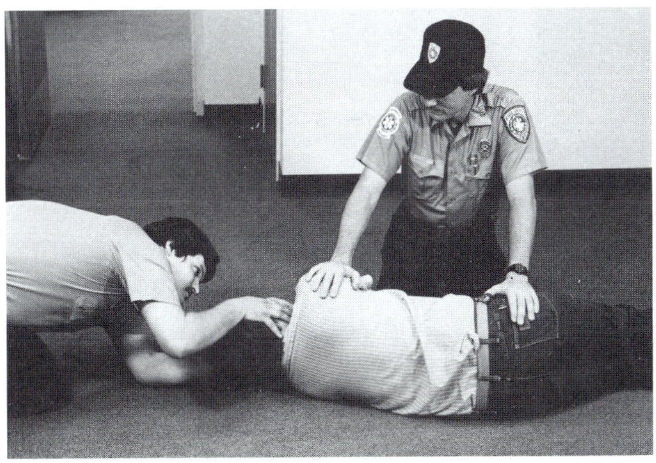

**Figure 5.63** If there are two rescuers, one rescuer can remain at the patient's head and provide axial traction during the move.

## Open the Airway

Open the patient's airway using the appropriate method from Section 1, Airway Care:

- Modified jaw-thrust maneuver
- Head-tilt chin-lift maneuver
- Head-tilt neck-lift maneuver
- Jaw-thrust maneuver
- Face-down maneuver

If the patient is an accident victim, you *must* suspect a spinal injury. Use *only* the modified jaw-thrust maneuver to open the patient's airway. The other four methods may be used *only* on patients in whom there is no reason to suspect a spinal injury.

### Assess Breathing

Once you have opened the patient's airway, you must determine whether or not the patient is breathing. To do this, lean over the patient's head facing toward the chest. Place your ear within an inch (25 mm) of the victim's mouth and nose, and

*Look* to see whether the patient's chest rises and falls.

*Listen* for air movement at the nose and mouth.

*Feel* for air movement on your cheek or ear (Figure 5.64).

The critical indications of breathing are feeling and hearing breathing at the mouth and nose. If a person is moving air into and out of the lungs, the air passes through the mouth and/or nose.

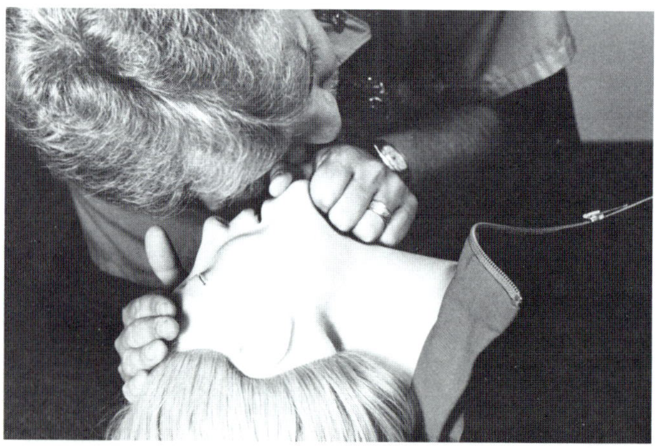

**Figure 5.64** Look, listen, and feel for the movement of air from the patient's mouth and nose.

If the patient *is* breathing, continue to maintain the airway in an open position. Monitor the patient's pulse and vital signs and arrange for rapid transport to a medical facility. It may be advisable to administer supplemental oxygen as well. If the patient is *not* breathing, begin rescue breathing immediately.

### Perform Rescue Breathing

Depending upon the size and physical condition of the patient, use one of the following rescue breathing techniques, as described in Section 2, Rescue Breathing:

- Mouth-to-mouth ventilation
- Mouth-to-nose ventilation
- Mouth-to-stoma ventilation
- Mouth-to-mask ventilation

Remember that the patient's airway must be kept in an open position or rescue breathing efforts will be futile. Do *not* take the time to look for foreign objects in the airway unless their presence is known or strongly suspected.

You will know that ventilation is adequate if you can

- *See* the patient's chest rise and fall.
- *Feel* the patient's lungs yield to your respirations.
- *Hear* and *feel* air escaping from the patient's lungs after each ventilation.

### Dislodge a Foreign Object from the Airway

If the patient's lungs do not yield relatively easily to your breath, reposition the patient's head and attempt to ventilate the lungs again. If you are still unsuccessful, you must suspect a foreign body obstruction and perform the Heimlich maneuver to try to dislodge the obstruction, as described in Section 1, Airway Care. If you cannot completely dislodge the foreign object, you may be able to move it enough to permit ventilation of the lungs.

### Assess Circulation

After giving two full breaths, determine quickly whether the heart has also stopped. To check for cardiac arrest, locate the carotid pulse in the neck. The carotid pulse is preferable because it is easily accessible and because it can be detected when other pulses are too weak to be felt. To check the carotid pulse,

Step 1: Maintain the airway by continuing the downward pressure of your hand on the forehead.

Step 2: Use the hand that is on the patient's chin to feel for the pulse. Slide your fingers down from the chin and find the Adam's apple with your fingertips about halfway between the patient's chin and collarbone.

Step 3: Draw your fingers back toward you into the groove beside the Adam's apple (Figure 5.65). Press *lightly* to feel the pulse with the most sensitive part of your fingertips. Feel very carefully to find a pulse. Take at least 5 seconds and up to 10 seconds if necessary.

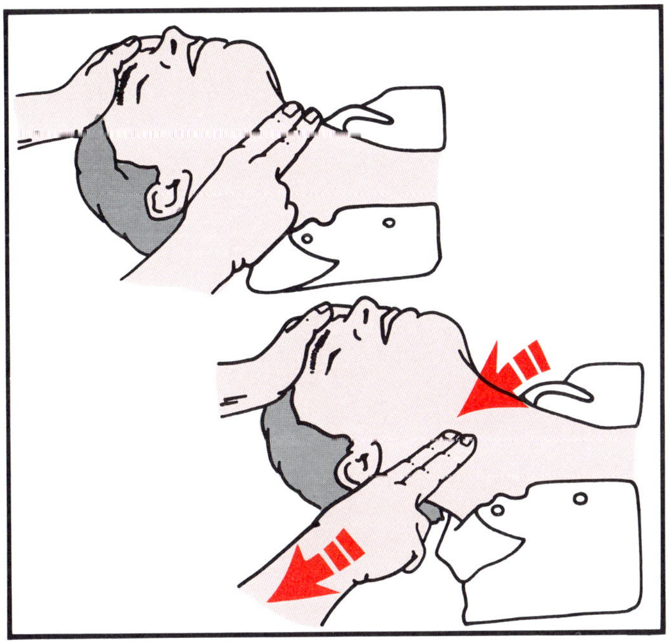

**Figure 5.65** Draw your fingers back toward you into the groove beside the Adam's apple.

**CAUTION: NEVER** begin chest compressions on someone whose heart is still beating — even if the pulse is weak or irregular. Performing compressions on a person whose heart is functioning causes the heart to stop.

#### PULSE PRESENT - RESCUE BREATHE

If the patient has a pulse, continue rescue breathing at a rate of once every 5 seconds, or 12 times per minute. If the victim is a child, breathe once every 4 seconds, or 15 times per minute. If the victim is an infant, breathe once every 3 seconds, or 20 times per minute.

Check the pulse once a minute to be sure that the heart is still circulating blood even though breathing has stopped. Continue to breathe for the patient as long as the breathing inadequacy persists or until additional help arrives. You may use adjunctive equipment (such as a bag-valve mask) to perform rescue breathing.

If the unconscious victim begins to breathe voluntarily while you are doing rescue breathing, discontinue rescue breathing but maintain the airway. Because vomiting may occur at this point, you may wish to turn the victim to one side as you continue to monitor breathing. If vomiting does occur, let the stomach contents drain from the mouth and wipe the mouth clean.

Always arrange to transport any victim who has required rescue breathing to the nearest medical facility. Even if the victim regains consciousness and claims to be fine, he or she must be evaluated by a physician as a safeguard against complications that may result from the respiratory emergency.

#### PULSE ABSENT - ADMINISTER EXTERNAL CHEST COMPRESSIONS

If the pulse check reveals that the victim is pulseless, administer artificial circulation (external chest compressions) as well as rescue breathing. If you are alone, stop briefly and make sure that an ambulance is on its way.

## TECHNIQUES FOR ADMINISTERING EXTERNAL CHEST COMPRESSIONS

### Hand Position

PROPERLY PERFORMED CHEST COMPRESSION IS ONLY ABOUT ONE-QUARTER TO ONE-THIRD AS EFFECTIVE AS NORMAL BLOOD FLOW; THEREFORE, IT IS CRITICAL THAT YOU USE THE PROPER TECHNIQUES WHEN ADMINISTERING CHEST COMPRESSIONS.

Before beginning chest compressions, you must locate the area of the sternum (breastbone) to which you can apply pressure without injuring the ribs or the organs under them. If extra people are available to help, and if there is no reason to suspect that the patient has a spinal injury, have someone elevate the patient's legs to improve circulation (if you are working with EMTs or paramedics, they may apply the MAST in order to help increase the patient's blood pressure). To locate the correct hand position for chest compressions,

Step 1: Remove the victim's clothing so that the sternum is exposed. This should be done for several reasons: (1) clothing makes it difficult to locate the correct hand position; (2) clothing may cause your hands to slip during compressions; (3) many layers of clothing may reduce the effectiveness of the compressions. Remove clothing quickly; there is no time to lose. If the patient has on a shirt that buttons up the front, tear it open. If the patient is a female and there are bystanders, particularly relatives, use some discretion. It is possible to expose the sternum without completely baring the chest.

Step 2: Kneel beside the patient and run your fingers up the rib cage until your middle finger fits right into the notch where the ribs and sternum meet, and your index finger is beside it across the lower end of the sternum. Then place the heel of your other hand on the victim's chest, centering it over the midline of the sternum, right beside your index finger (Figure 5.66). Now move your first hand and place it directly over the heel of the second hand, so that the heels of both hands are parallel to one another (Figure 5.67).

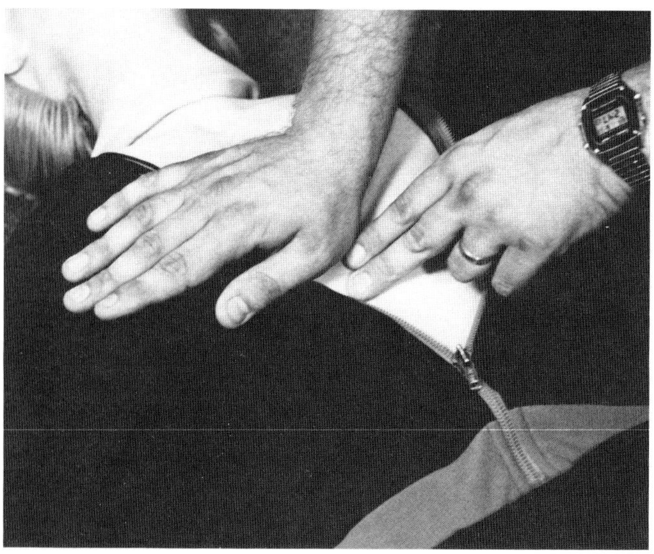

**Figure 5.66** Place your index and middle fingers just above the xiphoid process. Then place the heel of your other hand on the victim's chest and center it over the midline of the sternum, right beside your index finger.

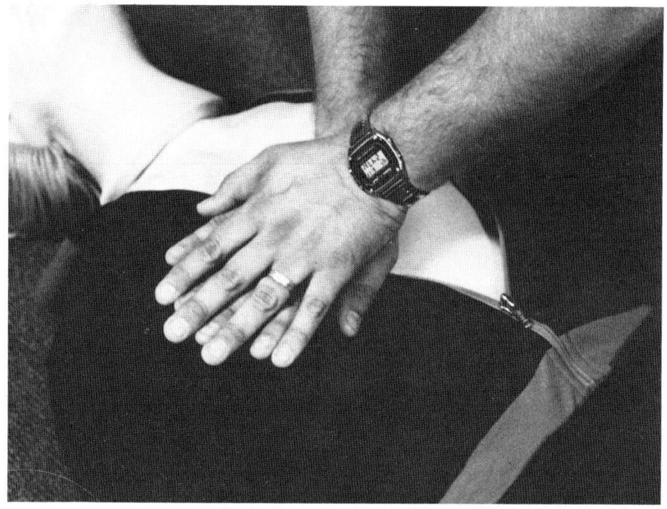

**Figure 5.67** Move your first hand and place it directly over the heel of the second hand, so that the heels of both hands are parallel to one another.

Step 3: Tip your fingers up off the chest or interlace them to avoid applying pressure to the ribs. The only point of contact between you and the patient should be between the heel of your hand and the flat lower half of the patient's sternum (Figure 5.68).

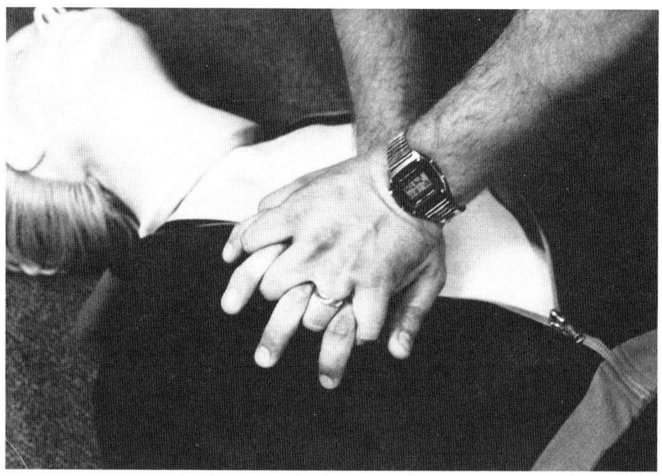

**Figure 5.68** Tip your fingers up off the patient's chest or interlace them so that only the heel of your hand rests on the lower half of the patient's sternum.

If your hands are correctly positioned to perform chest compressions, they rest over the lower half of the sternum, two or three fingers above the xiphoid process. Pressure *directly* over the xiphoid process is very dangerous: it may damage the liver and cause severe internal bleeding. In addition, pressure on the ribs can cause them to break and damage the organs beneath them. Proper hand placement decreases the possibility of rib fracture and increases compression effectiveness.

## Body Position

The position of the rest of your body is as important as your hand position for effective compressions. External chest compression requires considerable exertion, thus positioning your body properly allows you to maintain your energy and strength to keep the cardiac arrest victim alive.

With your hands in place on the chest, straighten out your arms so that your shoulders are directly over the patient's sternum (Figure 5.69). This position directs pressure straight down on the sternum rather than off at an angle. Your knees should be aligned below your shoulders; one knee should be near the victim's shoulders and the other knee near the patient's waist. Keep your arms straight and your elbows locked. Use your body weight to exert downward pressure. Bending your elbows or pushing with your arms or shoulders requires greater effort and is more tiring.

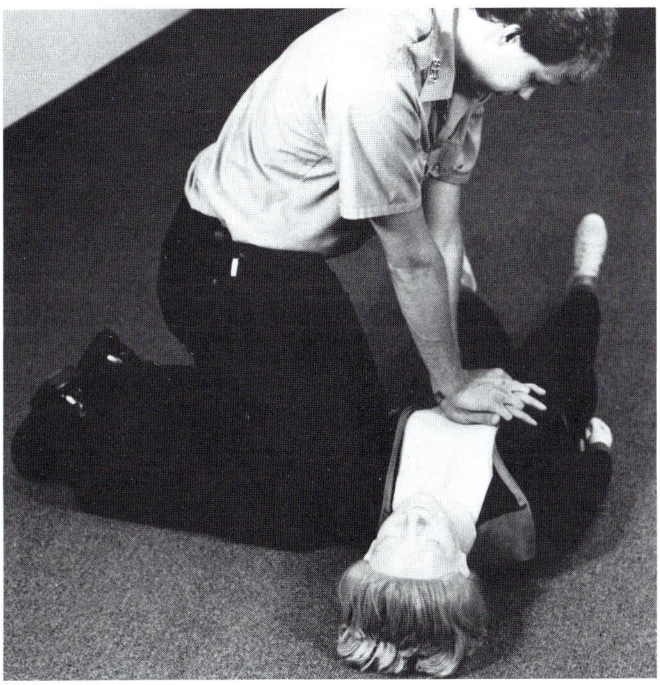

**Figure 5.69** With your hands in place on the chest, straighten out your arms so that your shoulders are directly over the patient's sternum.

With your hands and body in the proper position, lean forward with your shoulders directly over your hands until you feel as if you would fall forward if your hands and arms were not supporting you. Let the natural motion of your body falling forward provide the force to depress the victim's sternum. Bending at the hips allows your shoulders and arms to move straight up and down as a unit. DO NOT rock back and forth on your knees.

To compress the patient's sternum, DO NOT push with all of your strength, but with only enough force to depress the adult sternum 1½ to 2 inches (38 mm to 51 mm). This force provides sufficient pressure in the chest to circulate the oxygen-rich blood to maintain life.

After each compression, fully release the pressure to permit the chest to return to its normal position but do not remove your hand from the chest. This release in pressure allows blood to flow into the chest where it is oxygenated and is then available to be pumped out on the next compression. To release the pressure on the sternum, just bend up from your hips to shift the weight of your body up and away from the victim's chest. Avoid bouncing against the patient's chest and be careful not to change your hand position in any way. If you lose your hand position, take the time to relocate the landmark position properly, then begin again.

## Rhythm

The time required for compression (the downstroke) should equal the time allowed for release (the upstroke). Counting aloud, "One and two and three" helps maintain both speed and rhythm. You can keep the downward pressure time and the release time the same by compressing on "one" and releasing on "and," and compressing on "two" and releasing on "and," and so on. Avoid irregular, jabbing compressions. They increase the possibility of injury and may not produce adequate flow.

## Rate and Ratio

The rate at which you perform external compressions is the same for one and two-rescuer CPR: 80-100 compressions per minute. The ratio of compressions to ventilations depends upon whether you work alone or with another rescuer. A single rescuer must perform both rescue breathing and compressions. Two rescuers can divide these tasks.

## Single-Rescuer CPR

As a single rescuer treating an adult patient, the correct ratio of compressions to ventilations is 15:2. After the first two full breaths, if the pulse check indicates cardiac arrest, you must perform cycles of 15 deep, smooth compressions and 2 full breaths. For greatest effectiveness, you should complete 4 cycles of the 15:2 ratio in 52 to 73 seconds. This means you will do 60 compressions and 8 breaths in 60 seconds. Clearly, you will have to compress faster than once a second to allow time to give the 2 full breaths. In an average cycle, the 15 compressions take 9 to 11 seconds and the 2 breaths take 2 or 3 seconds. Remember, one compression includes both the downward pressure and the release. Compressions must be smooth, regular, and uninterrupted. Release of pressure must immediately follow compression and be of equal duration.

Compress an adult patient's chest 15 times as you count "One and two and three" and so on to 15. Compress on the numbers and release on the "and." Keep your knees in place, lean over from the waist, and perform rescue breathing. Open the airway, pinch the nose, give 2 full breaths, and allow the chest to deflate between breaths (Figure 5.70). Then repeat the cycle of compressions and rescue breathing. It may be useful to insert an oral airway in order to maintain the patient's airway in an open position.

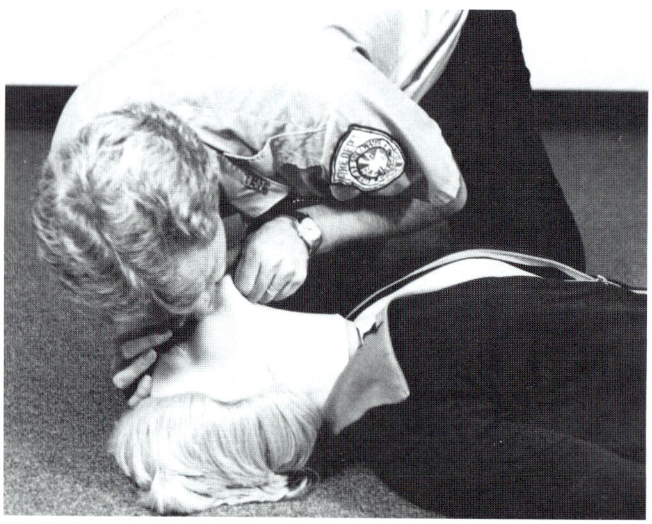

**Figure 5.70** Pinch the nostrils shut, make a seal over the patient's mouth with your own, and blow into the patient's lungs with two full breaths.

When you lean over to give rescue breathing, you lose your hand position for compressions. Since the proper location for compression is critical, both for safety and effectiveness, you must quickly locate the landmark area for compression on the lower half of the sternum every time you resume compressions.

After the first 4 cycles of 15 compressions and 2 ventilations, stop and check for a spontaneous pulse. After that, pause every few minutes to check for a spontaneous pulse. This pause should not take longer than 5 seconds. Remember that blood pressure and blood flow drop to zero when you stop!

**NOTE:** If you are alone and assistance is unlikely after one minute of CPR, you may briefly stop to call an ambulance if a phone is readily available. Rapid access to the EMS system improves the patient's chances of survival.

### Two-Rescuer CPR

Since rescue breathing must always accompany cardiac compressions, it is best to have two rescuers to divide the tasks in order to reduce rescuer fatigue. The compressor stays at the patient's side and performs external chest compressions while the ventilator, at the patient's head, keeps the airway open and performs rescue breathing (Figure 5.71). Rescuers work best on opposite sides of the patient, but two-person CPR is possible on the same side.

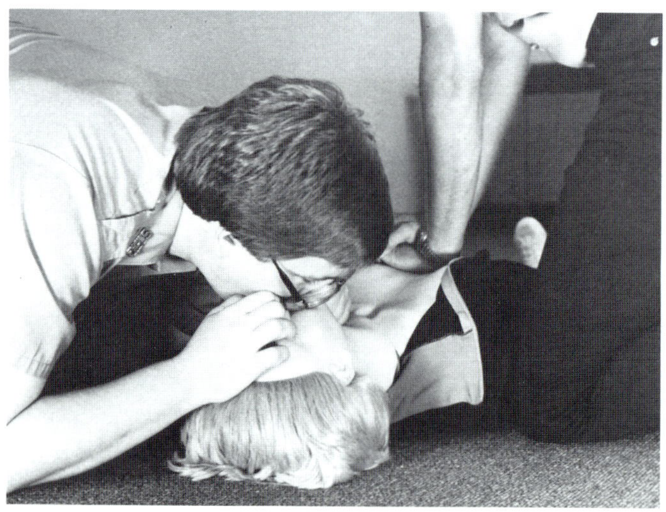

**Figure 5.71** The compressor stays at the patient's side and performs external chest compressions while the ventilator, at the patient's head, keeps the airway open and performs rescue breathing.

To begin two-rescuer CPR, the second rescuer indicates to the first rescuer that he or she is trained in CPR — that is, the second rescuer waits for the first rescuer to complete the current cycle, then says, "I know CPR, can I help?" If an ambulance is not already en route, the second rescuer should call for one immediately.

Some information needs to be exchanged between the two rescuers, but CPR must not be interrupted. After the second rescuer has called for an ambulance, the compressor accepts the offer to change to two-person CPR. While the second rescuer feels for the compression-created pulse (three or four beats so the rescuer will know that compressions are effective), he or she should indicate that there is a good pulse or that a pulse cannot be detected. If the second rescuer cannot detect a pulse, he or she should try to locate the pulse again. If the second rescuer still cannot detect a pulse, the compressions may not be effective. If this is the case, the compressor may need to check the hand position or press harder.

The first rescuer has been compressing and ventilating at a ratio of 15 compressions to 2 full breaths. After the single rescuer completes a cycle of 15 compressions, he or she gives 2 full breaths to complete the cycle and checks for a spontaneous pulse. The rescuer now stays at the patient's head and becomes the ventilator. If there is no pulse, the ventilator says, "Continue CPR." The second rescuer (the compressor) locates the correct hand position on the victim's sternum (Figure 5.72).

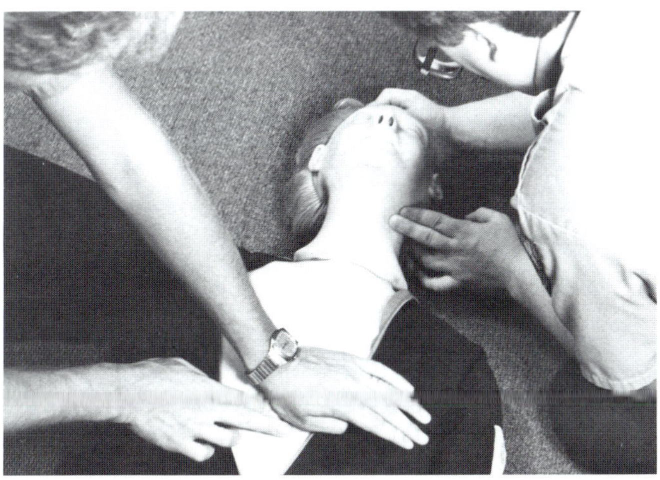

**Figure 5.72** During the pulse check, the compressor locates the proper hand position to resume compressions and waits for directions to continue.

The correct rate of compressions for single- or two-rescuer is 80-100 per minute. For two-rescuer CPR, the correct rate of compressions is 80-100 per minute, but the correct ratio of compressions to ventilations is 5:1. As the compressor pauses after the fifth compression, the ventilator is responsible for ventilating *once*, giving a full breath that lasts 1 to 1½ seconds.

The ventilator should check for a pulse during compressions to assure that compressions are adequate. The ventilator can keep one hand on the patient's forehead, with the palm pressing on the forehead and the thumb and index fingers maintaining the nose pinch. The fingers of the other hand can be used to check the victim's carotid pulse.

## Switching CPR Positions

Two rescuers should complete 10 cycles of compressions and ventilations before switching positions. To switch positions without any significant interruption in the 5:1 rhythm, the compressor signals the change. Instead of the usual count of "One and two and three and four and," he or she says, "CHANGE and two and three and four and," or similar words that maintain the rhythm.

The compressor (now the ventilator) quickly moves into position at the patient's head after the fifth compression. The rescuer who has been performing rescue breathing completes the cycle with one full breath and moves to the chest to become the compressor. The rescuer who is now the ventilator immediately opens the airway and checks for spontaneous pulse and breathing for 5 seconds. During the pulse check, the compressor locates the proper hand position to resume compressions and waits for directions to continue. If the victim is still pulseless, the ventilator breathes once and says, "Continue CPR."

## Assess Effectiveness of CPR

The primary indicators of effective CPR are a chest rise during rescue breathing and carotid pulse felt during chest compressions.

CPR is being performed correctly if the patient's skin color improves or if normal color is retained — this is especially noticeable around the lips and nailbeds. You may also notice that the patient's pupils react to light rather than remaining fixed and dilated. If these changes are not present, however, circumstances other than CPR may be involved.

### CPR Adjuncts

Several CPR adjuncts are commonly used to improve the effectiveness of CPR and to reduce rescuer fatigue. The CPR board provides a firm surface beneath the patient's shoulders and helps to ensure an open airway (Figure 5.73). Some ambulances carry external cardiac compression machines. After CPR is begun manually, these machines can be set to administer chest compressions and ventilations at the correct ratios (Figure 5.74).

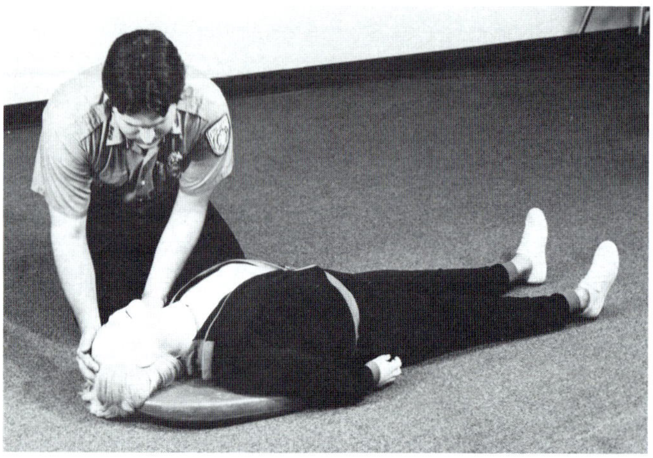

**Figure 5.73** A CPR board helps both to provide a firm surface beneath the patient and to keep the airway open.

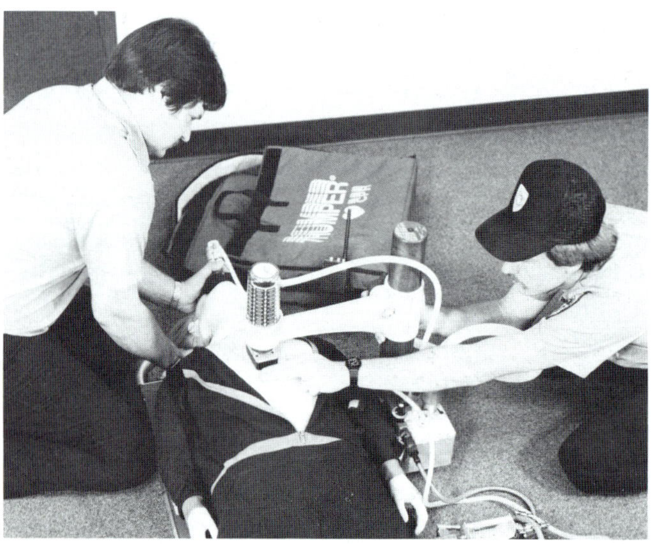

**Figure 5.74** A mechanical CPR device may be used by EMTs and paramedics to administer chest compressions and to ventilate the patient's lungs.

## CPR FOR INFANTS AND CHILDREN

The same *principles* govern CPR in infants, children, and adults, but the *techniques* differ somewhat according to the age and size of the patient. For the purposes of the following discussion, an *infant* is a baby less than one year old and a *child* is one to eight years old. Adult procedures apply to patients who are over eight years old.

### Causes of Respiratory and Cardiac Arrest in Infants and Children

For young patients, respiratory and cardiac arrest due to heart disease are rare. Cardiac arrest that follows a blocked airway is much more common. The most common causes of respiratory and cardiac arrest are as follows:

- Foreign body obstruction of the airway caused by food or small toys
- Near-drowning
- Trauma, such as an automobile accident
- Accidental poisoning
- Smoke inhalation
- Sudden Infant Death Syndrome (SIDS)
- Infection of the airway, such as epiglottitis

## TECHNIQUES OF CPR FOR INFANTS AND CHILDREN

As with adults, the steps of CPR for infants and children are as follows:

Step 1: AIRWAY
- Determine unresponsiveness
- Call for help
- Position the patient
- Open the airway

Step 2: BREATHING
- Assess breathing; determine breathlessness
- Perform rescue breathing
- Dislodge a foreign object from the airway

Step 3: CIRCULATION
- Assess circulation; determine pulselessness
- Activate EMS system
- Begin chest compressions

Step 4: ASSESS EFFECTIVENESS OF CPR
- Look for chest rise and improvement in color
- Determine pulselessness

Step 5: CONTINUE CPR

### Determine Unresponsiveness

Determine unresponsiveness by gently tapping or shaking the patient. You may also flick your fingers against the soles of the feet (Figure 5.75). If the patient is conscious and has an airway obstruction, you must determine whether there is good or poor air exchange or a complete obstruction, as well as the probable cause of the obstruction.

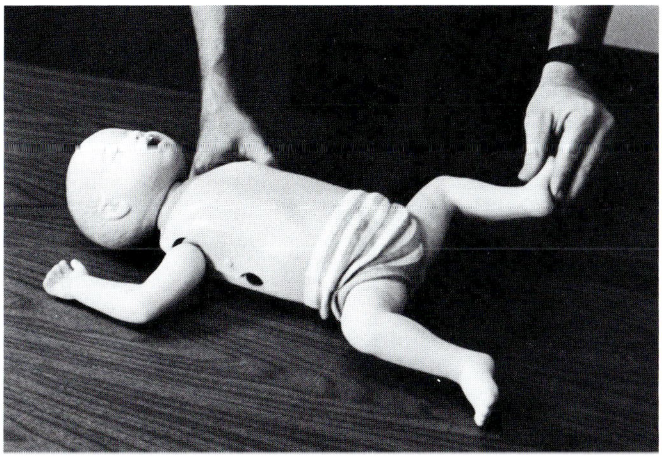

**Figure 5.75** If the patient is an infant or small child, you may establish unresponsiveness by flicking your fingers against the soles of the feet.

### Call for Help

As a first responder, you should make sure that EMTs or paramedics are on their way. If you are in a home or do not have access to a radio, enlist relatives or bystanders to telephone for additional help.

### Position the Patient

There are two methods for handling an infant (Figure 5.76). One is to support the infant on your forearm, tilting the head slightly as you support it in the palm of one hand. The other method is to place the infant lying face up on a firm surface, such as a table.

### Open the Airway

If you are holding the infant, tip the head back slightly so that the infant looks as though he or she is sniffing (see Figure 5.76). If the infant is lying on a firm surface, gently position the head using the head-tilt chin-lift method, again tilting the head only to the sniffing position (Figure 5.77). If the infant is lying on a firm surface and the head tilt

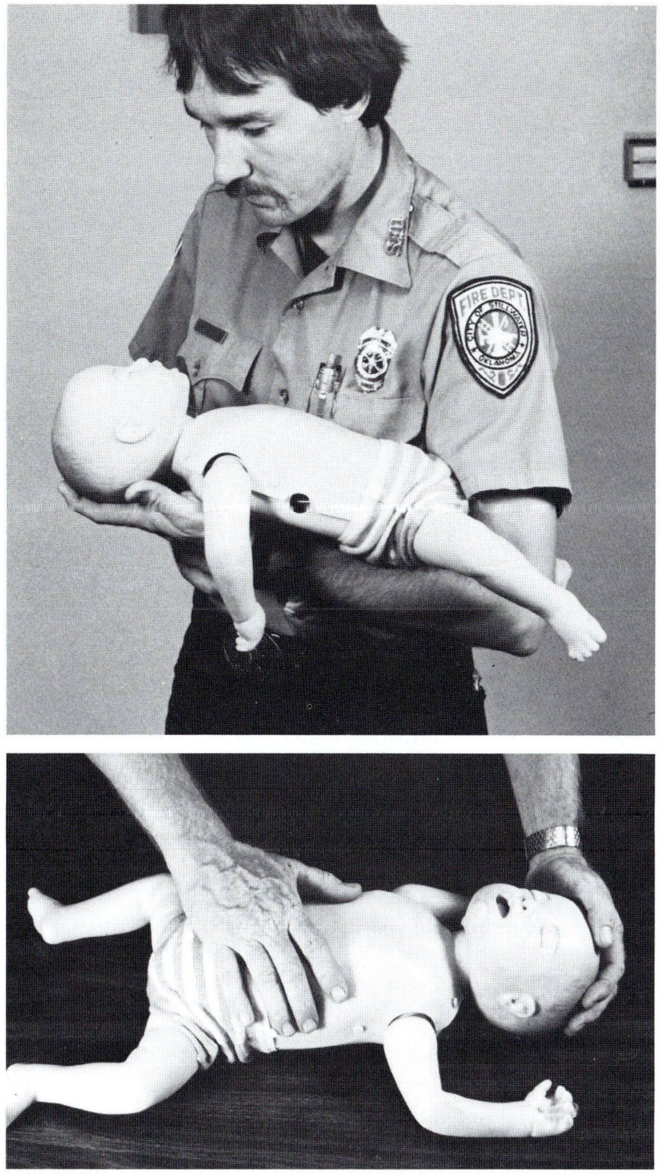

**Figure 5.76** Position an infant either on your forearm, supporting the head in the palm of one hand, or lying face up on a firm surface.

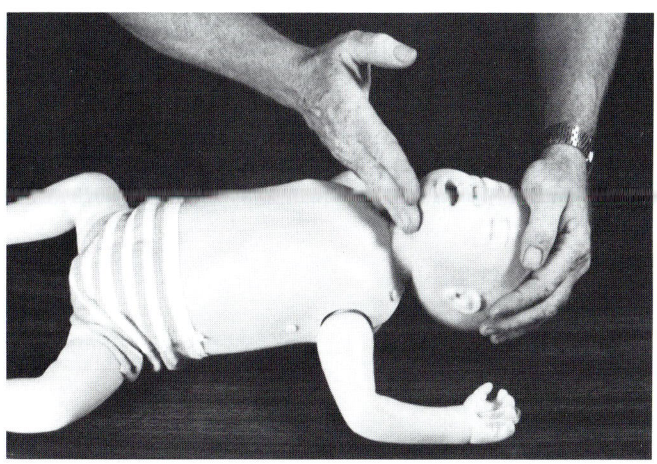

**Figure 5.77** Open the infant's airway by gently positioning the head using the head-tilt chin-lift method, tilting the head only to the sniffing position.

lifts the infant's shoulders, slip your hand under his or her back. Alternately, you may place a towel under the infant's shoulders to provide support. This action maintains the open airway position and provides a firm surface in the event that chest compressions are necessary.

### Assess Breathing

Assess breathing for infants in the same manner as you would for an adult or child: place your ear and cheek very close to the infant's mouth and nose and look, listen, and feel for movement of air. If the infant is breathing, maintain the airway in an open position and arrange for transportation to a medical facility.

### Perform Rescue Breathing

Remember the differences between adults and infants or very small children when you perform rescue breathing. Cover the infant's mouth *and* nose with your mouth. Be sure to adjust the volume of your breath to the size of the patient. For an infant, puffs of air from the cheeks usually provide adequate ventilation. You may choose to use the adult method of nose pinch and mouth seal for large children. Use larger breaths when you ventilate children, but not as large as you would use for an adult.

Watch the patient's chest to determine whether ventilation is adequate. After the first two full breaths, ventilate infants once every 3 seconds (20 breaths per minute), and children every 4 seconds (15 breaths per minute).

### Dislodge a Foreign Object from the Airway

If the infant or child's chest does not rise when you attempt to ventilate the lungs, reposition the head and try again. If you are still unsuccessful, you must suspect a foreign body obstruction and take steps to remove it (see Section 1).

### Assess Circulation

After you have given two full breaths and determined that the infant's chest rises as you perform rescue breathing, check the pulse at the brachial artery. If the pulse is present, continue rescue breathing at a rate of once every 3 seconds for infants and once every 4 seconds for children. If the pulse is absent, begin chest compressions.

### Begin Chest Compressions

Because the ventricles of an infant's heart lie higher in the chest than an adult's, the proper hand position for chest compression is slightly higher. To locate the landmark position for compressions on an infant, imagine a line across the infant's chest that intersects both nipples (the nipple line). Now, place your index finger just below this line where it intersects the sternum. The place where your middle and ring fingers touch the infant's chest is the compression area. Stated another way, the proper compression area on an infant is one finger's width below the nipple line, over the midsternum (Figure 5.78). DO NOT compress the *lower* sternum or xiphoid, since this action may lacerate the liver.

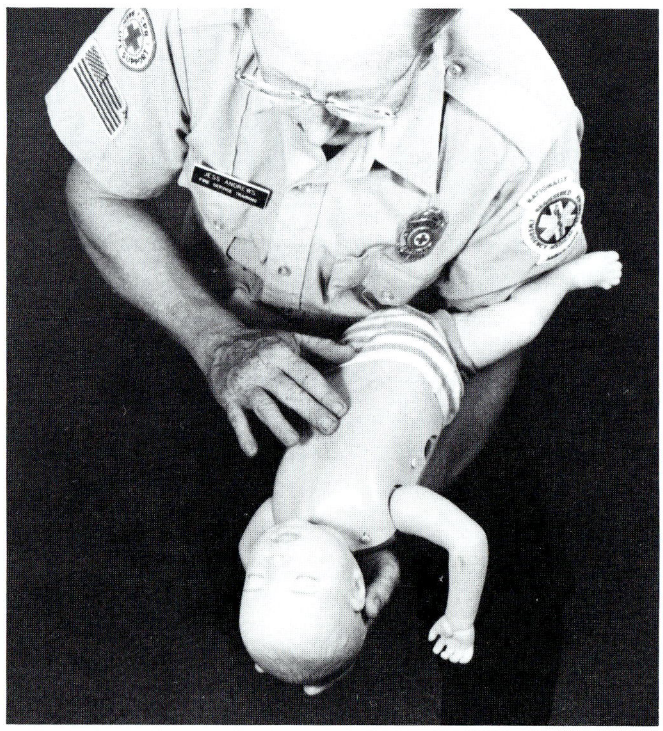

**Figure 5.78** The proper compression area on an infant is one finger's width below the nipple line, over the midsternum.

As the baby grows, the heart and upper abdominal organs take proportionally less space and descend gradually to their adult positions. Thus, for a *child*, the adult landmark method for determining proper hand placement is recommended.

The chest of an infant or child is smaller, of course, and more flexible than an adult's, so much less pressure is required to compress the sternum. For infants, use only the tips of your fingers to compress the sternum ½ to 1 inch (12 mm to 25 mm). For children, use only the heel of *one* hand to produce the required 1 to 1½ inch (25 mm to 38 mm) compression (Figure 5.79).

Compress an infant's chest at the rate of 100 compressions per minute. The correct ratio of compressions to ventilations is 5:1. A child's heartbeat is slightly slower; compress 80-100 times per minute, maintaining the 5:1 ratio. Table 5.1 lists different CPR techniques for adults, infants, and children.

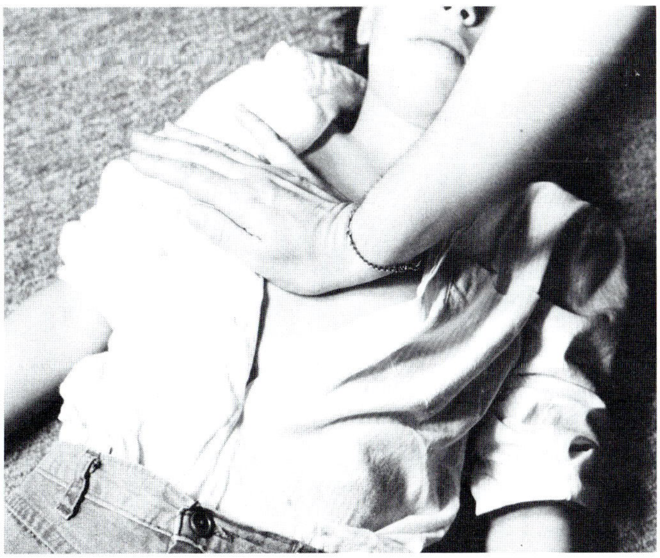

**Figure 5.79** When you administer CPR to children, use only the heel of one hand to administer chest compressions.

## SPECIAL SITUATIONS INVOLVING CPR

### Sudden Infant Death Syndrome (SIDS)

Sudden Infant Death Syndrome, also known as "crib death," kills more infants between one month and one year of age in this country than any other disease. Approximately 10,000 infant deaths are attributed to SIDS each year. The cause of the condition is unknown, although recent research indicates that it may be related to an immature breathing control center in the baby's brain.

While the death of an infant is devastating under any circumstances, SIDS cases are especially tragic because the condition kills apparently healthy babies; moreover, it kills them silently. There are no warning signs and, consequently, no preventive measures to be taken against the condition. Another tragic aspect of SIDS is the effect it has upon the child's parents. They typically blame themselves for the baby's death, although in almost every case the baby is simply put down to sleep and found dead later — usually well after resuscitative efforts are likely to be effective.

Nonetheless, when you are called to treat a SIDS victim, it is imperative that you begin CPR *immediately* (even if the baby is obviously dead) and continue CPR until additional help arrives. Bear in mind that the parents will, understandably, be highly distraught. Remain calm and dem-

**CPR TECHNIQUES**
**TABLE 5.1**

| | ADULTS | CHILDREN | INFANTS |
|---|---|---|---|
| AIRWAY | Head-tilt chin-lift maneuver; Modified jaw-thrust maneuver if spinal injury is suspected | Head-tilt chin-lift maneuver; Modified jaw-thrust maneuver if spinal injury is suspected | Head-tilt chin-lift maneuver to sniffing position |
| BREATHING | Tight seal over mouth; pinch nose. Two full breaths, each lasting 1 to 1½ seconds. Breathe every 5 seconds (12 times/minute) | Tight seal over mouth; pinch nose. Two breaths sufficient to cause normal chest rise, each breath lasting 1 to 1½ seconds. Breathe every 4 seconds (15 times/minute) | Tight seal over nose *and* mouth. Two breaths using puffs of air from the cheeks, each breath lasting 1 to 1½ seconds. Breathe every 3 seconds. (20 times/minute) |
| CHEST COMPRESSIONS | | | |
| METHOD | Both hands | Heel of one hand | 2-3 fingers |
| DEPTH | 1½ to 2 inches (38 mm to 51 mm) | 1 to 1½ inches (25 mm to 38 mm) | ½ to 1 inch (12 mm to 25 mm) |
| RATE OF COMPRESSIONS | 80-100/minute | 80-100/minute | 100/minute |
| RATIO OF COMPRESSIONS TO VENTILATIONS | 5:1 Two rescuers<br>15:2 One rescuer | 5:1 Two rescuers<br>15:2 One rescuer | 5:1 One rescuer |
| PULSE CHECK | Carotid artery | Carotid artery | Brachial artery |

onstrate by your actions that everything medically possible is being done for the baby. Ideally, one rescuer should administer CPR while another attends to the parents. This approach may help the parents to accept that they have done all that they could have done for the baby.

## Near-Drowning

Drowning is a type of asphyxia (concurrent decrease in oxygen and increase in carbon dioxide in the body) that is the result of prolonged submersion in water. Under such circumstances, of course, respiration cannot take place, and death is the result.

Normally, a drowning victim's first reaction when water enters the mouth and nose is to cough and swallow while trying to take a deep breath. If the head is under water, the victim may involuntarily inhale and swallow water. If water enters the trachea or larynx, an automatic muscular contraction called *laryngospasm* occurs. This spasm seals the airway, causing the victim to die of suffocation.

A 40-minute submersion time is the longest time recorded for survival with no neurological damage. Many physicians believe that there are two major factors involved in the extended survival times for some near-drowning victims. The first is hypothermia, a lowering of body temperature below 95°F (35°C). Hypothermia's life-preserving effects are basically decreases in blood flow to the brain and consumption of oxygen (see Chapter 14, Injuries and Illnesses from Heat and Cold). The second factor is a bodily reaction known as the mammalian dive reflex.

The diving reflex is triggered when the face is exposed to cold water, and the body reacts by shunting blood from the extremities to the core. In this way the diving reflex conserves oxygen, using it only where it is needed to immediately sustain life. This reflex, however, causes a near-drowning victim to appear lifeless, with apparent pulselessness and a greatly reduced heart rate, which may cause rescuers to assume that the victim is dead. Thus, it is critical that you begin basic life support for *all* drowning victims.

While it is essential to remove the victim from the water as soon as possible, take precautions so that you, too, do not become a victim. Ideally, a rescue unit or lifeguard should be at the scene when you arrive. If you must participate in the rescue, wear a life jacket and do not venture out onto ice or into the water without a rope around your waist that is securely tied off.

Many drowning and near-drowning incidents involve spinal cord injuries, especially in cases of diving accidents, so be prepared to immobilize the victim on a long backboard (see Chapter 8, Injuries to the Skull, Spine, and Chest).

### TREATMENT FOR NEAR-DROWNING

The emergency treatment for near-drowning victims is basic life support according to the ABC's. Cold-water drowning victims may appear to be clinically dead: the pupils may be widely dilated and unresponsive and the body may be cold and rigid. These signs do not mean that resuscitation is impossible, so begin basic life support at once.

Open the victim's airway with the head-tilt chin-lift or modified jaw-thrust maneuver and begin rescue breathing while the patient is still in the water, if possible (Figure 5.80). It is not necessary to try to expel water from the lungs; however, if you are unable to ventilate the patient's lungs, perform the Heimlich maneuver with the victim's head turned to the side, then attempt rescue breathing again. If the victim is pulseless, of course, CPR must be started as soon as the patient can be placed on a firm surface. Arrange for rapid transport to the nearest medical facility.

## Electric Shock

Electrical burns occur when the body comes between the source of an electrical charge and the grounding site. When this happens, the body becomes a conductor for the electricity as it flows to the ground. Electrical injuries can be caused by alternating current or direct current. Alternating current is more deadly because it causes severe muscle contractions that can immobilize the victim, causing him or her to be "frozen" to the source of the current.

Electricity does its major damage inside the body, not to the skin itself. This is because electric-

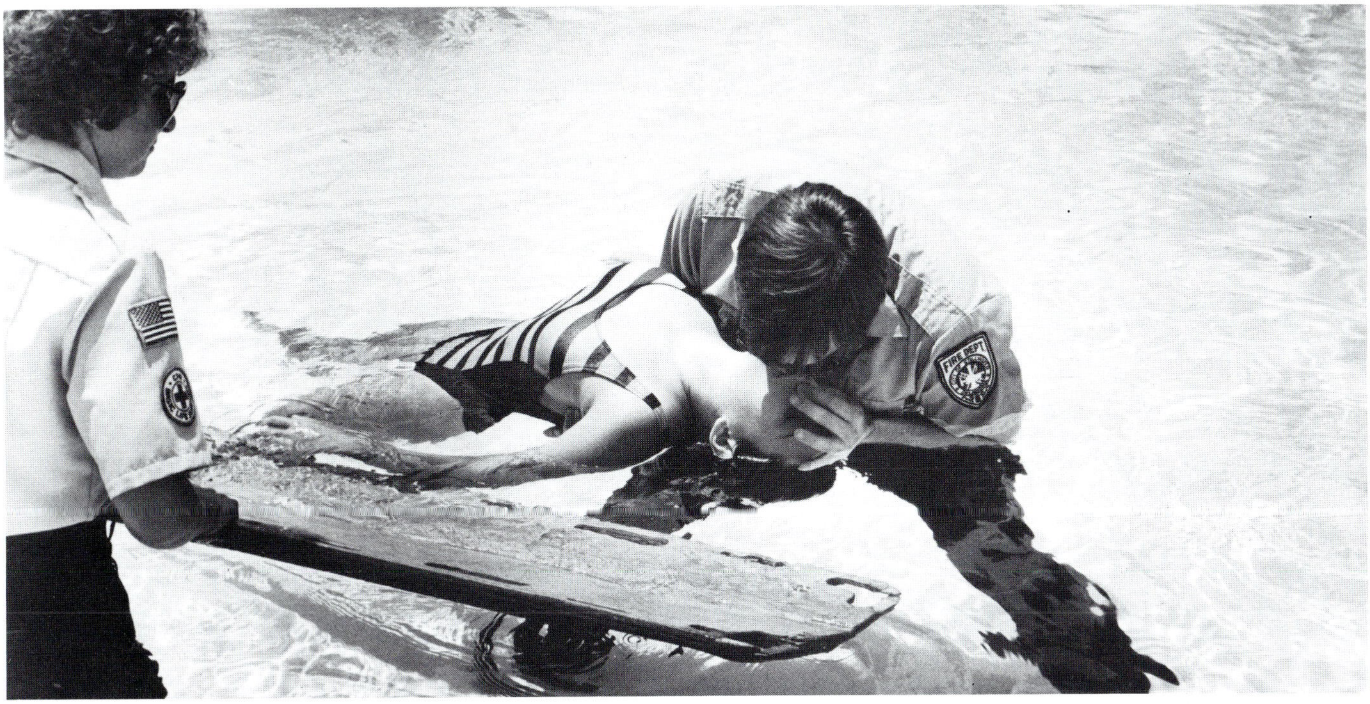

**Figure 5.80** Begin rescue breathing while the victim is still in the water.

ity is converted into extreme heat as it travels from the point of contact through the body. Massive internal injury to muscles, nerves, tissues, blood vessels, and internal organs is common.

In addition to internal damage, electricity often causes respiratory and/or cardiac arrest due to ventricular fibrillation (rapid, ineffective contraction of the heart). For this reason, the patient's ABC's must be stabilized before any electrical burns are evaluated.

### TREATMENT

If you are called to aid someone who has come into contact with an electrical current, your first impulse may be to rush to assist the patient. Be cautious or you may become a victim yourself. At the scene of the accident, keep the following safety points in mind:

- The patient may still be in contact with the source of the current. Do not endanger yourself by touching the patient, metal objects, water, or wet ground. Unless your department is trained in the use of hot sticks, lineman's gloves, and in moving electrical lines, do not try to provide medical assistance until all electrical hazards have been removed by the power company.
- Assume that all downed wires are live wires unless you are informed otherwise by a power company employee.
- Do not touch any wires, power lines, or other electrical sources until they have been deactivated by a power company employee.
- Instruct anyone who is trapped in an automobile by downed power lines to stay inside the car until the power company can turn off the power source and remove the lines.
- If the victim is lying on an electric cord, it may be possible to use a nonconducting object such as a broomstick to roll the victim away from the electrical hazard.

As soon as the patient can be safely moved from the source of the injury, look to the ABC's first before you look at the burns. It is more than likely that the patient has suffered respiratory or cardiac arrest from electric current passing through the body. Open the patient's airway using the modified jaw-thrust maneuver, determine whether he or she is breathing, and administer CPR if necessary. Arrange for immediate transportation to a medical facility. Often a patient who appears dead can be revived by rapid attention to the ABC's.

# 6

# Shock

**NFPA STANDARD 1001**
**EMERGENCY MEDICAL CARE**
**Fire Fighter II**

**4-4.4** The fire fighter shall identify the signs and symptoms of internal bleeding.

**4-4.5** The fire fighter shall demonstrate the emergency care for a person with known or suspected internal bleeding.

**4-4.15** The fire fighter shall identify symptoms and demonstrate emergency medical care of traumatic shock.

# Chapter 6
# Shock

The body needs a constant supply of oxygen and a carefully regulated amount of water to sustain life. The human body is chiefly water; it makes up 60 percent of the total body weight of an adult. Water is found both in the cells (intracellular fluid), and outside the cells (extracellular fluid). Water provides the environment in which the chemical reactions necessary for life take place. Water also provides a transport medium for nutrients, hormones, and waste materials. The liquid portion of the blood, known as plasma, carries red blood cells, white blood cells, and vital nutrients. The blood also carries waste materials (mostly carbon dioxide and acids) to the lungs, skin, and kidneys to be eliminated by the body.

Most important of all, the blood carries oxygen to all the body's cells. As oxygen is taken into the lungs, it combines with the blood, then the heart pumps the oxygenated blood to all parts of the body. An organ is *perfused* (receiving sufficient circulation of blood and, therefore, oxygen) if blood is entering it through the arteries and leaving it through the veins. Perfusion keeps body cells healthy by providing them with oxygen and other nutrients and by removing waste products.

To work properly, the body must have an effective pump (the heart), a closed network of tubes (arteries and veins), and the proper amount of fluid pumping through the system (Figure 6.1). If any one of these components fails to work (because of injury or illness, for example) body cells will not receive the amount of oxygen they need and will begin to suffocate. The condition that results from inadequate tissue perfusion is known as shock.

Shock can result from any injury or illness that leads to

- Failure of the heart to pump a sufficient amount of blood
- Severe blood or fluid loss so that there is insufficient blood traveling through the system
- Enlargement of blood vessels so that there is insufficient blood to fill them

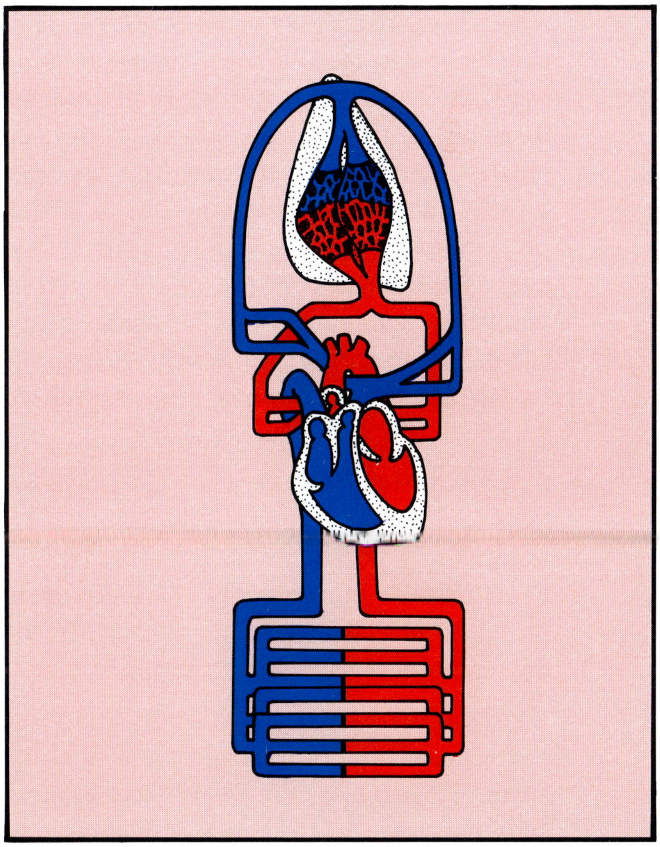

**6.1** The body needs fluid, a closed network of tubes, and a working pump in order to provide oxygen to all the body's cells.

- Breathing problems resulting in insufficient oxygen traveling through the system
- Severe allergic reaction
- Severe bacterial infection or untreated illness

Shock can follow severe injuries, untreated illness, or emotionally upsetting situations. Shock may be caused by profuse bleeding, traumatic injury, stroke, heart attack, heat exhaustion, severe burns, chemical or food poisoning, acute allergic reactions, or infection. No matter what the cause of shock, the consequences are the same: inadequate circulation of oxygenated blood, which leads to failure of the body systems and death if not treated.

## TYPES AND CAUSES OF SHOCK

The major types of shock are as follows:

- **Hypovolemic Shock** is caused by heavy loss of vital fluids from the body, such as blood, plasma, gastrointestinal fluids, and excessive sweating. The most common type of hypovolemic shock is *hemorrhagic shock*, which is caused by loss of whole blood. This loss leaves an insufficient amount of blood to fill the circulatory system. Blood volume may be reduced from external bleeding (open wounds); internal bleeding (injuries to internal organs); or severe burns, which produce extensive loss of plasma (the liquid part of the blood). Severe diarrhea and/or vomiting can cause loss of body fluids sufficient to bring on shock. Excessive sweating, unless replaced by increased water intake, can result in shock.
- **Cardiogenic Shock** occurs when the heart fails to pump or pumps inadequately, thus impairing circulation. A heart attack or heart disease may prevent the heart from pumping forcefully enough to provide the necessary perfusion of body organs.
- **Neurogenic Shock** results from an injury that causes loss of control of the nervous system. Normally, the blood vessels meet body demands for increases or decreases in blood flow by dilating or constricting. For example, during strenuous exercise more blood (and therefore more oxygen) flows to the large muscles doing the work and less to the digestive system, which does not need the extra blood flow then. This constant adjusting of the size of blood vessels, which is controlled by the nervous system, maintains the blood pressure at a steady rate and keeps blood flowing throughout the circulatory system. If the nervous system is damaged, the blood vessels may be temporarily or permanently paralyzed; they can no longer react to stimuli from the nervous system and remain widely dilated. Then, the blood circulating is not enough to fill the enlarged blood vessels, which causes the circulatory system to collapse.
- **Psychogenic Shock** (known as syncope, or fainting) occurs when blood vessels suddenly dilate, temporarily leaving the brain short of oxygen. This type of shock may be the result of anxiety, fear, joy, or the sight of blood. The effects of psychogenic shock are temporary because blood flow returns to the brain when the person faints. The chief danger to the patient from this type of shock is any injury the patient may suffer from falling, such as striking the head.
- **Septic Shock** occurs when severe bacterial infection causes toxins (poisons) to be released into the bloodstream. These toxins cause the blood vessels to dilate, which leaves an insufficient amount of blood to fill the circulatory system. The toxins also cause plasma to leak through the capillary walls, resulting in loss of fluid. Septic shock has elements of neurogenic shock (dilation of blood vessels) and hypovolemic shock (loss of fluid).
- **Metabolic Shock** is associated with drastic disturbance in body chemistry resulting from illness or disease. When disease causes serious loss of body fluids through vomiting, diarrhea, or excess urination (polyuria), metabolic shock is a type of hypovolemic shock.

- **Anaphylactic Shock** occurs when a person comes in contact with a substance to which he or she is extremely allergic. It is the most severe form of allergic reaction. Anaphylactic shock is indeed a true emergency and must be treated immediately. A severe reaction can result in a blocked airway due to constriction of the bronchial tubes and swelling of the larynx. The best the first responder can do is to provide basic life support, administer oxygen, and assist ventilations as necessary. For more information on anaphylactic shock, see Chapter 10, Medical Emergencies.

**ONE OF THE MOST IMPORTANT FUNCTIONS THE FIRST RESPONDER CAN PERFORM IS TO ASSUME AND TREAT FOR SHOCK IN ANY MEDICAL EMERGENCY OR FOR ANY SERIOUS INJURY.** Treating for shock will not harm the patient; however, anticipating shock and treating for it may save a patient's life. In particular, anticipate shock for the emergencies listed in Table 6.1.

## HOW THE BODY TRIES TO MAINTAIN ADEQUATE CIRCULATION

Remember that the body must maintain a careful balance of fluid and oxygen to keep all its cells adequately perfused. If the body's cells do not receive enough oxygen, they must turn to other sources for fuel, such as fats. Using other fuel sources than oxygen is an inefficient way to create energy and causes acid waste materials to build up in the blood. The body seeks to remove these waste materials in several ways. First, a buffer system in the body tries to neutralize the acids chemically. The buffer system is automatic and reacts to excess acid almost immediately. If there is still too much acid in the blood, respiratory centers in the brain are stimulated to increase the rate and depth of respiration. Breathing more rapidly and more deeply brings in more oxygen and eliminates more carbon dioxide. If both the buffer and respiratory systems fail to restore the body to normal, the kidneys act as a third line of defense; however, the kidneys take several hours to days to begin filtering and eliminating waste materials.

### TABLE 6.1
### COMMON CAUSES OF SHOCK

**INTERNAL BLEEDING DUE TO TRAUMA**

CHEST TRAUMA - suspected pneumothorax, hemothorax, pericardial tamponade; flail chest; bruises on the chest, mechanism of injury that suggests blunt trauma to the chest

ABDOMEN - evidenced by rigidity, bruising, severe pain

FRACTURES - particularly of the femur or pelvis; two or more fractures

**INTERNAL BLEEDING DUE TO ILLNESS**

Gastrointestinal bleeding, such as from an ulcer

Bleeding associated with disorders of the female reproductive system, such as ectopic pregnancy or predelivery hemorrhage

**SEVERE EXTERNAL BLEEDING**

**FLUID LOSSES**

Dehydration due to excessive vomiting, urination or diarrhea

Fluid losses due to severe infection, especially in elderly people

**BURNS**

The brain is very demanding: it is the organ most sensitive to lack of oxygen. If the brain still does not receive enough oxygen, it signals the body to release epinephrine. Epinephrine causes the pulse to increase and the blood vessels near the skin to constrict, causing the skin to cool but preserving oxygen flow to the brain and kidneys. Epinephrine also causes the skin to sweat, giving the shock patient clammy skin. As less and less oxygen reaches the brain, the body's compensatory mechanisms begin to fail: the blood vessels dilate, blood pressure drops, and the patient dies unless oxygen and vital fluids can be replaced.

## SIGNS AND SYMPTOMS OF SHOCK

The most common signs and symptoms of shock are as follows (Figure 6.2):

- Restlessness or anxiety
- Extreme thirst
- Dull, vacant-looking eyes; dilated pupils
- Nausea or vomiting
- Cold and clammy skin
- Pale or cyanotic face
- Rapid, shallow breathing; possibly labored, irregular, or gasping
- Weak, rapid pulse
- Falling blood pressure

Often, before showing any other signs of shock, a patient will appear anxious or frightened. He or she may be restless and appear unable to get comfortable. The patient may complain of thirst (the body is short of fluids) yet feel nauseated or even vomit. Because the blood vessels near the skin constrict in an effort to channel blood flow to vital organs, the skin feels cool and clammy. The patient breathes more rapidly in an effort to bring in more oxygen and eliminate waste materials, so respirations are rapid and shallow. Likewise, the heart is pumping faster to circulate the oxygenated blood, so the pulse is rapid and weak.

The vital organ most susceptible to lack of oxygen is the brain, so when oxygen levels in the body begin to drop, the patient's level of consciousness is affected. The patient may be sleepy, disoriented, or unconscious. Falling blood pressure, which is a relatively late sign of shock, indicates that the circulatory system is collapsing. Blood pressure may fall gradually or may drop suddenly. This is another reason why it is important to monitor vital signs frequently for change.

Signs of shock may not develop for an hour or more after an injury. The patient may show few signs of shock at first, leading you to believe that there is little cause for concern. But a patient's condition can deteriorate very rapidly, so **DO NOT WAIT TO SUSPECT SHOCK UNTIL THE PATIENT'S BLOOD PRESSURE FALLS.** Pay particular attention to elderly people and to children. The aged and the weak do not withstand shock as well as others, and an injury or illness that ordinarily would not be fatal may be if it is complicated by shock. Watch children carefully because they do not exhibit signs of shock until they are already in deep shock. Treat shock signs in a child as an emergency.

Not all types of shock exhibit the same signs (see Table 6.2). Neurogenic shock is a good case in point. Since the blood vessels are dilated rather than constricted, the skin does not cool like it does

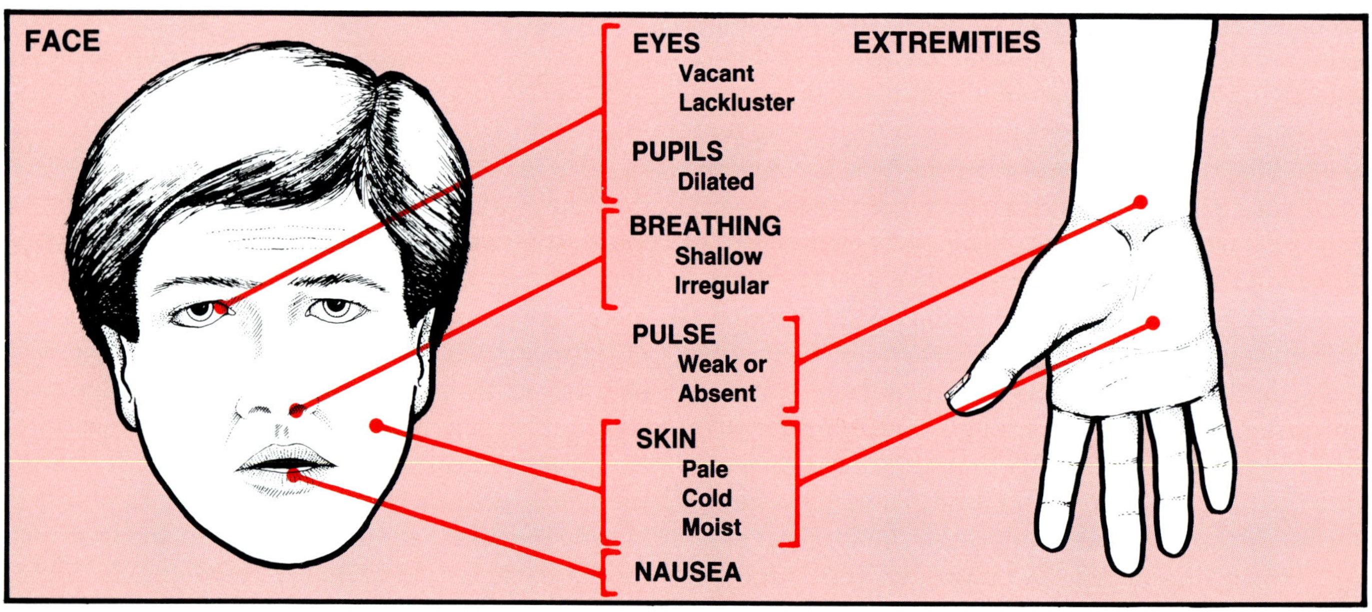


**Figure 6.2** All first responders should know how to evaluate a patient for signs of shock. Pay special attention to level of consciousness, respirations, pulse, and skin condition.

**TABLE 6.2**
**SIGNS AND SYMPTOMS OF SHOCK**

| TYPE | CAUSE | SIGNS AND SYMPTOMS | TREATMENT |
|---|---|---|---|
| **Hypovolemic Shock** | Loss of fluid due to severe bleeding, burns, vomiting, diarrhea, excessive sweating | Restlessness; anxiety<br>Pale, cold, clammy skin<br>Rapid, weak pulse<br>Rapid, shallow breathing<br>Nausea or vomiting<br>Falling blood pressure | Position patient lying down; elevate legs<br>Establish an airway<br>If hemorrhagic shock (caused by severe bleeding), control bleeding by direct pressure or pressure points<br>Administer oxygen<br>Maintain body temperature<br>Give nothing to eat or drink<br>Monitor vital signs and level of consciousness frequently<br>Arrange for transport to a medical facility |
| **Cardiogenic Shock** | Damage to the heart, leaving it unable to pump adequately<br>Examples: heart attack, congestive heart failure | Restlessness; anxiety<br>Pale, cold, clammy skin<br>Rapid, weak pulse<br>Rapid, shallow breathing<br>Nausea or vomiting<br>Falling blood pressure | Position patient lying down unless there is difficulty breathing<br>Establish an airway<br>Administer oxygen<br>Maintain body temperature<br>Give nothing to eat or drink<br>Monitor vital signs and level of consciousness frequently<br>Arrange for transport to a medical facility |
| **Neurogenic Shock** | Injury causing loss of control of nervous system, resulting in dilated blood vessels<br>Example: spinal cord injury | Pulse may be normal or even slow<br>Warm, dry skin<br>Low blood pressure | Position patient lying down; elevate legs<br>NOTE: Take extra care handling someone with a suspected spinal cord injury; immobilize the head and neck first<br>Establish an airway<br>Administer oxygen<br>Maintain body temperature; dilated blood vessels increase loss of body heat<br>Give nothing to eat or drink<br>Monitor vital signs and level of consciousness frequently<br>Arrange for transport to a medical facility |
| **Psychogenic Shock** (also known as fainting or syncope) | Short-term neurogenic shock: Blood vessels suddenly dilate, leaving the brain temporarily short of oxygen<br>Examples: sudden emotional upset, fear, joy, sight of blood | Sudden unconsciousness<br>Pulse may be regular and full<br>Breathing may be normal | Position patient lying down; elevate legs<br>Establish an airway<br>Administer oxygen<br>Maintain body temperature<br>Give nothing to eat or drink<br>Monitor vital signs and level of consciousness frequently<br>Keep patient lying down when he or she regains consciousness<br>Arrange for transport to a medical facility |
| **Septic Shock** | Bacterial infection in the bloodstream<br>Examples: diabetes, cancer, intestinal or urinary tract infections, infection following childbirth or abortion | Skin may remain warm and dry<br>Elevated body temperature due to infection<br>May have chills<br>Rapid, weak pulse<br>Rapid, shallow breathing<br>Falling blood pressure | Position patient lying down; elevate legs<br>Establish an airway<br>Administer oxygen<br>Maintain body temperature<br>Give nothing to eat or drink<br>Monitor vital signs and level of consciousness frequently<br>Arrange for transport to a medical facility |
| **Metabolic Shock** | Severe disturbance in body chemistry and loss of body fluids caused by illness or disease | Similar to hypovolemic shock:<br>Restlessness; anxiety<br>Pale, cold, clammy skin<br>Rapid, weak pulse<br>Rapid, shallow breathing<br>Falling blood pressure | Position patient lying down; elevate legs<br>Establish an airway<br>Administer oxygen<br>Maintain body temperature<br>Give nothing to eat or drink<br>Monitor vital signs and level of consciousness frequently<br>Arrange for transport to a medical facility |
| **Anaphylactic Shock** | Severe allergic reaction to food, drugs, insect stings, or chemicals<br>Examples: penicillin, bee stings, shellfish, nuts | Flushed, red skin, or very pale, ashen skin<br>Swelling, especially around eyes, lips, ears, hands and feet<br>Intense itching; hives<br>Difficulty breathing, accompanied by sneezing, wheezing, or coughing<br>Feeling of tightness in the chest<br>Nausea, vomiting, cramps, diarrhea<br>Rapid, weak pulse<br>Falling blood pressure | Position patient lying down unless there is difficulty breathing<br>Establish an airway<br>Administer oxygen<br>Arrange for *immediate* transport to a medical facility |

with other types of shock. Similarly, the heart does not receive signals to speed up pumping. So the patient may feel warm and dry, have a normal or even slow pulse, yet have falling blood pressure. The patient suffering from septic shock usually has an elevated temperature because of the underlying infection. In the case of anaphylactic shock, the patient has difficulty breathing (dyspnea), may break out in hives, and may exhibit swelling of the face and hands. If the reaction is very swift, the larynx may swell enough to block the airway.

## TREATMENT FOR SHOCK

Shock can be controlled if it is recognized and treated promptly. Shock cannot be reversed but proper treatment can keep it from worsening. The major steps for treating shock are as follows:

- **ESTABLISH AN OPEN AIRWAY.** This is always the first step of any emergency treatment. All your care will be ineffective if the patient cannot breathe.
- Make sure the patient is breathing and administer oxygen. Since shock is caused by inadequate oxygenation of tissues, it is vitally important that the patient be able to take in as much oxygen as possible. Provide artificial ventilation if necessary.
- Treat the cause of shock:
  — Control bleeding
  — Splint fractures as necessary
- Position the patient to put the least stress on vital systems and to provide maximum blood flow to vital organs, usually lying down with legs elevated.
- Prevent loss of body heat.
- Avoid rough handling of the patient.
- Do not give the patient anything to eat or drink.
- Monitor vital signs and level of consciousness frequently.
- Arrange for immediate transport to a medical facility.

### Position the Patient to Increase Blood Flow to Vital Organs

Generally, the patient should be lying down (supine) with the legs elevated 8 to 12 inches (203 mm to 304 mm) (Figure 6.3). This position favors the flow of blood to the head and chest where it is

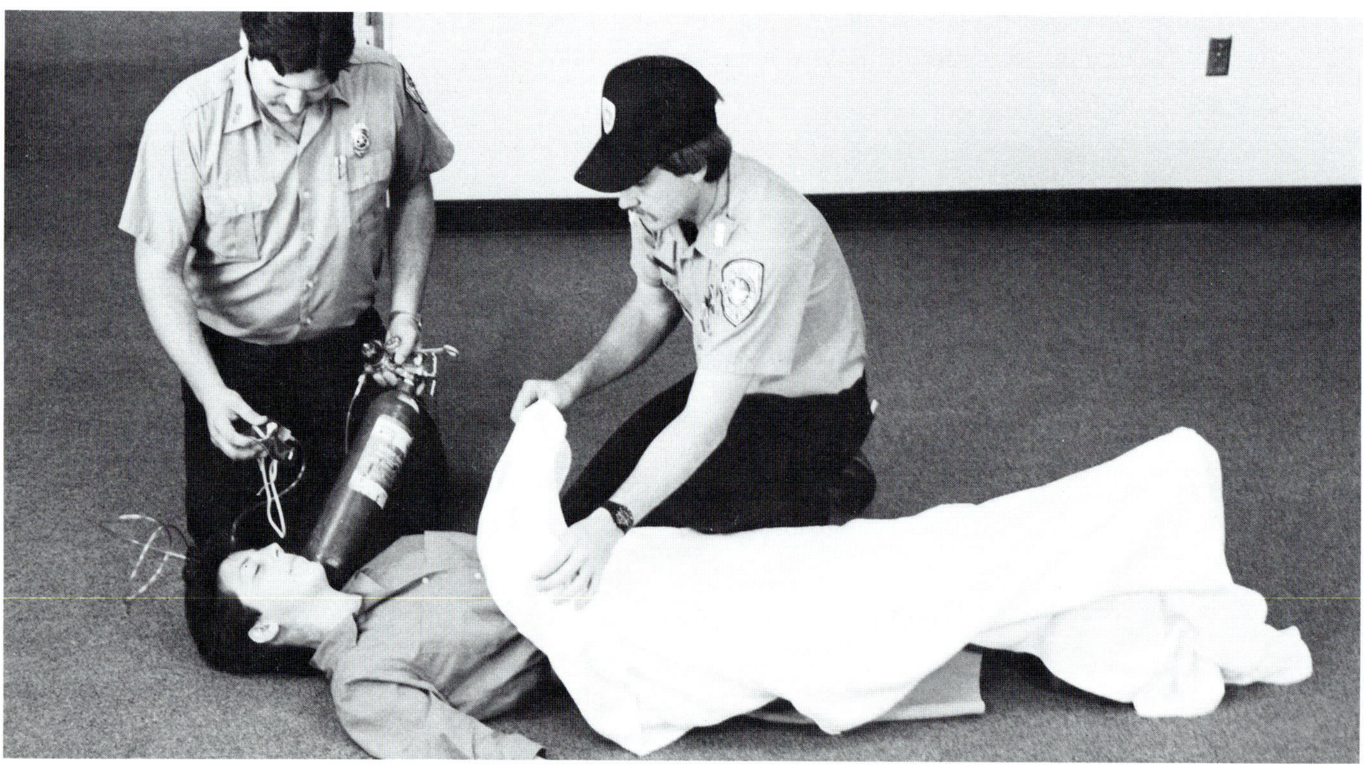

**Figure 6.3** Unless injuries or breathing difficulties make it inadvisable, keep the patient in shock lying down with legs elevated.

needed most. A patient who has severe wounds to the jaw or lower face or who is unconscious should be placed on his or her side. This position allows fluid to drain and keeps the airway from being blocked by blood or vomit. The patient who is also having difficulty breathing due to a heart attack, lung condition, or anaphylactic reaction may be more comfortable in a semisitting or sitting position. Place a pillow or folded object under the patient's head and shoulder. Position a pregnant woman on her left side to avoid supine hypotensive syndrome. For more information about supine hypotensive syndrome see Chapter 15, Emergency Childbirth. **CAUTION:** As always, take extra care with the patient who may have spinal cord injuries. This type of patient will have to be immobilized first on a long backboard. Then the backboard may be slanted to ease breathing or prevent a blocked airway.

### Oxygen

Administer oxygen to aid the patient's breathing and circulation. Naturally, a patient who is having difficulty breathing needs oxygen. If oxygen cannot be taken into the lungs in the first place, it cannot be circulated. But giving oxygen is beneficial for another, equally important, reason: it enriches the blood so that as much oxygen as possible can be circulated. The patient is already trying to compensate for inadequate circulation by breathing more rapidly. Administering oxygen will make the patient's efforts more productive and help keep shock from worsening.

### Handle the Patient Gently

Avoid rough handling of the patient since any type of motion tends to aggravate the shock condition. Handle the patient as gently and as little as possible.

### Fluids

Do not give the patient anything to eat or drink, even if the patient complains of thirst. A patient suffering from internal bleeding or other serious wounds may need emergency surgery, which requires an empty stomach. In addition, a common sign of shock is nausea; giving fluids may cause the patient to vomit.

### Keep the Patient Warm

It is important to maintain the patient's normal body temperature. Cover the patient if the weather is cool. Place a blanket under the patient unless you suspect spinal injuries. Be careful not to overheat the patient or cause the patient to sweat. The rule is, do not add heat: simply prevent a loss of body heat.

### Monitor Vital Signs Frequently

The patient in shock is in a very serious and unstable condition. Monitor vital signs and level of consciousness frequently to obtain as complete and accurate a record as possible of the patient's condition. Level of consciousness is an excellent indicator of the amount of oxygen reaching the brain, so assume that a patient whose level of consciousness is worsening is slipping into deeper shock.

# 7

# Bleeding Control and Soft-Tissue Injuries

**NFPA STANDARD 1001**
**Emergency Medical Care**
**Fire Fighter I**

**3-4.8** The fire fighter shall identify three types of external bleeding, and the characteristics of each type.

**3-4.9** The fire fighter shall demonstrate techniques for controlling bleeding.

**Fire Fighter II**

**4-4.4** The fire fighter shall identify the signs and symptoms of internal bleeding.

**4-4.5** The fire fighter shall demonstrate the emergency care for a person with known or suspected internal bleeding.

**4-4.8** The fire fighter shall identify the emergency medical care for chemical burns, including chemical burns of the eyes.



**U.S. DEPARTMENT OF TRANSPORTATION**
**First Responder Training Course**

**Objectives:**

- Given a description of a wound type, describe management procedures and special considerations. Wound types will include:
  - Avulsed parts
  - Impaled objects
  - Protruding organs
  - Face and scalp wounds
  - Cheek wounds
  - Nosebleeds
  - Lacerated eye
  - Eye with penetrating object
  - Extruded eyeball
  - Arterial bleeding in the neck
  - Severe venous bleeding in the neck
  - Abdominal injuries
  - Genitalia injuries
- Given a "patient," dress and bandage wounds of the following body parts:
  - Arm/leg
  - Elbow/knee
  - Forehead/scalp
  - Neck
  - Shoulder/hip
  - Eye (with protruding eyeball)
  - Ear

# Chapter 7
# Bleeding Control and Soft-Tissue Injuries

Soft-tissue injuries are caused by accident or violence in which the tissue beneath the skin or the skin itself is damaged. Soft-tissue injuries cause internal or external bleeding, which can be serious enough to lead to shock or death.

This chapter begins with a brief overview of the skin and its functions, followed by a discussion of bleeding control and basic dressing and bandaging techniques. The section on soft-tissue injuries begins with an overview of types of soft-tissue injuries, followed by specific soft-tissue injuries and their management.

## THE SKIN

The skin is the body's largest organ and serves many functions. Skin is waterproof and acts as a protective covering for the body, keeping out harmful bacteria. The skin assists in regulating body temperature and, along with the kidneys and lungs, excretes waste material from the body. It controls the flow of fluids, keeping external fluids from passing into the tissues and preventing the loss of critical body fluids from the tissues. In addition, the skin acts as a sensory organ, detecting changes in temperature and body position, and sensations of pain. When this protective covering is damaged, the body is open to invasion by bacteria, to marked temperature changes, and to major disturbances in fluid balance.

The skin is composed of two principal layers, the epidermis and the dermis (Figure 7.1). The epidermis, or outermost layer, is the body's first line of defense. The outer cells of the epidermis are constantly being shed. The deeper layers of the epidermis contain melanin, which is the pigment responsible for skin color.

Below the epidermis is a tough, highly elastic layer of connective tissue called the dermis. The dermis contains many specialized skin structures, including nerve endings, blood vessels, sweat glands, sebaceous glands (oil glands), and hair follicles. Bleeding can be external, that is, visible from the outside, or internal, within the body. Both internal and external bleeding, if heavy, can cause shock or death, so it is very important that bleeding be controlled promptly. Even bleeding that is not serious needs to be controlled and treated to minimize entry of bacteria into the wound.

The average adult male has about twelve pints (6 L) of blood. The loss of two pints (1 L) is considered life-threatening. In a child, the loss of one pint (0.5 L) is extremely dangerous. Obviously, unless severe bleeding is stopped as soon as possible, the

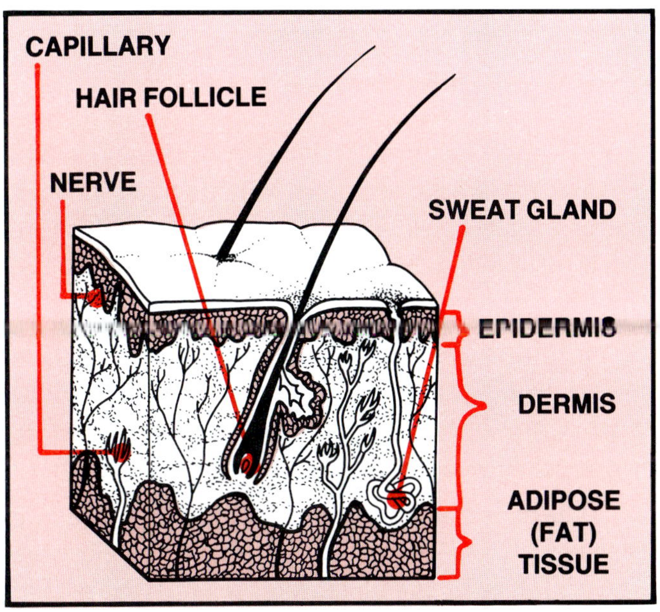


**Figure 7.1** The skin is composed of two principal layers: the epidermis and the dermis.

patient will die. Remember, too, that rapid loss of large amounts of blood is more serious than slower bleeding.

## EXTERNAL BLEEDING

Bleeding is classified as arterial, venous, or capillary, depending upon the type of blood vessel that has been injured.

Arterial bleeding spurts with the rhythm of the heartbeat and is bright red because it is rich in oxygen (Figure 7.2). Blood loss is rapid and profuse.

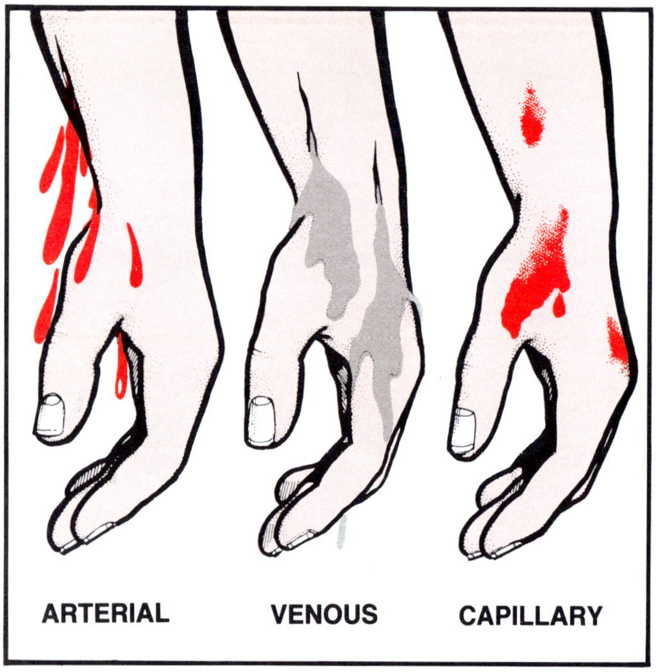


**Figure 7.2** Bleeding is classified as arterial, venous, or capillary, depending upon which type of blood vessels have been broken.

Because veins carry blood containing carbon dioxide and waste products, venous blood is dark red or bluish in color. Although venous bleeding can be profuse, it does not spurt, but oozes from the wound at an even rate.

Capillary bleeding oozes blood only slightly and is usually present in abrasion wounds. The color of the blood may be bright red or dark red. Capillary bleeding often stops by itself.

The body has a system for controlling bleeding that is not too serious, which is known as clotting. The platelets in the blood release substances that combine with the proteins in the blood to form a clot, which closes the wound and stops the bleeding. However, if bleeding is profuse (very heavy), the clots are washed away by the force of the blood and bleeding will continue unless steps are taken to stop it.

### Control of External Bleeding

There are three ways to control external bleeding that does not stop by itself, and they should always be attempted in this order: 1) direct pressure, 2) pressure points, and, as a last resort, 3) tourniquet.

#### DIRECT PRESSURE TO THE WOUND

Most bleeding can be controlled by direct pressure. Direct pressure means just that — pressure applied directly over an open wound. Place a sterile dressing over the wound, then apply pressure to the wound using your fingers or the heel of your hand (Figure 7.3). If a sterile dressing is not available, use a clean cloth, handkerchief, or sanitary napkin. If you have no dressing at all, press your hand on the wound to stop the bleeding. Maintain pressure for three to five minutes. If the wound happens to be in an arm or leg, elevate it to decrease the flow of blood to the area. Do not elevate the limb if there is a possibility that it is fractured, if it has an object embedded in it, or if the patient has a possible spinal cord injury.

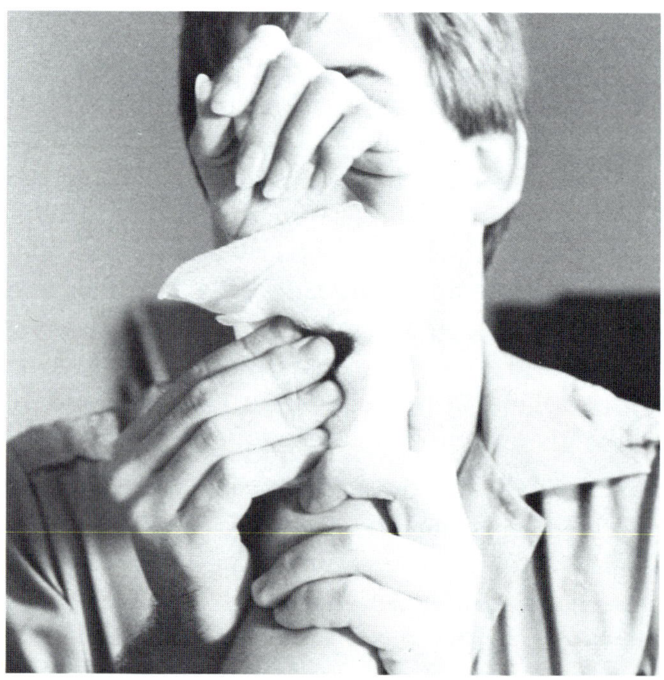

**Figure 7.3** To control bleeding, cover the wound with a sterile gauze dressing and apply direct pressure.

Once the bleeding is under control, apply a pressure bandage so you can free your hands for other patient care. Place a universal dressing or other bulky dressing over the original dressing, then wrap the wound firmly with a roller-type bandage. Begin wrapping the bandage below the wound, cover the entire dressing, and finish wrapping the bandage above the wound (Figure 7.4). The bandage needs to be wrapped firmly enough to help stop the bleeding but not so tight that it cuts off circulation. If the bandage is on an arm or leg, leave fingertips or toes exposed so they can be checked for changes in circulation.

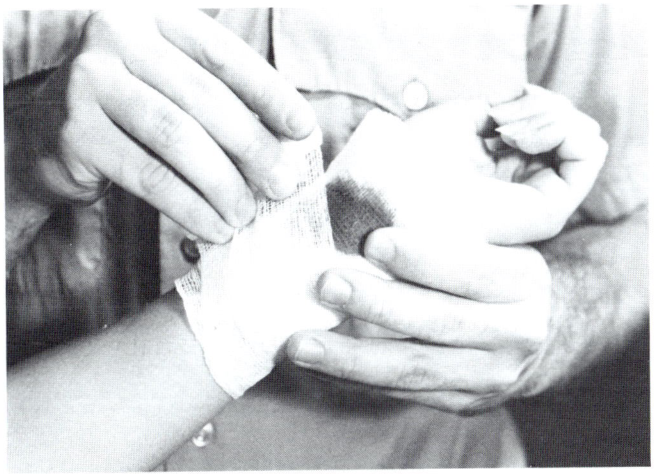

**Figure 7.4** Place a bandage over the dressing and wrap securely.

Do not remove the dressing once it is in place. If the patient has no pulse below the dressing site, loosen the bandage until you can detect a pulse. Do not take off the bandage in order to check if the bleeding has stopped. Removing the bandage interferes with the clotting that has already taken place and increases the chances of bacteria entering the wound. If the patient bleeds through the bandage, place another dressing and bandage on top of the first one. It may be necessary to apply additional manual pressure to slow the bleeding.

## PRESSURE POINTS

Another way to slow bleeding is to compress an artery that supplies the bleeding area. Compressing an artery will slow circulation to the tissues supplied by the artery, so this technique is used only when direct pressure and elevation are not proving effective. If bleeding is serious, using pressure points may help slow the blood flow enough to make direct pressure effective. The principal pressure points are the brachial artery in the arm, the femoral artery that supplies the leg, and the carotid and temporal arteries, which supply the head. See Figure 7.5 for more pressure points on the body.

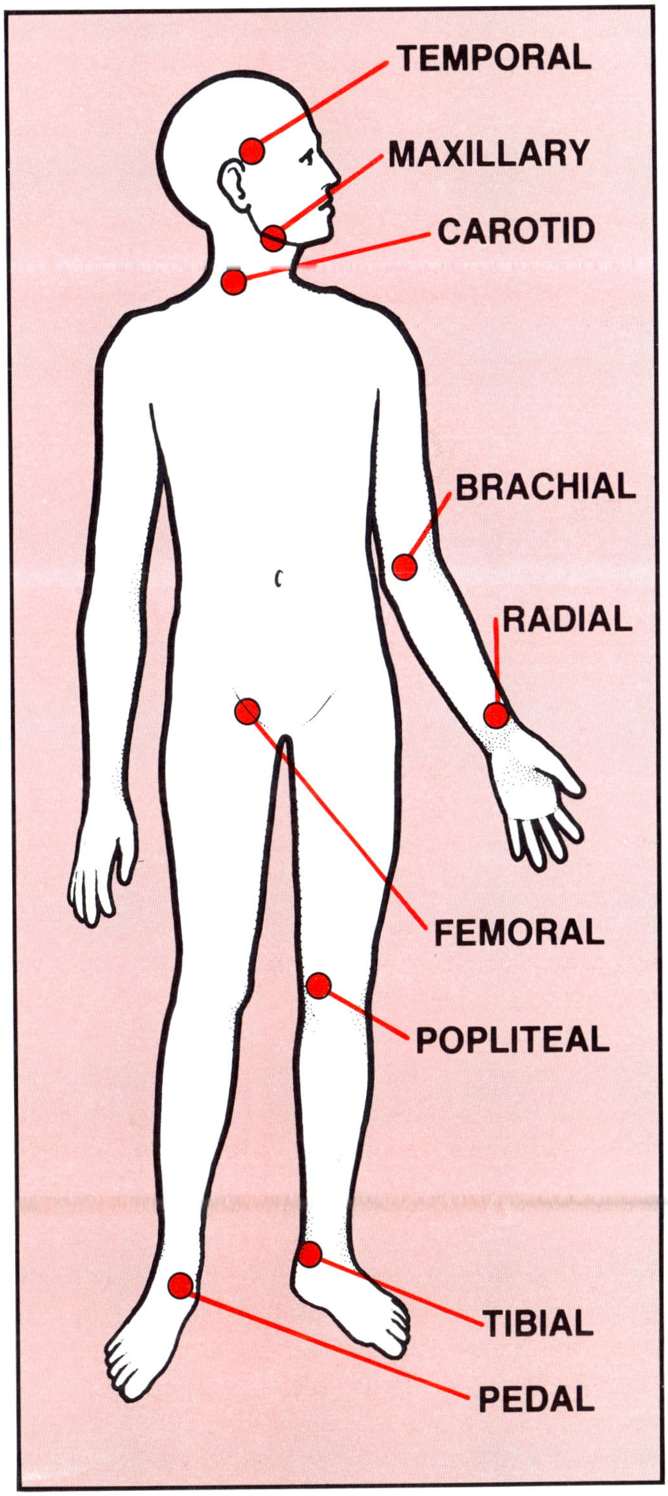


**Figure 7.5** There are a number of pressure points on the body that can be compressed to restrict the flow of blood to an area.

The first of these pressure points is against the brachial artery on the upper arm. The shoulder and arm are supplied with blood by an artery from the chest cavity running just behind and along the upper edge of the collarbone into the armpit. Bleeding in the arm may be controlled by pressing the artery against the humerus (upper arm bone) about two or three inches (50 mm to 76 mm) below the armpit (Figure 7.6).

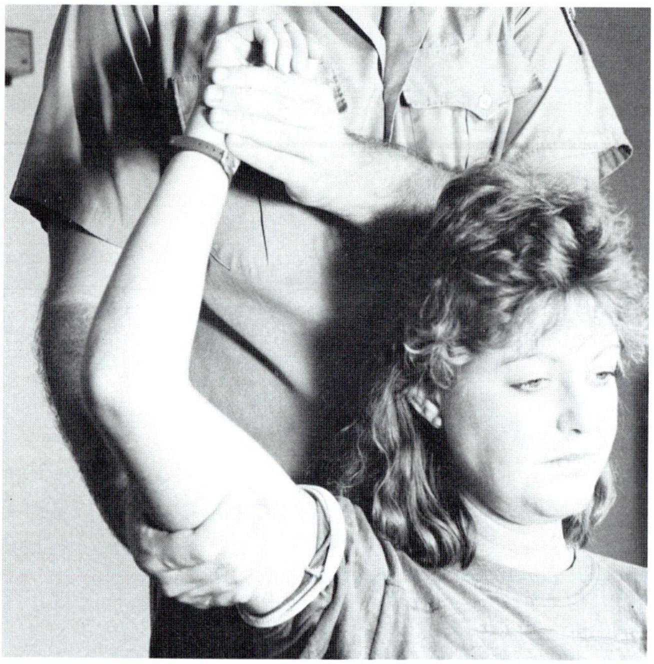

**Figure 7.6** Compress the brachial artery to restrict the flow of blood to the arm.

The second of these pressure points is against the femoral artery on the thigh. The leg is supplied with blood from the femoral artery, which emerges from the interior of the body at the groin, then passes to the underside of the knee and divides to supply the lower leg. To stop blood flow from the leg, press the heel of your hand deep into the groin midway between the crotch and the crest of the hip (Figure 7.7). This action will compress the artery against the thigh bone.

It may be necessary to use the carotid and temporal pressure points to control bleeding in the neck and face. If it is necessary to compress the carotid artery, press straight back against the spinal column, not against the trachea, or the patient will not be able to breathe (Figure 7.8). Because the brain is so sensitive to lack of oxygen, do not compress both carotid arteries at the same time.

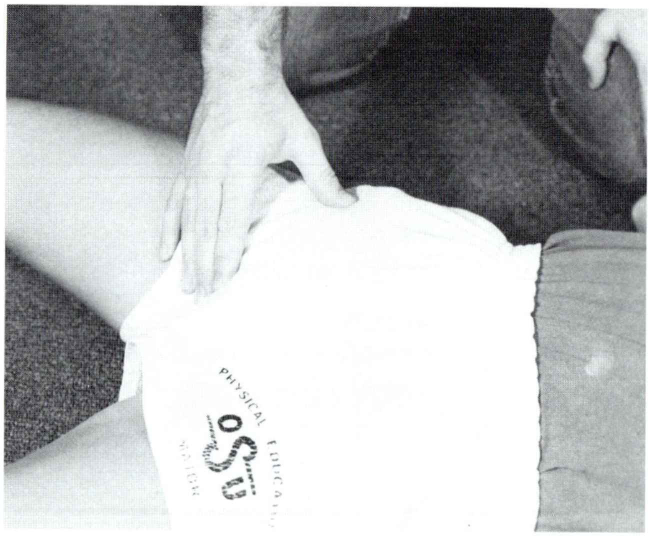

**Figure 7.7** Compress the femoral artery by pressing deep into the groin.

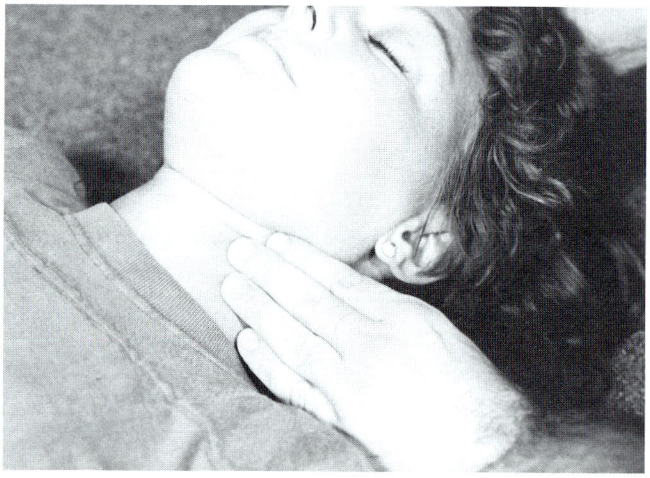

**Figure 7.8** If it becomes necessary to compress a carotid artery, do so only on one side, taking care not to press against the trachea.

Do not apply pressure at a site where there may be a bone fracture. Additional pressure in such a case will cause more tissue damage and increased bleeding.

## TOURNIQUET

It is very rare that bleeding cannot be stopped or controlled by direct pressure or pressure points. However, if a patient is suffering severe, uncontrolled hemorrhage from an arm or leg, and all other measures to stop the bleeding have failed, a tourniquet can be justified by the principle that saving a life is more important than saving a limb. Tourniquets can do serious damage to nerves and blood vessels; because all blood supply is cut off below the tourniquet site, the patient may lose the entire limb.

**A TOURNIQUET SHOULD BE USED ONLY FOR LIFE-THREATENING HEMORRHAGE THAT CANNOT BE CONTROLLED BY OTHER MEANS.**

The steps for applying a tourniquet are as follows:

Step 1: Apply a pad over the artery to be compressed.

Step 2: Place a folded or rolled cloth pad on the artery at that point.

Step 3: Use a wide, flat material, such as a cravat or folded handkerchief. Never use rope, wire, or any narrow material that might cut into the skin. Do not use a rubber tourniquet because it is not likely to be effective.

Step 4: Wrap the tourniquet twice around the extremity (about four inches [101 mm] below the armpit or groin) and tie a half knot (Figure 7.9).

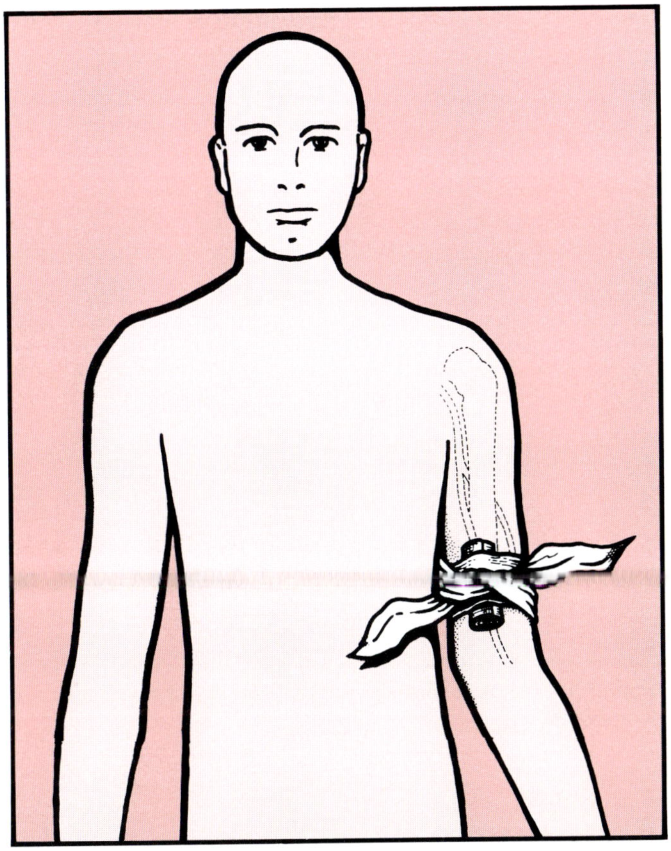

**Figure 7.9** To tie a tourniquet, first pad the artery to be compressed. Then wrap a cravat or similar strip of material around the extremity and tie it into a half knot.

Step 5: Place a stick, pencil, or similar object on top of the half knot. Tie the ends of the tourniquet in a square knot above the stick.

Step 6: Twist the stick just enough to stop the bleeding and tie the ends of the tourniquet in place (Figure 7.10).

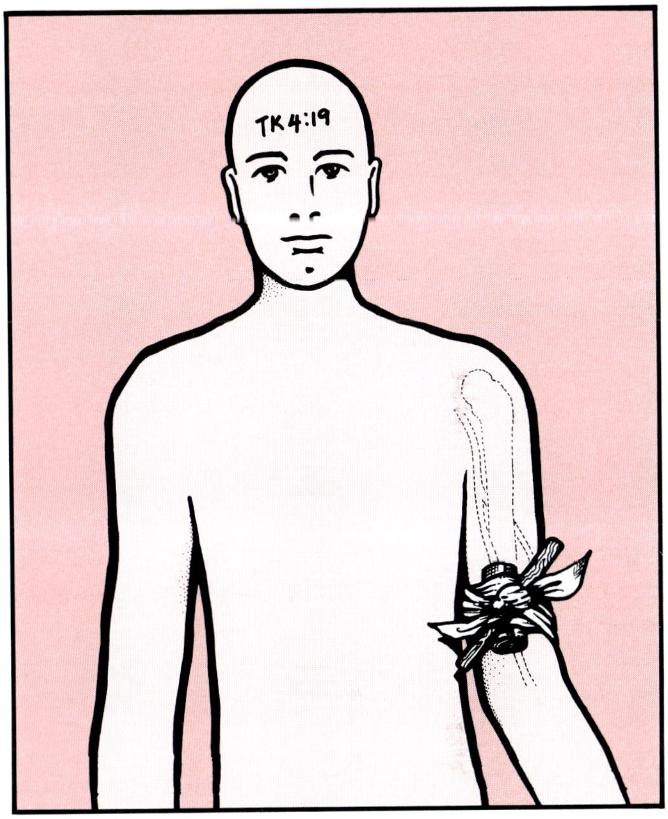


**Figure 7.10** Place a stick over the half knot and tie a full knot. Twist the stick until the bleeding stops. Write TK and the time on the patient's forehead.

Step 7: Mark TK and the time the tourniquet was applied on the patient's forehead. Do not cover up the tourniquet, or other emergency medical personnel may miss it. Be sure to notify other emergency personnel who take charge of the patient that a tourniquet is in place.

The patient should be taken to a medical facility as soon as possible after a tourniquet has been applied. **NEVER REMOVE A TOURNIQUET ONCE IT HAS BEEN APPLIED.** Physicians or medical personnel who are prepared to control hemorrhage and replace blood volume are the only ones who should be permitted to release a tourniquet.

### INTERNAL BLEEDING

Internal bleeding is just as serious a condition as external bleeding; in fact, it can be more dangerous to the patient because it may be overlooked. Severe external bleeding is hard to miss, but a patient can quietly bleed to death internally without any blood showing outside the body.

Trauma, particularly to the abdominal cavity, can cause massive internal bleeding because the abdominal cavity is filled with organs rich in blood vessels. A lacerated liver or spleen can result in a person dying from shock due to heavy blood loss. Another example of an injury that can result in serious internal blood loss is a fractured femur, which can cause a person to lose as much as three units (2 pints or 1 liter) of blood.

The signs and symptoms of internal bleeding are similar to those for shock because they *are* shock: serious loss of blood and vital fluids lead to hypovolemic shock (see Chapter 6, Shock). The patient suffering from internal bleeding typically exhibits pale, cool, clammy skin; increased heartbeat and respirations; nausea; altered level of consciousness; and falling blood pressure. In addition, the patient who is bleeding in the abdominal cavity often has a tender and/or rigid abdomen that is enlarging. The abdomen may also be bruised. The patient may cough up bright red blood, vomit dark blood (the color of coffee grounds), pass blood through the rectum, or have bloody urine.

**IF YOU SUSPECT THAT A PATIENT IS SUFFERING FROM INTERNAL BLEEDING, TREAT FOR SHOCK AND ARRANGE FOR IMMEDIATE TRANSPORT TO A MEDICAL FACILITY.** Internal bleeding cannot be controlled in the field, so do not delay. To treat the patient with suspected internal bleeding

- Establish an open airway.
- Make sure the patient is breathing and administer oxygen.
- Position the patient lying down; elevate the patient's legs.
- Handle the patient gently.
- Maintain the patient's body temperature.
- Monitor vital signs and level of consciousness frequently.

### WOUND CARE: DRESSING AND BANDAGES

Since one of the purposes of the skin is to prevent germs from entering the body and causing infection, any break in the skin should be considered potentially serious. An important part of the treatment of open wounds involves controlling bleeding and applying dressings and bandages. Together, dressings and bandages perform three functions:

- They protect an open wound from outside contamination and infection.
- They help to stop or control bleeding.
- They help to immobilize the injured part and surrounding tissues.

Dressings are used to control bleeding and to prevent contamination. Bandages are used to hold dressings in place (Figure 7.11). There are many different kinds of dressings: the most commonly used are gauze squares, known as 4 x 4s, and bulky dressings. Ideally, dressings should be sterile, but if no sterile dressings are available, nonsterile substitutes such as sanitary napkins, bed sheets, towels, or handkerchiefs are acceptable. There are also many different kinds of bandages.

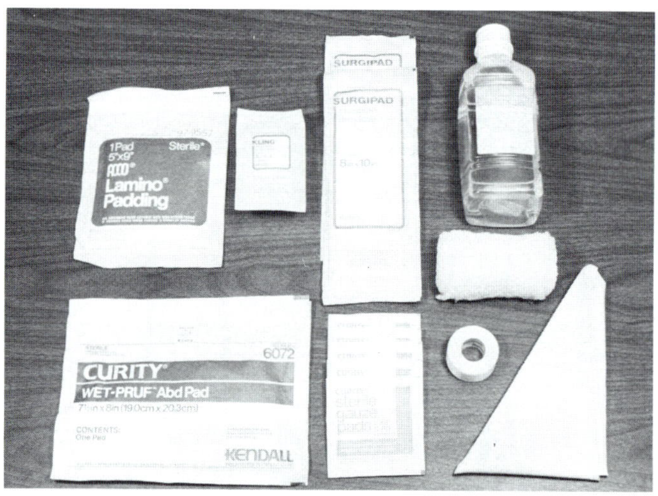


**Figure 7.11** The most common types of dressings and bandages are shown above.

## Dressings

### GAUZE SQUARES

Gauze squares, known as 4 x 4s, are made from many layers of folded gauze, and are available in different sizes. These squares are sealed in individual packages and remain sterile until the package seal is broken.

### BULKY DRESSINGS

Bulky dressings are made of many layers of absorbent material. They may be referred to as universal dressings, multitrauma dressings, or abdominal dressings. They are available in many sizes and are useful for controlling bleeding, covering large wounds, and for stabilizing impaled objects. Sanitary napkins may also be used as bulky dressings; although they are not sterile, they are very clean and absorbent. Bulky dressings can also be improvised by using many layers of gauze squares.

### BURN DRESSINGS

Patients with extensive burns need a large, sterile dressing. A bed sheet that has been sterilized and sealed in plastic makes a good burn dressing. Commercial burn dressings are also available. Never cover a burn victim with any dressing that may stick to the skin, such as one that has been impregnated with petroleum jelly.

### OCCLUSIVE DRESSINGS

Occlusive dressings are used when it is necessary to seal a wound, such as a sucking chest wound or eviscerated (exposed) abdominal organs. Some examples of occlusive dressings are gauze impregnated with petroleum jelly, plastic, or aluminum foil. Aluminum foil can be obtained in sterilized packages. Occlusive dressings still need to be taped down and covered with a bandage.

## Bandages

### ADHESIVE STRIP

An adhesive strip consists of a pad of sterile gauze that has been placed in the middle of a strip of adhesive. Adhesive strips are available in various sizes for special purposes and are very useful as both a dressing and bandage for small cuts or scratches.

### BANDAGE COMPRESS

The bandage compress is made to be used for the same purpose as the adhesive compress, except that it can be applied to much larger wounds. Instead of being held by adhesive tape, the compress is fastened in the middle of a strip of gauze or muslin. The bandage compress can also be converted into a four-tailed bandage compress by splitting each end of the gauze or muslin toward the center. Combine dressings are often used as bandage compresses. They are made of gauze with cotton inserted and sewn to the edges. This type of dressing can be obtained in rolls up to 19 yards (17 m) long and in various widths that can be cut to size. Combine dressings can also be obtained in precut, sterilized packaged sheets varying in size from 4 x 4 inches to 20 x 26 inches (101 mm by 101 mm to 508 mm by 660 mm).

### GAUZE ROLLER BANDAGE

Gauze roller bandages are rolls of cotton gauze, usually five yards (5 m) long and from one to six inches (25 mm to 152 mm) in width. They can be obtained in sterile or nonsterile form. The roller bandage is well suited for the extremities because it can be applied neatly and snugly to irregular surfaces. Roller gauze can be held in place with adhesive tape, or the end of the gauze can be cut lengthwise, wrapped around the injured part, and tied (Figure 7.12).

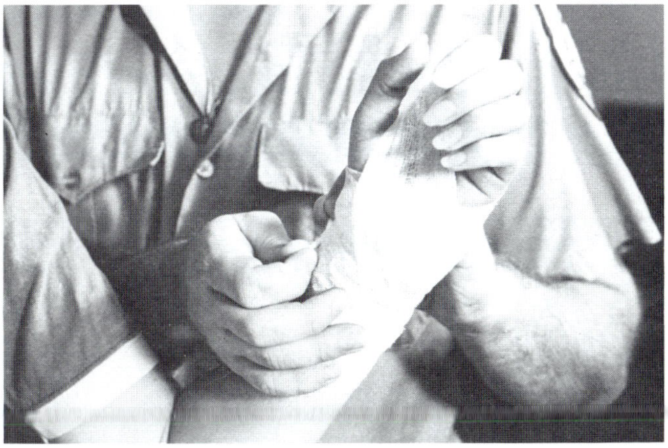

**Figure 7.12** To secure a bandage, cut the gauze lengthwise, wrap it around the wound, and tie it.

### SELF-ADHERING ROLLER GAUZE BANDAGES

Self-adhering roller gauze bandages are slightly elastic multilayered gauze. This type of bandage is being used by many departments and medical personnel to replace the original roller gauze. Because it is self-adhering, a roller gauze bandage seldom requires tying or taping of the ends as does a regular roller gauze bandage.

### TRIANGULAR BANDAGE

Triangular bandages are used to support and cover wounds. A triangular bandage is a piece of cloth approximately 55 inches (1 397 mm) across the base and 36 to 40 inches (914 mm to 1016 mm) along the sides. Although these bandages can be purchased in individual packages, they can be made by purchasing cloth of adequate width. The triangular bandage can be folded into a cravat bandage of varying widths. One method of converting a triangular bandage into a cravat is illustrated in Figure 7.13.

To form a smooth-edged cravat, first fold a hem along the base side of the triangle. Bring the apex to the center of the base side and continue to fold from the apex toward the base until the desired width is obtained.

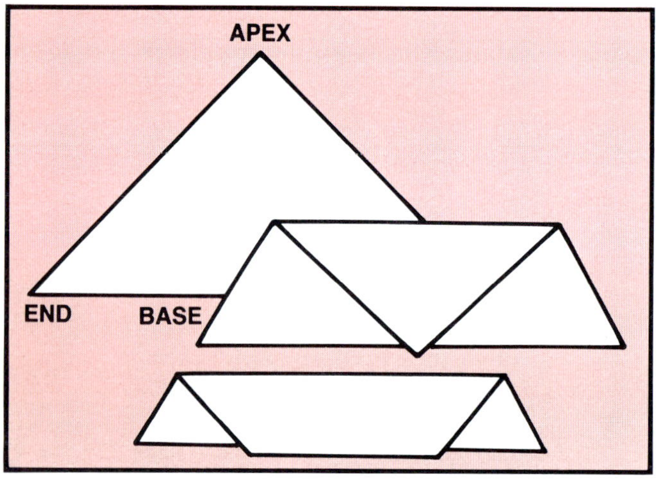


**Figure 7.13** Fold a triangular bandage into a cravat in the manner shown above.

## Applying Dressings and Bandages

At the scene of an emergency where several victims may require dressings and bandaging, it is most important to bandage efficiently and quickly. Bandages do not need to be applied perfectly as long as they hold the dressings in place. Some general guidelines to keep in mind when learning bandaging techniques are as follows:

- Use a dressing that is large enough to extend an inch (25 mm) or more beyond the edge of the wound. Lower a dressing onto the wound; do not slide it onto the wound from the side (Figure 7.14).
- Take special care to preserve the sterility of the gauze square when it is removed from its envelope. To remove a gauze square from its envelope, secure a small corner of the dressing between your thumb and index finger, or grasp the gauze in the center (Figure 7.15). Do not touch or breathe on the side that is to be placed over the wound because this will contaminate it. After the dressing is in place, hold it over the wound and secure it with a bandage.

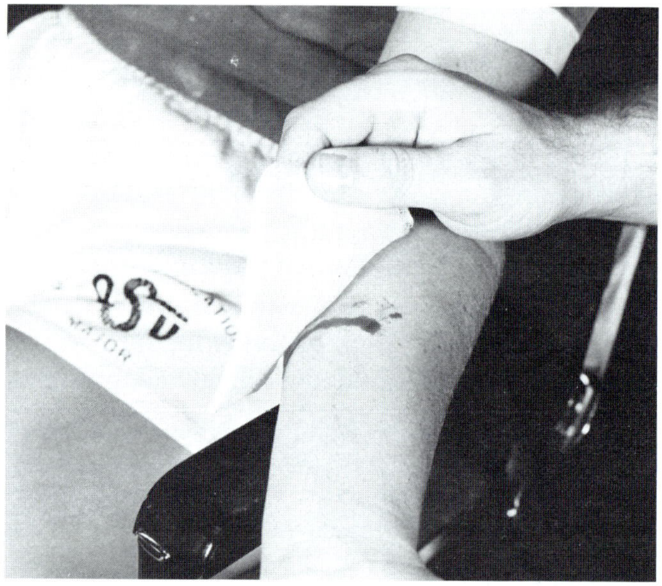

**Figure 7.14** Lower a dressing carefully onto the wound.

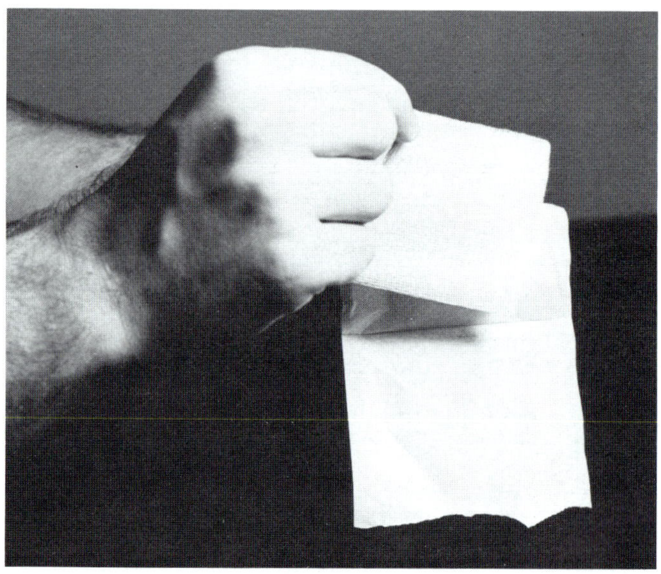

**Figure 7.15** When you remove a sterile gauze square from its envelope, grasp it by the corner to avoid contaminating it.

- Do not apply bandages too tightly or too loosely. Bandages that are too tight will restrict the flow of blood, and bandages that are too loose will not hold the dressing in place. For this reason, when bandaging extremities, leave the tips of the fingers or toes exposed. Watch for changes in color or swelling.
- When pressure is needed on the dressing to control bleeding, turn the bandage when crossing the dressing (Figure 7.16).

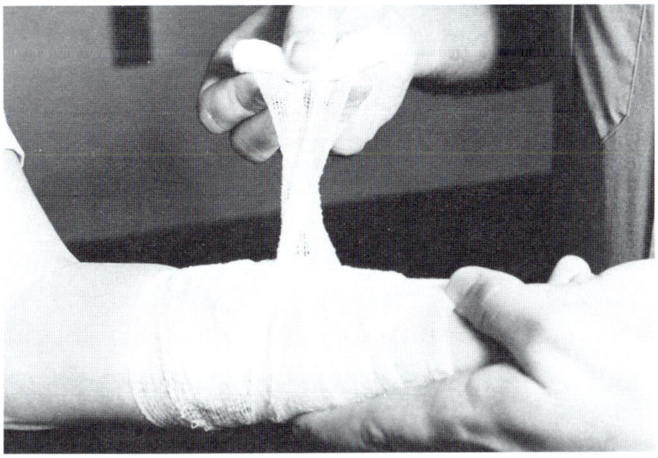

**Figure 7.16** To provide a little extra pressure to control bleeding, turn the bandage as you wind it over the dressing.

- When bandaging an extremity, always start bandaging at the lower part of the extremity.

Methods of applying dressings and bandages vary greatly and will differ according to the specific types used and the injured part to which they are applied. Because there are many good bandaging techniques, only a few examples are shown on the following pages for consideration (Figure 7.17 a-h).

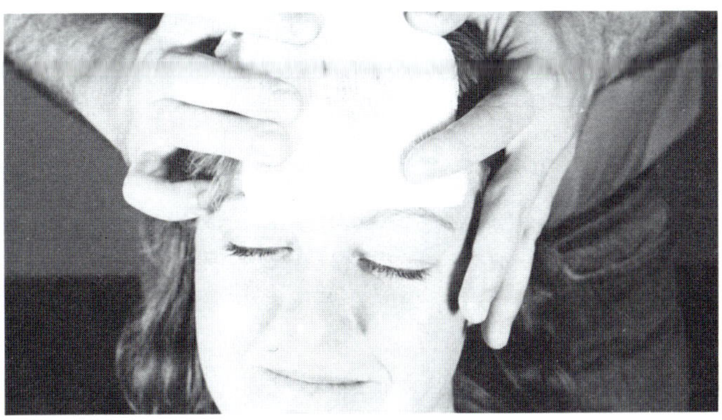

**Figure 7.17a** Place the dressing directly over the wound.

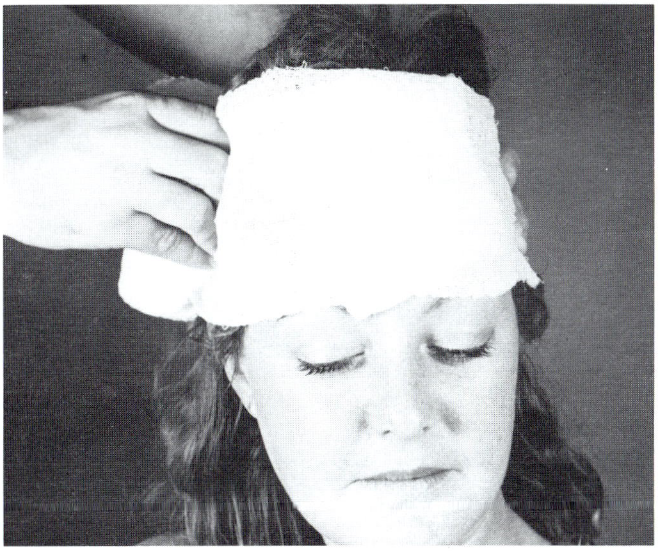

**Figure 7.17b** Begin bandaging over the dressing.

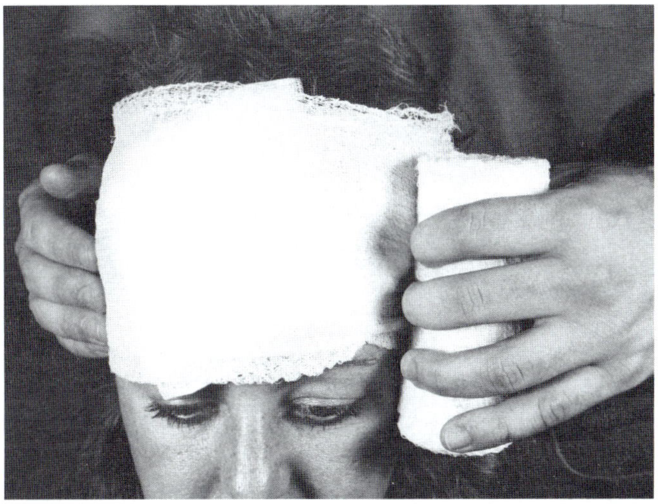

**Figure 7.17c** Wrap the bandage around the forehead several times to ensure adequate bandage thickness.

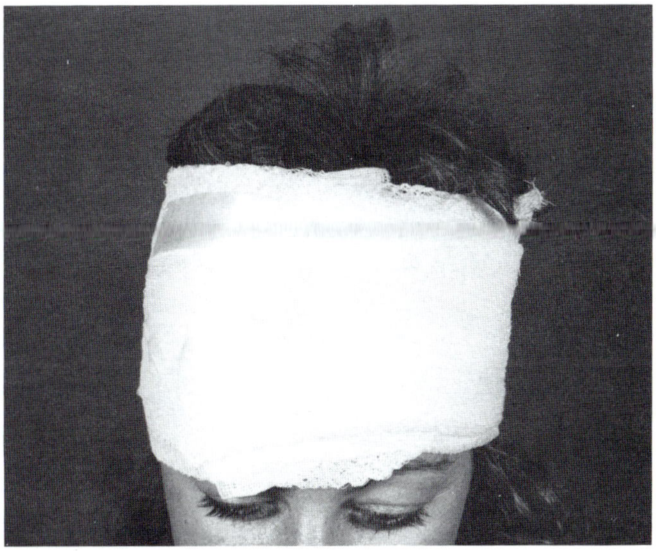

**Figure 7.17d** Tape the bandage to secure it.

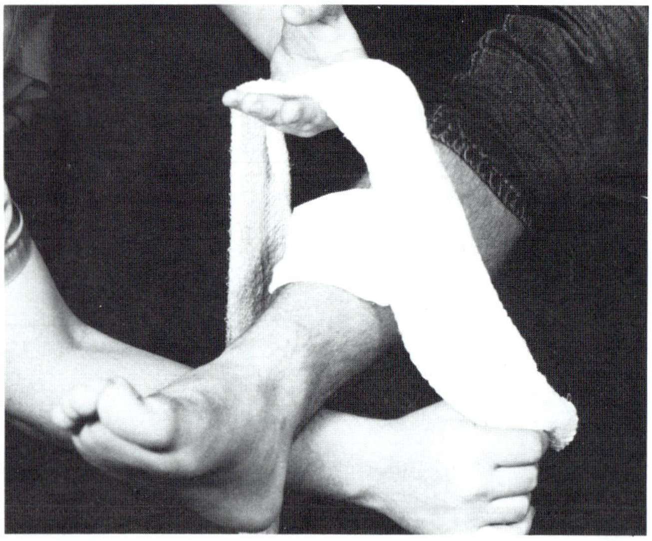

Figure 7.17e First place the dressing over the wound and then begin to bandage.

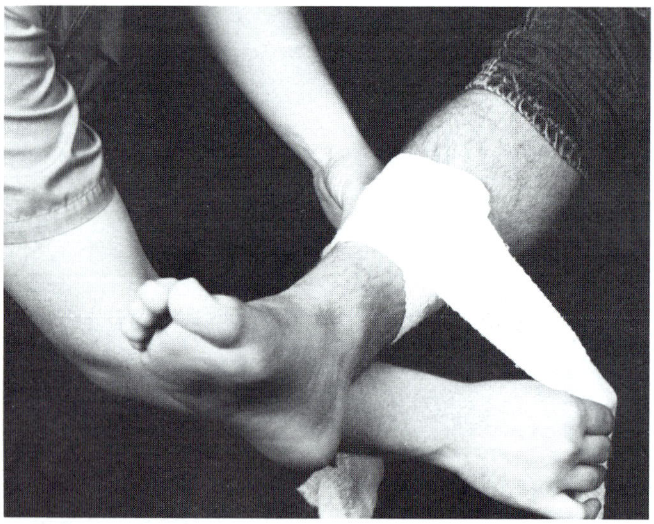

Figure 7.17f Wrap the bandage around the leg several times.

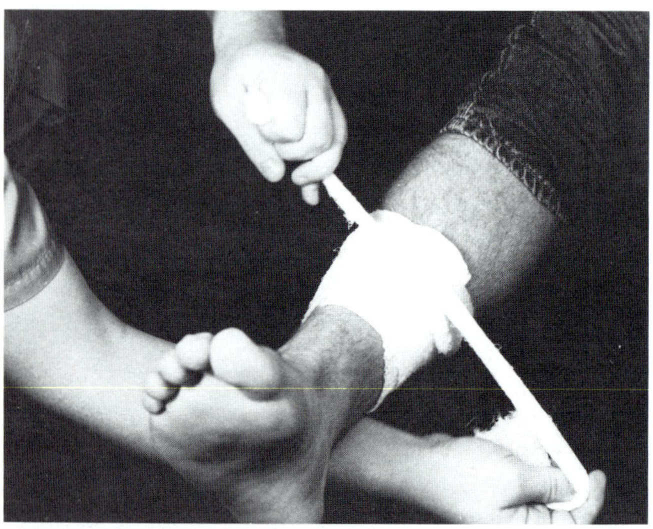

Figure 7.17g If the bandage is not self-adhering, it will be necessary to tie or tape it. Here, the bandage is being tied.

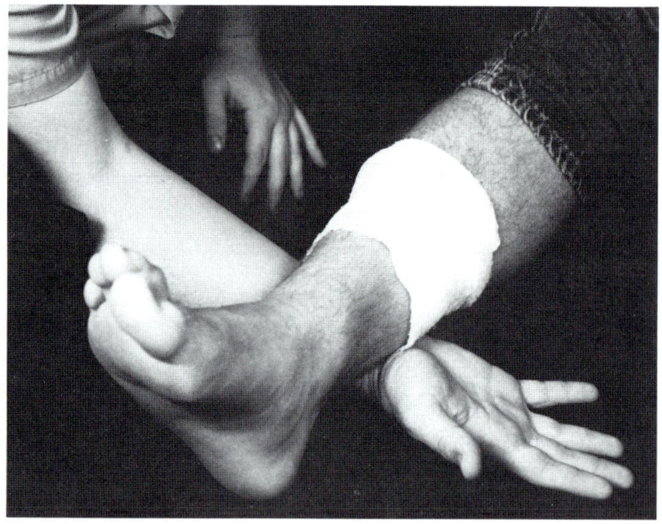

Figure 7.17h A completed bandaged leg.

## SOFT-TISSUE INJURIES

Soft-tissue injuries are caused by accident or violence in which the tissue beneath the skin or the skin itself is damaged. Soft-tissue injuries are classified as closed or open. With a closed injury there is damage to the soft tissue beneath the skin but no actual break in the skin. Contusions (bruises) are marked by local pain and swelling. If small blood vessels beneath the skin have been broken, there will be ecchymoses (black and blue marks) as well. If large vessels have been torn beneath the contused area, a hematoma, or collection of blood beneath the skin, will be evident as a lump with bluish discoloration. Treat these types of closed wounds by applying ice packs to reduce swelling and relieve pain.

Just because the skin is not broken during a closed injury does not mean that the injury may not be serious. Bruises are not life-threatening, but a closed injury to the neck can result in a fractured trachea and a blocked airway, necessitating an all-out effort to establish and maintain an open airway. Closed abdominal injuries are particularly dangerous because they may be overlooked while the patient suffers massive internal hemorrhage.

With an open wound the skin is broken, leaving the body susceptible to external hemorrhage and contamination. Open wounds may be of several types (Figure 7.18 a-d).

- An *abrasion* is a superficial wound caused by rubbing or scraping, such as happens

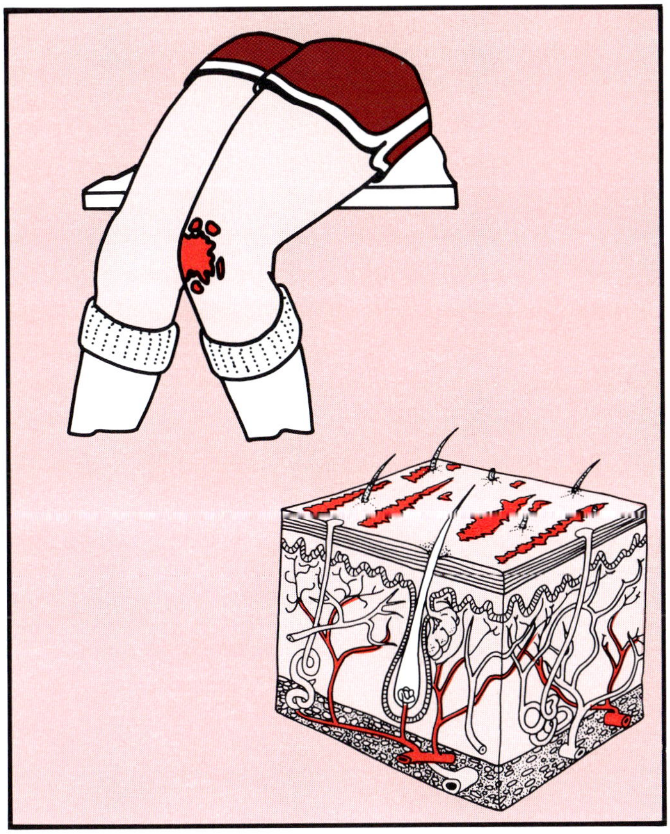

**Figure 7.18a** An abrasion is a superficial wound that causes partial loss of the skin surface.

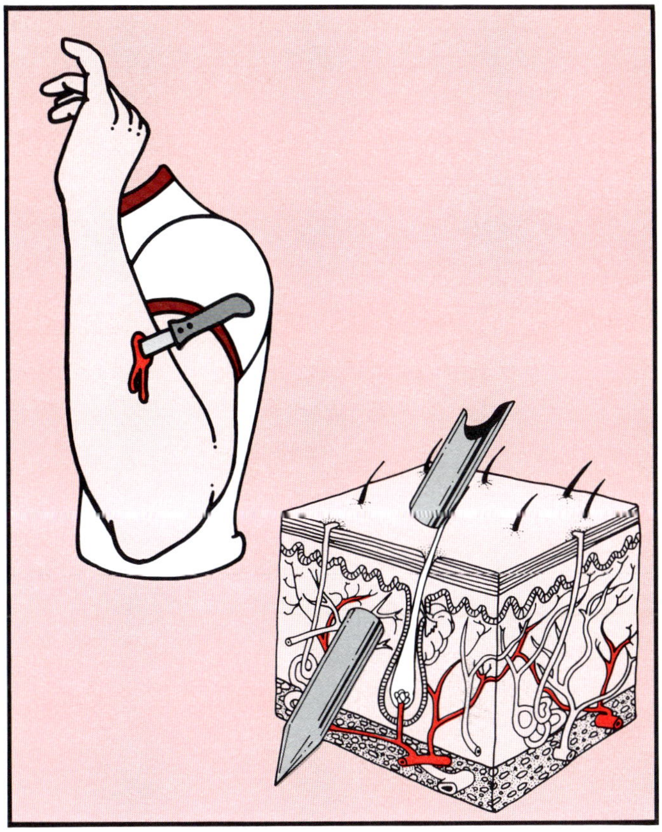

**Figure 7.18c** Puncture wounds often do not bleed heavily; however, they still carry the risk of infection.

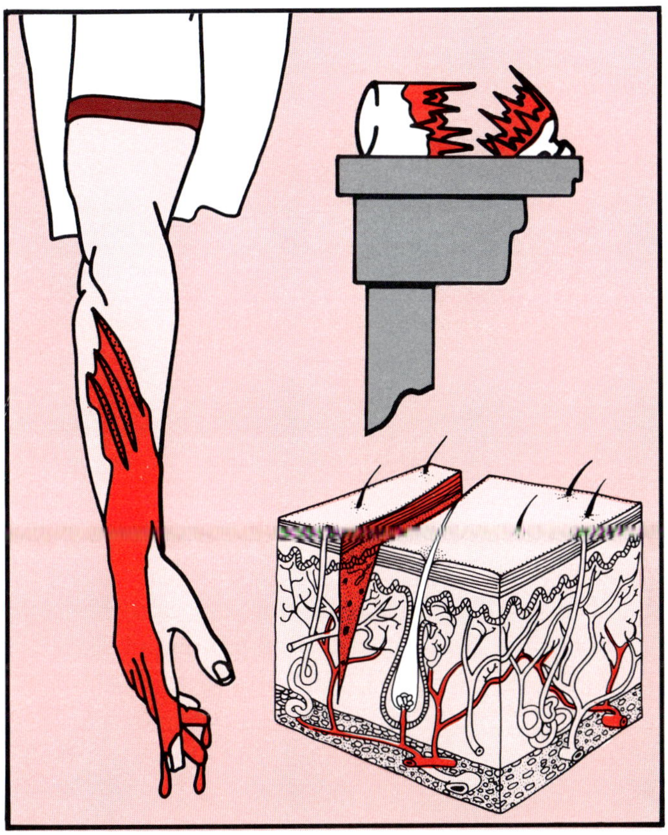

**Figure 7.18b** A laceration is a sharp or jagged cut through the surface of the skin.

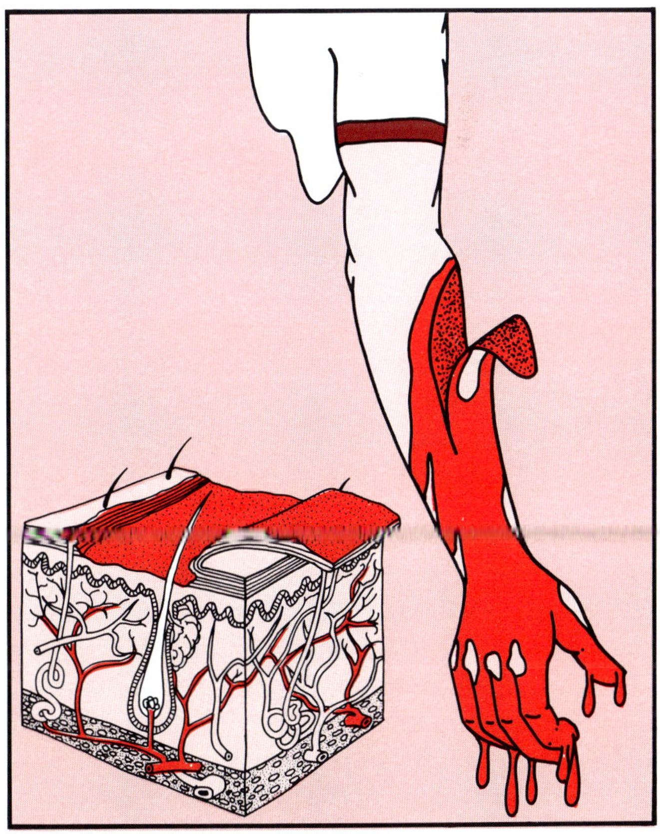

**Figure 7.18d** An avulsion results in the partial or complete tearing away of the skin surface.

with a skinned knee. Abrasions often look like burns. Any bleeding that occurs will be capillary bleeding. The greatest concern with this type of injury is the possibility of infection.

- A *laceration* is a cut made by a sharp instrument, such as a knife or razor blade, that produces a clean or jagged incision through the skin surface and underlying tissue. A laceration can also cause serious bleeding if the sharp instrument penetrates a major blood vessel such as an artery.
- A *puncture wound* is a stab from a pointed object, such as a nail, ice pick, or knife. Special treatment is required when the object remains in the wound.
- An *avulsion* is the tearing of a patch of skin or other tissue that if not totally torn from the body creates a loose, hanging flap.

## General Principles for Management of Open Wounds

Treat open wounds AFTER you have evaluated and stabilized the patient's ABC's. It is easy to get distracted by bleeding injuries and forget that what the patient needs first and foremost is an open airway. Remember, ALWAYS evaluate the patient's ABC's first.

Once the patient's ABC's are stable, treat open wounds by controlling bleeding and by applying dressings (preferably sterile) to prevent further contamination of the wound. Control hemorrhage by applying direct pressure to the wound. If bleeding is severe, place a sterile pressure dressing over the wound and apply compression manually, with bandages, or with an air splint inflated over the dressing.

Keep the wound as clean as possible. It may be necessary to cut away any clothing covering the wound. Irrigate the wound with large amounts of sterile saline or water to remove any loose dirt and debris; however, do not try to pick out foreign matter that is embedded in the wound. Do not irrigate the wound if it has already clotted. Cover the wound with a dry, sterile dressing.

### IMPALED OBJECTS

Stabilize open wounds in which foreign objects are impaled (Figure 7.19). In almost all cases, do not attempt to remove an impaled object. Efforts to remove an impaled object can cause severe hemorrhage and do further injury to the skin and underlying tissues. Control hemorrhage by direct compression, but do not apply pressure to the impaled object itself. Stabilize the impaled object with bulky dressings and bandage it in place. If necessary, use splints for further stability.

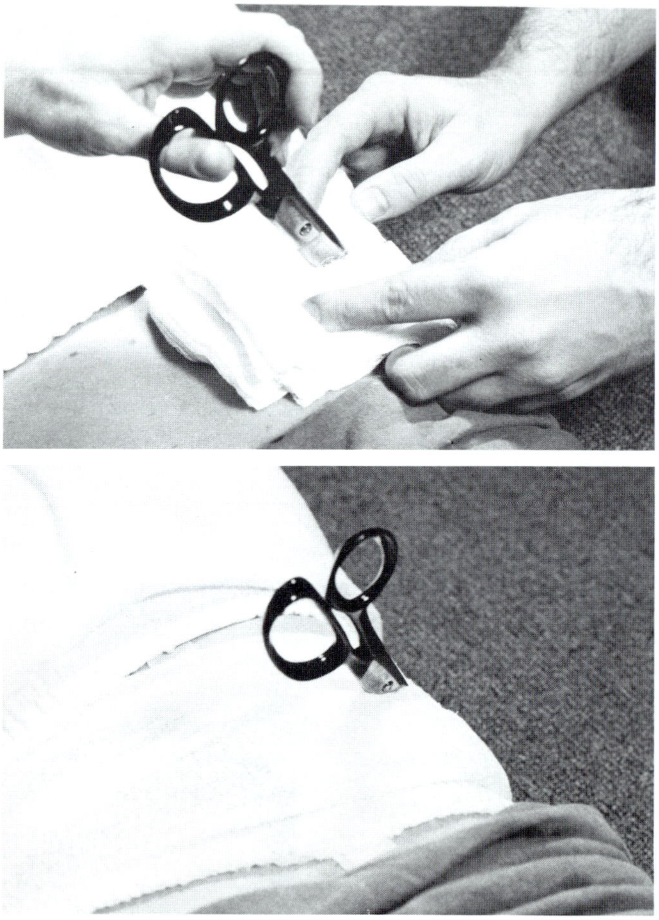

**Figure 7.19** If a foreign object is impaled in a wound, stabilize the object with bulky dressings and bandage it in place.

### AVULSIONS

Flaps of skin should be carefully folded back to their normal position and then bandaged. If a part is completely avulsed, such as an ear or finger, wrap it in gauze soaked in sterile saline. Then place the part in a plastic bag and place the plastic bag on a bed of ice. Do not immerse the bag in the ice. The part needs to be kept cool but will be damaged if it is frozen.

#### EVISCERATED (PROTRUDING) ORGANS

Do not try to replace protruding organs; it will only do more damage than already has been done. Cover the protruding part with gauze that has been soaked in sterile saline. Protruding organs, such as intestines, should also be covered with an occlusive dressing such as aluminum foil, which will help keep the organs moist.

### Injuries to the Face

The face and scalp are heavily supplied with blood by a great number of arteries and veins, and injuries to these areas frequently bleed profusely. Treatment centers on maintaining an open airway, controlling hemorrhage, and applying a dressing and bandage.

First of all, handle the patient carefully! Wounds to the head may also be accompanied by injury to the brain or neck, so do not move the patient any more than necessary. As always, establish an open airway first. Bleeding from the nose, mouth, chin, or other open facial wounds may make it difficult to keep the airway clear. In addition, blood draining into the throat may cause the patient to vomit, further complicating airway management. It may be necessary to turn the patient on his or her side and provide suction. (**CAUTION:** If you have stabilized the patient's head and neck with a cervical collar or padding, turn the patient as a unit).

Cover facial wounds with a sterile dressing, apply direct pressure to control bleeding, and secure the dressing with a bandage. Replace partially avulsed skin as nearly as possible in its normal position before dressing and bandaging. Save any completely avulsed skin by wrapping it in gauze that has been soaked in sterile saline. Have the EMS team transport it with the patient to a medical facility.

If an object is impaled in the patient's cheek, attempt to remove it. **NOTE:** This is one of the few times that an impaled object should be removed. The steps for removing an object impaled in the cheek are as follows:

Step 1: Check the penetration of the object on the inside of the cheek wall.

Step 2: If the object has penetrated the cheek wall, carefully pull the object out from the direction of entry. If this proves difficult, leave the object in the cheek and stabilize it with dressings and bandages.

Step 3: If you do succeed in removing the object, pack a sterile dressing between the wound and the patient's teeth. Apply a sterile dressing and bandage over the outside of the wound.

Step 4: If bleeding is profuse, position the patient so that blood will drain out the mouth and not into the throat.

### Injuries to the Mouth and Jaw

A person who suffers significant trauma to the face may have a fractured jaw and damaged or lost teeth. When the mandible (lower jaw) is fractured, it is likely to be broken in at least two places. The patient suffering mandibular fracture will complain of pain and will have an uneven bite. The patient may also show bruising and swelling. Fracture of the maxilla (upper jaw) is often accompanied by a "black eye." The face appears elongated, swollen, and the patient's bite is no longer even.

Treat injuries to the mouth and jaw by maintaining an open airway, controlling bleeding, and by caring for the mouth in a way that facilitates repair of the mouth and teeth.

- Establish an airway. Insert an oral airway if the patient is unconscious. Inspect the mouth for small fragments of teeth or dentures that can be aspirated (drawn into the throat or lungs). Remove any fragments and suction blood from the mouth or throat.
- Inspect the mouth for any broken or loose teeth. If a tooth has been avulsed, wrap the tooth in a sterile gauze pad soaked in sterile saline. If not too much time has elapsed since the patient lost the tooth, an oral surgeon may be able to reattach it.
- Save dentures or pieces of dentures for transport with the patient. Dentures are needed to establish proper alignment when wiring a fractured jaw.

- Stabilize the patient's jaw by applying a four-tailed bandage or elastic gauze wraps (Figure 7.20). Fasten the bandage so that it can be removed quickly if the patient vomits.

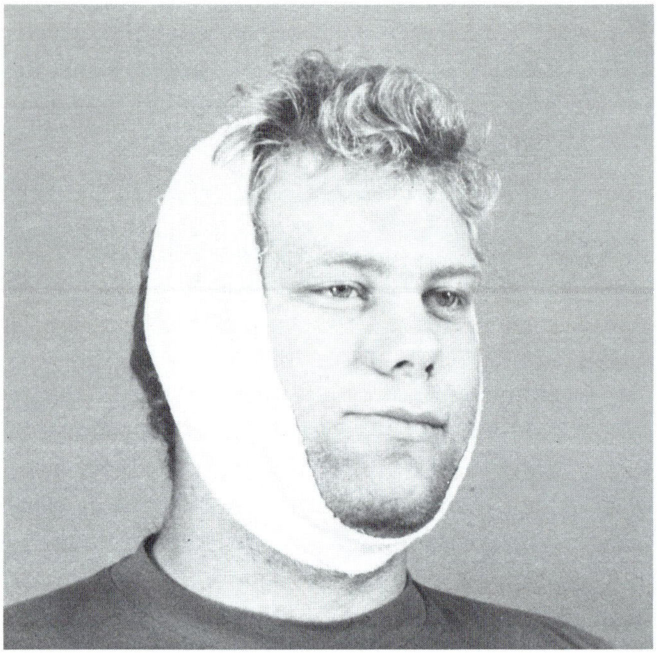

**Figure 7.20** Elastic gauze wraps can be used to stabilize a fractured jaw.

## Emergencies Involving the Ear

The ear is one of our important sense organs. The ear serves two functions: first, it amplifies and reproduces sound waves, enabling us to hear; second, the semicircular canals of the inner ear provide a sense of balance, enabling us to stand, walk, and move.

The ear is divided into three parts: the external, middle, and inner ear (Figure 7.21). The external ear is mainly cosmetic but also helps direct sound waves into the ear canal. The ear canal penetrates approximately one inch (25 mm) into the ear with the tympanic membrane (eardrum) at its end.

The middle ear is an air-filled cavity on the other side of the eardrum. The middle ear has an opening leading to the mastoid bone and a tubular passage (eustachian tube) that opens into the throat. The eardrum vibrates when sound waves strike it. These vibrations are amplified by three tiny bones called the ossicles. Individually, the ossicles are the malleus (hammer), incus (anvil), and stapes (stirrup).

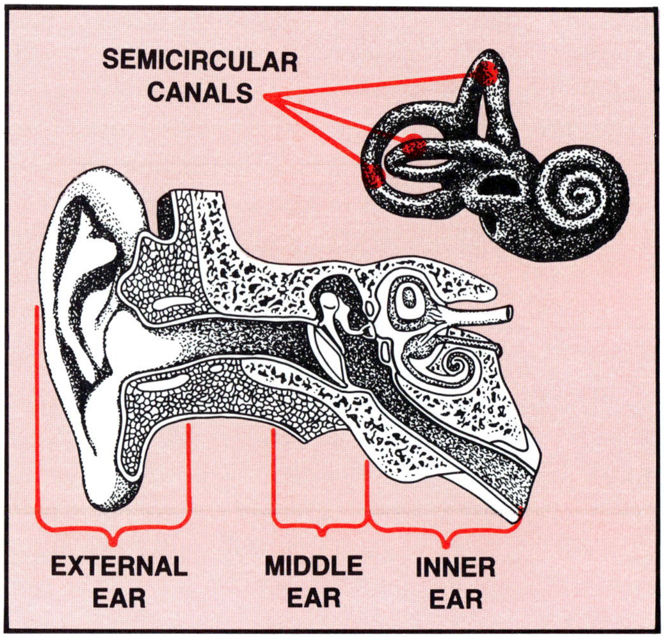


**Figure 7.21** The ear's many structures amplify and reproduce sound waves. The semicircular canals are responsible for our sense of balance.

The vibrations from the stirrup strike the membrane off the inner ear. Inside the inner ear is a tiny, snail-shaped tube called the cochlea. As the stirrup vibrates, the fluid inside the cochlea also vibrates. The vibrating fluid stimulates special nerve endings, which send impulses to the auditory center of the brain. Near the cochlea are three semicircular canals, which are the organs of equilibrium.

The external ear (known as the pinna) and the eardrum are particularly susceptible to injuries. The external ear may be lacerated or avulsed due to trauma, and the eardrum can be ruptured by a very loud noise, such as an explosion, or by a sharp blow to the head.

Treat lacerations of the external ear the same way as any other soft-tissue injury. Use direct pressure to control bleeding, then apply a bulky dressing and bandage. If the ear is completely avulsed, wrap it in gauze soaked in sterile saline and place it on a bed of ice.

A patient who complains of a clogged ear or an inability to hear may have wax or fluid in the ear, or a damaged eardrum. Discourage the patient from hitting the side of his or her head in an effort to "clear" the ear. Cover the ear lightly with a sterile dressing and advise the patient to see a physician.

Blood or clear fluid coming from the ear is a sign of skull fracture. **DO NOT** try to stop the bleeding or fluid drainage or pressure may build up in the patient's skull. Apply sterile dressings lightly to the outside of the ear to catch the fluid.

Foreign objects in the external ear are a common problem among children, who often put such small objects as beans and peanuts in their ears. LEAVE THE EAR ALONE. Do not poke in anyone's ears or you may do some real damage. Foreign objects should be removed by a physician, who has access to the proper lighting and instruments.

### Injuries to the Eye

The eyes are globe shaped and approximately one inch (25 mm) in diameter. The globe shape is maintained by a jelly-like mass called vitreous humor. This fluid cannot be replaced. If it is lost, the eye will be lost.

The important structures of the eye are shown in Figure 7.22. The cornea is transparent to allow light to enter the eye. The white, opaque portion of the eyeball is called the sclera. A thin membrane, called the conjunctiva, covers the anterior sclera and the inner surface of the eyelids. The iris gives the eyes their color. The pupil is a central opening in the iris that regulates the amount of light that enters the eye by constricting or dilating. The lens, located behind the iris, focuses light rays to form an image on the retina. The retina lines the back of the eye and receives visual images.

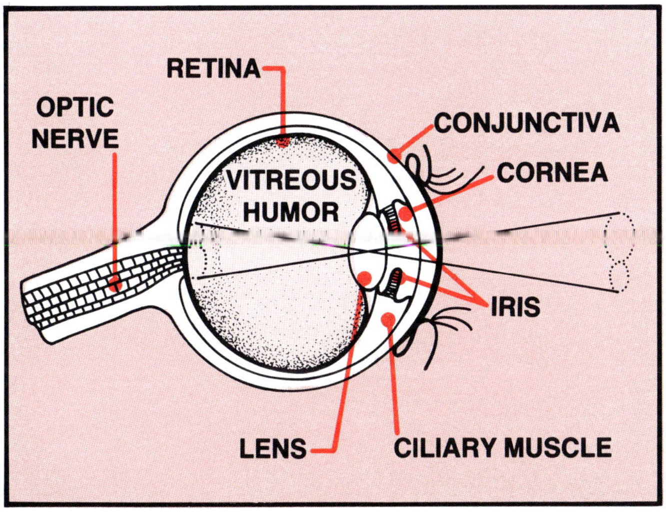


**Figure 7.22** Light enters the eye through the cornea and then passes to the lens. The lens focuses images on the retina; these images are then transmitted to the brain along the optic nerve.

Light enters the eye through the cornea and then passes through the iris, which adjusts to the amount of light. Light then passes through the lens, and the muscles in the eye change the shape of the lens to focus the image on the retina. The light rays strike the retina, providing an upside-down image. The optic nerve then transmits upright sensory images to the brain.

The eye is protected in a number of ways. It is located in a bony socket, or orbit, of the skull, which helps protect it from impact. Tears lubricate the eye and help wash away any foreign matter that may enter the eye. Blinking, which is a reflex action, also helps clean the eyes and protects them from foreign particles. Eyelashes act as a further screen for irritants. The eyebrows act as a moisture guard, much like the eave on a house.

Injuries to the eyes can be caused by fractured orbits, foreign objects in the eye, lacerations of the eyelid or globe, impaled objects or avulsions, and chemical, heat, or light burns. Eye injuries can be both painful and frightening to the patient, who naturally fears the loss of sight. Because eyes are the organs of sight, treat any eye injury seriously.

#### EXAMINATION OF THE EYE

Handle the patient with an eye injury carefully; be sure your hands are clean. Ask the patient when the pain or accident occurred, what symptoms were noticed first, and whether both eyes were affected. Physical examination of the eyes should include the following:

- The orbits — for bruising, swelling, laceration, and tenderness.
- The lids — for bruising, swelling, or laceration.
- The conjunctivae — for redness, pus, or foreign bodies.
- The globe — for redness, abnormal color, or laceration.
- Eye movements in all directions — for dysconjugate gaze (eyes that do not move together), paralysis of gaze, or pain on movement.

- A rough assessment — for visual acuity. Ask the patient to read newsprint or some other simple test. Knowing how much vision the patient had at this point can be a great help to the emergency physician.

Trauma to the face can result in fracture of one or several of the bones of the skull that form the orbits. A patient with an orbital fracture may complain of double vision and may have loss of sensation above the eyebrow or over the cheek due to associated nerve damage. Some patients may have a heavy nasal discharge of mucus, and others report markedly decreased vision. Ask the patient to follow your finger as you move it 90 degrees left, right, up, and down. If the inferior (lower) orbit is fractured, the patient may not be able to look upward. If there does not seem to be any injury to the globe (eyeball), apply ice packs to the orbital area to lessen swelling. **DO NOT** use ice packs if a globe injury is even suspected.

Lacerations of the eyelid tend to bleed heavily because the area is richly supplied with blood vessels. Check to make sure that the eyeball is not lacerated before applying any direct pressure to control the bleeding. Pressure applied to a lacerated eyeball will cause the vitreous humor to be squeezed out and the patient will lose the eye. If there is any doubt about the condition of the eyeball, apply a sterile dressing loosely over the eyelid. If just the eyelid is lacerated, gently apply a pressure dressing and bandage.

## FOREIGN OBJECTS IN THE EYE

Most foreign objects are introduced into the eye by flying particles and lodge under the eyelid or on the globe (eyeball). These objects are often very painful and the body's natural reaction is to try to flush them out by tearing. However, this does not always work, and the first responder may have to help locate and remove the object. The steps for removing a foreign object from the eye are as follows:

Step 1: First, try to flush object out by rinsing the eye gently with water or sterile saline (Figure 7.23). You may have to help hold the eye open. Instruct the patient to move the eye as it is rinsed.

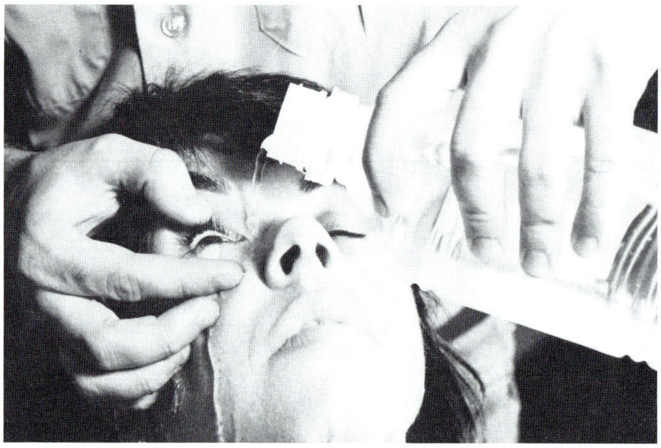

**Figure 7.23** Remove a foreign object from the eye by gently flushing the eye with water. If necessary, help hold the patient's eye open.

Step 2: If rinsing does not work, the object is probably stuck under the upper or lower lid. To examine the lower lid, pull it down gently. If you see the object, flush the eye with water or sterile saline. To examine the upper lid, grasp the lashes of the upper lid, place a cotton-tipped applicator horizontally across the upper lid and roll the lid upward over the applicator (Figure 7.24). If you see the object, remove it with a moistened, sterile applicator or gauze square.

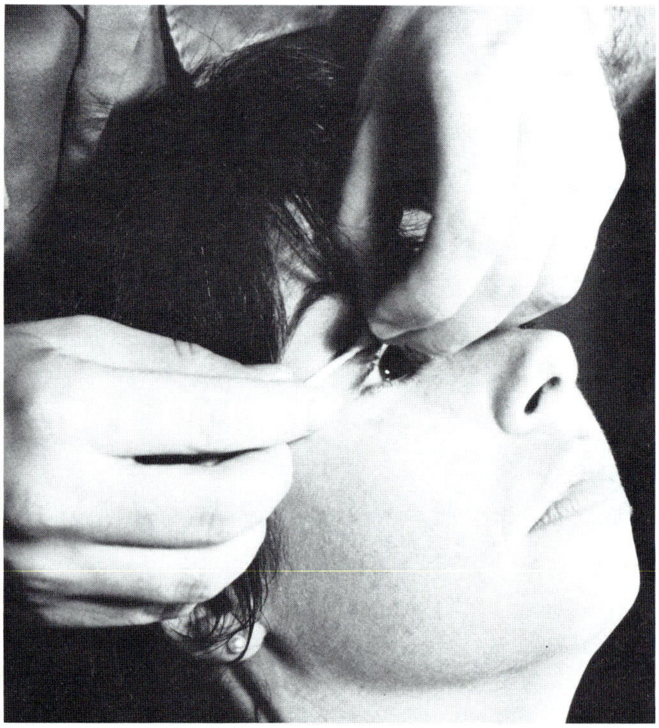

**Figure 7.24** To examine the upper eyelid, grasp the patient's eyelashes and gently roll the lid over a cotton-tipped applicator.

Step 3: If the foreign object is on the sclera (white part of the eye), have the patient look down while you rinse the eye with sterile saline.

Step 4: If the foreign object is on the surface of the cornea, rinse the eye with sterile saline. DO NOT touch the cornea with an applicator or gauze.

### FOREIGN OBJECT IMPALED IN THE EYE

A foreign object impaled in the eye should not be removed; stabilize the object in place. Stabilize a foreign object impaled in the eye in the following manner.

Step 1: Cut a hole in several thicknesses of gauze large enough to pass over the impaled object.

Step 2: Position the dressing over the injury site, taking care not to move the impaled object.

Step 3: Place an inverted paper cup over the object and the dressing (the cup should be large enough to fit over the object without touching it).

Step 4: Fasten the cup in place with self-adhering roller bandages (Figure 7.25).

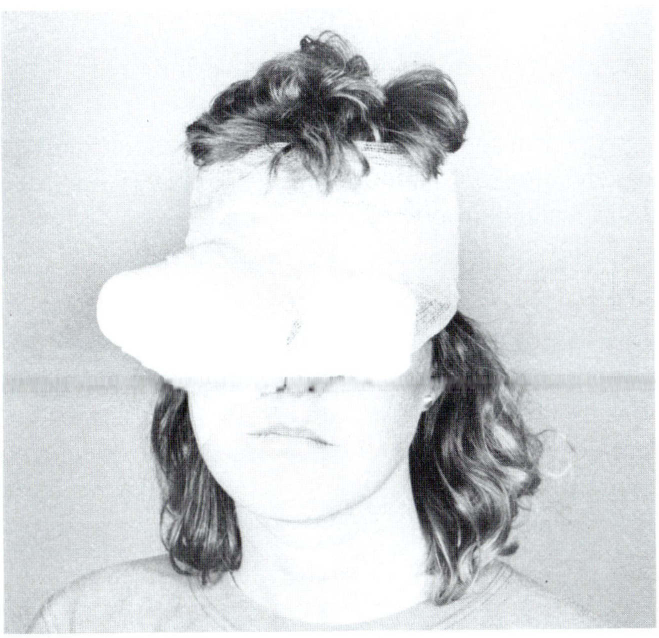

**Figure 7.25** If an object is impaled in the eye, stabilize the object with bulky dressings, then place a paper cup over the eye. Fasten the cup in place with self-adhering roller bandages. Cover the other eye to lessen eye movement.

Step 5: Cover the other eye. Because the eyes move together, covering both eyes lessens eye movements. It is frightening not to be able to see, so explain to the patient what you are doing and why.

### EXTRUDED (AVULSED) EYE

Severe trauma to the face can on occasion cause an eye to be torn from its socket and hang outside the orbit. Do not attempt to push the eye back into its socket, but rather stabilize it in place in the same manner as an impaled object in the eye. Cover the avulsed eye gently with gauze dressings that have been moistened with sterile saline. Place a paper cup over the avulsed eye and bandage in place. Cover the other eye to reduce eye movements.

### BURNS TO THE EYE

CHEMICAL BURNS. Chemical burns of the eyes, especially alkaline burns, can lead to blindness. **DO NOT WASTE TIME TRYING TO FIND OUT WHAT CHEMICAL IS IN THE EYE.** Immediately begin flushing the eyes with large amounts of gently flowing water, and continue flushing for at least 20 minutes. You may need to help hold the patient's eyelids open, particularly if he or she is in great pain.

THERMAL BURNS. Thermal burns are the result of exposure to intense heat. The patient may have singed eyelashes and red, swollen eyelids. Do not attempt to open the patient's eyes, but cover them with sterile, moist dressings (Figure 7.26a).

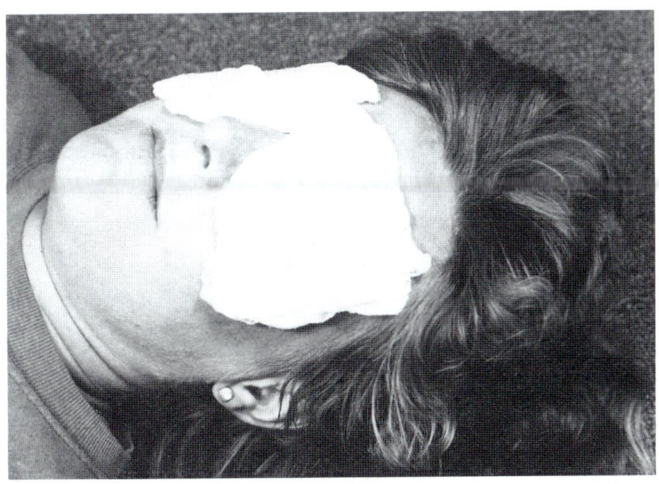

**Figure 7.26a** If the patient is suffering from thermal burns to the eye, cover the eyes with sterile, moist dressings.

LIGHT BURNS. Light burns can result from exposure to ultraviolet light, such as happens with the "arc welder's burn," or overexposure to sunlight. The patient may be in severe pain. Patch both eyes with cold, moist compresses and cover with material dark enough that no more light can reach the patient's eyes (Figure 7.26b).

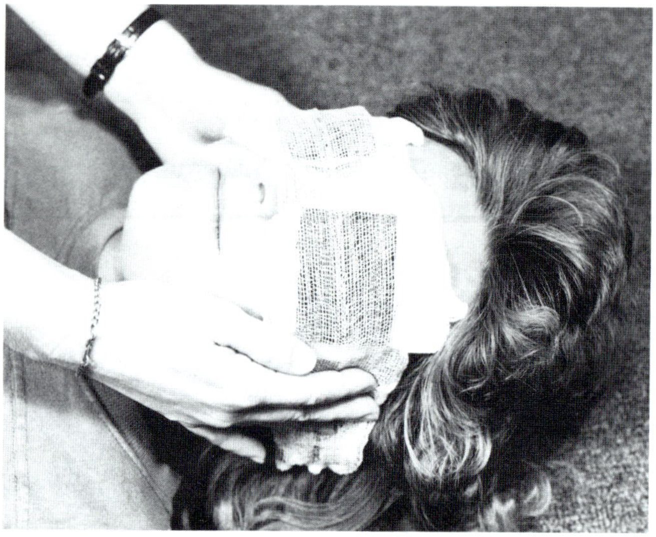

**Figure 7.26b** If eyes have been damaged by exposure to intense light, cover them with sterile, moist dressings. Then apply dark patches to keep light from entering the eyes.

A person may become unconscious with his or her eyes open. This situation is dangerous because eyes need to be kept moist; if the corneas dry out, ulcers that can lead to blindness may result. To maintain the natural moisture of the eyes, close the eyelids, cover them with moist dressings, and tape the eyelids shut. Take care that the tape does not touch the eyeball. If the patient is wearing contact lenses, remove them first.

### EYE CARE FOR THE PATIENT WEARING CONTACT LENSES

Approximately 14 million people in the United States wear contact lenses, so it is not unusual to encounter a patient who is wearing contact lenses. In most emergency situations, contact lenses can safely be left in place. Merely note the presence of the lenses and notify other emergency care personnel. Ask the patient if he or she is carrying a contact lens case and lens solution. Allow the patient to remove his or her own lenses if possible: the patient will be able to remove the lenses more quickly and the lenses will be stored properly.

Contact lenses should be removed if the patient has suffered chemical burns to the eyes or if there will be a lengthy delay in transporting an unconscious patient to a medical facility.

If a patient has been splashed in the eyes with a chemical, immediately flush the eyes with water to dilute the chemical and to wash as much of it away as possible. If the victim is wearing contacts, the contacts will probably wash off the eyes as they are flushed; however, check the patient's eyes afterward because the lenses may still be there.

Check to see if an unconscious patient is wearing contact lenses by gently opening the patient's eyelids and looking at the eyes from the side. Use a flashlight or penlight if it is dark. Examine both eyes: some people wear only one lens. In addition, look for contact lenses on the eyes of patients wearing glasses. Some people, such as those who have had cataracts removed, wear both contacts and glasses.

If the lens is in position, it will be riding on the cornea over the iris and pupil. A hard lens is slightly smaller in diameter than the iris; a soft lens is slightly larger than the iris. A few people today may wear a scleral lens, which is about one inch (25 mm) in diameter and covers most of the visible part of the eye. Check under both upper and lower eyelids for a stray contact lens. Soft lenses usually stay in place, but a hard lens may have slipped off the cornea onto the sclera. If the lens is on the sclera, leave it there. Contact lenses are much more likely to damage the eyes if they are left on the corneas.

If the victim has suffered an eye injury, do not attempt to remove contact lenses. Furthermore, do not attempt to remove contact lenses if the patient's cornea is not visible when you open the patient's eyelids. Patch both eyes loosely and alert other members of the EMS team about the contact lenses.

### REMOVING CONTACT LENSES

For manual removal of contact lenses, the American Optometric Association recommends the following procedures, which can be performed with the patient standing, sitting, or lying down.

### Hard Contact Lenses

A contact lens remover, which has a small suction cup at one end, is very handy for removing hard contact lenses. To use it, moisten the suction cup and apply it gently to the contact lens (Figure 7.27). Then lift gently, moving your hand slightly up or down (Figure 7.28). If you have no contact lens remover, remove hard contacts in the following manner:

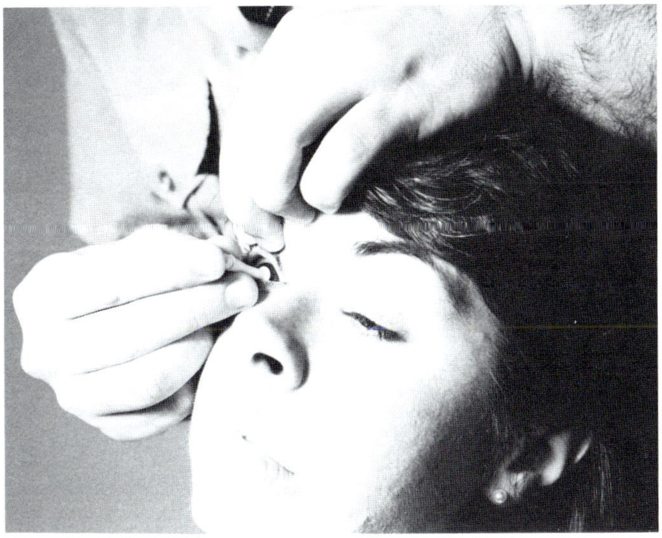

**Figure 7.27** Moisten the suction cup and apply it to the contact lens.

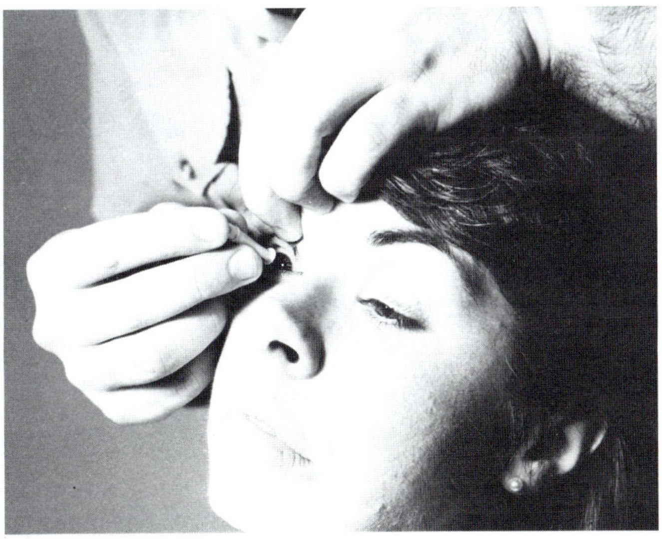

**Figure 7.28** Lift the remover gently, moving your hand slightly up or down. The lens will adhere to the suction cup.

Step 1: With clean hands, position one thumb on the upper eyelid and one thumb on the lower eyelid, with thumbs near the margin (edge of each eyelid).

Step 2: Gently separate the eyelids.

Step 3: A visible lens should slide easily with a gentle movement of the eyelids. If the lens is not over the cornea, slide it to this position with an appropriate movement of the eyelids.

Step 4: With the lens over the cornea, widen the opening of the eyelids beyond the top and bottom edges of the lens (Figure 7.29). Maintain this opening.

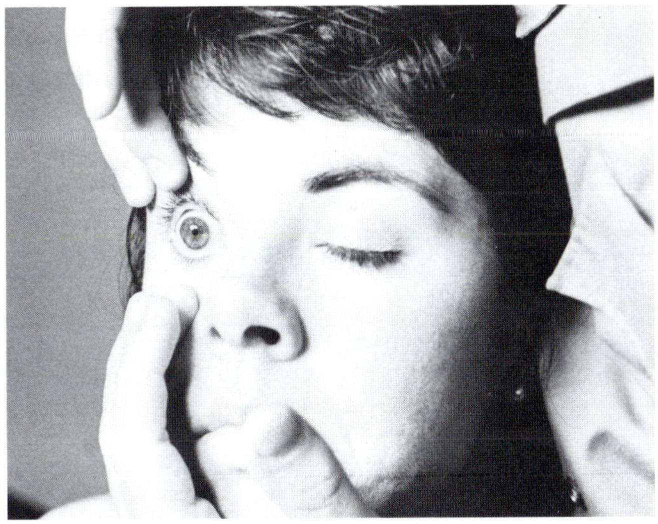

**Figure 7.29** Widen the opening of the eyelids beyond the top and bottom edges of the lens.

Step 5: Press both eyelids gently but firmly on the eye.

Step 6: Move the lower eyelid margin to a position barely touching the bottom edge of the lens (Figure 7.30).

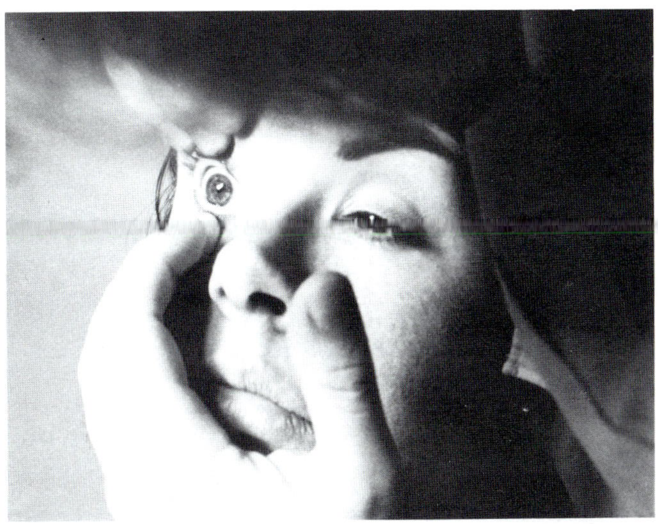

**Figure 7.30** Move the lower eyelid margin to a position barely touching the bottom edge of the lens.

Step 7: Now bring the upper eyelid margin down to the top edge of the lens, with both eyelids still pressed firmly on the eye.

Step 8: By pressing slightly harder on the lower eyelid, move it underneath the bottom edge of the lens. This movement should cause the lens to tip outward from the eye by pivoting on the top edge and flipping out on the bottom edge.

Step 9: When the lens has tipped slightly, begin moving both eyelids toward one another. The lens should slide out between the eyelids where it can be retrieved (Figure 7.31).

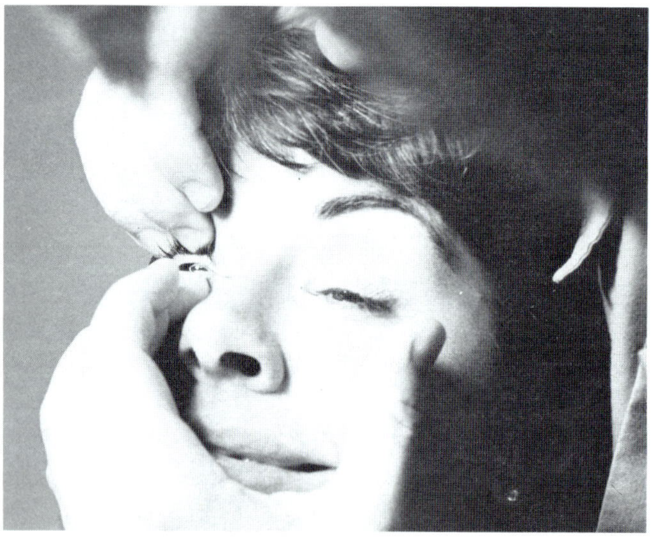

**Figure 7.31** When the lens has tipped slightly, move both eyelids together. The lens should slide out.

### Soft Contact Lenses

Step 1: With clean hands, pull down the lower lid with the middle finger and place the index fingertip on the lower edge of the lens (Figure 7.32).

Step 2: Slide the lens down to the white part of the eye.

Step 3: Compress the lens lightly between the thumb and index finger.

Step 4: Bring thumb and index finger together in a "pinching" motion causing the lens to double up between fingers, allowing air underneath (Figure 7.33).

Step 5: Remove the lens from the eye.

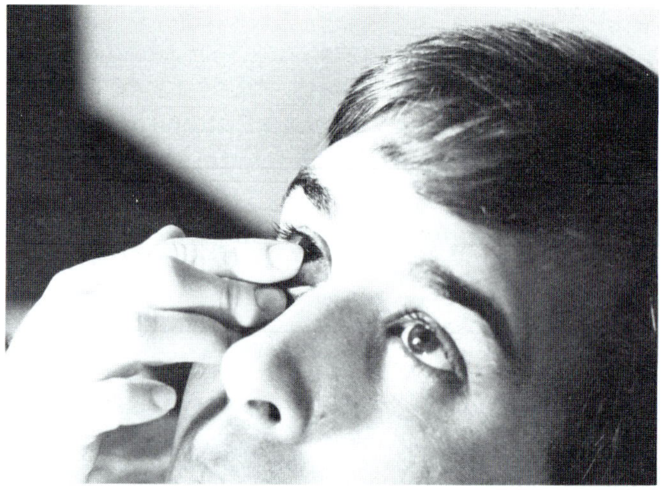

**Figure 7.32** Pull the lower lid down with your middle finger and place your index finger on the lower edge of the lens.

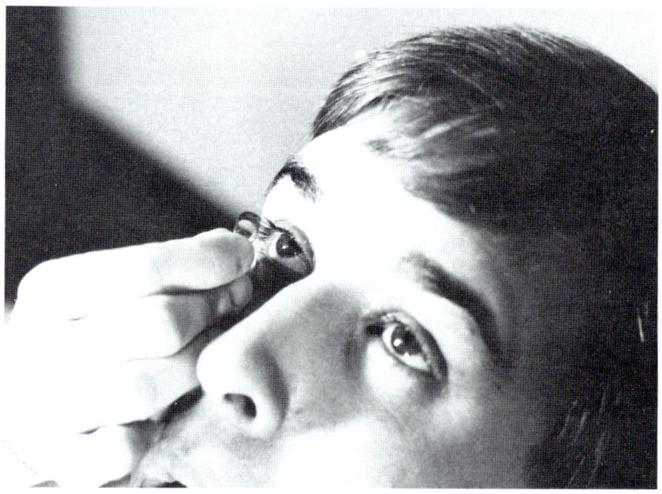

**Figure 7.33** Bring thumb and index finger together in a pinching motion and remove the lens from the eye.

Never use force when trying to remove contact lenses; it can cause more harm than leaving the lenses on the eyes. Never attempt to pry a lens loose with fingernails, swabs, or other instruments. Instead, try washing the eye with water to dislodge the lens.

After contact lenses have been removed, place them in a case or bottle with a little water and note the victim's name on the outside. If possible, use two containers, one for the left lens and one for the right lens.

### Injuries to the Nose

Nosebleeds are usually caused by a blow to the face, but can also be triggered by high blood pressure, overexertion, sinus infection, bleeding disorders that interfere with clotting, or skull fracture.

Nosebleeds are usually more annoying than dangerous, but can be serious if bleeding is profuse and prolonged.

With a simple nosebleed, the bleeding area is in the anterior (front) part of the nose. Have the patient sit quietly, leaning slightly forward. Discourage the patient from walking about, talking, or blowing his or her nose. Pinching the patient's nostrils together is often enough to stop the bleeding. Another treatment is to place a small dressing between the patient's teeth and upper lip and apply pressure to the upper lip. If ice is available, wrap some in a towel and hold it over the patient's nose or against the back of the patient's neck.

Nosebleeds that originate from the posterior (back) part of the nasal cavity are more difficult to control. The patient may be bleeding entirely down the back of the throat, with no blood coming out of the nostrils. Bleeding down the throat may cause the patient to vomit. Posterior nosebleeds are more common in older people, particularly those who have high blood pressure. The treatment for this type of nosebleed is to pack both the anterior and posterior nasal passages with dressings, and this must be done by a qualified EMT/Paramedic or a physician. Keep the patient sitting up, leaning forward, if vital signs are stable. If the patient shows signs of shock, have the patient lie down with the head to the side to aid drainage.

Any nosebleed that is difficult to stop or that starts again after stopping should be evaluated by a physician.

If you have any reason to suspect that a patient may have a fractured skull, DO NOT try to stop a nosebleed. To stop the bleeding may cause pressure to build up in the brain. If the patient is the victim of trauma, immobilize the head and neck. Arrange for immediate transport to a medical facility.

A fractured nose is often characterized by bruising, swelling, and deformity. The only treatment in the field is to place an ice pack on the nose in order to lessen the swelling and to provide some pain relief.

Foreign objects in the nose are usually a problem with small children, who have a tendency to put beans, peanuts, and small toys into their mouths, noses, and ears. Do not try to remove anything from anyone's nose. To make such an attempt without the proper tools and lighting could cause a real injury. The foreign object needs to be removed by a physician.

## Neck Wounds

Soft-tissue injuries involving the neck must be considered critical until proven otherwise. The neck is a very vulnerable part of the body, as it contains the airway, the major blood vessels to and from the head, and the spinal cord.

### CLOSED NECK INJURIES

The chief danger with closed neck injuries is a blocked airway due to collapse of the trachea. Therefore, check these patients immediately to make sure that air exchange is adequate. Remember that any accident serious enough to cause blunt — or sharp — trauma to the neck may also produce cervical spine injury. Keeping this in mind, immobilize the patient's head and neck. Avoid any unnecessary movement of the neck.

Blunt injury to the neck, such as happens in automobile accidents or falls against sharp objects, can damage the trachea enough to cause it to collapse. Blunt neck injury is signaled by pain, swelling, and ecchymoses (black and blue marks). The patient may be unable to speak because of damage to the larynx, and may be struggling to breathe. A fractured trachea will leak air into the surrounding tissues, producing a condition known as subcutaneous emphysema. The signs of subcutaneous emphysema are swelling of the neck and perhaps the chest. The skin crackles when touched because of all the air trapped in it.

**A COLLAPSED TRACHEA IS A DIRE EMERGENCY.** This patient needs to be transported to a medical facility as soon as possible. In the meantime, instruct the patient to breathe slowly in order to create less pressure on the trachea. Administer high-flow oxygen.

### OPEN NECK INJURIES

Open neck injuries, such as lacerations or punctures, have two special hazards: death from blood loss and air embolism. Heavy bleeding, of course, needs to be controlled. Keep the patient supine with the legs slightly elevated. Control arterial bleeding by placing a bulky sterile dressing on the wound and applying manual pressure. Be careful not to press against the trachea or the patient will not be able to breathe (Figure 7.34). In addition, do not compress both carotid arteries at the same time or circulation to the brain will be impaired. Likewise, do not use circumferential bandages to hold dressings in place. Circumferential bandages can interfere with blood flow in the uninjured side of the neck, making it difficult for the patient to breathe.

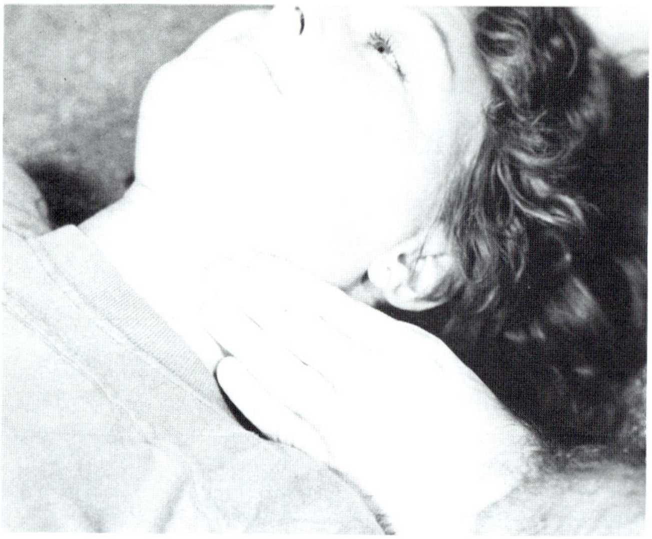

**Figure 7.34** If you must use direct pressure to control bleeding from the neck, be careful not to press against the trachea or the patient will not be able to breathe.

Venous bleeding in the neck is not as heavy as arterial bleeding, but carries the special hazard of air embolism. Air embolism occurs when air is sucked into the open wound and travels through the veins. If the air embolism travels to the heart, the patient may die.

To treat venous bleeding in the neck, position the patient on his or her left side with the feet slightly higher than the head. This position helps to trap any air bubbles that have already entered the circulatory system. Apply manual pressure using bulky dressings both above and below the wound. Cover the wound with an occlusive dressing, such as aluminum foil or plastic, and tape it down so that no air can enter the wound. Continue to apply manual pressure, administer oxygen, and treat for shock.

## Chest Injuries

The ribs offer a good deal of protection to the organs in the thoracic (chest) cavity; however, blunt or penetrating trauma can cause bruising, laceration, or puncture wounds to the lungs and heart. Motor vehicle accidents frequently result in deceleration injuries, which occur when the body strikes a seat belt, steering wheel, or other part of a vehicle with great force. Deceleration injuries can cause cardiac contusion (bruising of the heart) or cardiac tamponade (blood in the pericardial sac). A patient suffering cardiac contusion will exhibit the same signs and symptoms as those for a heart attack. The patient with pericardial tamponade will likely have distended jugular veins and signs of shock.

The lungs can be punctured internally, by broken ribs, or externally, by penetrating chest wounds. A penetrating chest wound will result in a sucking chest wound, which must be covered with an occlusive dressing as part of the primary survey. Remember that air can become trapped in the chest, causing tension pneumothorax. If this happens, remove the dressing for a few seconds in order to let the trapped air escape. (For more information about injuries to the chest and their management, see Chapter 8, Injuries to the Skull, Spine, and Chest.)

## Abdominal Injuries

Abdominal injuries, like other soft-tissue injuries, can be classified as closed or open. The abdominal area, unlike other parts of the body, is not well cushioned by the skeleton. Injuries, whether blunt or penetrating, can cause rapid and severe damage to the abdominal organs. The solid organs, such as the liver, spleen, and pancreas, will bleed profusely. The hollow organs, such as the stomach, bladder, and intestines, will spill their contents into the abdominal cavity, causing inflammation and pain. The stomach contains concentrated hydrochloric acid; if this acid is emptied into the abdominal cavity, it causes almost instant, severe pain. Organs that are full at the time of injury, such as the stomach or bladder, will rupture much more easily than if they are empty.

### CLOSED ABDOMINAL INJURIES

Severe abdominal injuries can occur without the patient showing any external signs of injury. Knowing the mechanism of injury is an important first step in determining the patient's likely injuries. Automobile accidents, whether or not the victim wore a seat belt, and beatings are frequent causes of closed abdominal injuries. Pay special attention to the patient who is known to have suffered trauma to the abdominal area.

Another clue to the presence of abdominal injuries is the behavior and position of the patient. The patient whose peritoneal cavity is inflamed due to spilled digestive juices will be in severe pain and will lie very still with the legs drawn up, a position known as abdominal guarding. The patient also may vomit.

After checking the patient's ABC's and ruling out spinal cord injury (or stabilizing the patient's neck and spine), take vital signs. Suspect that the patient who is restless or whose pulse is rapid is going into shock. If the patient exhibits signs of shock and shows no other signs of injury, suspect internal bleeding. Remember that internal bleeding leads to loss of vital fluids and hypovolemic shock (Chapter 6, Shock).

Examine the patient's abdomen by placing the patient supine with the legs flexed to relax the abdominal muscles. Open the patient's clothing and inspect the chest and abdominal area for bruises, welts, seat belt marks, and rib or pelvic fractures. The patient who is bleeding into the abdomen often has a rigid, boardlike abdomen that is enlarging. Ask the patient to describe the pain: Where is it? Is it steady? Does it radiate? Do any movements make it feel better or worse?

GENTLY palpate (feel) the abdominal and pelvic area by touching areas away from the area of pain first. If you touch the painful area first, the patient will tense the stomach muscles and you will not be able to determine if the abdomen is rigid.

**TREAT ANY PATIENT WITH SUSPECTED CLOSED ABDOMINAL INJURIES FOR SHOCK**

To treat the patient with suspected closed abdominal injuries,

- Check and correct the ABC's first
- Place the patient supine with the legs elevated or slightly flexed. Administer oxygen. Given nothing to eat or drink. Continue to monitor vital signs and level of consciousness frequently. Arrange for transportation to a medical facility.

### OPEN ABDOMINAL WOUNDS

Open abdominal wounds are those in which the abdomen has been penetrated by a foreign object, such as a knife, bullet, or tool. The abdomen may also be torn open as a result of trauma, such as an automobile or industrial accident. Penetrating abdominal wounds are especially serious because they not only break the skin, but can do major damage to vital organs beneath the skin. As with closed injuries, lacerated hollow organs will spill their contents into the peritoneal cavity, and lacerated solid organs will bleed profusely, sometimes fatally.

Open abdominal wounds, by their nature, are obvious on patient examination. However, if the wound is the result of a bullet, look for an exit wound as well. Treat open abdominal wounds by first checking and correcting the ABC's, controlling bleeding, applying sterile dressings and bandaging the wound, and treating for shock. Two special types of abdominal wounds, those with impaled objects in them and eviscerated abdominal organs, require special treatment.

If an object is impaled in the abdomen, such as a knife or screwdriver, do not try to remove it. Stabilize the object in place with bulky dressings and apply pressure bandages to help control bleeding.

Sometimes an abdominal injury causes organs, such as the intestines, to protrude or hang out of the abdominal cavity. An injury of this type is known as an evisceration. **DO NOT TRY TO REPLACE EVISCERATED ORGANS.** Cover the organs with a universal dressing that has been soaked in sterile saline. Place an occlusive dressing, such as aluminum foil or plastic wrap, over

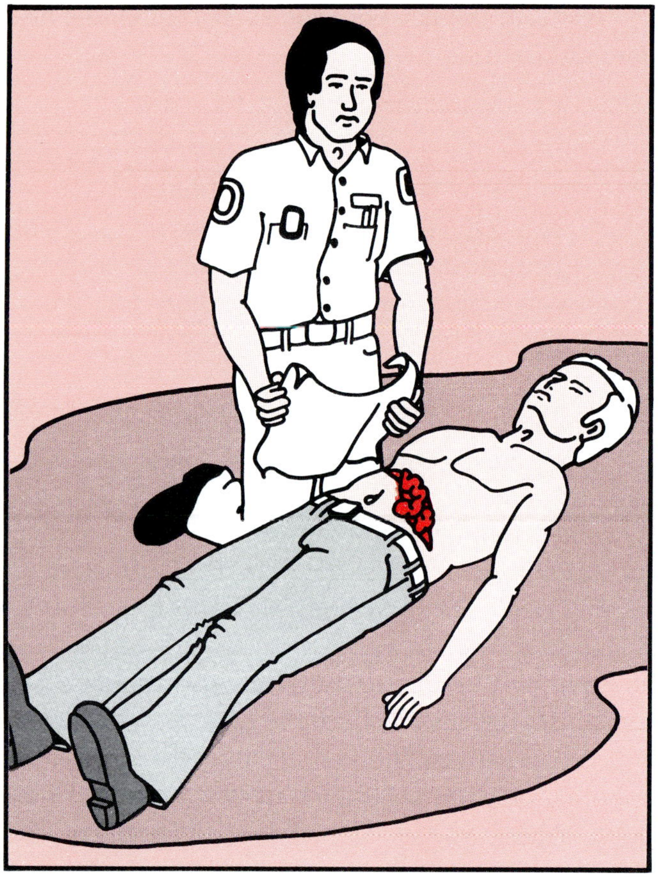

**Figure 7.35a** Do not try to replace organs that protrude from the abdominal cavity. Cover the wound with a large dressing that has been soaked in sterile saline.

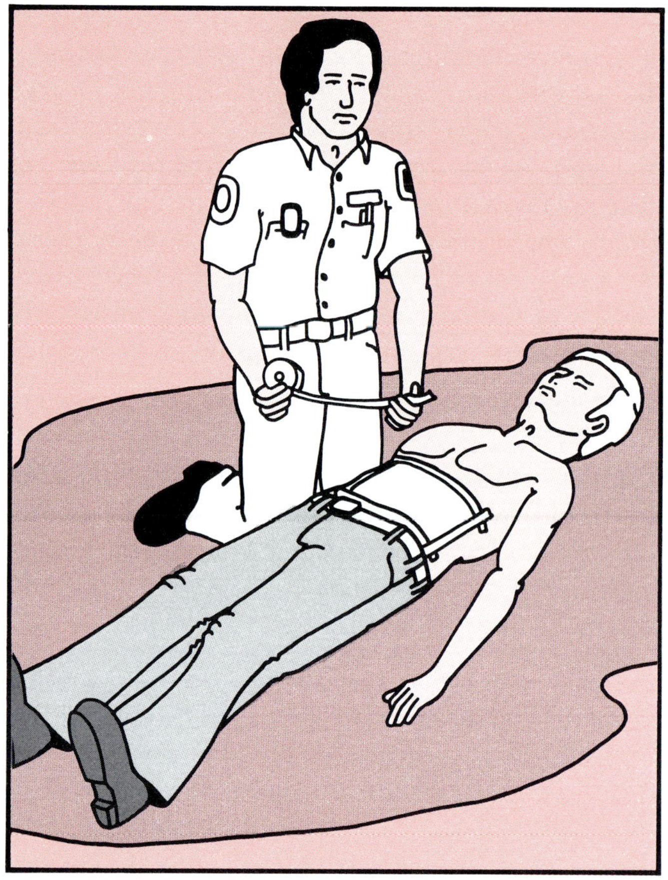

**Figure 7.35b** Cover the moist dressing with an occlusive dressing, such as aluminum foil. Tape the occlusive dressing down on all sides.

the moist dressing (Figures 7.35a, b). Tape the occlusive dressing down on all sides. Sealing the wound this way will keep the dressing moist and will prevent air from getting into the wound.

## Injuries to the Genitalia

Because the male genitalia are external, they are more vulnerable to soft-tissue injuries, which can be extremely painful. As with other soft-tissue injuries, injuries to the genitalia involve abrasions, lacerations, blunt trauma, avulsions, and impaled objects. Although injuries to the genitalia are rarely life-threatening, they are naturally of concern to the patient. First responders need to act in a calm, professional manner. Provide some measure of privacy during the examination, particularly if the patient is outside.

Abrasions and lacerations should be managed the same as other soft-tissue injuries. Apply a sterile dressing and then bandage the wound. Blunt trauma to the genital area may cause injury to both the penis and scrotum. The scrotal area will be bruised, swollen, and extremely painful. Administer ice packs to help reduce the swelling and relieve pain. Treat an avulsion by controlling bleeding and applying sterile, moist dressings. If the penis or any part of it is completely avulsed (amputated), control bleeding by applying firm pressure with a moist dressing. Wrap the amputated part in sterile, moist saline, and keep it cool. If an object is embedded in the urethra or any other part of the genitalia, DO NOT attempt to remove it, but rather stabilize it in place.

The only external part of the female genitalia is the vulva, the soft tissue that includes the labia majora, labia minora, and clitoris. Of course, this area of the body is subject to soft-tissue injuries as a result of trauma or accident. If a woman is bleeding in the genital area, apply sterile pressure dressings to control bleeding. Bleeding that originates from the internal genitalia can be massive; however, do not pack dressings into the vagina. Continue to apply manual pressure with bulky dressings.

While trauma may be due to an accident, it may also be a result of sexual assault. The woman who reports that she has been raped must be handled very carefully and professionally. The patient may find it extremely difficult to discuss what has happened and may fear or feel hostile toward a male first responder. If at all possible, have a female first responder conduct the patient examination. The examiner needs to make every effort to understand the patient's feelings and to respond with kindness and reassurance. If the patient chooses to talk about the assault, record her words on the patient care form. Do not record your opinions.

After conducting a primary survey, observe whether the patient's clothes are torn or in disarray. Check for signs of trauma elsewhere on the patient's body, especially around the thighs, lower abdomen, and buttocks. If the patient does not want to be disrobed and is not bleeding significantly, leave out this part of the examination. If vaginal or rectal bleeding is significant, apply sterile pressure dressings. Encourage the patient to report the assault to the police and to the nearest rape crisis center. Also encourage her not to change her clothes or to wash, which will destroy physical evidence of the assault.

Men also can be and are sexually assaulted. They need the same calm, concerned, professional level of care as do women. Conduct the physical examination in an atmosphere of privacy and calm. Physical care for the male victim of sexual assault should consist of a primary assessment, control of any bleeding, and examination and treatment of any associated injuries.

# 8

# Injuries to the Skull, Spine, and Chest

**U.S. DEPARTMENT OF TRANSPORTATION**
**First Responder Training Course**

**Objectives:**

- Identify the two main parts of the skull and describe their functions.
- Given descriptions of "patients" with injuries of the skull, spine and chest, identify the condition and describe appropriate emergency care.
- Given "patients," perform an examination for injuries of the skull, spine and chest, explaining aloud what is being checked for and why.
- Given "patients," describe appropriate emergency care for any injuries to the spine.
- Given "patients," perform appropriate emergency care for injuries to the skull and chest.

**NOTE:** It is assumed that the first responder will *not* have primary responsibility for splinting spinal injuries.

# Chapter 8
# Injuries to the Skull, Spine, and Chest

Skull and spine injuries are potentially very serious and, unfortunately, very common in accident situations. Injuries to the skull and spine commonly occur as a result of automobile accidents, falls, and direct blows to the head and the back in sports-related accidents. Skull injuries can result in brain injuries, and, in turn, the failure of vital body functions, while spinal injuries can cause paralysis. Between 10,000 and 15,000 accidents involving spinal injuries result in paralysis every year in the United States: statistically, most of these victims are young men between the ages of 15 and 30. For the victim, of course, paralysis is devastating physically, emotionally, and financially. For family members, too, the paralysis is tragic and traumatic, for they have the responsibility of caring for the victim for the rest of his or her life.

The initial assessment and treatment of the patient with head or spinal trauma often determines whether he or she will walk again. While it is important to know how to recognize and manage injuries to the skull and spine, it is equally important to know what *not* to do: improper treatment often causes permanent disability or death.

## INJURIES TO THE SKULL AND SPINE

On the following pages, injuries to the skull and spine are treated together in one section, followed by a discussion of injuries to the chest. This arrangement reflects the importance of a rule that you will see repeated many times in this section: **SUSPECT SPINAL DAMAGE IN ANY PATIENT WHO HAS SUSTAINED AN INJURY TO THE HEAD OR SKULL, AND HANDLE THE PATIENT ACCORDINGLY.** Similarly, anytime you encounter a patient who is unconscious due to unknown causes, suspect spinal injury and treat the patient accordingly. Patients will not be harmed by unnecessary spinal immobilization, but they can be seriously injured if they do have spinal injuries and are not immobilized.

### Airway

If the trauma patient is unconscious, pay special attention to maintaining an open airway. As you know, the tongue often relaxes and drops against the back of the throat in unconscious patients, thereby obstructing the airway. In a patient who has facial injuries, blood may flow into the airway and be aspirated into the lungs. Similarly, if an unconscious patient vomits, stomach contents, including swallowed blood, can also be aspirated because these patients lack the protection usually provided by the gag reflex. Patients with facial fractures may have bone fragments or teeth lodged in the back of the throat, causing partial or complete airway obstruction. Because all trauma victims must be assumed to have cervical spine injuries until proven otherwise, use the modified jaw-thrust maneuver to open the airway (see Chapter 5, Basic Life Support: the ABC's).

#### HELMET REMOVAL

If the patient has been injured during a sports activity or while riding a motorcycle, he or she may be wearing a helmet. If this is the case, you must make the decision whether or not to remove the helmet. The general rule is this: Unless the helmet interferes with efforts to maintain the patient's ABC's, leave it on. If the patient has a blocked airway, is bleeding heavily into the airway, or requires rescue breathing, you will probably have to remove the helmet, particularly if it is a full-face helmet.

A helmet *can* be removed without aggravating (worsening) the patient's injuries, but it is critical that you practice proper helmet-removal tech-

## Types of Helmets

Full face coverage—motorcycle, auto racer

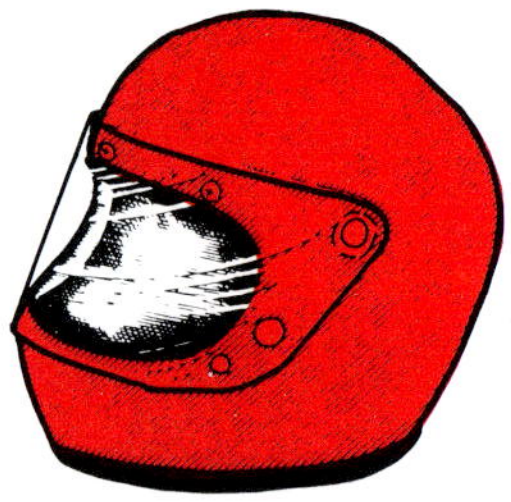

Full face coverage—motocross

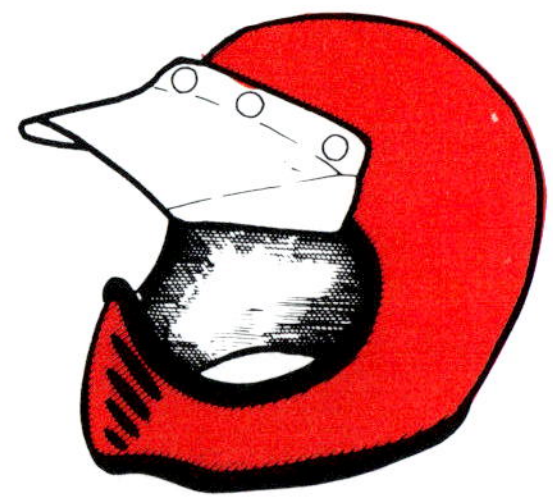

## Helmet Removal

1

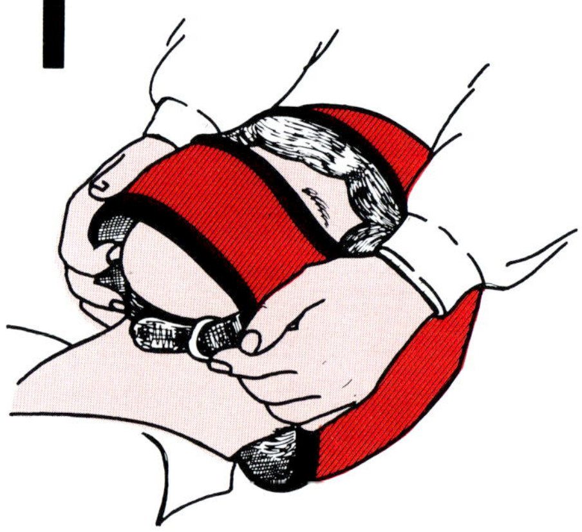

One rescuer applies inline traction by placing his or her hands on each side of the helmet with the fingers on the victim's mandible. This position prevents slippage if the strap is loose.

2

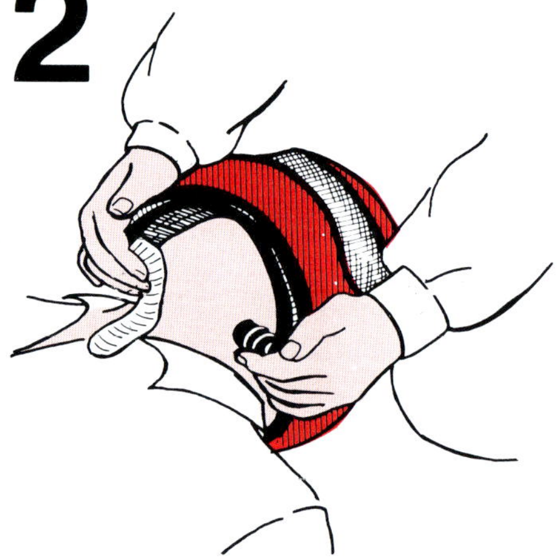

The rescuer cuts or loosens the strap at the D-rings while maintaining inline traction.

The varying sizes, shapes, and configurations of motorcycle helmets necessitate some understanding of their proper removal from victims of motorcycle accidents. The rescuer who removes a helmet improperly might inadvertently aggravate cervical spine injuries.

The Committee on Trauma believes that physicians who treat the injured should be aware of helmet removal techniques. A gradual increase in the use of helmets is anticipated because many organizations are urging voluntary wearing of helmets, and some states are reinstating their laws requiring the wearing of helmets.

American College of Surgeons
Committee on Trauma
July 1980

5

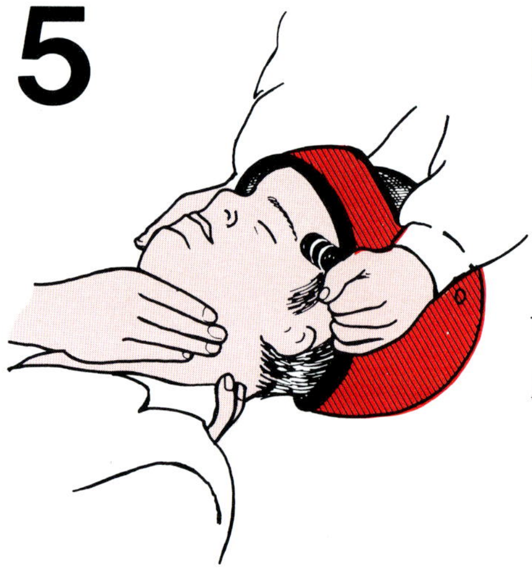

Throughout the removal process, the second rescuer maintains inline traction from below in order to prevent head tilt.

6

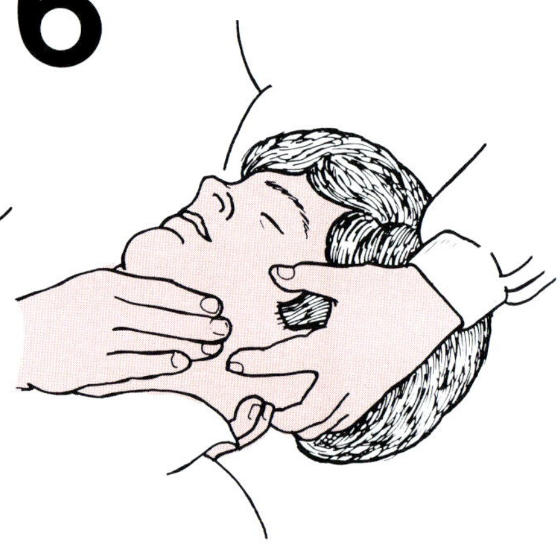

After the helmet has been removed, the rescuer at the top replaces his hands on either side of the victim's head with his palms over the ears.

niques before trying to remove a helmet from an actual patient. These techniques are described in Figure 8.1.

**Figure 8.1** (pages 168 and 169) Practice the correct procedures for helmet removal before attempting to remove a helmet from an actual patient. *Courtesy of American College of Surgeons.*

**Partial face coverage—motorcycle, auto racer**

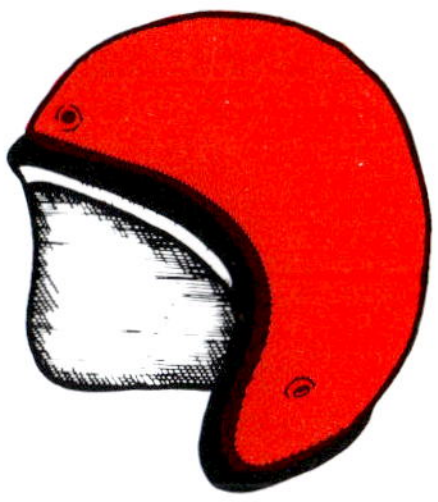

**Light head protection—bicycle, kayak**

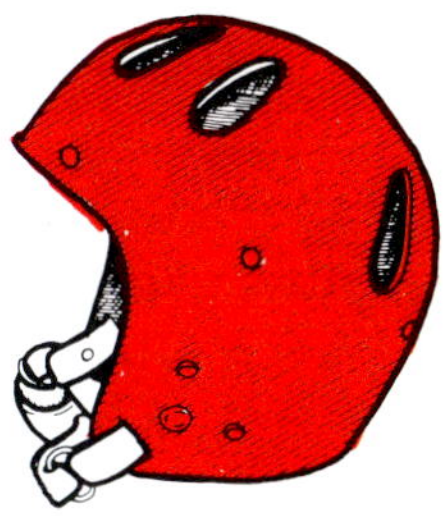

**Football**

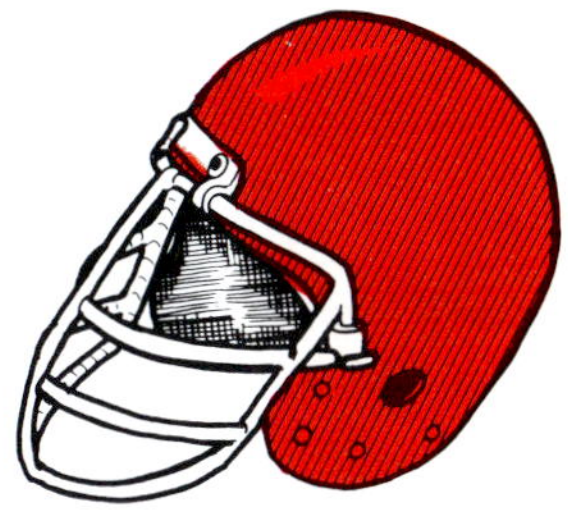

**3**

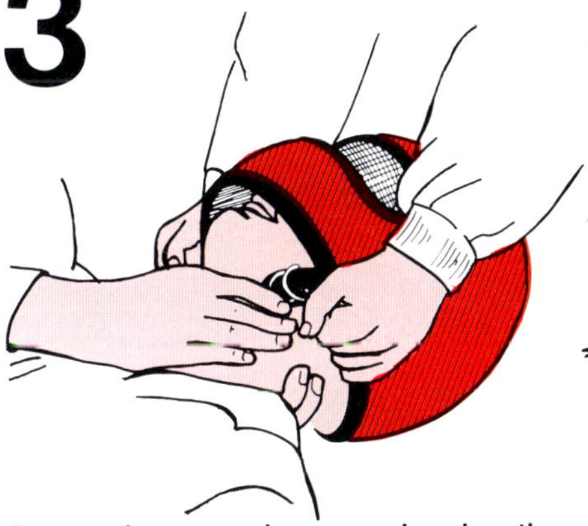

A second rescuer places one hand on the mandible at the angle, the thumb on one side, the long and index fingers on the other. With his other hand, he applies pressure from the occipital region. This maneuver transfers the inline traction responsibility to the second rescuer.

**4**

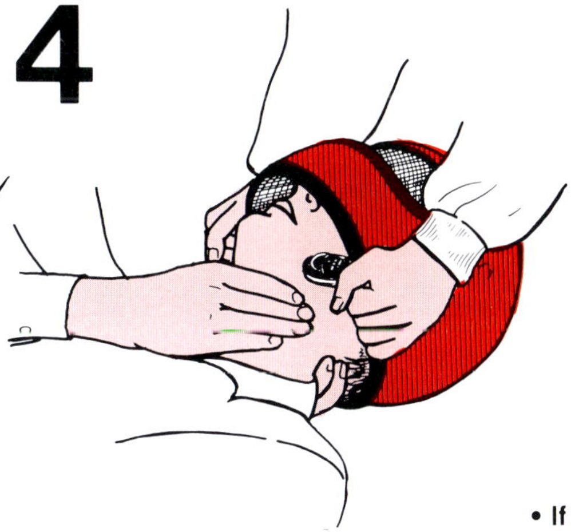

The rescuer at the top removes the helmet. Three factors should be kept in mind:

- The helmet is egg-shaped, and therefore must be expanded laterally to clear the ears.
- If the helmet provides full facial coverage, glasses must be removed first.
- If the helmet provides full facial coverage, the nose will impede removal. To clear the nose, the helmet must be tilted backward and raised over it.

**7**

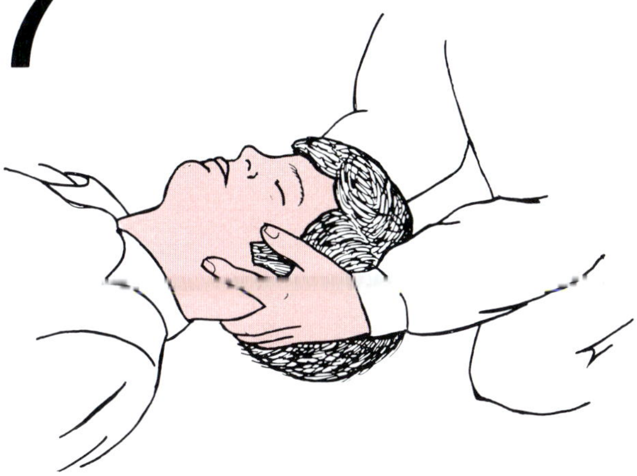

Inline traction is maintained from above until a backboard is in place.

Summary

The helmet must be maneuvered over the nose and ears while the head and neck are held rigid.

- Inline traction is applied from above.
- Inline traction is transferred below with pressure on the jaw and occiput.
- The helmet is removed.
- Inline traction is re-established from above.

NOTE: "Techniques of Helmet Removal from Injured Patients" was designed for use by *medical and allied health professionals,* including emergency medical technicians and paramedics.

Untrained lay persons not serving as qualified members of rescue squads or ambulance crews are not encouraged to use these techniques to manipulate injured helmeted victims unless trained personnel are present. This is further borne out by consideration of the next step, which is proper fixation of the injured person's head and neck to a backboard.

The fact that techniques of helmet removal have been described is not an indication that helmets must be removed in every instance, or by any person. The decisions should be made by suitably trained persons.

Because you must assume that the patient has suffered a spinal cord injury, helmet removal requires two persons — one to maintain axial traction and one to remove the helmet (see Applying In-Line Traction later in this chapter.) Remember that the helmet must be spread slightly to fit over the patient's ears, and take care not to catch the chin piece on the patient's nose.

### Breathing

Patients with major head or spinal trauma and serious neurological injury frequently stop breathing. Increased *intracranial pressure* (pressure within the skull) caused by bleeding within the skull can exert pressure on vital control centers and can decrease the patient's ability to breathe. Direct injury to the breathing centers of the medulla can also create breathing difficulties.

The trauma patient's rate and quality of breathing may vary according to the nature and extent of brain or spinal injury. The breathing pattern may be normal, or the patient may exhibit *Cheyne-Stokes respiration*, a cyclic type of irregular breathing that occurs as a result of some grave head injuries. It is characterized by respirations that are first shallow, then quite deep and rapid, and then shallow once again, followed by a period of 5 to 30 seconds during which the patient stops breathing.

Some trauma patients may exhibit *central neurogenic hyperventilation*, a sustained pattern of very deep and rapid breathing. After central neurogenic hyperventilation, the patient's breathing may become irregular and ineffective, and the patient may eventually stop breathing altogether.

Cervical spinal cord injuries can also impair respirations. "High" cervical cord damage, that is, damage around the first four vertebrae, can produce complete respiratory paralysis. Damage at the level of the next two vertebrae paralyzes the diaphragm, but allows the *intercostal muscles* (those between the ribs) to continue to function. Breathing in this manner is very inefficient, however, and the patient will be struggling to breathe.

### Circulation

Assess the patient's circulation and note any signs of shock, especially cool, clammy skin and a weak, rapid pulse. Shock rarely occurs as a result of a head injury, so its presence usually means that the patient has a major source of bleeding elsewhere in the body. If the patient shows signs of shock and has no major external bleeding, assume internal bleeding.

If you cannot find a pulse, begin chest compressions at once. If the patient is pulseless, he or she is clinically dead, so possible spinal or internal injuries are secondary to beginning CPR (see Chapter 5, Basic Life Support: the ABC's). **NEVER** begin chest compressions on someone whose heart is still beating, even if the pulse is very weak.

### Severe Bleeding

Bleeding from the head is usually from ruptured blood vessels in the scalp. These wounds may bleed heavily enough to cause hypovolemic shock, particularly in children. Control bleeding from the scalp with direct pressure unless there is evidence of a skull fracture beneath the wound, such as a depression in the skull, visible bone fragments, or exposed brain tissue. Direct pressure under these circumstances may drive bone fragments into the brain. Simply cover the wound with a bulky dressing and secure it with a roller bandage. When direct pressure is ineffective in controlling bleeding from an uncomplicated scalp wound, compressing the temporal artery may slow or stop the flow of blood (Figure 8.2).

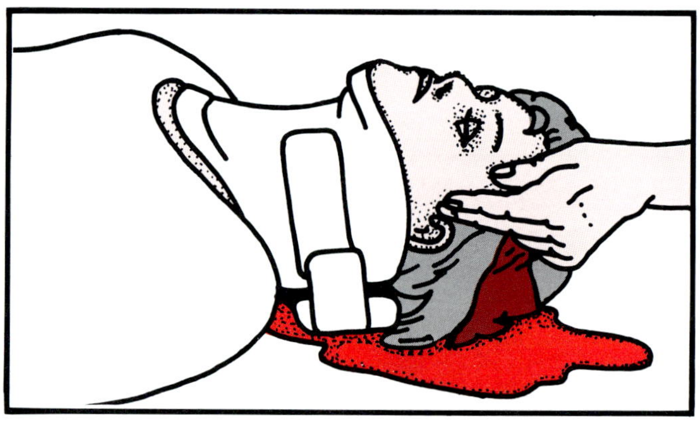

**Figure 8.2** Compressing the temporal artery may help slow the flow of blood from a head wound.

### Vital Signs

Patients with skull and spine injuries may have vital signs that change over time. Check vital signs every 5 to 10 minutes.

If the patient has low blood pressure and a rapid pulse, he or she may be suffering from hemorrhagic, cardiogenic, or neurogenic shock (see Chapter 6, Shock). Falling blood pressure is rarely caused by head injury; if it accompanies head injury, look for a source of major hemorrhage elsewhere in the body.

Rising blood pressure is often the result of increasing intracranial pressure. During the early stages of increasing intracranial pressure, the pulse slows and the blood pressure and temperature rise. Later, as the pulse rate increases, the blood pressure falls to normal or below-normal (hypotensive) levels while the temperature remains elevated. As these changes develop over time, it is especially important to make frequent observations of the patient's vital signs.

Note the rate and rhythm of respirations. Determine whether an abnormal pattern, such as Cheyne-Stokes respiration, is present. Note whether the patient breathes normally, or only with difficulty, using the accessory muscles.

### Patient History

It is often difficult to assess patients who have injuries to the skull or spine. Because their mental functioning is often impaired, they may be unable to give a history or to cooperate in physical examinations. In such cases, you must obtain information from careful observation, not only of the patient, but also of the scene of the accident.

If the patient is a trauma victim, answers to the following questions are particularly important:

- *What* happened?
- *When* did the accident occur?
- *How* did it occur? What were the mechanisms of injury? Was the spine flexed, extended, or twisted? If the patient was involved in an automobile accident, was he or she wearing a seat belt? Did the patient sustain a direct blow to a specific part of the head or spine? Was there a rapid deceleration?
- Was the patient unconscious at any time? For how long? Did unconsciousness occur immediately after the accident, or later?
- If the patient is able to communicate, what is the chief complaint? Does the patient experience any pain, numbness, tingling, or paralysis? Have the symptoms changed since the accident?
- Are there possible complicating factors such as significant underlying medical problems?
- Has the patient moved or been moved since the accident?
- Did the patient vomit? (Children frequently vomit after head injury, but vomiting in adults may indicate serious intracranial problems.)
- What symptoms does the patient have now? Headache? Dizziness? Double or blurred vision? Nausea? Weakness? Can the patient move all extremities? Does the patient have any pain in the head, neck, or spine? Does the patient have numbness or a tingling sensation?
- Has the patient used any alcohol or drugs in the past few hours?

### Head-To-Toe Examination

After taking a patient history, conduct a head-to-toe survey, paying particular attention to skull injuries, which may be open or closed. *Closed* and *open*, as they are used to describe head injuries, refer to the skull. Thus, if the skull is fractured, the head injury is termed *open*, whether or not the skin is broken. If the skull is not fractured, the head injury is termed *closed*, even if the skin is lacerated.

A scalp laceration may bleed profusely. On the other hand, a patient with a skull fracture may not have obvious signs of such an injury upon first inspection. It is critical that you touch the skull carefully, feeling for deformities or depression of the skull bones. Blood coming from the nose most often flows from a nasal injury, but it can also be the result of a skull fracture. Assume that clear fluid coming from the ears or nose is cerebrospinal fluid, an indicator of major skull fracture. If clear or bloody fluid is leaking from the ears or nose, DO NOT attempt to block the flow; simply cover the ear or nose with sterile gauze. Attempting to stop the flow of blood and/or cerebrospinal fluid from the ears or nose may increase intracranial pressure if the patient's skull is fractured.

Purple discoloration (ecchymosis) behind the ears, known as "Battle's sign," or around the eyes, usually called "coon's eyes," also suggests a basal skull fracture.

Next, check the patient's pupils. Note whether they are the same size and if they react quickly to direct light. In patients who have increased intracranial pressure, compression of the nerve that controls pupil constriction causes the pupil to dilate widely — a condition known as a "blown" pupil (Figure 8.3).

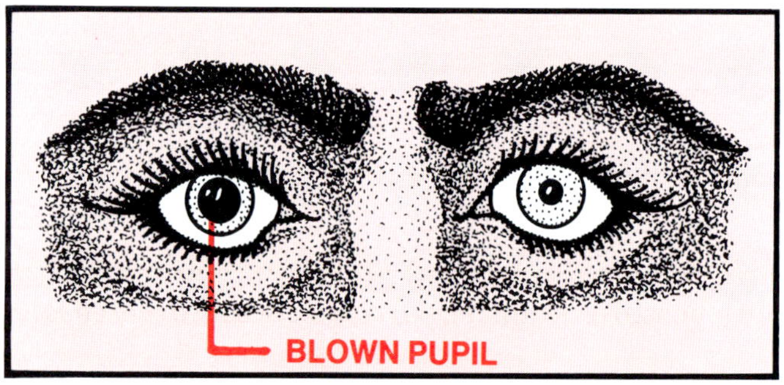


**Figure 8.3** A "blown" pupil results when a head injury damages the nerve that controls dilation and constriction of the pupil, causing the pupil to dilate widely.

The conscious patient's ability to move his or her eyes is also an important part of the assessment. Inability to move the eyes in a coordinated manner indicates damage to the nerves leading to the eyes or to the part of the brain stem that controls these nerves.

Next, assess the patient's neck. Have your partner maintain in-line (axial) traction while you check the patient's neck for vertebral irregularities or tenderness, then apply a cervical collar or otherwise immobilize the neck (see Applying In-Line Traction later in this section).

After examining the head and neck, check the patient for spinal injury. **SUSPECT SPINAL DAMAGE IN ANY PATIENT WHO HAS SUSTAINED AN INJURY TO THE HEAD OR SKULL, AND HANDLE THE PATIENT ACCORDINGLY.** If the patient is positioned in such a way that his or her back is readily accessible for examination, look for cuts and bruises near or over the spine and note any obvious deformity of the spine. If the patient is supine, either move your hand gently under the patient to palpate the spinal column, or do it as the patient is logrolled onto a backboard (Figure 8.4). Any open injuries of the spinal column should be covered immediately with sterile dressings. If bony deformity or pain is present, immobilize the patient before you continue the assessment.

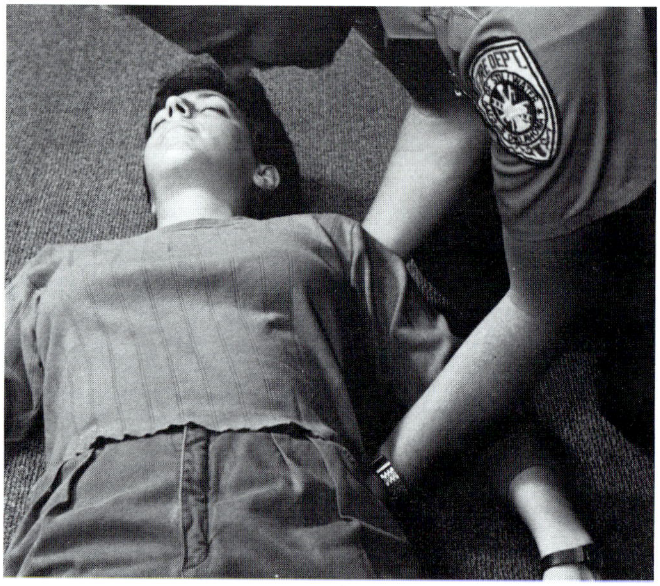

**Figure 8.4** If the patient is lying supine, move your hand gently under the patient to examine the spinal column.

One obvious indication of spinal injury is a condition known as *priapism*. Priapism is a sustained, painful erection of the penis. The presence of this condition is unmistakable and should not be overlooked. Of course, the most common signs of spinal injury are tingling sensations and paralysis. (See Testing for Paralysis later in this section.)

Complete the physical exam in the usual head-to-toe order, and look for fractures or lacerations. Keep the airway clear, and be sure that the patient is breathing adequately. Check the patient's vital signs every 5 to 10 minutes.

## Seizures

It is not uncommon for patients who have suffered an injury to the head to have seizures after the accident. As a result of automobile accidents alone, 540,000 Americans suffer head injuries each year. Almost 20,000 of these people develop persistent epileptic seizures. A seizure after an accident, then, is a good indication that the brain has been injured. Do not attempt to restrain a convulsing patient: it is virtually impossible to do so anyway. As soon as the seizure ends, talk to the patient in a soothing voice and apply a cervical collar if you have not already done so. Be prepared to suction blood or vomit from the patient's airway. (See Chapter 10, Medical Emergencies, for more information about seizures and their management.)

## The Neurological Examination

After finding and correcting life-threatening problems and immobilizing the patient to prevent further spinal injury, assess the patient's level of consciousness. Any change in level of consciousness, whether good or bad, is important and must be noted. These changes can occur rapidly, so reassess the patient's level of consciousness every 5 to 10 minutes.

First, assess the patient's verbal response and sense of orientation. Note whether the patient is alert and oriented to person, place, and time (alert and oriented times three), or whether he or she seems confused. Is the patient's speech normal, incomprehensible, or absent?

The Glasgow Coma Scale was developed to enable emergency personnel to quickly assess a patient's neurological function (Figure 8.5). As you test a patient's eye-opening, verbal, and motor responses, assign a number from the Glasgow scale that corresponds to the patient's reaction. The total from the three categories of assessment is the patient's "score." The highest score on the Glasgow Coma Scale is 15, and the lowest score is 1.

Note whether the patient opens his or her eyes spontaneously, in response to the sound of your voice, in response to a painful stimulus, or not at all.

The patient's motor response to a painful stimulus is also an important indicator of mental functioning. The standard painful stimulus consists of pressing your knuckles into the patient's sternum with varying degrees of pressure. If the patient attempts to push your arm away, he or she is said to "localize" pain. If the patient moves away from a painful stimulus, he or she is said to "withdraw" in response to pain.

**Glasgow Coma Scale**

| | | | Total Glasgow Coma Scale Points |
|---|---|---|---|
| **Eye Opening** | Spontaneous | 4 | 14-15 = 5 |
| | To Voice | 3 | 11-13 = 4 |
| | To Pain | 2 | 8-10 = 3 |
| | None | 1 | 5- 7 = 2 |
| **Verbal Response** | Oriented | 5 | 3- 4 = 1 |
| | Confused | 4 | |
| | Inappropriate Words | 3 | |
| | Incomprehensible Words | 2 | |
| | None | 1 | |
| **Motor Response** | Obeys Command | 6 | |
| | Localizes Pain | 5 | |
| | Withdraw (pain) | 4 | |
| | Flexion (pain) | 3 | |
| | Extension (pain) | 2 | |
| | None | 1 | |

**Figure 8.5** The Glasgow Coma Scale is used to assess a patient's eye-opening, verbal, and motor responses. *Courtesy of Dr. Howard Champion.*

If the patient has suffered a major neurological injury, he or she may respond to painful stimuli with postures known as *decorticate* and *decerebrate* (Figure 8.6). In decorticate posturing, the arms are

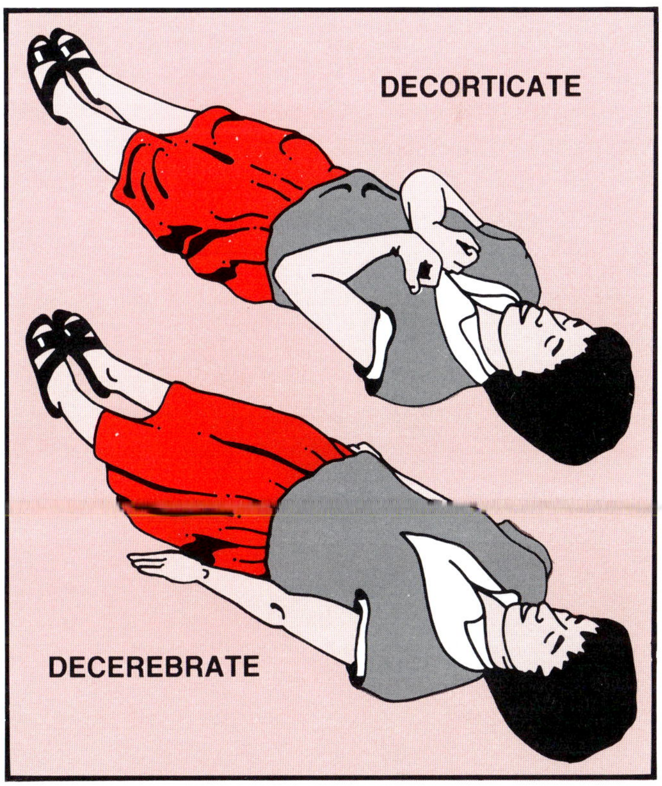


**Figure 8.6** In decorticate posturing, the arms are flexed but the legs remain extended. In decerebrate posturing, both the arms and the legs are extended.

flexed but the legs remain extended; this is termed "flexion." In decerebrate posturing, both arms and legs are extended; this is termed "extension." Patients may either exhibit these postures in response to a painful stimulus, or may assume and maintain them indefinitely.

Reassess the patient's eye-opening, verbal, and motor responses in accordance with the Glasgow Coma Scale every 10 minutes to keep track of any changes in the patient's neurological status.

## Testing for Paralysis

The most reliable sign of spinal cord damage is paralysis, but this sign may not be present despite cord damage. Even if the patient shows no signs of paralysis or neurological injury, immobilize the patient until hospital examination can rule out spinal cord damage.

Because loss of function occurs below the injured segment of the spinal cord, start at the lowest point of the lower extremities, the feet. If the patient can communicate, ask if he or she can feel the feet and legs being touched. Cover the area you are testing to avoid giving the patient misleading clues. Also, ask if he or she can wiggle the toes or raise the legs. Move the patient's toes up and down without the patient seeing and ask the patient to tell in which direction the toes are being moved (Figure 8.7) If the patient can respond only to a limited degree and with pain, there may be pressure on, or damage to, the cord. Inability to move on command is a strong indication of severe damage to the spinal cord.

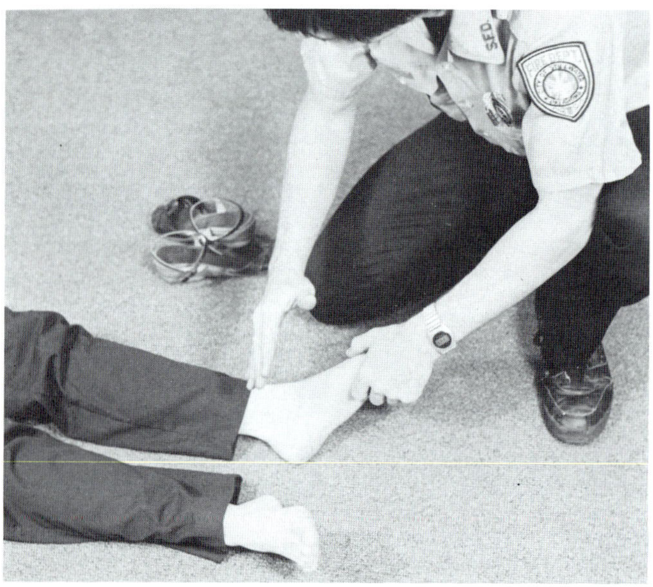

**Figure 8.7** Using your hand as a shield, move the patient's toes up and down and ask if he or she can tell in which direction the toes are being moved.

Check the function of the upper extremities to see whether there is damage to the cervical spine. Follow the same basic procedures used to assess the function of the lower extremities. Touch the patient's hands and arms and ask whether the touch can be felt. Move the patient's finger up and down to determine whether he or she knows in which direction it is being moved. Ask the patient to squeeze your fingers tightly. The average adult should be able to squeeze tightly enough so that it is difficult for you to remove your fingers. In addition, note whether the pressure exerted is equal on both sides.

When you check for paralysis, test all extremities, left and right. Paralysis in both legs (paraplegia) or in both arms and both legs (quadriplegia) indicates spinal cord damage. Paralysis of the arm and leg on one side of the body (hemiplegia) may indicate a stroke.

Continue to monitor the patient's vital signs, level of consciousness, and pupillary reflexes. Watch carefully for the development of shock.

## Injuries to the Skull and Brain

Head trauma can injure the scalp, the skull, or the brain. The scalp bleeds easily and profusely when it is injured, but the brain usually is not affected by superficial scalp lacerations. It is important to remember that the brain can be damaged without any apparent damage to the scalp or skull.

### SKULL FRACTURES

Skull fractures are common in accident victims, yet their seriousness depends upon the degree of injury to the brain. Serious brain injury, in fact, is much more common when there is no skull fracture. Still, you *must* suspect at least minimal brain injury in any patient who has a skull fracture. In addition, suspect spinal damage in any patient who has suffered an injury to the head or skull, and handle the patient accordingly.

Skull fractures may be either open or closed, and they may be further classified as

- *Linear* — A linear fracture is a line fracture or crack in the skull. Most skull fractures are of this type.
- *Comminuted* — A comminuted fracture is basically a crushed bone. A comminuted skull fracture has multiple cracks in the skull that radiate from the center of impact.
- *Depressed* — A depressed skull fracture is similar to a comminuted fracture except that pieces of bone are pushed inward. These bone fragments press upon brain tissue and sometimes tear it.
- *Basal* — A basal fracture is a linear, comminuted, or depressed fracture of the base of the skull. Common signs are Battle's sign and coon's eyes.
- *Penetrated* — The skull may also be fractured by an object such as a bullet or knife that penetrates the skull and lodges in the brain.

In extremely severe head injuries, the skull may be fractured and pieces of bone driven into the brain matter, thereby destroying brain cells. If the skull is fractured in such a way that the brain is exposed, significant damage to brain tissue usually occurs very quickly. These patients are susceptible to serious infections of the brain (cerebritis) and meninges (meningitis).

## CONCUSSION

When the brain is forced to move rapidly within the skull, as it does when a patient sustains a blow to the head, the areas in the brain stem that control consciousness may be damaged. When this happens, the victim usually loses consciousness. This injury is called a *concussion*. A concussion usually causes unconsciousness, either temporary or prolonged, and the patient may regain consciousness gradually or quite suddenly. Many patients who sustain concussions suddenly draw their knees up toward the chest and vomit.

The symptoms of a concussion vary according to the location and extent of the injury: the patient may experience symptoms that range from mild dizziness to various paralyses. The signs of concussion include unequal pupils, unconsciousness, and shock.

## EPIDURAL HEMATOMA

An epidural hematoma occurs when blood vessels located between the skull and the dura mater (the membrane covering the brain) are torn by a skull fracture (Figure 8.8). The resulting accumulation of blood within the skull causes increased intracranial pressure and compresses vital structures of the brain and brain stem. With such an injury, the patient often loses and then regains consciousness, but his or her condition begins to deteriorate as blood collects in the skull.

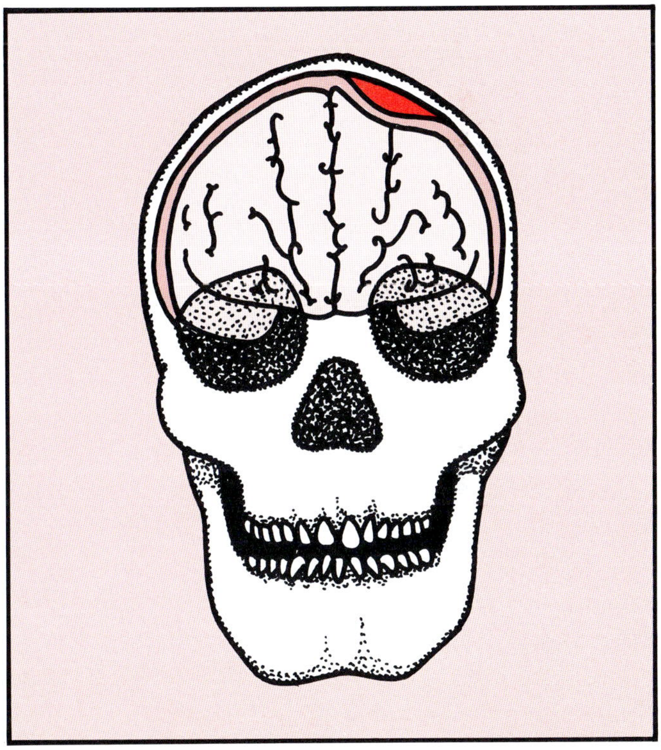

**Figure 8.8** An epidural hematoma occurs when blood vessels between the skull and the membrane covering the skull are torn by a skull fracture.

## SUBDURAL HEMATOMA

In a subdural hematoma, bleeding occurs from torn vessels between the dura mater and the arachnoid mater (Figure 8.9 on next page). The subdural hematoma usually develops more slowly than the epidural hematoma, and the patient's condition deteriorates more gradually. When the resulting blood clot is large enough, intracranial pressure increases, and respiratory and other centers are affected.

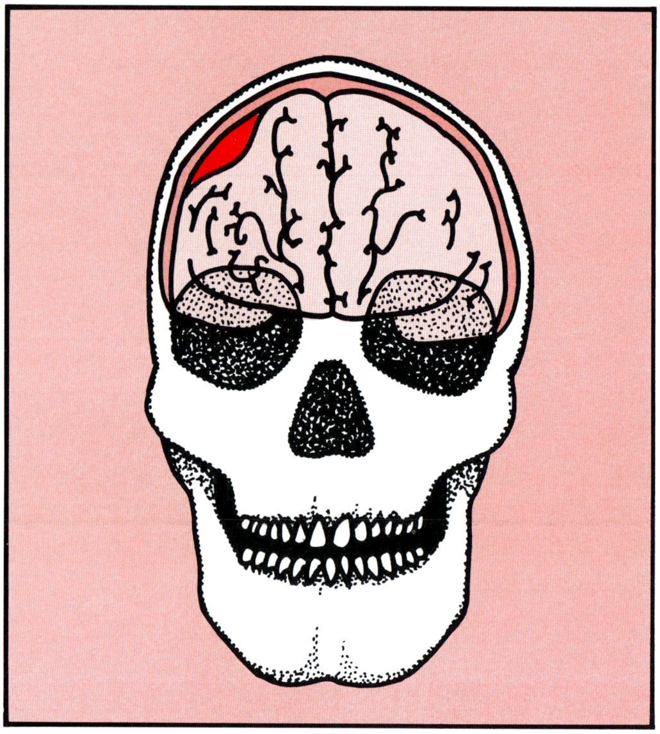

**Figure 8.9** In a subdural hematoma, bleeding occurs from torn vessels between the dura mater and the arachnoid mater.

Often a hematoma damages the nerve that controls dilation and constriction of the pupil. This damage causes the pupil to dilate widely, a condition known as a "blown" pupil.

The signs of a hematoma may take up to two hours to develop. Suspect a possible hematoma in a patient who has suffered head trauma several hours earlier. Because the patient's condition worsens as blood collects inside the skull, it is very important to monitor the patient's vital signs and neurological function every 5 to 10 minutes.

## Emergency Treatment for Head Injuries

In the field, there is relatively little specific treatment for the patient with head injury. Try to maintain the patient's ABC's, prevent further injury, and monitor the patient's neurological status by

- Keeping the patient in a supine position
- Establishing an airway, being careful not to aggravate (worsen) possible cervical spine injury
- Maintaining axial traction on the neck, and applying a cervical collar
- Administering oxygen and assisting ventilations if necessary
- Monitoring vital signs frequently

### APPLYING IN-LINE (AXIAL) TRACTION

In-line, or axial, refers to an imaginary line that runs along the main axis of the body, that is, a line that roughly corresponds to the spine. Traction refers to an act of drawing or pulling. Thus, maintaining in-line traction means keeping the head and spine of an accident victim aligned with a gentle pulling action. If an unconscious victim's neck is flexed or bent when you arrive at the scene, DO NOT straighten it to apply traction, unless you must open the airway to enable the victim to breathe. Instead, immobilize the patient in the position in which you find him or her.

To apply in-line traction, kneel above the patient's head and position your hands on both sides of the head, so that your palms are over the patient's ears. Your thumbs should be in the temporal region on each side of the head, index fingers along the cheekbones, middle fingers along the jaw, ring fingers along the muscle below the jaw, and little fingers along the back of the skull (Figure 8.10). *Gently* pull the patient's head toward you without turning the head in either direction. **Do not release manual traction until a cervical collar is applied and the patient's head is securely strapped to a KED, short backboard, or long backboard** (see Immobilizing Patients for Transportation later in this chapter). Be sure that the pulling force you exert is constant and not excessive: only slight pressure is required.

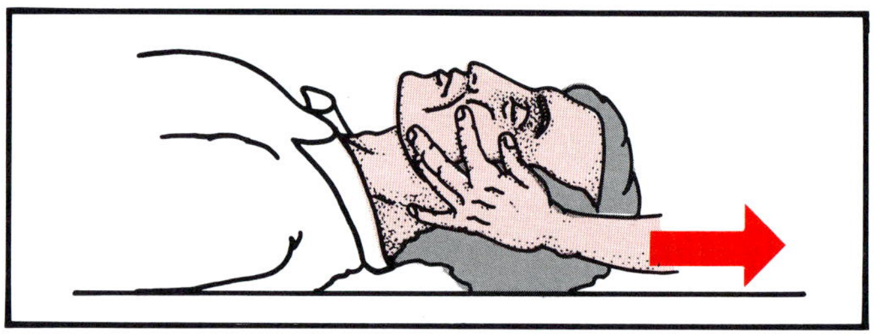

**Figure 8.10** To apply in-line (axial) traction, position your hands on both sides of the patient's head in the manner shown above. *Gently* pull the patient's head toward you without turning the head in either direction.

## Injuries to the Spine

Like the brain, the spinal cord can be damaged by direct or indirect injury. The spine, however, has less protection than the brain because its bony protection is flexible (Figure 8.11). The thoracic vertebrae are protected by the ribs and associated muscles, so injury to the thoracic spine is relatively rare. The neck lacks even this support and is the most flexible part of the spine, so injuries to the cervical spine are quite common. The size and muscular protection of the lumbar spine make it somewhat more resistant to injury than the cervical spine, but it is still more vulnerable than the thoracic spine.

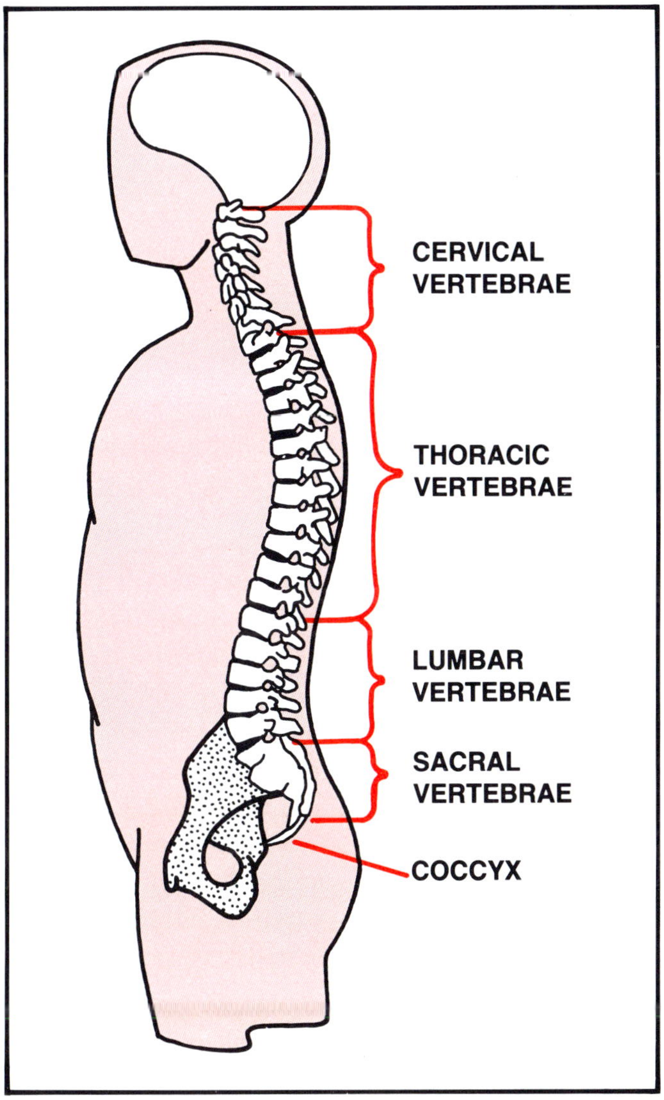


**Figure 8.11** The cervical (neck) vertebrae are most susceptible to injury because they form the most flexible part of the spine and are not well protected by associated muscles.

The spinal cord may be injured by compression from flexion or twisting, laceration or compression from bony fragments of the spine in spinal fractures, protrusion of the cartilage discs between vertebrae into the spinal canal, dislocation of one vertebra from the vertebra below it, or bleeding into the spinal canal (Figure 8.12).

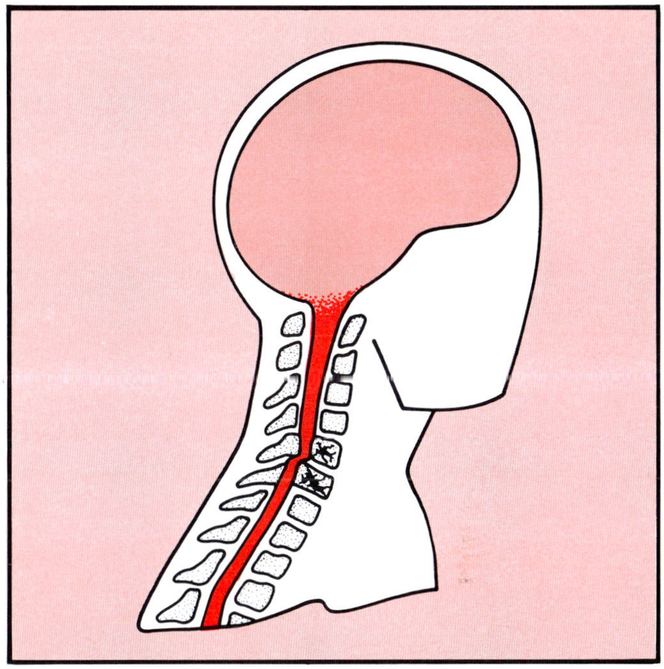

**Figure 8.12** The spinal cord may be compressed from flexion or twisting.

When the spinal cord is lacerated or compressed, nerve fibers that carry impulses to and from the brain are disrupted. There is a direct relationship between the location of a spinal cord injury and any loss of body function. This relationship is based on the distribution of nerves that branch away from the spinal cord. When a specific nerve pathway is interrupted, the part of the body served by that nerve is affected. In other words, when the pathway is interrupted, the message cannot be carried. For this reason, paralysis is a common sign of injury to the spinal cord.

The initial care given to the patient with spinal injury can determine whether he or she regains normal function or is permanently crippled. In few other areas of emergency care is early treatment so critical to the patient's future.

Suspect spinal injury in patients who are injured in automobile, sledding, or diving accidents, and in falls. Try to determine the precise circumstances of the accident. Was the neck flexed, extended, or twisted? When did the accident occur? Does the patient have localized pain in the neck or back? Is there numbness or tingling in any extremity? Are the extremities weak? If the patient is unable to move, find out whether the patient was able to move at any time after the accident. Because the patient who has any movement at all after spinal injury has a fair chance of recovering nerve function, it is important for the physician to know this. Has the patient been moved since the accident? Have symptoms changed since the injury?

As with head injury, management of spinal injuries is aimed at supporting vital functions and preventing further spinal cord damage. To manage spinal injuries

- Establish and maintain an airway, being careful not to aggravate possible cervical spine injury. Use the modified jaw-thrust maneuver to open and maintain the airway.
- Administer oxygen and assist ventilations as needed.
- Apply axial traction and immobilize the neck with a cervical collar (Figure 8.13).
- Immobilize the patient on a long backboard whenever a spinal injury may have occurred. Paticnts will not be harmed by unnecessary spinal immobilization, but they can be seriously injured if they do have spinal injuries and are not immobilized.
- Keep the patient covered to avoid heat loss.

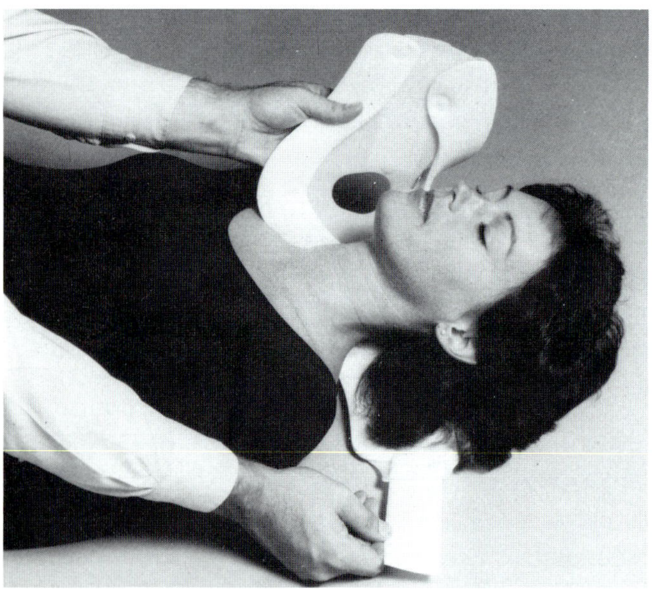

**Figure 8.13** After ensuring that the patient has an open airway, immobilize the neck with a cervical collar. *Photo courtesy of Dyna Med.*

## Immobilizing Patients for Transportation

Any patient who has a suspected spinal cord injury must be immobilized for transportation to a medical facility. To do this, use a KED-type device or a short backboard and a long backboard, since these devices offer rigid support for the patient's head, neck, and back (Figure 8.14). An orthopedic (scoop) stretcher can be used when rescuers have very little room in which to work.

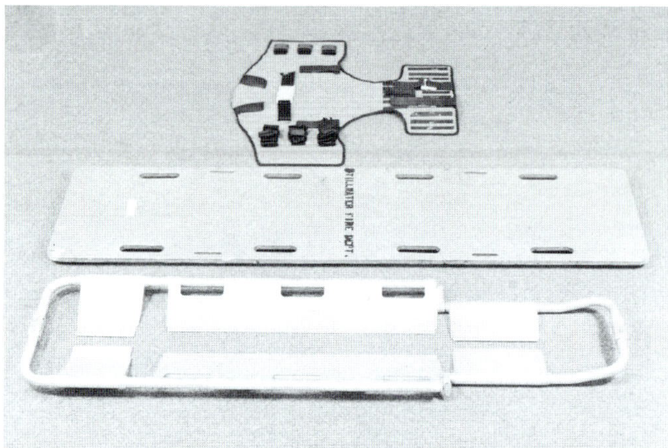

**Figure 8.14** To prepare a patient with a suspected spinal injury for transportation, use a KED-type device or short backboard, and a long backboard.

### LONG BACKBOARD

Immobilizing a patient on a long backboard requires four rescuers, one to maintain axial traction throughout the process, and three to actually move the patient to the board. It is critical that the patient with a suspected spinal injury be moved in such a way as to avoid any unnecessary jolting or twisting of the spinal column. For this reason, the rescuer who applies and maintains axial traction directs the other rescuers in their actions to ensure that the patient's head and body are moved as a unit. When dangers at the scene are life-threatening to the patient and rescuers, this process may be performed with only two rescuers — one to maintain axial traction, and one to move the patient.

Step 1: The first rescuer applies axial traction.

Step 2: A second rescuer applies a cervical collar, then prepares the long backboard by placing the straps through the side slots of the board. Once the board is prepared, the rescuer places it alongside and parallel to the patient (Figure 8.15).

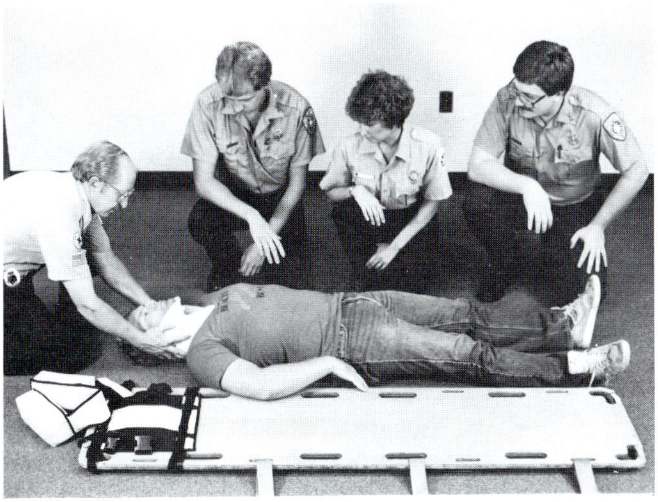

**Figure 8.15** After placing the straps through the side slots of the backboard, the second rescuer places the backboard alongside and parallel to the patient.

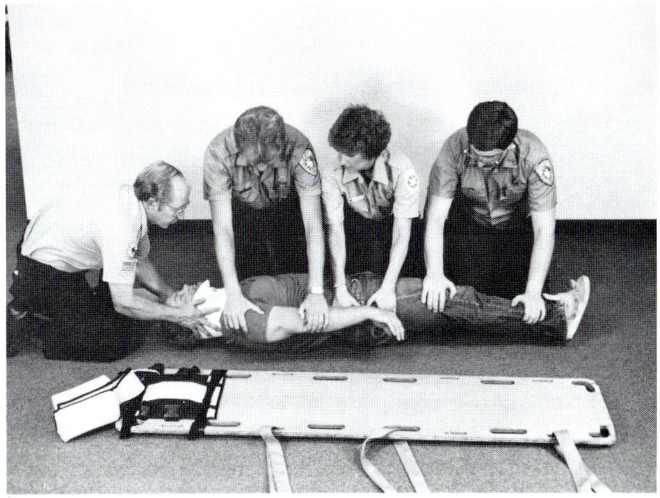

**Figure 8.16** The first rescuer remains at the patient's head and applies axial traction. The other three rescuers grasp the patient's shoulders, waist, and legs.

Step 3: Three rescuers kneel on one side of the patient — one at the head, one at the waist, and one at the feet. The first rescuer continues to maintain axial traction throughout the lift. The rescuer at the patient's head is in charge of moving the patient; all other rescuers move on this person's command.

Step 4: The rescuer at the patient's shoulder grasps the patient's opposite shoulder and upper arm. The rescuer at the waist grasps the patient's waist and buttocks on the opposite side. The rescuer at the patient's knees grasps the patient's lower thigh and calf on the opposite side (Figure 8.16).

Step 5: At the direction of the first rescuer, the three rescuers gently roll the patient toward them as a unit (Figure 8.17).

Step 6: The rescuer who is at the patient's waist reaches across the patient's body with one hand and pulls the backboard into position against the patient.

Step 7: The first rescuer directs the other three to roll the patient onto the board, again making sure that the patient's head and body are rolled as a unit (Figure 8.18). (**NOTE:** The patient will not be completely on the backboard at this point.)

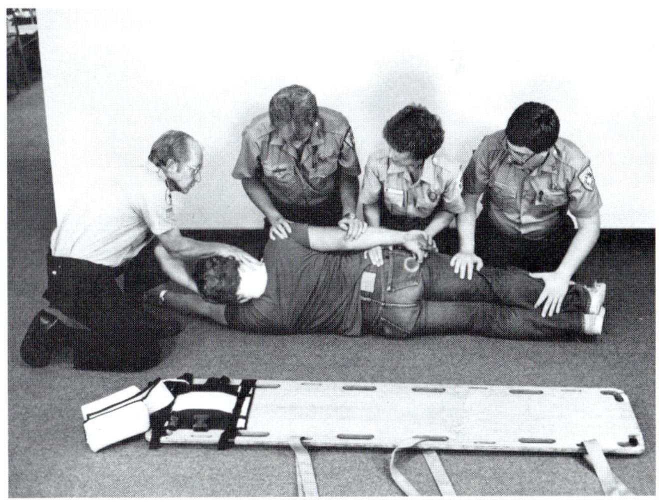

**Figure 8.17** At the direction of the first rescuer, the other three rescuers gently roll the patient toward them as a unit.

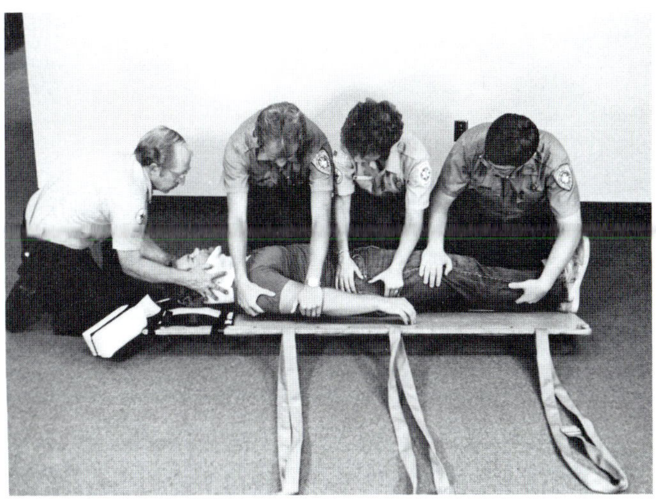

**Figure 8.18** On command, the three rescuers roll the patient onto the backboard as a unit. The rescuer at the patient's head continues to maintain axial traction.

Step 8: On the command of the first rescuer, the three rescuers gently push the patient so that he or she is centered on the backboard (Figure 8.19). **CAUTION:** This step must be carefully coordinated in order to move the patient's head and body as a unit. All rescuers *must* move only at the command of the first rescuer, who continues to maintain axial traction. Alternate method: while the rescuer at the patient's head maintains axial traction, the other three rescuers stand and straddle the patient. Again, one rescuer grasps the patient's shoulders, one grasps the patient's hips, and the third rescuer grasps the patient's legs. On command, all slide the patient and center the patient on the backboard (Figure 8.20).

Step 9: The rescuer who is at the patient's shoulders places rolled towels, blankets, or sandbags on both sides of the patient's head. These items and the patient's head must be secured to the board with a cravat or tape that passes over the forehead. If a head immobilizer is used, place the sides in position and secure the chin and forehead straps as shown in Figure 8.21.

Step 10: Each of the three rescuers fastens the patient to the board with the appropriate strap — one across the chest, one above the hips, and one above the knees (Figure 8.22).

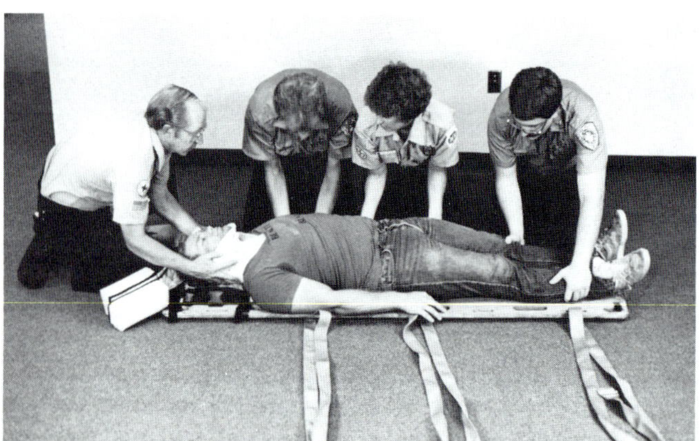

**Figure 8.19** On the command of the first rescuer, the three rescuers gently push the patient so that he or she is centered on the backboard.

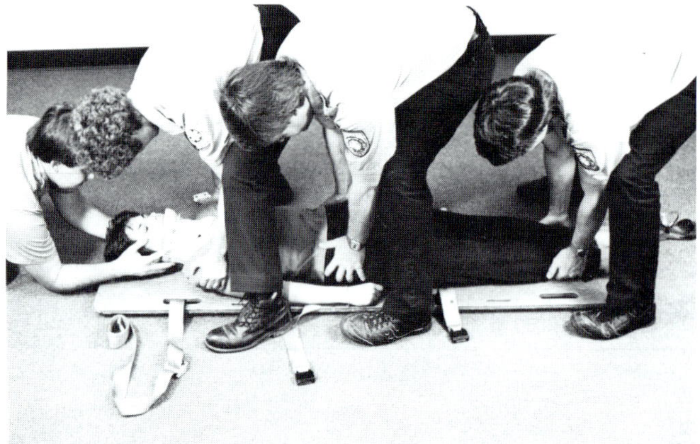

**Figure 8.20** The three rescuers stand and straddle the patient, grasping the shoulders, waist, and legs. On command of the first rescuer, all slide the patient to center him or her on the backboard.

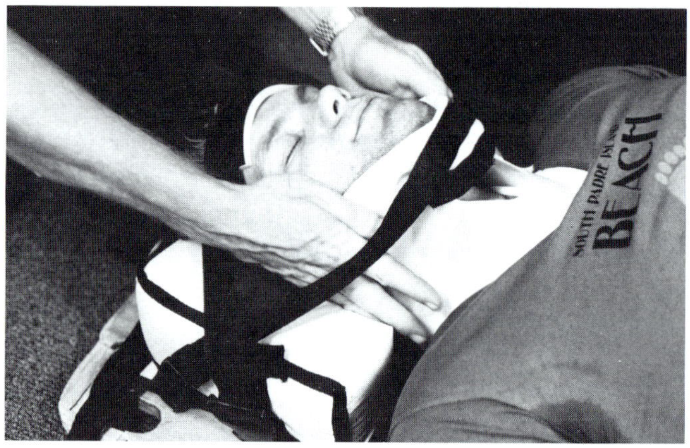


**Figure 8.21** After padding both sides of the patient's head, the rescuer at the patient's shoulders secures the patient's head to the backboard with a cravat or tape. If a head immobilizer is used, the straps are secured across the patient's head and chin.

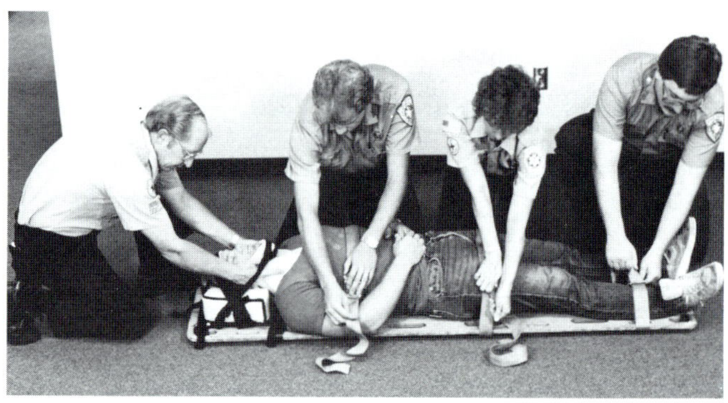

**Figure 8.22** Each of the rescuers fastens the patient to the backboard with the appropriate strap.

## ORTHOPEDIC (SCOOP) STRETCHER

An orthopedic (scoop) stretcher is used for temporary spinal immobilization or for lifting a patient while moving the patient as little as possible. This is useful for a patient in severe pain. Immobilizing a patient on a scoop stretcher requires at least two rescuers — one to apply and maintain axial traction, and one to prepare and position the stretcher.

Step 1: The first rescuer applies axial traction.

Step 2: The second rescuer applies a cervical collar, then prepares the scoop stretcher by adjusting the length to fit the patient (Figure 8.23).

Step 3: The second rescuer then separates the stretcher halves and places one half along each side of the patient (Figure 8.24).

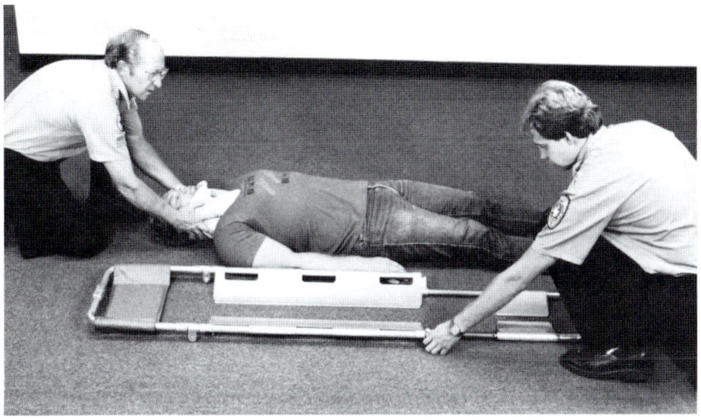

**Figure 8.23** While the first rescuer maintains axial traction, the second rescuer adjusts the stretcher to fit the patient.

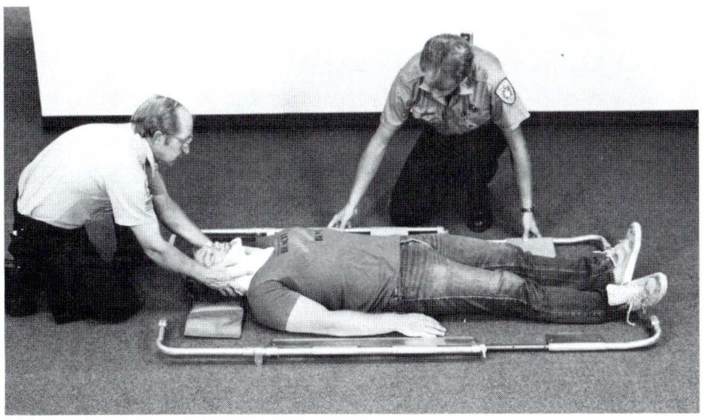

**Figure 8.24** The second rescuer separates both halves of the stretcher and places one-half along each side of the patient.

Step 4: The second rescuer slides the stretcher under the patient, one half at a time. (The patient may have to be logrolled a very small amount, so a third rescuer at the patient's hips or shoulders is very useful.)

Step 5: The second rescuer fastens the latches at both the head and foot of the stretcher, making sure that the stretcher halves are securely locked together (Figure 8.25).

Step 6: The second rescuer places rolled towels, blankets, or sandbags on both sides of the patient's head, then secures the patient's head to the stretcher with a cravat or tape. The first rescuer is free to release axial traction (Figure 8.26).

Step 7: Both rescuers cover the patient with a blanket if necessary, then move the stretcher to an ambulance cot.

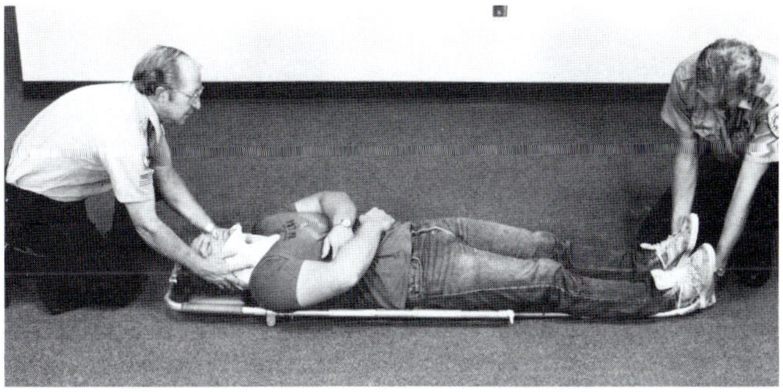

**Figure 8.25** After fastening the latches at the head and foot of the stretcher, the second rescuer checks to make sure that the latches are securely locked together.

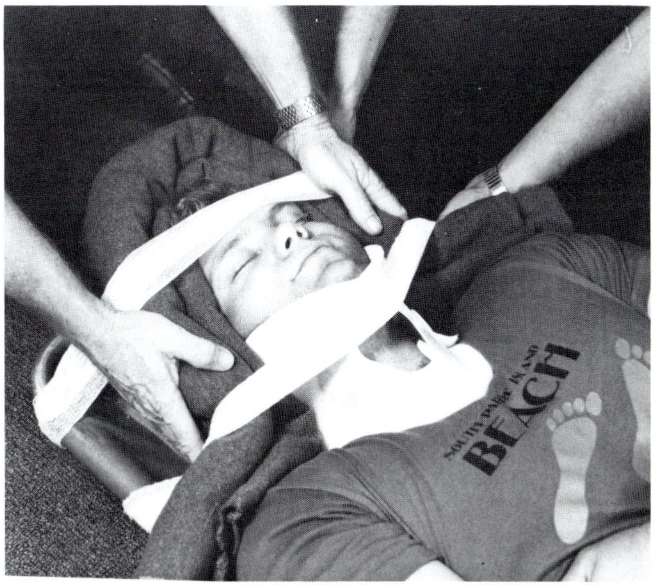


**Figure 8.26** Rolled towels, blankets, or sandbags are placed on both sides of the patient's head and the patient's head is secured to the stretcher with tape or a cravat.

### KENDRICK EXTRICATION DEVICE (KED)

The most common cause of spinal injury is trauma suffered during an automobile accident. After such an accident, the goal is to remove the patient from the vehicle without further damaging the spinal cord. This is best accomplished with a Kendrick Extrication Device (KED) or KED-type device (Figure 8.27). Applying the KED requires at least two rescuers: one to maintain axial traction throughout the procedure, and one to strap the patient into the KED.

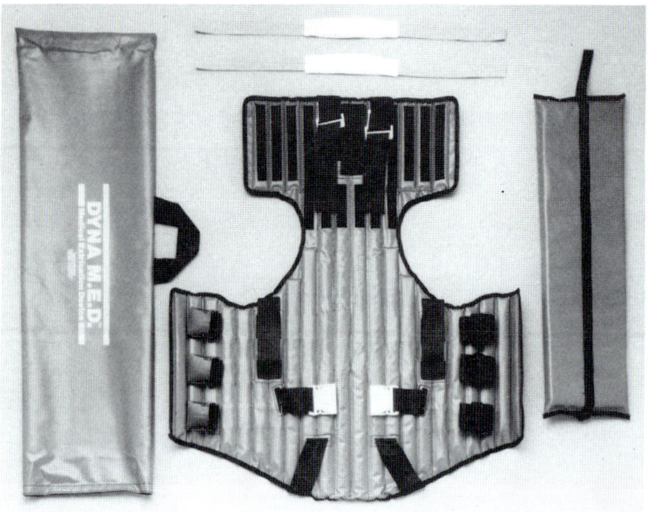


**Figure 8.27** A KED-type device is very useful for immobilizing patients who are injured in automobile accidents. *Photo courtesy of Dyna Med.*

Step 1: Have your partner position himself or herself behind the patient (usually in the back seat) and apply axial traction.

Step 2: Apply a cervical or extrication collar as your partner maintains axial traction (Figure 8.28).

Step 3: Slide the KED behind the patient either from the side or from above. It is best not to undo the straps until you are ready to strap the patient into the KED; otherwise, you will find that the straps get tangled up.

Step 4: Pull the chest straps across the patient's chest and buckle them (Figure 8.29).

Step 5: Bring one white buckle from behind the patient and up between the patient's legs to fasten it into the white buckle receiver. Repeat the process for the other leg.

Step 6: Secure the patient's head to the KED with the head straps or with self-adhering roller gauze (Figure 8.30).

Step 7: Remove the patient from the car and to a long backboard (These steps are under Short Backboard below.)

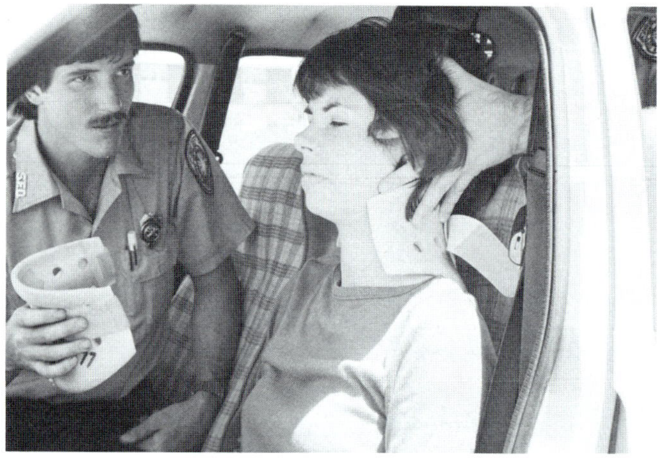

**Figure 8.28** While one rescuer maintains axial traction, another rescuer applies a cervical collar.

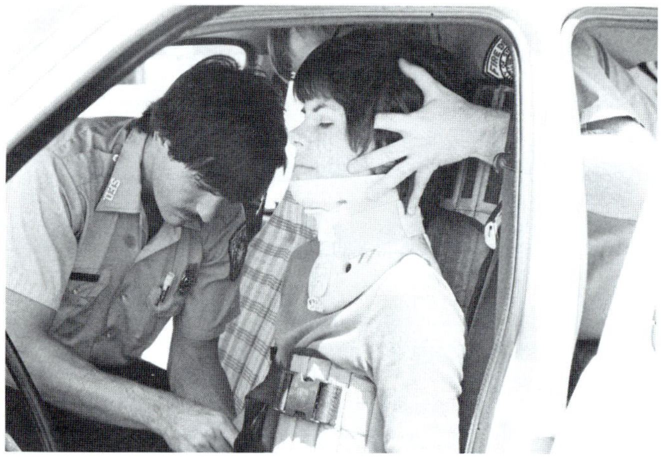

**Figure 8.29** The second rescuer fastens the chest straps.

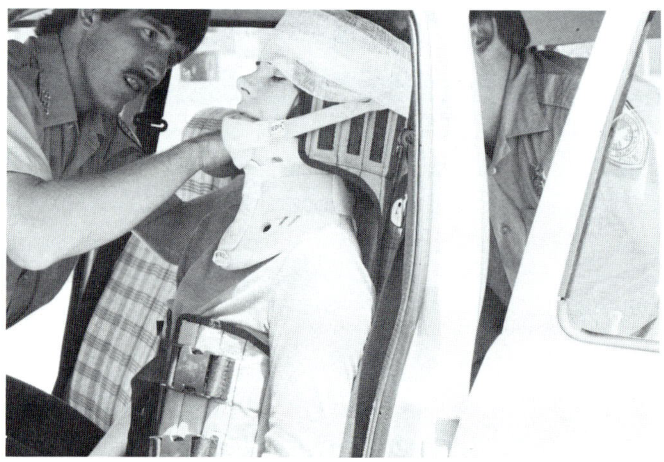

**Figure 8.30** Secure the patient's head to the KED with the head straps or with self-adhering gauze.

## SHORT BACKBOARD

Although KED-type devices are flexible and easier to handle within the limited space that rescuers usually encounter inside accident vehicles, some departments still use short backboards rather than the KED or similar extrication device. Immobilizing and removing a patient using a short backboard also requires at least two rescuers — one to maintain axial traction throughout the procedure, and one to strap the patient to the short backboard. A third rescuer may be needed to help lift the patient.

Step 1: One rescuer positions himself or herself behind the patient (usually in the back seat) and applies axial traction.

Step 2: The second rescuer applies a cervical collar, then prepares the short backboard by placing the straps through the side slots of the board (Figure 8.31).

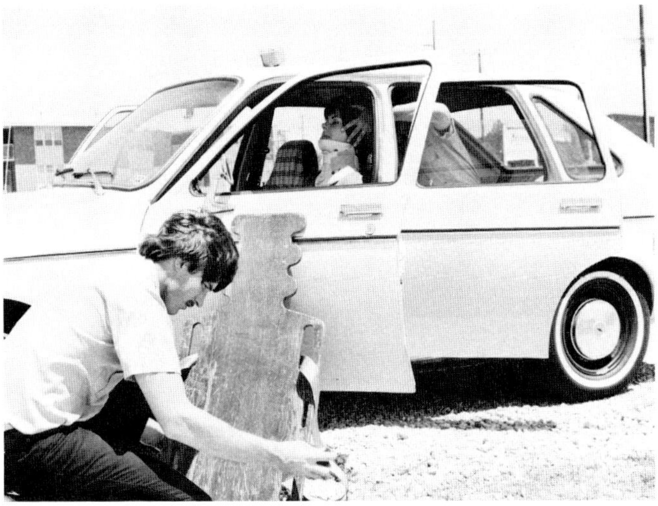

**Figure 8.31** The second rescuer prepares the short backboard by placing the straps through the side slots of the board.

Step 3: The second rescuer slides the board behind the patient and aligns the patient's head with the head extension of the backboard. If the automobile seat is curved, both rescuers may need to move the patient slightly forward so the board will fit between the patient and the seat (Figure 8.32). When moving the patient in this manner, both rescuers must coordinate their movements to ensure that axial traction is maintained. For this reason, the rescuer who is maintaining axial traction directs the other rescuer in this movement. Both rescuers determine that the board is pushed well down into the seat, so that the patient's lower spine is well supported.

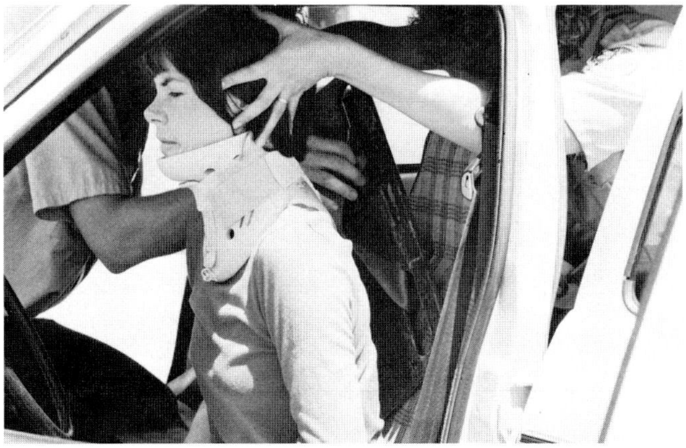

**Figure 8.32** Both rescuers may have to move the patient forward a little in order to slide the backboard between the patient and the seat.

Step 4: When the backboard is in position behind the patient, the second rescuer fills the gap between the patient's neck and the backboard with an air splint or a towel.

Step 5: The second rescuer then straps the patient's torso to the backboard. The second rescuer must adjust the straps so that the buckles are high on the patient's chest, near the shoulders — buckles placed over the mid-chest inhibit CPR. Since the buckles are usually the quick-release type, it is best to tape them to prevent accidental release (Figure 8.33).

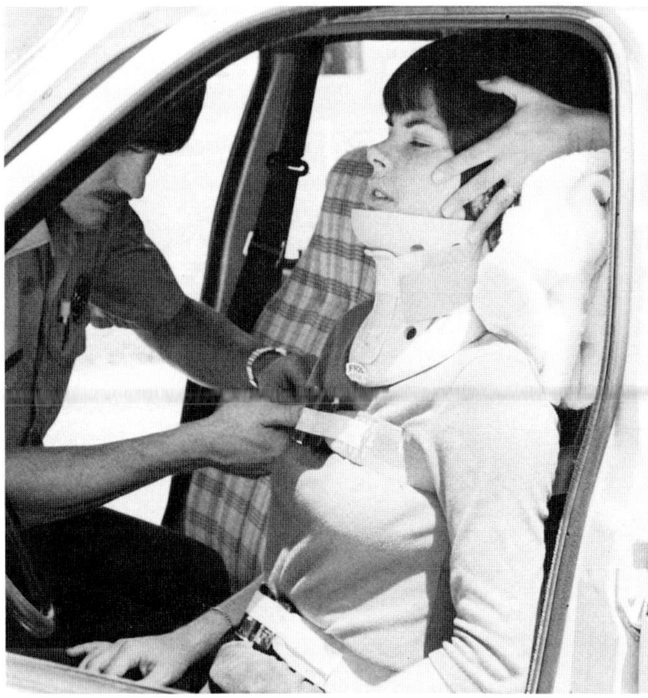

**Figure 8.33** After strapping the patient to the backboard, tape the buckles to prevent accidental release.

Step 6: Finally, the second rescuer straps the patient's head securely to the head extension (Figure 8.34).

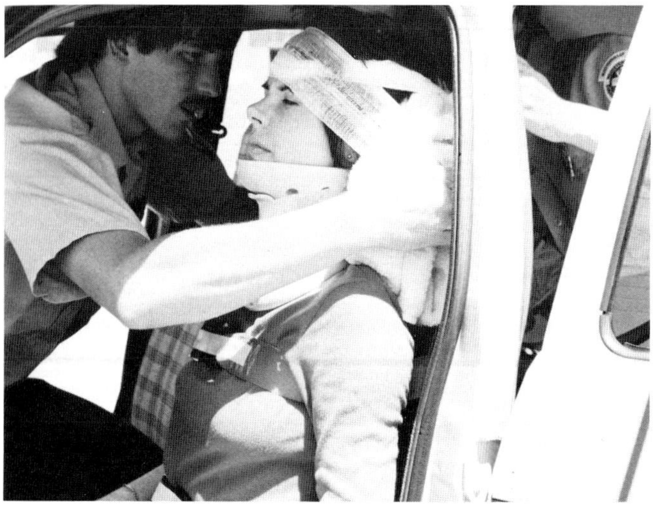

**Figure 8.34** Strap the patient's head to the head extension with roller gauze or cravat.

Step 7: After the patient is securely strapped to the short backboard, the patient can be removed from the vehicle with a long backboard. To remove the patient, both rescuers rotate the patient into a supine position. One rescuer holds one end of the long backboard parallel to the ground with the other end resting firmly on the vehicle seat (Figure 8.35). While the second rescuer barely lifts the short backboard up, the first rescuer slides the long backboard underneath the short backboard and the patient. If the patient is in a KED or KED-type device, loosen the leg straps between the patient's legs so that they can rest on the long backboard.

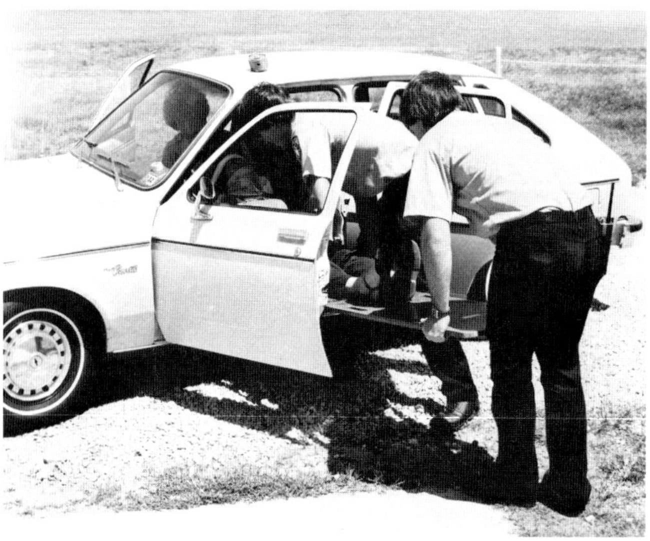

**Figure 8.35** After the patient is rotated to a supine position, the first rescuer slides the long backboard underneath the short backboard and the patient.

Step 8: With one rescuer lifting on each end of the long backboard, and one rescuer in the middle to help lift the patient, all remove the patient from the vehicle (Figure 8.36).

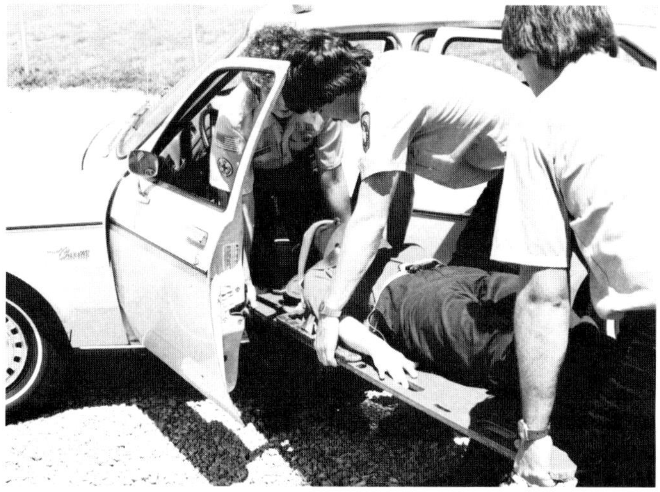

**Figure 8.36** The patient is carefully removed from the vehicle.

Patients injured in different types of accidents require different measures for extrication and spinal immobilization, but the basic principles are the same. The patient injured in a diving accident, for example, often has a cervical spine injury and must be approached with that possibility in mind. If the patient is still in the water, the procedure is as follows:

Step 1: The first rescuer places one arm under the patient's body so that the patient's upper body is supported on the rescuer's hand and the head is supported on the rescuer's upper arm. The rescuer places the other arm across the patient's head and back, immobilizing the patient's head and neck between the rescuer's arms (Figure 8.37).

Step 2: The rescuer turns the patient smoothly into the supine position while maintaining support on the head and neck. If the patient is not breathing, the rescuer begins mouth-to-mouth resuscitation immediately, while the patient is still in the water.

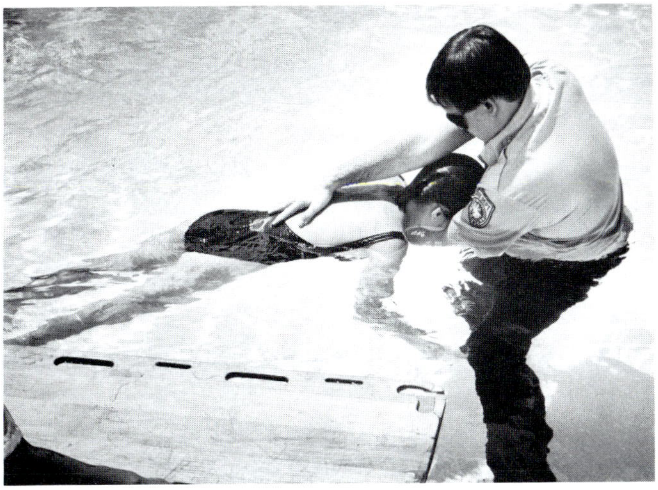

Figure 8.37 The first rescuer supports the patient's neck and upper body between both arms.

Step 3: The second rescuer slides a rigid device — such as a long backboard, surfboard, door, or wooden plank — under the patient (Figure 8.38). The second rescuer then applies a cervical collar to stabilize the neck further. Both rescuers float the board to the edge of the water and lift it out. One rescuer should stabilize the patient on the board to keep from jostling the patient too much.

Step 4: After the board is removed from the water, the second rescuer straps the patient to it, then further stabilizes the patient's head with roller bandages or sandbags.

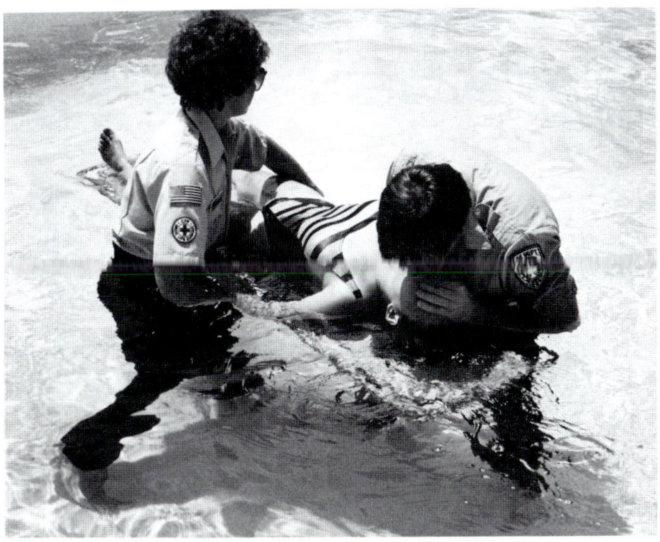

Figure 8.38 As the first rescuer begins rescue breathing, the second rescuer slides a long backboard or other rigid device underneath the patient.

## INJURIES TO THE CHEST

Severe chest trauma most commonly results from deceleration injuries, decompression injuries, or violence. Deceleration and decompression injuries most often occur during automobile accidents. Just as the front of an automobile is damaged when it collides with a tree or a bridge abutment, the chest and the contents of the chest cavity can be damaged when the chest forcefully strikes an obstruction. Likewise, the chest wall can be penetrated as the result of an accident or by violence, such as a stabbing incident.

Certain injuries to the chest, such as a sucking chest wound or a tension pneumothorax, are life-threatening emergencies. Failure to recognize and correct these conditions when assessing the patient's ABC's makes any further treatment useless.

### Airway

The patient who sustains a serious chest injury may have airway problems due to blood, mucus, or vomitus blocking the airway. If the patient is unconscious, the airway may also be blocked by the tongue, so maintain a close watch on the airway. Provide suction as needed and insert an oral airway if necessary.

### Breathing

The patient with severe chest trauma will more than likely be showing signs of respiratory distress: rapid, shallow breathing, flaring nostrils, use of accessory muscles trying to breathe, and possibly cyanosis. Pain from fractured ribs may cause the patient to breathe very shallowly, which leads to inadequate oxygenation of tissues. Administer high-flow oxygen by mask and assist ventilations if necessary. An open chest injury, such as a sucking chest wound, must be covered *immediately*.

### Circulation

Since shock frequently accompanies chest trauma, the patient is likely to have a weak, rapid pulse. Although chest trauma usually does not produce serious external bleeding, internal bleeding can be very serious. If the patient shows any signs of shock, suspect internal bleeding. Administer high-flow oxygen by mask and arrange for immediate transportation to a medical facility.

Injuries to the chest, like injuries to other parts of the body, are commonly classified as either open or closed, depending upon whether the chest wall has been penetrated or is intact.

## Open Chest Injuries

An open chest injury is an injury in which the chest wall is penetrated, which may be the result of an accident or violence. The chest may also be penetrated from within, such as when a fractured rib pierces the chest.

When the chest or lung surface is punctured, air is pulled into the pleural space and effective breathing becomes impossible. Under normal circumstances, the lungs are held in expansion by the negative pressure within the chest cavity, and when the pressure balance within the chest is upset, the lungs can no longer inflate properly.

### SUCKING CHEST WOUNDS

When the chest wall is penetrated, air is drawn into the chest through the wound. This movement of air into the chest causes a sucking noise with each inhalation, thus the name "sucking chest wound." As the patient exhales, some or all of the air that is drawn into the chest cavity flows back out of the wound.

A sucking chest wound severely threatens respiration since sufficient negative pressure to expand the lung cannot develop within the pleural space. As a result, the lung expands and contracts very little during respiration (Figure 8.39). Consequently, the lung on the affected side rapidly becomes depleted of oxygen.

The recommended emergency treatment for a sucking chest wound consists of covering the wound with an occlusive dressing (such as petrolatum gauze, cellophane, or plastic wrap), and administering supplemental oxygen to the patient.

**NOTE:** Closing a sucking chest wound can lead to the development of a tension pneumothorax. Tension pneumothorax is covered later in the chapter under Closed Chest Injuries.

### IMPALED OBJECTS IN THE CHEST

When a patient has an impaled object in the chest, treat it as you would any impaled object: **LEAVE IT IN PLACE.** (See Chapter 7, Bleeding Control and Soft-Tissue Injuries.) Stabilize the object with bulky dressings and arrange for transportation to the nearest medical facility. Administer oxygen and assist ventilations as necessary.

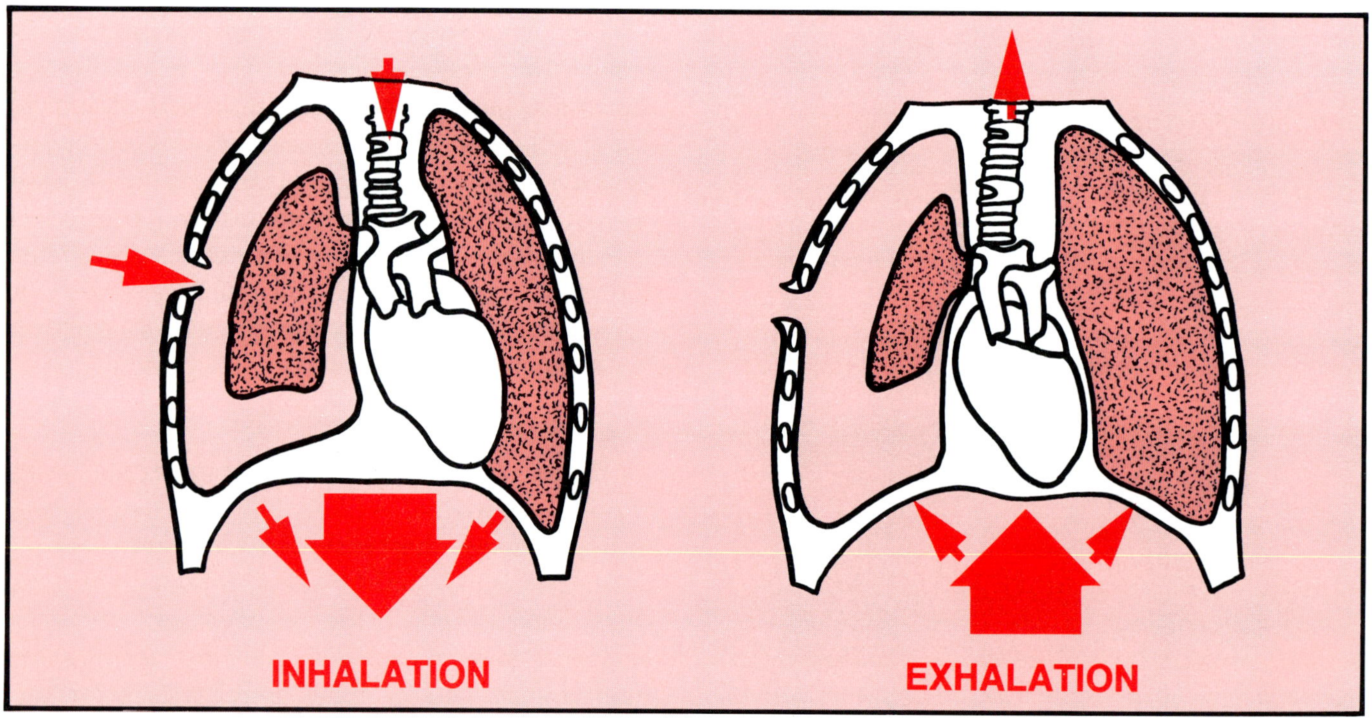


**Figure 8.39** When the chest wall is penetrated, air is drawn into the chest cavity during inhalation and normal lung expansion becomes impossible.

## Closed Chest Injuries

The forceful compression of the chest cavity by a stationary object, such as an automobile steering wheel or dashboard, is the most common cause of chest injuries.

In a closed chest injury, the skin of the chest wall is intact. One danger of closed injuries to the chest, of course, is that the severity and extent of injury may be overlooked by the rescuer.

### RIB FRACTURES

When the chest cavity is damaged, ribs may be broken. The damage may be limited to a simple fracture occurring near the point of impact, but because the ribs are part of a ring, a break at one point without a bend or fracture at another point is unlikely.

A fractured rib, of course, can lacerate internal organs, but fractured ribs alone create problems because of the pain associated with this type of injury. This pain causes the patient to splint that portion of the chest — that is, it causes the patient to decrease lung expansion on the injured side(s) of the chest. The decrease in lung expansion means a decrease in the amount of oxygen entering and circulating within the body. This condition can ultimately lead to the collapse of the lung, and later to pneumonia.

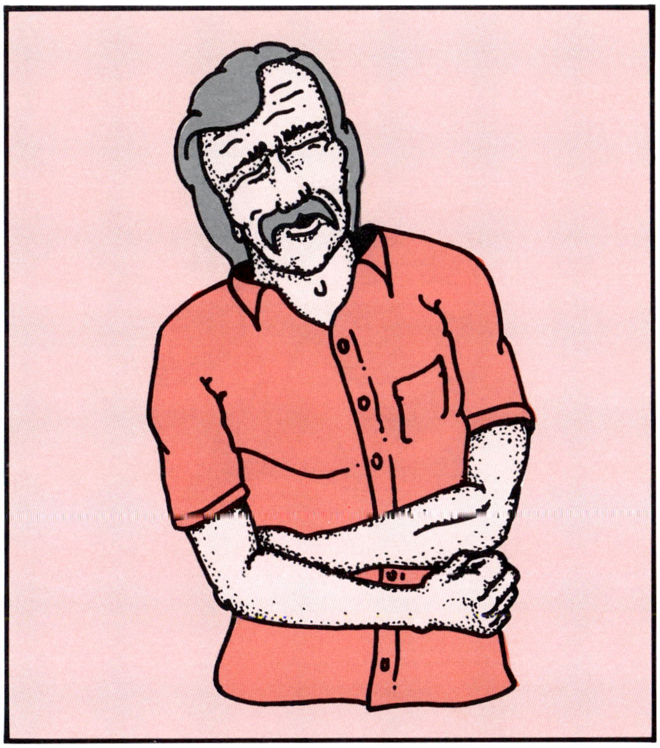

**Figure 8.40** The pain from rib fractures causes patients to display a characteristic splinting posture, hugging the chest and breathing shallowly.

Aside from the characteristic splinting posture of the conscious patient with a fractured rib or ribs (Figure 8.40), the most reliable indication of rib fracture is pain. The patient will report pain at the site of the fracture(s), and increased pain associated with movement, including deep breathing or coughing.

The treatment for rib fractures aims to reduce the associated pain, thereby enabling the patient to breathe more effectively. If the patient has only one or two fractures, he or she may obtain some pain relief from hugging a pillow against the chest. If the patient is in severe pain or has multiple fractures, immobilize the chest. Have the patient place the arm on the injured side across his or her chest and tie several cravats over the arm and around the trunk. Add a third cravat to support the patient's arm at the elbow (Figure 8.41).

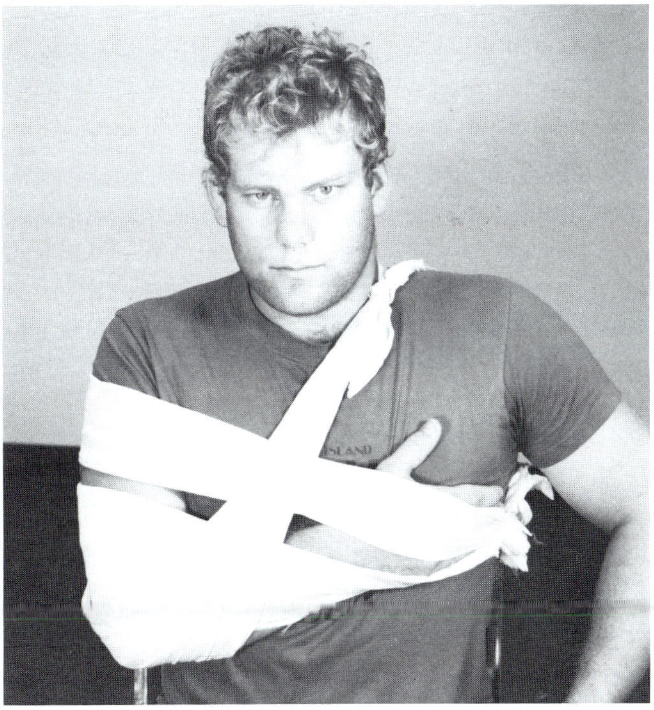

**Figure 8.41** Immobilize the chest by tying several cravats over the arm and around the chest. Add a third cravat to support the patient's arm at the elbow.

### FLAIL CHEST

Flail chest occurs when two or more adjacent ribs on the same side of the chest are fractured in two or more places. The result of such an injury is

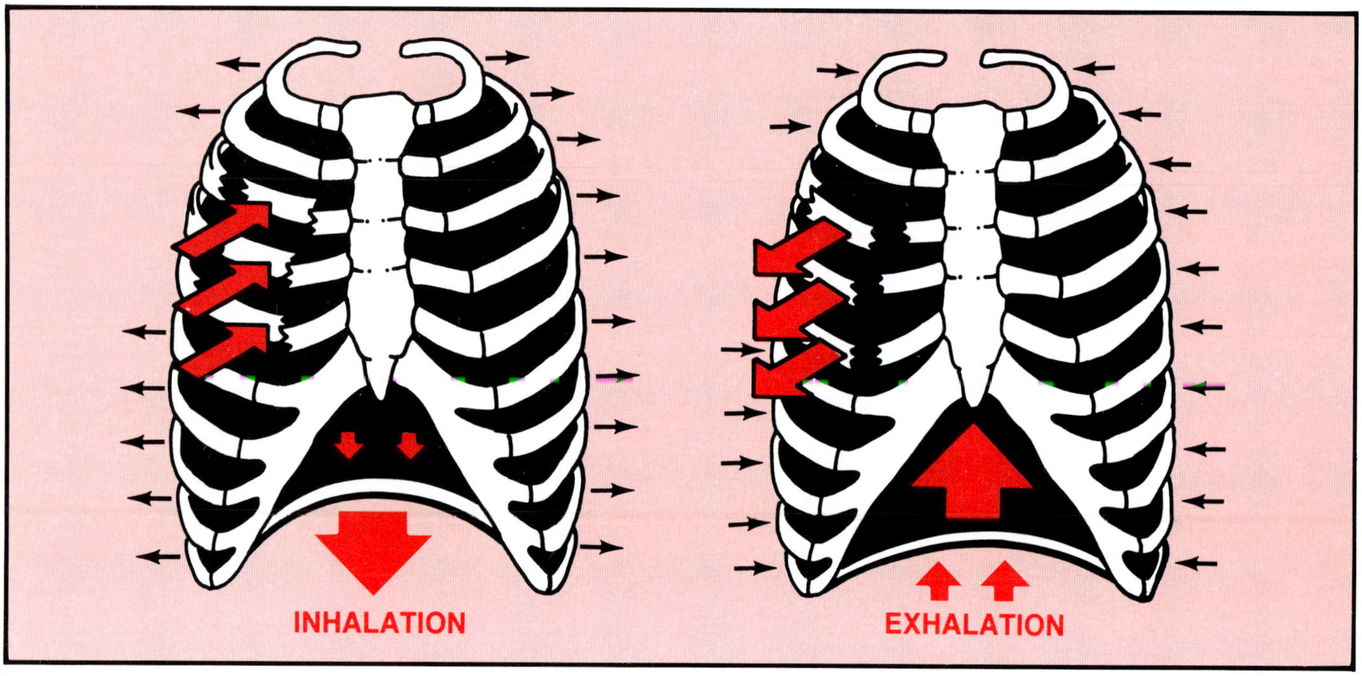


**Figure 8.42** In flail chest, a portion of the thoracic cage becomes detached; when this happens, the flail segment moves inward during inhalation and outward during exhalation.

that a segment of the thoracic cage becomes detached. The loose (flail) segment moves inward as the patient inhales and moves outward as he or she exhales (Figure 8.42). This condition, known as *paradoxical respiration*, interferes with the oxygenation of the body and severely affects respiration.

The diagnosis of flail chest can be made only by removing the patient's clothes from the waist up and by carefully examining the chest. Gently locate the edges of the flail segment with your fingers, and use your hand to immobilize the segment in its inward position until you can tape a thick dressing, pillow, or lightweight sandbag over it (Figure 8.43). Administer supplemental oxygen and arrange for immediate transportation to a medical facility.

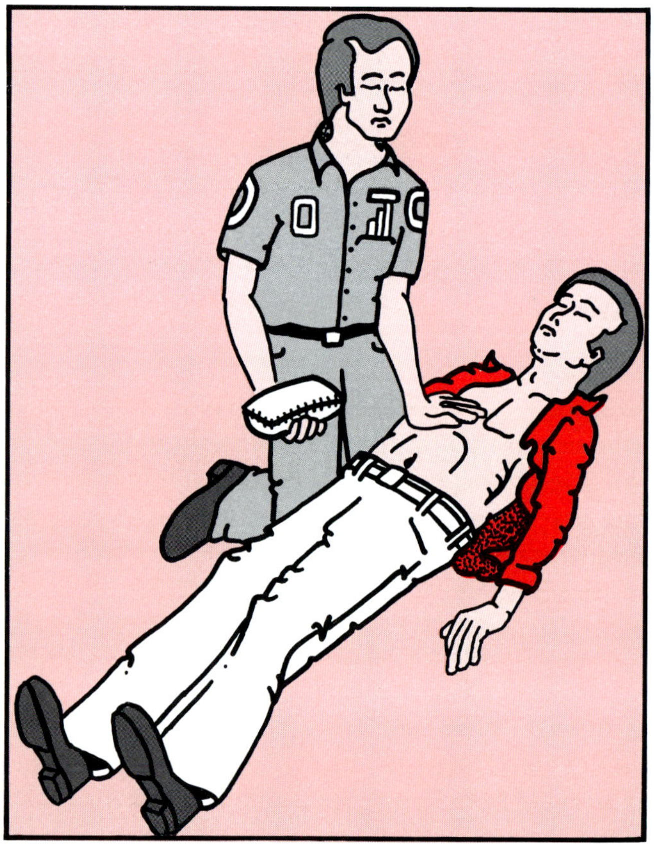

**Figure 8.43** Use your hand to immobilize the flail segment in its inward position until you can tape a pillow or lightweight sandbag over it.

### PULMONARY CONTUSION

A pulmonary contusion is a bruise to the lung tissue that causes swelling and hemorrhage within the affected part of the lung. Perhaps as many as 75 percent of patients who have suffered blunt chest trauma sustain a pulmonary contusion.

It is often difficult to determine the severity of the contusion based on the outward appearance of the chest alone. Children, for example, may have massive lung contusion without having even a single broken rib because of the pliability of the young rib cage. In addition, a patient suffering pulmonary contusion usually shows little signs of respiratory distress at first, but gradually develops severe respiratory problems as more blood and fluid collect within the lung.

Signs and symptoms of pulmonary contusion may take several hours to develop, so you must suspect pulmonary contusion in every patient who has sustained blunt trauma to the chest and arrange for immediate transportation to a medical facility. Administer supplemental oxygen and assist ventilations as needed.

### PNEUMOTHORAX

Pneumothorax is defined as an accumulation of air in the pleural space. Recall from Chapter 2 that there are two pleural layers within the chest cavity: one layer lines the lungs and one layer lines the chest cavity. Between these layers is an extremely small "space." If either of these layers is torn, usually as a result of injury, air can accumulate in the pleural space. This air can come either from outside the chest cavity or from within the chest cavity. Pneumothorax usually occurs as the result of trauma, but sometimes occurs spontaneously.

Generally, the tear in the pleura seals itself off and stabilizes. But if the space does not seal itself or enlarges, ventilation in the opposite lung may also be affected. Regardless of its cause, the effect of pneumothorax is the same: if a portion of the pleural cavity is filled with air, the lung cannot expand into it, and respiration is impaired.

There are several types of pneumothorax, depending upon whether the chest wall has been penetrated or is intact.

A *simple* pneumothorax occurs when air enters the pleural space from within the chest cavity, such as when a fractured rib pierces a lung. The patient will be in respiratory distress and the trachea will deviate (pull) toward the side of the pneumothorax. If you tap the affected side of the chest it will sound hollow, since the chest cavity is filled with air rather than lung tissue. Allow the patient to sit up unless he or she shows signs of shock and splint any rib fractures. Administer supplemental oxygen by mask and be ready to assist ventilations if necessary. Arrange for rapid transport to a medical facility.

An *open* pneumothorax results when air enters the pleural space from outside the chest cavity. A penetrating chest wound, for example, such as a gunshot wound or stab wound, may cause an open pneumothorax. A sucking chest wound is an open pneumothorax. To treat an open pneumothorax, seal the opening in the chest with an occlusive dressing, such as petrolatum gauze or plastic wrap, and administer supplemental oxygen by mask. Arrange for rapid transport to a medical facility and **watch for the development of a tension pneumothorax.**

A *tension* pneumothorax occurs when air accumulates in the pleural space under tension, or pressure. Generally, the tear in the lung that causes a pneumothorax seals itself off and stabilizes. Tension pneumothorax develops when the tear in the lung fails to seal itself and acts as a one-way valve in the affected part of the chest. Air is drawn into the pleural space as the patient inhales, but none escapes as he or she exhales.

This steady accumulation of air impairs ventilation as the air begins to fill the space into which the unaffected lung normally expands (Figure 8.44). The accumulation of air also pushes the heart towards the unaffected side, further limiting expansion of the unaffected lung. Pressure within the chest can be so severe that it presses against the vena cava, reducing the return of blood to the

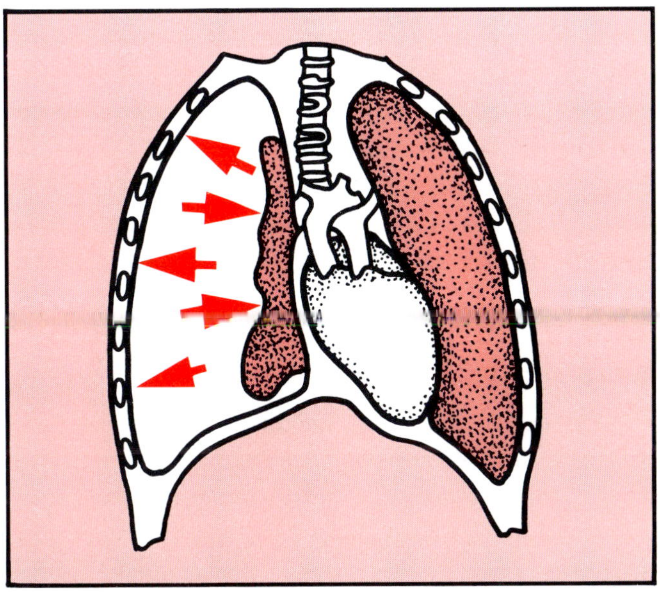

**Figure 8.44** In a tension pneumothorax, air accumulates in the pleural space under pressure. This air begins to fill the space into which the unaffected lung normally expands.

heart. The signs and symptoms of tension pneumothorax are as follows:

- Severe respiratory distress; possible cyanosis
- Tracheal deviation towards the opposite side of the pneumothorax
- Distended neck veins
- Shock signs due to reduced blood flow: rapid, shallow breathing and weak, thready pulse
- Subcutaneous emphysema

Subcutaneous emphysema occurs when air accumulates in the subcutaneous tissues. Touching the chest of a patient who has subcutaneous emphysema produces a crackling sound as small bubbles of air move from one compartment to another. This sign indicates that there is a great deal of air trapped within the tissues and the patient may have a bloated appearance.

Tension pneumothorax can result from the closing of a sucking chest wound as air is trapped within the chest cavity. If a patient with a sucking chest wound shows signs of deterioration after the wound is sealed, open a corner of the dressing as the patient exhales to allow air to escape, and reapply the dressing as the patient inhales.

The only treatment for tension pneumothorax consists of inserting a needle or tube into the affected side of the chest to relieve the air pressure that has built up within the chest cavity. This procedure can only be performed in the hospital or by authorized EMTs or paramedics. **TENSION PNEUMOTHORAX IS A DIRE EMERGENCY AND THE PATIENT WILL DIE WITHIN MINUTES UNLESS HE OR SHE IS TREATED. GET THIS PATIENT TO A HOSPITAL AS RAPIDLY AS POSSIBLE.** In the meantime, administer high-flow oxygen by mask.

Pneumothorax can occur spontaneously — that is, not as the result of accident or injury to the lung. *Spontaneous* pneumothorax occurs in people who have weak areas in the lung tissue. Typically, the patient is a thin young man who reports that he was sitting quietly when he developed a sudden pain in the chest. Spontaneous pneumothorax can also occur as a result of changes in atmospheric pressure, as, for example during air travel. The signs and symptoms of spontaneous pneumothorax are the same as for a simple pneumothorax, and recommended treatment is the same. Allow the patient to sit up, administer supplemental oxygen, and arrange for rapid transport to a medical facility.

### HEMOTHORAX

Hemothroax is the presence of blood in the pleural space. A laceration of any blood vessel within the chest, including the vessels in lung tissue, can cause blood to accumulate within the pleural space. Hemothorax often accompanies pneumothorax caused by trauma.

The accumulation of blood within the pleural space has the same effect as the accumulation of air — the lung on the affected side cannot expand normally (Figure 8.45). If the accumulation of blood is significant, the patient develops the signs and symptoms of tension pneumothorax. Further, the blood that pools in the pleural space is not available to the circulatory system, and the patient develops shock. The patient who is suffering with hemothorax, must be transported to a medical facility without delay. Administer high-flow oxygen by mask and monitor vital signs.

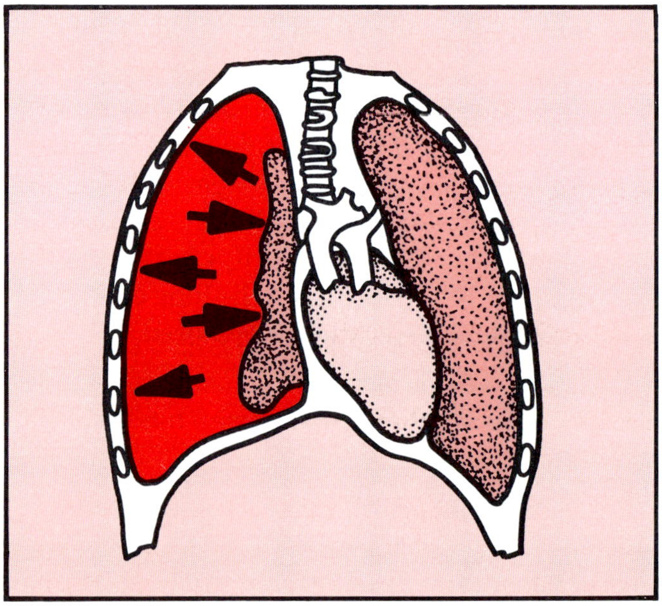

**Figure 8.45** Hemothorax is accumulation of blood in the pleural space. The effect is the same as with a tension pneumothorax — the lung on the affected side cannot expand normally.

## TRAUMATIC ASPHYXIA

Traumatic asphyxia can develop as a result of a very sudden, severe compression injury to the chest. The impact causes a sudden rise in pressure within the chest cavity, which forces blood out of the heart and up into the victim's shoulders, neck, and head. This life-threatening syndrome has unmistakable signs:

- Caved-in chest wall with fractures of the ribs and sternum
- Distended veins above the shoulders
- Bulging, bloodshot eyes
- Swollen, cyanotic tongue and lips
- Blue or purple head, neck, and shoulders
- Extreme respiratory distress
- Shock

The victim of traumatic asphyxia may also be vomiting or coughing up blood. **TRAUMATIC ASPHYXIA IS A DIRE EMERGENCY. GET THIS PATIENT TO A HOSPITAL AS RAPIDLY AS POSSIBLE.** Try to keep the patient's airway open and administer high-flow oxygen by mask.

## INJURIES TO THE HEART (Myocardial Trauma)

Chest injuries can also injure the heart and related blood vessels. Trauma to the heart (myocardial trauma) and vessels of the heart can result from chest trauma. Automobile accidents, especially steering wheel injuries, are the main cause of myocardial trauma. Two of the most common types of myocardial trauma are myocardial contusions and pericardial tamponade.

Myocardial contusion is a bruising of the heart tissue. It is often caused by front-impact collisions where the chest is severely compressed against the steering wheel. The signs of myocardial contusion are often the same as those for a heart attack: chest pain, difficulty breathing, and heavy sweating. (For more information about heart attacks [acute myocardial infarction], see Chapter 10, Medical Emergencies.)

Treat the patient with myocardial contusion by administering oxygen by mask or cannula, allowing the patient to sit up if this position eases breathing, and arranging for rapid transport to a medical facility.

Pericardial tamponade is an accumulation of blood in the pericardial sac, which is the tissue that surrounds the heart (Figure 8.46). Severe myocardial contusion or a tear in a blood vessel at a point where it leaves the pericardial sac can result in a pericardial tamponade. When blood fills the pericardial sac the heart is unable to pump effectively, and the patient quickly develops signs of cardiogenic shock. The signs of this condition are as follows:

- Distended jugular veins
- Shock signs - weak, rapid pulse, falling blood pressure

**PERICARDIAL TAMPONADE IS A DIRE EMERGENCY AND THERE IS NO EFFECTIVE TREATMENT OUTSIDE OF A HOSPITAL. ADMINISTER HIGH-FLOW OXYGEN BY MASK AND GET THE PATIENT TO A HOSPITAL AS RAPIDLY AS POSSIBLE.**

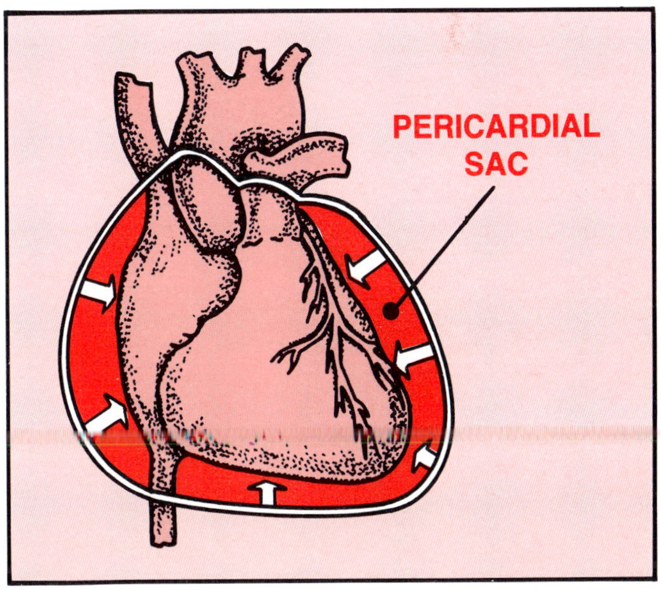


**Figure 8.46** Pericardial tamponade is an accumulation of blood in the pericardial sac, which surrounds the heart. The heart is unable to pump effectively and the patient quickly develops signs of shock.

# 9

# Injuries to the Extremities and Splinting

**NFPA STANDARD 1001**
**Emergency Medical Care**
**Fire Fighter II**

**4-4.9** The fire fighter shall define the types of fractures and describe the differences.

**4-4.10** The fire fighter shall identify three general signs and symptoms of fractures.

**4-4.11** The fire fighter, given an identified fracture, shall demonstrate the emergency medical care necessary to transport the victim.



**U.S. DEPARTMENT OF TRANSPORTATION**
**First Responder Training Course**

**Objectives:**

- Define functions of the skeletal system.
- Define and identify types of fractures, dislocations and sprains.
- Given a list of symptoms, identify those associated with fractures and dislocations.
- Given a sign that differentiates fractures from dislocations, identify the injury as a fracture or dislocation.
- State the primary reason for splinting.
- Given a list of statements, select general rules for splinting.
- Given "patients," perform an examination for extremity injuries explaining aloud what he or she is doing and why.
- Given descriptions of "patients" with injuries of the extremities, identify the injury and describe appropriate emergency care.
- Given "patients," perform appropriate emergency care for fractures and dislocations of the extremities.

**NOTE:** It is assumed that the first responder will have minimal equipment and that most actual splinting will be done by EMTs or paramedics.

Chapter 9

# Injuries to the Extremities and Splinting

Fractures, dislocations, and sprains seldom present an immediate threat to life, although they are often quite painful and may present gross deformity. It is critical, therefore, that you identify and immobilize these musculoskeletal injuries **only after you have checked the patient's ABC's and corrected life-threatening conditions.** While it is true that first responders have only limited access to most of the splinting equipment described in this chapter, we have included the material on the assumption that first responders will assist EMTs in mass casualty incidents. Keep in mind, then, as you read this chapter, that most of the actual splinting described here will be carried out by EMTs as they arrive on the scene.

## FRACTURES

A fracture is a break in the continuity of bone, usually accompanied by a muscular spasm in the area of the fracture. Fractures are classified as either closed (simple) or open (compound), depending upon whether or not the overlying skin is intact. In a closed fracture, the overlying skin is intact, while in an open fracture, there is a wound over the fracture site. Bone ends may or may not be protruding from the wound in an open fracture. Significant blood loss may occur as a result of either type of fracture, but open fractures are potentially more serious because the risks of contamination and infection are far greater than in closed fractures.

The signs and symptoms of fracture include

- Deformity — the injured extremity may be angled unnaturally.
- Pain — the injured limb will very likely be tender or sore.
- Crepitus — you may hear a grating sound (crepitus) when the patient moves the injured extremity. This sound arises from the broken bone ends rubbing together, and indicates a strong likelihood that surrounding nerves and blood vessels may be damaged by the bone fragments. Thus, it is important to urge the patient to keep the extremity as still as possible.
- Swelling and discoloration — these signs are due to fluid in the tissues surrounding the fracture, but they may not be apparent until several hours after the accident.
- Loss of function — while it is unlikely that the patient will be able to move a fractured limb without extraordinary pain, this symptom is not definitive in impacted fractures since the ends involved are jammed together and may function as if no fracture were present.
- Exposed bone fragments — this sign is, of course, definitive.

Fractures are further classified according to the severity and angle of the break, but this classification, of course, can only be determined by x-ray. These fracture types (Figure 9.1) include

- Transverse — A transverse fracture, such as that of the tibia, for example, is often the result of a direct injury. In this type of fracture, the bone is broken at right angles to its long axis.
- Greenstick — A greenstick fracture is similar to a transverse fracture in that the bone, usually as the result of a direct blow, is bro-

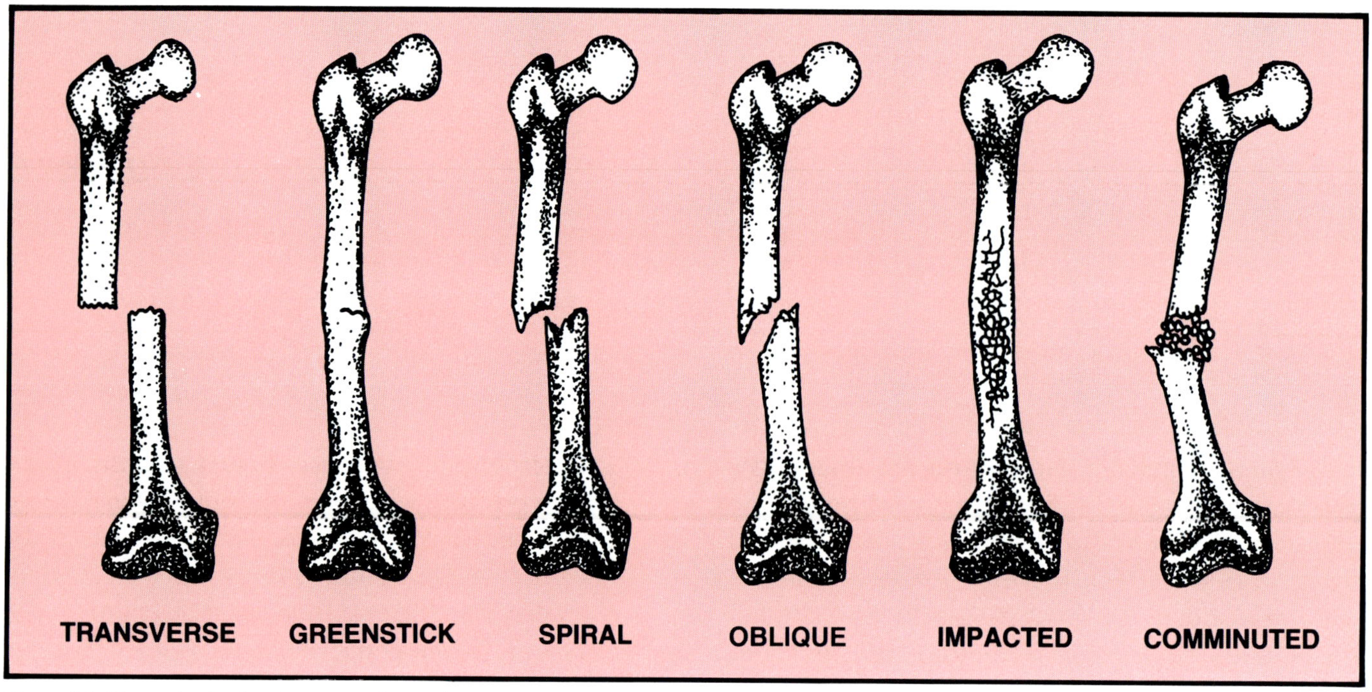


**Figure 9.1** The major fracture types are shown above.

ken at right angles to its long axis. A greenstick fracture, however, is an *incomplete* fracture that commonly occurs in children, whose bones (like greensticks) are still pliable and bend considerably without breaking.

- Spiral — Spiral fractures usually result from twisting injuries, and are so named because the fracture line spirals around the bone.
- Oblique — The fracture line of an oblique fracture crosses the bone at an oblique angle, or in a slanting direction. Oblique fractures are usually the result of a direct blow to the involved extremity.
- Impacted — In impacted fractures, the ends of the involved bone are jammed together and may function as if no fracture were present. This type of fracture occurs indirectly, such as when a patient falls forcefully onto his or her own outstretched arm. The resulting fracture along the shaft of the humerus is an impacted fracture.
- Comminuted — A comminuted fracture is one in which the bone is fragmented into two or more splintered or crushed pieces. This type of fracture is usually the result of an extraordinarily forceful direct blow.

## DISLOCATIONS

A dislocation is the displacement of a bone end from its joint surface, accompanied sometimes by tearing of the ligaments that normally hold the bone end in place, and also by muscular spasm in the area of dislocation. While it is possible that any joint may be dislocated, the shoulder, elbow, fingers, hips, and ankles are the joints that are most frequently dislocated.

The principal symptoms of dislocation are either pain or a feeling of pressure over the involved joint and loss of motion of the joint. The principal sign of dislocation is deformity. If the dislocated bone end presses on nerves or blood vessels, there may also be numbness or paralysis below the dislocation.

## SPRAINS

Sprains are injuries in which ligaments are partially torn, and usually occur when a joint is suddenly twisted beyond its normal range of motion. Sprains most commonly affect the knees and ankles and are characterized by pain, swelling, and discoloration over the injured joint. Unlike fractures and dislocations, sprains usually do not cause deformity.

## GENERAL PRINCIPLES OF SPLINTING

Splinting is done for the following reasons:

- To prevent a closed fracture from becoming an open one
- To prevent damage to surrounding nerves, blood vessels, and other tissues caused by broken bone ends
- To lessen bleeding and swelling
- To diminish pain

Because splinting is intended to immobilize and to protect an injured extremity from further injury, it is important that you splint all fractures and possible fractures *before* moving the patient. The exception to this rule, of course, is a situation in which the patient's life is in danger if he or she is *not* moved.

When preparing to splint an extremity, first remove or cut away clothing from the injured extremity. If the patient has an open (compound) fracture, you will most likely be instructed to irrigate the wound with large amounts of normal saline to remove dirt and debris before dressing and splinting the wound. **NEVER** attempt to push broken bone ends back into place in an open fracture—just irrigate, dress, and splint the extremity as it is. **NEVER** attempt to push dislocated bones back into place before splinting — simply splint the extremity in the position in which you find it.

For splinting to be effective as a system of immobilizing an injured extremity, the joint above and below the injury must be immobilized. A splint that does not immobilize the joints both above and below the fracture actually worsens the injury. If a patient, for example, has a suspected fracture of the radius or ulna, you must immobilize the patient's elbow and wrist as well as the shaft of the radius or ulna.

**REMEMBER, AN EXTREMITY SHOULD BE SPLINTED IN THE POSITION IN WHICH IT IS FOUND. DO NOT ATTEMPT TO PUSH BROKEN BONES BACK INTO PLACE OR TO STRAIGHTEN THE EXTREMITY.**

Finally, always note and record the patient's pulse and sensation distal to the injury both before and after applying a splint. Splinting must be done firmly, of course, but not so tightly as to occlude circulation in the injured extremity. Check the distal pulse periodically after the splint is in place to be certain that the circulation is still adequate. If the pulse disappears, loosen the splint until you can feel the pulse once more.

## TYPES OF SPLINTS

Any device that is used to immobilize a fracture or dislocation (or possible fracture or dislocation) is a splint. A splint may be improvised, such as a rolled newspaper, a cane, a triangular bandage, or virtually any other object that can provide stability, including the patient's own body; or it may be one of the several commercially available wooden, inflatable, or traction splints. The lack of a commercially made splint should never prevent you from properly immobilizing an injured patient; multiple casualties may tax the resources of even the best-equipped ambulance, and ingenuity is often necessary to render adequate care. Whether a splint is improvised or commercial, be sure that each splint is well padded to prevent unnecessary pressure and discomfort to the patient.

### Sling and Swathe

An arm fracture can usually be managed by simply immobilizing the arm against the patient's chest with a sling and swathe. Even when a rigid splint is applied, it may be appropriate to add a sling and swathe to support the weight and prevent movement of the injured part. The following instructions for applying a sling and swathe are written for someone who uses two triangular bandages, but a sling and swathe can be made from sheets, towels, pieces of clothing, or anything else that is handy.

Step 1: Ask the patient to place the injured arm in a comfortable position across his or her chest. If the patient cannot hold his or her own arm in place, have your partner hold the patient's arm until you are ready to tie the sling.

Step 2: Slip a triangular bandage (the sling) between the injured extremity and the patient's chest with a long edge of the bandage laid along the patient's side opposite the injury and with one point of the triangular bandage extending beneath the elbow on the injured side (Figure 9.2).

Step 3: Bring the bottom edge of the bandage up over the forearm and tie it to the other end of the bandage to one side of the patient's neck (Figure 9.3). Tying the bandage against the back of the patient's neck is likely to be very uncomfortable for the patient.

Step 4: Tie or pin the pointed edge of the sling at the elbow to form a cradle for the patient's elbow (Figure 9.4).

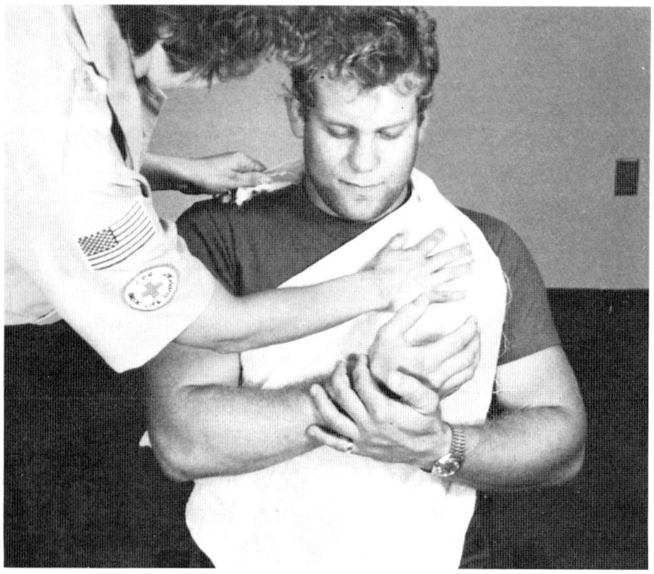

**Figure 9.2** Place the bandage between the patient's arm and chest so that the point extends beyond the elbow on the injured side.

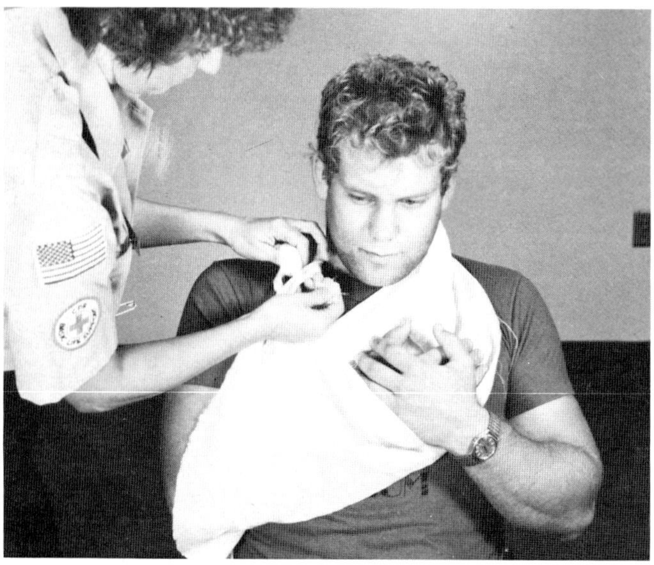

**Figure 9.3** Tie the bandage to one side of the patient's neck.

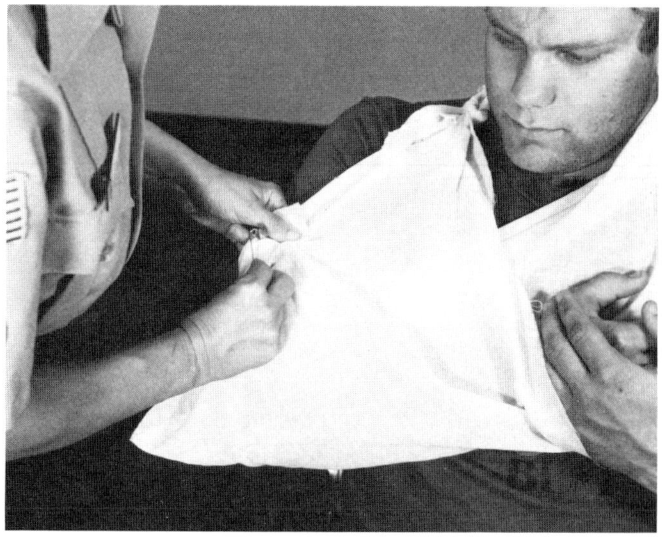

**Figure 9.4** To support the patient's elbow, tie or pin the pointed edge of the sling.

Step 5: Put another triangular bandage (this one is the swathe) around the patient's chest and injured arm, over the sling. Bring the swathe ends together under the arm on the uninjured side, and put padding beneath the arm to protect the patient's armpit before you tie the swathe (Figure 9.5).

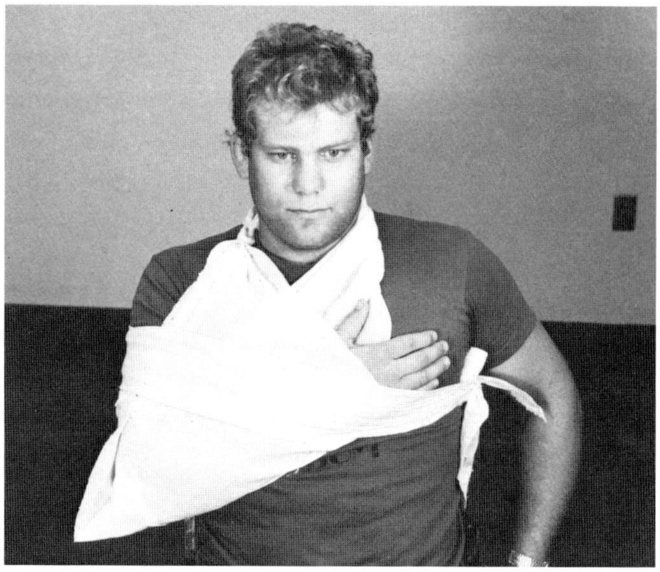

**Figure 9.5** Tie another triangular bandage over the sling, over the patient's chest and injured arm.

An alternate method for making an arm sling is illustrated in Figure 9.6. This method is quick and easy, as long as the patient is wearing a shirt that has reasonably long shirt tails and that buttons down the front.

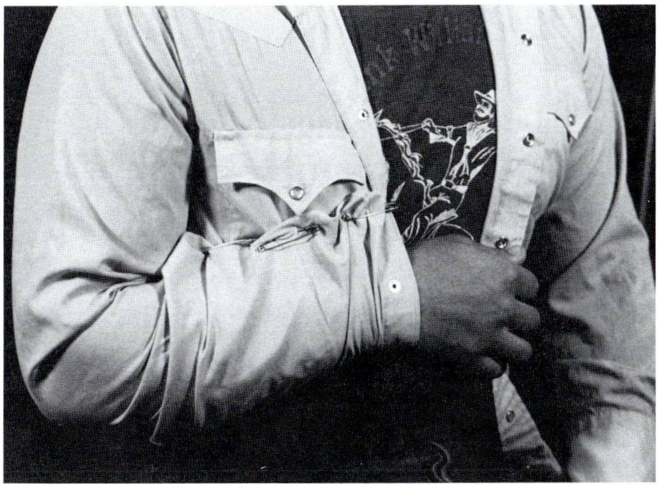

**Figure 9.6** A sling can be made quickly if the patient is wearing a shirt that buttons down the front.

## Pillow Splint

The best way to immobilize an injured foot is to splint it with an ordinary pillow. To apply a pillow as a splint, simply mold the pillow around the injured area and fasten it with safety pins or with several cravats (Figure 9.7).

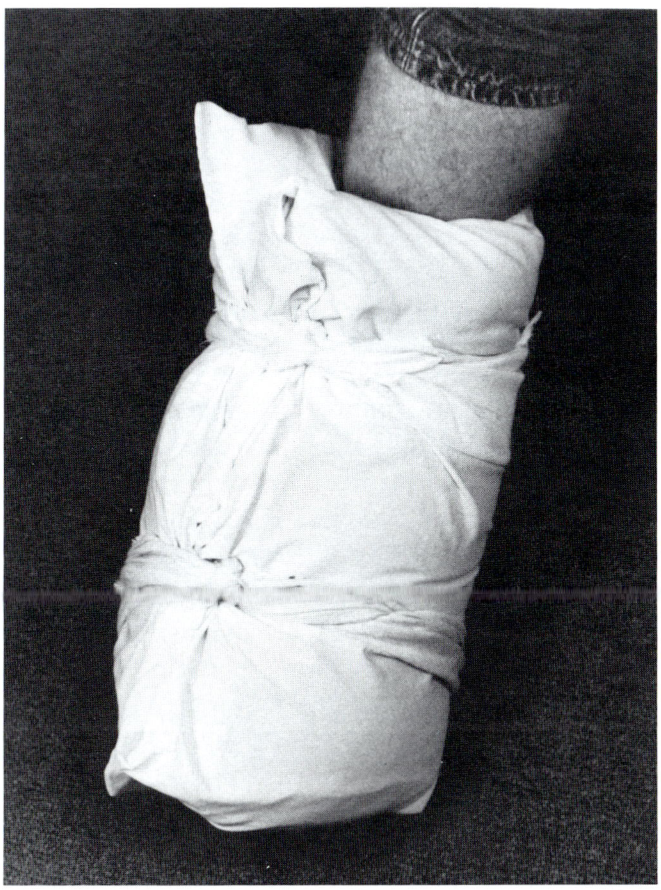

**Figure 9.7** To make a pillow splint, simply mold the pillow around the injured area and fasten it with safety pins or cravats.

## Rigid Splints

A rigid splint is an inflexible splint that is designed to maintain stability in an injured limb. It may be a padded board, a piece of heavy cardboard, or an aluminum splint that can be molded to fit the extremity (Figure 9.8). Whatever its construction,

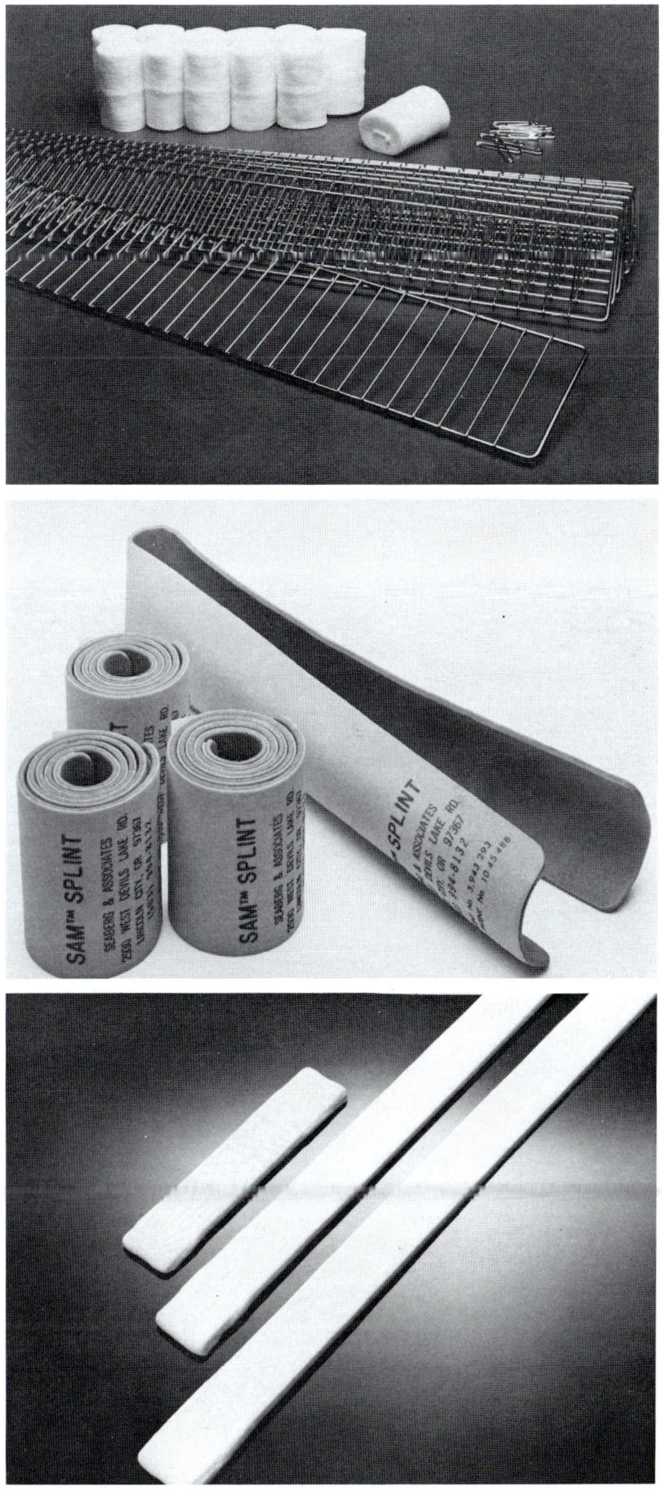


**Figure 9.8** Shown are several types of rigid splints. *Courtesy of Dyna Med.*

a rigid splint, like all splints, must be long enough to extend to the joint above and to the joint below the fracture site. Because the proper application of a rigid splint requires pulling traction on the injured extremity, you will be assisting an EMT with its application. To apply a rigid splint

Step 1: Attach the splint to the injured extremity as the EMT grasps the extremity above and below the fracture site and applies gentle traction (Figure 9.9).

Step 2: Wrap the limb and splint in self-adhering bandages as the EMT continues to maintain traction (Figure 9.10). Wrap the bandages tightly enough to hold the splint firmly to the extremity, but not so tight as to occlude circulation in the limb.

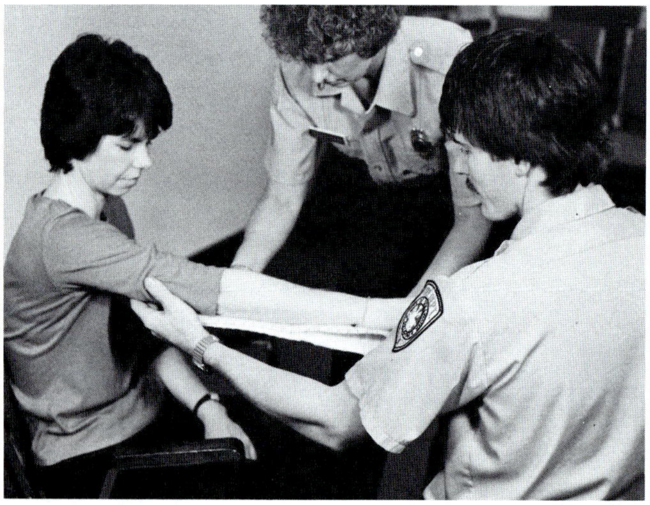

**Figure 9.9** Attach the splint to the injured extremity as the EMT applies traction.

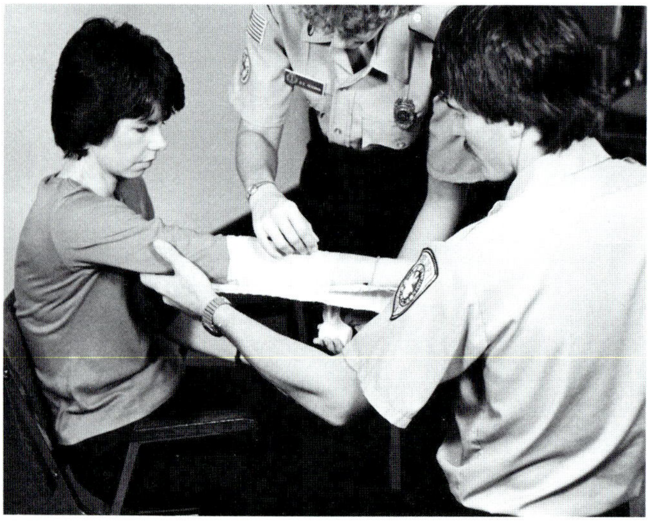

**Figure 9.10** Wrap the limb and splint in self-adhering bandages.

## Air Splints

Air splints are useful primarily for immobilizing fractures that involve the lower leg or forearm. Although they are widely used, air splints have certain disadvantages of which you should be aware. The possibility of overinflation is a dangerous complication of using air splints since overinflating the splint causes damaging levels of pressure to be exerted upon the injured limb. This is particularly a danger when the splinting is applied in low temperatures and the patient is later moved to a warmer area, where the air in the splint expands. Furthermore, hemorrhage into the fracture site can increase splint pressure. To avoid overinflating the splint initially, it is critical that you ALWAYS inflate the splint by mouth, NEVER with a pump. Inflate the splint just to the point that your finger pressed against it makes a slight dent. You should be able to fit two fingers under the splint if it is inflated properly (Figure 9.11).

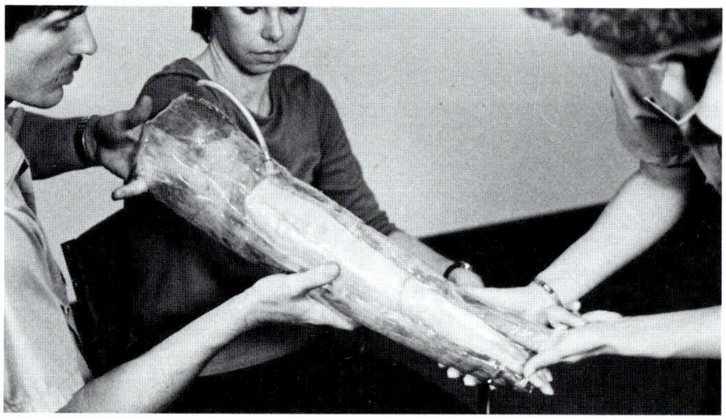

**Figure 9.11** You should be able to fit two fingers under the splint if it is inflated properly.

Aside from the dangers associated with overinflating air splints, there are also dangers associated with the fact that air splints tend to leak. An air splint that loses its rigidity, of course, fails to immobilize the injured extremity effectively and increases the likelihood that nerve and vascular damage will result from the movement of broken bone ends. In addition, the application of an air splint makes it impossible to monitor the pulse distal to the injury, a situation that could result in further damage to the injured extremity. Finally, air splints do not allow for application of cold packs, which are commonly used to reduce pain and swelling in fractures, dislocations, and sprains.

The instructions that follow are for the application of an air splint to a patient's forearm, but the process is essentially the same for application to a lower leg. Again, because the process involves applying traction to the injured extremity, you will be assisting an EMT.

Step 1: The EMT gathers the splint over his or her own arm so that the bottom edge is just above the wrist (Figure 9.12).

Step 2: With the hand that is covered by the splint, the EMT grasps the hand of the patient's injured arm and applies gentle traction, then instructs you to apply countertraction from above the elbow (Figure 9.13).

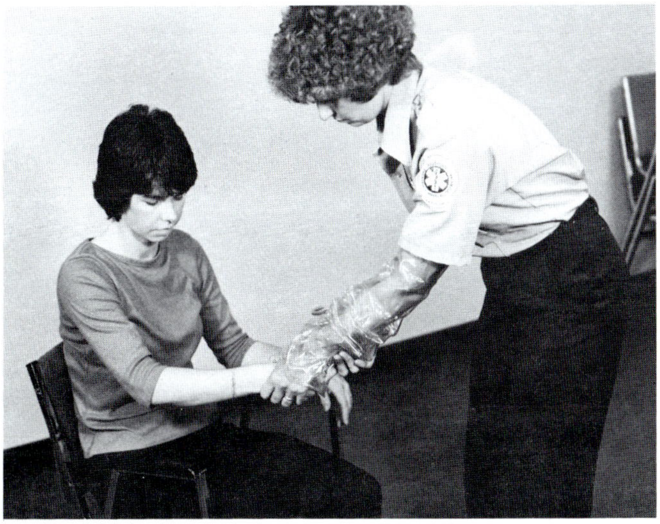

**Figure 9.12** The EMT gathers the splint over his or her own arm.

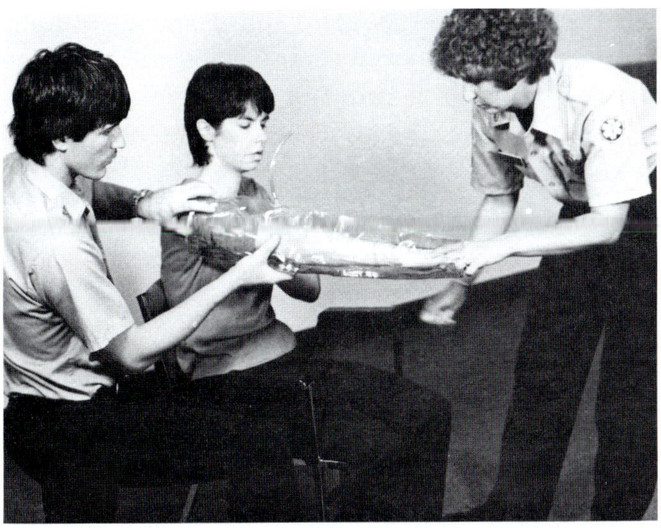

**Figure 9.13** The EMT applies gentle traction to the patient's arm while the first responder applies countertraction from above the elbow.

Step 3: As you both continue to maintain traction, the EMT slides the air splint from his or her arm onto the patient's arm and makes sure that the air splint is free of wrinkles and that the patient's fingers do not protrude beyond the end of the air splint (if they do, the splint may act as a tourniquet).

Step 4: Finally, the EMT will instruct you to inflate the air splint as he or she maintains traction. The EMT will tell you when the splint is properly inflated.

Some air splints are equipped with zippers to simplify the procedure for applying them. If you use an air splint that has a zipper, an EMT will maintain traction on the injured extremity proximally and distally while you wrap the splint around the injured area and zip it up. The EMT will continue to pull traction while you inflate the splint.

After the air splint has been applied, the EMT will check the skin color and the patient's capillary refill return in the fingers or the toes and ask the patient if the pain has been partially relieved by stabilization of the fracture. The EMT may ask you to check the skin color through the transparent splint every five minutes to guarantee continued good circulation. Make sure that the patient has sensation and movement in the fingers and toes and monitor the splint carefully to be sure that it does not lose pressure or become overinflated.

### Traction Splints

Traction splints, like all splints, are used to immobilize fractures and to prevent further injury to surrounding tissues. Traction splints are so named, however, because once they are applied they also provide constant traction to the injured extremity. This traction is developed by affixing the proximal end of the splint to the proximal end of the injured extremity — specifically, to the pelvis, since traction splints are used only for injuries of the femur or hip. Traction splints do not realign the broken bone ends, but simply immobilize them. Immobilization is a critical aspect of treating a fractured femur or hip because of the powerful muscle spasms that surround fractures in these areas.

The most commonly used traction splints are the Thomas half-ring splint and the Hare traction splints. The basic principles of application are the same for both, and both require manual traction initially, thus traction splints are always applied by EMTs.

The application of a traction splint basically involves attaching the splint to the distal and proximal ends of the injured extremity and developing traction by tightening the winding device (Figure 9.14). You may be asked to assist an EMT in this process by securing the splint to the leg with straps or cravats and by checking the pulses proximal and distal to the fracture.

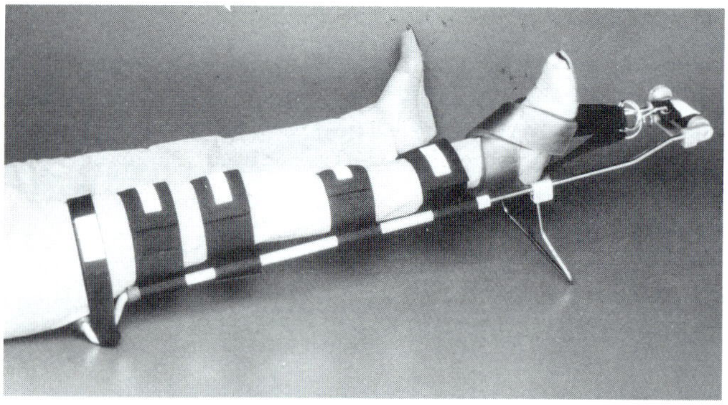

**Figure 9.14** Traction splints are attached to the proximal and distal ends of the injured extremity. Traction is developed by tightening the winding device. *Courtesy of Dyna Med.*

## Medical Anti-Shock Trousers (MAST)

MAST are, in effect, a type of air splint. They are commonly used for lower extremity trauma and are especially useful for pelvic fractures. When they are inflated to their maximum, MAST reduce vascular capacity in the abdomen and legs sufficiently to compensate for blood loss as great as 30 percent. This is enough to restore adequate perfusion to the oxygen-sensitive tissues in the heart-brain-lung circulation until adequate whole blood can be added to restore the cardiovascular fluid volume.

In addition, the external pressure of MAST can indirectly apply enough extra vascular pressure to decrease blood loss from either external or internal hemorrhage. This makes the device extremely useful in controlling intra-abdominal blood loss or the blood loss associated with pelvic or femoral fractures. The trousers are also used to immobilize fractures of the femur and pelvis, since they can be applied to extend above and below the fracture.

First responders are not involved in the decision to apply the trousers, but may assist EMTs in their application, especially in monitoring the patient's blood pressure. Essentially, the process consists of positioning the MAST on the patient, and slowly inflating first the leg compartments, then the abdominal compartment. The patient's blood pressure must be closely monitored and constantly reevaluated both during and after application (Figure 9.15).

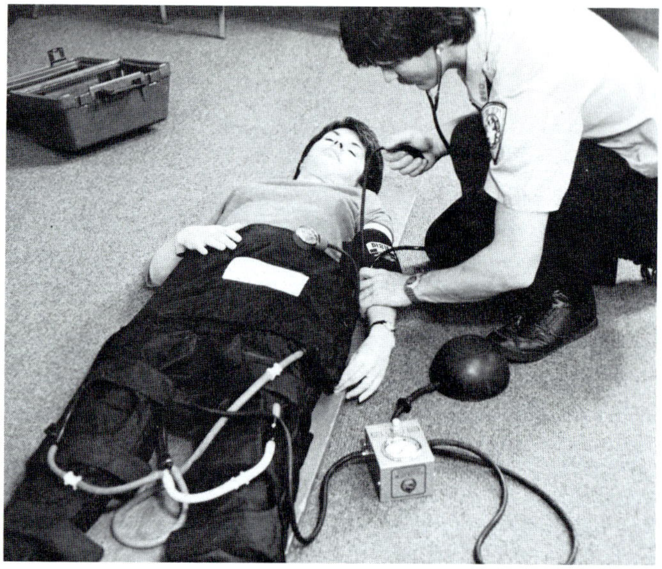

**Figure 9.15** The patient's blood pressure must be closely monitored both during and after application of MAST.

When the patient's blood pressure returns to within normal limits, inflation is stopped. Because the trousers are a type of air splint, similar complications may arise from their use, especially those associated with leaking or overinflation in response to changes in atmospheric pressure or temperature.

## MANAGING INJURIES TO THE EXTREMITIES

Because a fracture, dislocation, or sprain can only be positively diagnosed by x-ray, you must assume that a fracture is present when a patient complains of pain, tenderness, or loss of function in an extremity, and treat the injured limb accordingly. This means that the emergency treatment for fractures, dislocations, and sprains is essentially the same: this treatment consists of immobilizing and splinting the injured extremity. Remember, NEVER attempt to replace protruding bone ends or dislocations. Simply immobilize and splint the extremity in the position in which you find it and arrange for these patients to be transported to the nearest medical facility for x-rays and further evaluation and treatment of their injuries.

## Clavicle

Fractures of the clavicle (collarbone) are relatively easy to detect by palpation and observation since the clavicle lies close to the skin. Stabilize this fracture with a sling and swathe to prevent shoulder motion.

## Shoulder

Deformity and restricted motion identify this dislocation. Immobilize the arm in a sling and a swathe, and be sure to pad the armpit. It is often necessary to use a pillow or blanket between the arm and the chest wall because the arm is fixed away from the chest.

## Humerus

Fractures of the humerus are usually caused by falling on an outstretched arm. Diagnosis may be difficult because the broken parts are frequently impacted. Fractures of the shaft usually cause gross deformity, swelling, loss of function, and pain. The most effective way to stabilize this fracture is to sling and swathe the arm against the chest. Rigid splints can be added for protection, but cannot be used alone because they do not immobilize the joint above the fracture.

## Elbow

Pain and loss of motion signal an elbow fracture or dislocation. This type of injury is particularly serious because of the proximity of bone ends or fragments to nerves and blood vessels. Elbow fractures are often associated with loss of circulation, and surgery is frequently necessary to reestablish blood flow to the extremity. Immobilize an elbow fracture or dislocation by splinting it in the position in which you find it. Use either a sling and swathe or a long arm padded splint, depending upon the degree to which the arm is flexed.

## Forearm

Fractures of the forearm are usually caused by a fall on the outstretched arm. Even though mid-shift fractures usually produce great deformity, it is not uncommon for fractures (particularly in the elderly) to be impacted and relatively stable. Therefore, an x-ray is necessary to confirm that no fractures exist.

Frequently, the best method of managing this fracture is to apply a sling and swathe along with a ladder splint or short board splint to stabilize the wrist. Complete immobilization must include the joint above the fracture, the elbow. This means, of course, that air splints or long rigid splints must immobilize the arm in full extension.

## Wrist

Again, a fracture or dislocation of the wrist is most often caused by a fall on the outstretched arm. Splint the wrist in the position in which you find it with an air splint or a long rigid splint. Be sure to immobilize the joint above the fracture or dislocation (the elbow) as well.

## Hand

Fractures of the carpals and metacarpals may be either impacted or greenstick. Frequently, the diagnosis is based on pain alone. To splint a hand, immobilize the hand in its position of function. That is, have the patient hold something round — a roll of gauze, for instance — so the fingers are slightly flexed, then secure the hand in that position with self-adhering gauze (Figure 9.16). Add a padded rigid splint to immobilize the wrist and forearm.

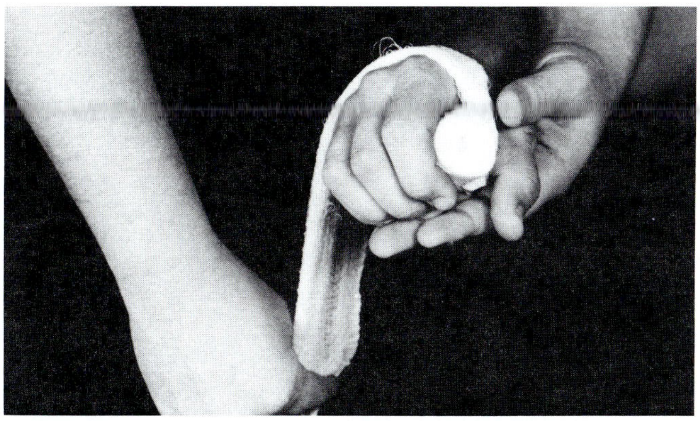

**Figure 9.16** To immobilize a hand fracture, have the patient hold something round, then secure the hand with self-adhering gauze.

## Fingers

Fractures and dislocations of the fingers are identified by obvious deformity and painful movement. Immobilize the injured finger in the position of function with a small, rigid splint. These injuries swell considerably, so be sure to tape the splint to the finger in such a way that the tape does not interfere with the swelling (Figure 9.17).

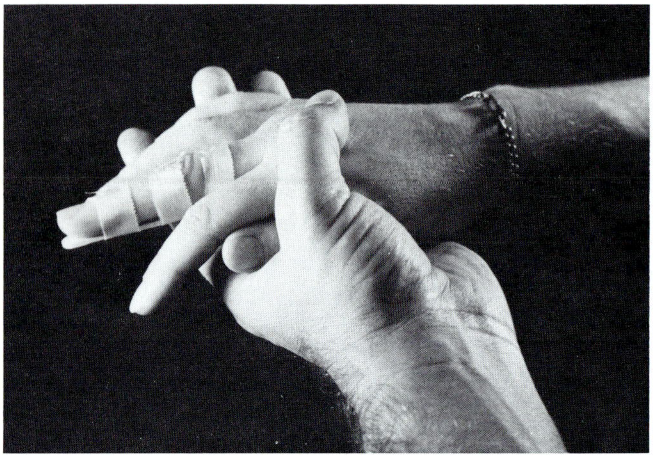

**Figure 9.17** Do not wrap the tape all the way around the finger — finger fractures swell considerably.

## Pelvis

A fractured pelvis commonly results from compression injuries and falls. This fracture can be diagnosed in a conscious patient by pressing straight down on the hip bones, then by squeezing the hip bones together. If these tests are painful to the patient, you must assume a fracture of the pelvis.

Blood loss from pelvic fractures and accompanying rupture of abdominal organs is probably the most extensive of all fractures. As much as 2½ liters of blood can be lost, and shock can develop from this fracture alone. MAST are especially beneficial in the management of these patients and provide the added benefit of controlling severe bleeding.

## Hip

Fractures and dislocations of the hip are generally caused by a fall or some other type of trauma, such as hitting the dashboard with the knees in a head-on automobile crash. The leg on the injured side of the hip may appear to be shorter than the other leg. Rotation of the leg and pain when moving the extremity are also common in both fractures and dislocations of the hip (Figure 9.18).

Traction splints are preferred for the management of this type of fracture, although MAST may be used. Alternately, the patient may be placed on a long backboard with pillows to immobilize the leg in its rotated position.

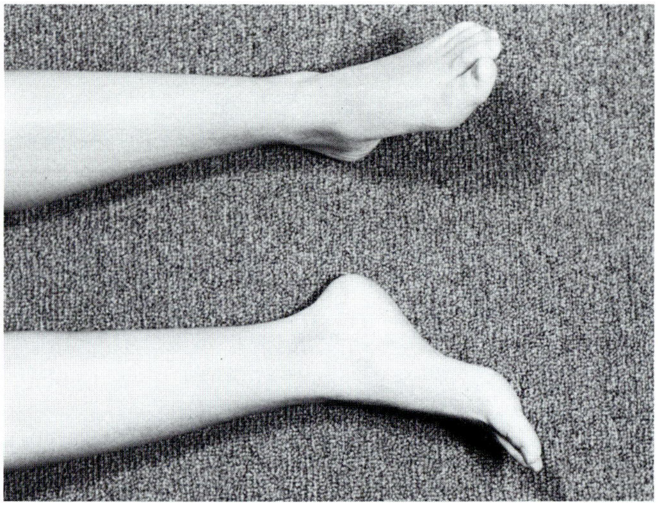

**Figure 9.18** If a patient's hip is fractured or dislocated, the leg may be rotated either inward or outward.

## Femur

Tenderness and deformity are the most common physical findings in a fracture of the femur. Shortening of the extremity is also possible (Figure 9.19).

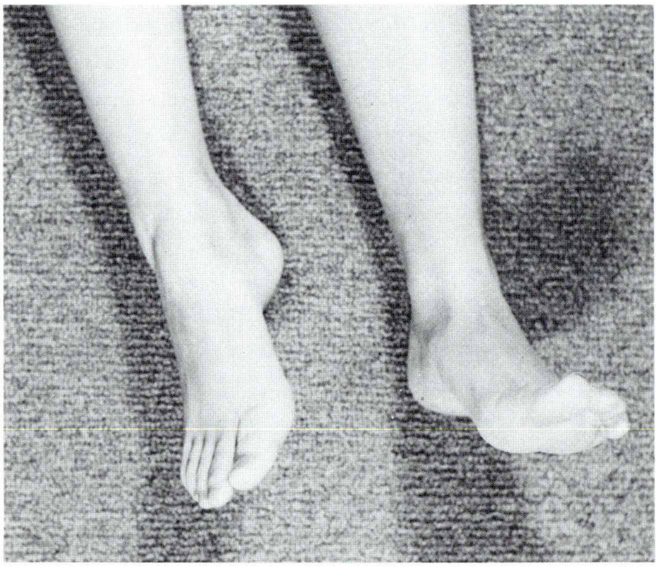

**Figure 9.19** If a patient has a fractured femur, the injured leg may appear shorter than the other leg.

Management of this fracture is similar to management of hip fractures; traction splints are preferred. If necessary, a traction splint and MAST may be used together for severe hip or femur fractures when hypovolemic shock — caused by a drastic reduction in the body's plasma — is present or is likely to develop. When this is necessary, the MAST is applied over the traction splint.

### Knee

Impaction may make these fractures difficult to identify, except by testing for tenderness. When treating a fracture of the knee, as in all femoral fractures, the knee must be immobilized. Therefore, similar management techniques as with the hip and femur are used. However, pain and occasional angulation of this fracture may prevent the use of traction splinting. Therefore, splinting the knee in the position most comfortable to the patient may require the use of wire splints, such as the ladder splint.

The position of the fracture may cause vascular complications similar to those in elbow fractures.

### Tibia and Fibula

Fractures of the tibia and fibula, particularly those near the ankle, resemble a sprain or strain and can be difficult to identify. Although angulation may be present in the midshaft, pain and tenderness may be the only evidence of injury.

Long leg air splints, traction splints or board splints are all acceptable methods of immobilizing this fracture. The MAST do not immobilize the ankle and, therefore, cannot be used as immobilization for below-the-knee fractures.

Vascular complications, particularly around the ankle, are not uncommon, especially if a fracture or dislocation at the ankle has occurred.

### Ankle

Dislocations of the ankle are frequently associated with fractures. Generally, there is gross deformity of the ankle, but often it is not possible to distinguish a fracture from a dislocation.

Treat ankle dislocations as if they were fractures — immobilize the ankle with leg splints, air splints, or a pillow splint.

### Foot

Like fractures of the hand, fractures of the foot may be detected by palpation, but the diagnosis may be based on pain alone. Use a pillow splint to immobilize the foot. Complications rarely occur with these fractures. However, patients with heel fractures from falls should be examined for fractures of the hip or spine, since a force sufficient to fracture the heel is usually transmitted upward to the hip or lower spine.

### Toe

Diagnosis of a fracture or dislocation of the toe is usually made on the basis of pain and swelling. Tape the injured toe to the adjacent toe to immobilize it.

### Amputated Extremities

If the patient has sustained a traumatic amputation of a body part, search for the part at the accident scene and have it transported with the patient to the emergency room. Rinse the amputated part with sterile saline and wrap it gently in a bulky sterile dressing and soak the dressing and the part together in cool saline. Finally, seal the wrapped part in a plastic bag, and place it on ice. **NEVER** place amputated parts directly on ice or in dry dressings, and never use any solution other than sterile saline to moisten the dressing.

# 10

# Medical Emergencies

**U.S. DEPARTMENT OF TRANSPORTATION**
**First Responder Training Course**

**Objectives:**

- Define heart attack, angina, heart failure, stroke, diabetic coma, insulin shock, grand mal seizures and petit mal seizures.
- Given patients simulating heart attacks, angina, heart failure, stroke and diabetic and epileptic conditions, examine the patient, note appropriate signs and perform or describe appropriate care.

## Chapter 10
# Medical Emergencies

Anything that threatens a person's airway, breathing, or circulation is an emergency. Although many emergencies result from trauma or accident, other emergencies result from illness or disease. In this chapter, medical emergencies are defined as those emergencies resulting from illness or disease that pose a serious threat to the patient's life.

Some emergencies are more commonly seen in older persons, such as chronic obstructive pulmonary disease, heart attack, and stroke. Other emergencies, such as diabetic states, seizures, and anaphylactic shock, are found in all age groups. Medical emergencies require rapid treatment and transport to a medical facility so that the patient can be further evaluated and treated.

## RESPIRATORY DISTRESS

Respiratory distress may result from trauma or illness. Most patients in respiratory distress complain of dyspnea (difficulty breathing), although some may have serious respiratory problems without dyspnea. When called to any patient who is in respiratory distress, obtain answers to the following questions:

- How long has the patient had difficulty breathing? Is this a long-standing problem, for example, Chronic Obstructive Pulmonary Disease (COPD), or is it recent?
- Have symptoms developed gradually or abruptly? Breathing difficulties associated with asthma or congestive heart failure may take hours to develop, while pulmonary embolism often causes sudden, severe dyspnea.
- Does any position make the pain better or worse?
- Has the patient been coughing? If so, is the patient coughing anything up (productive cough)? What does the sputum look like? Patients with COPD often have a chronic cough associated with thick, white sputum. If their condition worsens, their sputum may increase and become yellow-green and thick.
- Does the patient have pain? What is the nature of the pain (sharp, dull, for example)?
- Has the patient suffered any medical problems in the past? The patient may give a history of heart trouble, heavy smoking, or chronic cough.
- What medications does the patient take regularly?

When taking the patient history, note whether the patient appears anxious or uncomfortable. Is the patient having difficulty speaking? Do your questions easily distract the patient from symptoms? Are the patient's answers appropriate or does the patient seem disoriented? All of these observations are an essential part of assessing the patient's general appearance and mental status.

After completing the primary survey, take the patient's vital signs, paying special attention to the rate and quality of respirations. During the secondary survey, look for signs of respiratory distress, including the following:

- Nasal flaring: the nostrils open wide on inspiration

- Tracheal tugging: the Adam's apple pulls upward on inspiration
- Retraction of the intercostal muscles (the muscles between the ribs) during inspiration
- Use of the diaphragm and neck muscles during breathing
- Cyanosis, which indicates lack of oxygen

Respiratory distress may be the result of a chronic condition, such as Chronic Obstructive Pulmonary Disease, or an acute condition. *Chronic* refers to a long-standing condition; *acute* refers to a condition that develops suddenly. Some acute conditions that result in respiratory distress are pulmonary embolism, pneumonia, and, in children, croup and epiglottitis.

## COPD

Chronic Obstructive Pulmonary Disease, or COPD, is the term given to several chronic conditions of the lungs that cause narrowing and obstruction of the lower airways. Obstructive airway diseases are very common: it is estimated that 10 to 20 percent of adults have COPD. The most often-encountered chronic conditions are emphysema, chronic bronchitis, and asthma.

### EMPHYSEMA AND CHRONIC BRONCHITIS

Emphysema and chronic bronchitis are much more common in men than in women, and they strike city dwellers more often than rural inhabitants. Cigarette smoking is the most important contributing factor to both diseases. Many people have symptoms of both emphysema and chronic bronchitis.

Emphysema is a progressive lung condition in which the bronchioles are damaged and some of the alveolar walls are broken down or destroyed. Because alveolar walls are destroyed, the lungs hold more air, which remains in the lungs even after exhaling. As emphysema advances, breathing becomes more difficult and the person's activities become more restricted.

The typical emphysema patient is thin, even somewhat emaciated, but has normal, even pink, skin. Coughing is not severe. Because emphysema patients tend to purse their lips when exhaling, they are often referred to as "pink puffers."

Chronic bronchitis is a lung condition characterized by production of mucus in the bronchial tubes. The patient also has a chronic cough, which produces a large amount of sputum. The typical patient is a heavy smoker, overweight, and has had many respiratory tract infections. Because these patients often have a bluish cast to their complexions, they are frequently called "blue bloaters."

Chronic bronchitis results in poor exchange of respiratory gases, lowered oxygen levels in the blood, and retention of carbon dioxide. The increased carbon dioxide levels hinder pulmonary circulation (the circulation from the heart to the lungs), which increases the work of the right ventricle. This strain on the heart can lead to right heart failure. (See Congestive Heart Failure later in this chapter.)

The patient with chronic bronchitis finds it difficult to both inhale and exhale. Because respiration is barely adequate, any extra strain on the system, such as a cold, can lead to respiratory failure. The patient becomes increasingly short of breath, so much so that sleep is disturbed. Lack of oxygen (hypoxia) leads to confusion, agitation, cyanosis, and sometimes muscle twitching.

More than anything else, patients suffering from acute respiratory failure need oxygen. However, you must take extra care when administering oxygen because persons with advanced COPD are stimulated to breathe by a different mechanism than people with healthy lungs. Healthy people are stimulated to breathe when recepters in the brain sense a high level of carbon dioxide in the blood. In patients with COPD, however, carbon dioxide levels in the blood increase over time; eventually, the brain is constantly receiving high carbon dioxide messages. The brain learns to ignore these messages, accepting only *low oxygen* messages from the blood. When oxygen levels in the blood become low, the brain receives a low oxygen message and sends a stimulus to breathe. This is known as breathing by hypoxic (low in oxygen) drive.

Administering high levels of oxygen decreases the patient's stimulus to breathe because the brain no longer receives low oxygen messages from the blood. The patient's breathing may slow down or stop entirely. Do be aware that you may have to coach the patient to breathe or to assist ventilations with a bag-valve-mask or with artificial respiration.

**NEVER WITHHOLD OXYGEN FROM A PATIENT WHO NEEDS IT, EVEN IF YOU HAVE TO ASSIST RESPIRATIONS.**

The treatment for patients with COPD is as follows:

- Establish an airway.
- Place the patient in a sitting or semisitting position to make breathing easier. Ask the patient if he or she is having more difficulty breathing than normal. If the patient reports increased difficulty breathing, administer oxygen at a rate of approximately 2 to 4 liters per minute. If the patient is in severe respiratory distress, administer oxygen by mask and be prepared to assist ventilations.
- Monitor vital signs frequently.
- Arrange for immediate transport to a medical facility.

#### ASTHMA

Approximately 6 million Americans suffer from asthma, and 4,000-5,000 people die from it each year. Asthma is an allergic or psychogenic reaction that causes spasms of the bronchial tubes. Asthma attacks can be brought on by an allergic reaction to inhaled irritants, by respiratory infection, or by emotional stress. During an acute asthma attack, the bronchial tubes become constricted, the membranes lining the tubes swell and congest, and bronchial secretions increase. These changes cause pools of stale air to remain in the lungs and make full breaths impossible. The oxygen shortage that results causes a slowing down of bodily processes.

A person suffering from an acute asthma attack is usually found sitting up, often leaning forward, and struggling to breathe. The patient will be using accessory muscles in the neck and chest in an attempt to move air in and out. Because the patient finds it especially difficult to exhale, you will be able to hear whistling or wheezing sounds. As air remains trapped in the lungs, the patient's chest becomes enlarged, or hyperinflated. The patient may cough without bringing up any sputum. Because air hunger is extremely frightening, the patient may become increasingly apprehensive, which makes breathing even more difficult.

Reassure the patient to help relieve anxiety. Attempt to make the patient as comfortable as possible. A sitting position is most conducive to breathing. Most asthma sufferers are under a physician's care and will have prescribed medication in the form of inhalers or pills. Find out if the patient has already taken medication; if not, help the patient do so. Be sure the patient has an open airway, and administer humidified oxygen. Pure oxygen is very dry and may make the thick secretions in the lungs worse. Arrange for immediate transport to a medical facility.

Status asthmaticus is a severe, prolonged asthmatic attack that cannot be relieved by the usual medications. The patient is usually exhausted, dehydrated, and may act sleepy from lack of oxygen. The patient will make heavy use of chest and neck muscles in a desperate attempt to move air through the obstructed airways. The chest will be very distended due to trapped air in the lungs. Wheezing is absent; the patient is moving very little air at all.

The treatment for status asthmaticus is the same as for a standard acute asthma attack, except that the need for care in a hospital is much more urgent.

**STATUS ASTHMATICUS IS A SERIOUS MEDICAL EMERGENCY AND THE PATIENT NEEDS TO BE TRANSPORTED TO A MEDICAL FACILITY IMMEDIATELY.**

### Pulmonary Embolism

An embolism is a blood clot or other undissolved particle that breaks loose and is carried through the circulatory system. A pulmonary embolism is usually caused by a blood clot that blocks a pulmonary artery or one of its branches. Several conditions make a person more prone to pulmonary embolism:

- Prolonged bed rest, which causes blood to become stagnant in the lower extremities.
- Thrombophlebitis (inflammation of the veins), especially those in the arms and legs.
- Certain drugs, especially oral contraceptives.

The typical patient with pulmonary embolism experiences sudden, severe dyspnea. The patient may also have sharp chest pains made worse by coughing and deep breathing. There may be no other symptoms. On examination, the patient will probably be laboring to breathe, have a very fast heartbeat (tachycardia), and may have falling blood pressure.

Anyone with a pulmonary embolism needs to be hospitalized, so treatment consists of the following:

- Establish an airway.
- Allow the patient to assume the position of greatest comfort.
- Administer oxygen.
- Monitor vital signs frequently.
- Arrange for immediate transport to a medical facility.

## Pneumonia

Pneumonia is caused by bacteria, viruses, or fungi. Pneumonia results in pus or fluid accumulating in the alveoli, which prevents proper oxygenation of the blood.

The pneumonia patient usually reports several hours to several days of fever, weakness, productive cough, and sometimes chest pain worsened by coughing. Pneumonia can begin abruptly, with a shaking chill, or set in gradually, progressively weakening the patient. The elderly and those with chronic diseases are more prone to pneumonia than are younger, healthier persons. The pneumonia patient is often feverish, with hot, dry skin, and has a productive cough. He or she may exhibit respiratory distress, especially rapid, shallow breathing.

The patient with pneumonia needs to be hospitalized. The only treatment in the field is to allow the patient to assume the position of greatest comfort and administer oxygen. Monitor vital signs and arrange for transportation to a medical facility.

## Respiratory Distress in Children

Because children's airways are very small, any condition that causes the airway to swell can cause serious airway problems. Croup and epiglottitis are two upper respiratory infections that can cause life-threatening airway problems in children.

### CROUP

Croup is a viral infection of the upper airways that occurs in children between six months and four years of age. It rarely occurs in older children. Croup causes swelling and narrowing of the airway just below the larynx. The child with croup typically has a cold or is hoarse during the day, and develops respiratory distress during the night. The signs and symptoms of croup are as follows:

- Loud, barking cough ("seal bark" cough)
- Wheezing or whooping during inhalation or exhalation
- Fever
- Signs of respiratory distress:
  - flared nostrils
  - use of chest and neck muscles trying to breathe
- Restlessness and tachycardia (rapid heartbeat) as oxygen levels fall

Let the child assume the position of greatest comfort. Do not try to take the child away from his or her parents; such action will only frighten the child, making breathing even more difficult. Breathing can be eased by placing the child by a cold steam vaporizer or in a bathroom with the shower turned on. If breathing is extremely labored, administer oxygen by mask. Arrange for immediate transport to a medical facility.

### EPIGLOTTITIS

Epiglottitis is an inflammation of the epiglottis, the flap of skin that covers the larynx during swallowing. Epiglottitis is caused by a bacterial infection and is found in children between three and seven years of age. The onset of epiglottitis can be very rapid, with the child developing the following:

- High fever
- Severe pain while swallowing
- Drooling
- Signs of respiratory distress:
  - flared nostrils during inhalation
  - use of chest and neck muscles trying to breathe
- Restlessness and tachycardia (rapid heartbeat) as oxygen levels fall

Keep the child sitting up; you probably will not be able to get a child with epiglottitis to lie down anyway because breathing is so difficult. Drooling is common because the child's throat is so swollen and sore that he or she cannot swallow. DO NOT try to look in the child's mouth because it can cause laryngospasm, which will close off the airway completely. DO NOT try to suction the mouth. Do administer oxygen with a pediatric mask.

**THE CHILD WITH EPIGLOTTITIS IS IN SERIOUS DANGER OF COMPLETE AIRWAY OBSTRUCTION DUE TO SWOLLEN TISSUES. GET THIS CHILD TO A MEDICAL FACILITY AS RAPIDLY AS POSSIBLE.**

Many children with epiglottitis require tracheostomy (insertion of a breathing tube into the throat), so do not delay.

### Anaphylaxis (Anaphylactic Shock)

Anaphylactic shock occurs when a person comes in contact with a substance to which he or she is extremely allergic. Anaphylaxis results from a breakdown of the immune system. Normally, when people are exposed to foreign substances (called antigens), the immune system develops antibodies to protect against further exposure. This production of antibodies is the principle behind immunization. During immunization, a harmless form of a disease (another antigen) is introduced into the body so that the immune system can develop antibodies to that particular antigen. If the immune system again comes in contact with that antigen, the individual is protected.

In the case of allergic reactions, however, the immune system offers no protection (anaphylaxis means "without protection"). Rather than developing antibodies to a particular antigen, the body becomes extremely sensitive to it. The next time the individual is exposed to the antigen, he or she has an allergic reaction. Anaphylaxis is the most severe form of allergic reaction.

Some of the more common substances that cause anaphylactic reactions are listed below (Figure 10.1):

- Insect stings — bees, wasps, hornets, and yellow jackets
- Injected substances — drugs such as morphine, penicillin, or tetanus antitoxin
- Ingested substances — certain foods such as nuts, berries, and shellfish; oral medications such as penicillin

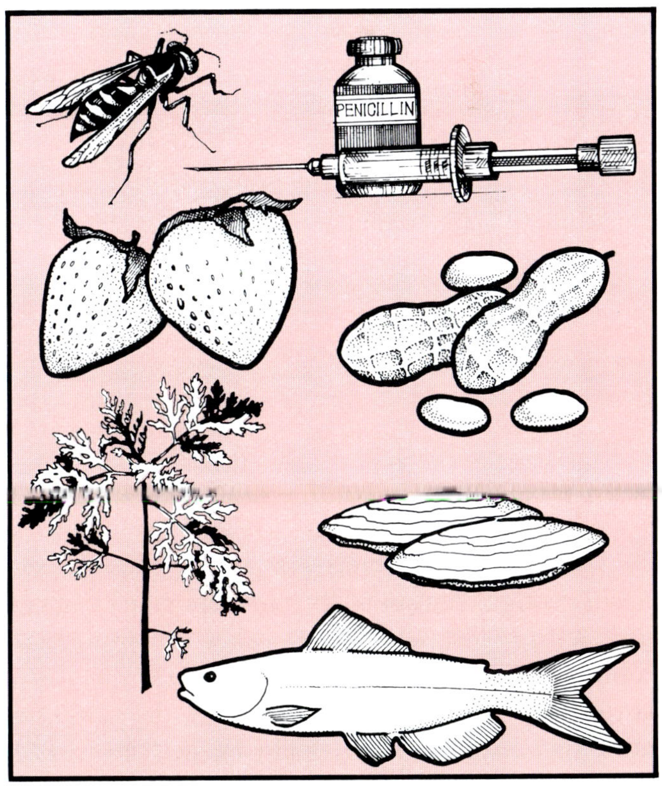


**Figure 10.1** Substances to which people are allergic are numerous and various; some of the more common ones are shown here.

The classic signs of anaphylactic shock are as follows:

- Dyspnea (difficulty breathing)
- Flushed or ashen skin
- Swelling (edema), especially of the face, hands, and feet
- Intense itching
- Hives
- Abdominal cramps, nausea, and diarrhea
- Rapid pulse (tachycardia)
- Falling blood pressure (hypotension)

During an anaphylactic reaction, the bronchial and laryngeal muscles constrict, the arterioles dilate, and the capillaries leak fluid into the surrounding tissues, causing edema (swelling). As the airways narrow and the surrounding tissues swell, it becomes increasingly difficult to breathe. The patient frequently complains of tightness in the chest or a sensation that his or her throat is closing. The patient is often sneezing, wheezing, or coughing up blood-tinged sputum. The patient's face may be flushed or ashen, with marked swelling, especially around the eyes. The patient may complain of severe itching, either generalized or in the throat. The patient often has hives or the skin may simply become red and inflamed. Abdominal cramps, followed by nausea, vomiting, and diarrhea, are common. Blood pressure falls and the heart beats faster as the circulatory system starts to collapse.

**WASTE NO TIME SUMMONING EMTS OR PARAMEDICS WHO CAN ADMINISTER EPINEPHRINE TO A PATIENT SUFFERING FROM ANAPHYLACTIC SHOCK.**

The patient suffering from anaphylactic shock needs prompt treatment with epinephrine by injection or inhaler, which will relax the bronchial tubes and ease breathing. In the meantime, keep the patient lying down with the legs elevated and administer high-flow oxygen by mask. However, if the patient finds it easier to breathe in a semisitting or sitting position, allow him or her to sit up.

## HEART DISEASE

Heart disease causes more deaths per year in the United States than any other illness. Approximately 4 to 5 million Americans have heart disease, and more than 500,000 people die from it every year.

Like all other organs of the body, the heart requires a continuous flow of oxygenated blood in order to function properly. The coronary arteries are blood vessels that supply the heart with nutrients and oxygen. When a coronary artery becomes blocked, the part of the heart muscle it supplies is rapidly deprived of oxygen. Coronary arteries become blocked by a disease known as atherosclerosis. During childhood, fatty deposits begin to accumulate in the coronary arteries. Over many years, these fatty deposits leave scars and eventually lead to hardening of the arteries (Figure 10.2).

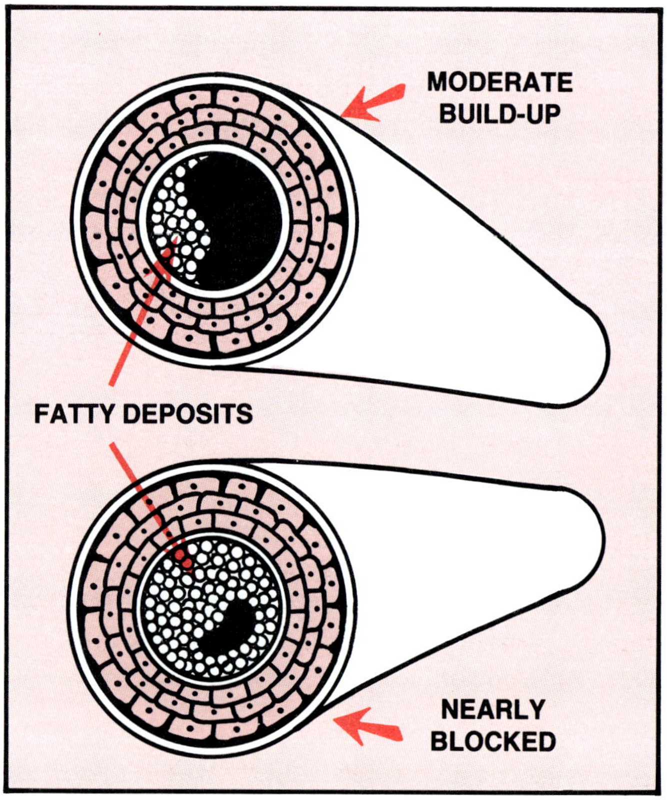


**Figure 10.2** Atherosclerosis causes fatty deposits to accumulate in the coronary arteries. Eventually these arteries become partially or completely blocked.

Certain factors increase a person's risk of developing atherosclerosis. They are

- Hypertension (high blood pressure)
- Cigarette smoking

- Diabetes
- High serum cholesterol
- Obesity
- Poor physical fitness
- Being a male
- Family history of heart disease
- Birth control pills (especially if taken by women over 35)
- Aggressive, competitive, Type A personality

Normally, when the body is under physical or emotional stress, the arteries dilate to allow more oxygen to get to the heart. However, in people with atherosclerosis dilation is no longer possible and the heart suffers from a lack of oxygen. Lack of oxygen causes chest pain (angina pectoris), heart attack (acute myocardial infarction), congestive heart failure, cardiogenic shock, or even cardiac arrest.

## Angina Pectoris

The principal symptom of coronary artery disease is angina pectoris, which literally means "choking in the chest." Patients usually describe the pain of angina as a heavy weight or squeezing of the chest. Sometimes the pain radiates to the neck, jaw, or arms, particularly the left arm. Angina may be brought on by stress, exertion, excitement, or heavy eating.

An angina attack typically lasts three to five minutes. The pain of angina is not affected by deep breathing, coughing, or change in body position. Angina is relieved by resting or by taking the drug nitroglycerin.

When taking a patient history, try to determine whether the angina is stable or unstable. Stable angina follows a standard pattern: the patient regularly experiences pain after a certain amount of physical exertion or stress. The pain occurs in the same area of the body and for a predictable period of time.

Unstable angina is more serious because it indicates further obstruction of the coronary arteries and often signals an impending acute myocardial infarction (AMI). The patient with angina who calls for emergency help usually does so because of a change in the pattern of the anginal attacks. The patient often states that over the past several days or weeks the anginal attacks have grown more frequent or severe, or that they occur during periods of rest.

Ask the patient who complains of chest pain if he or she has a history of chronic angina. If the answer is yes, the patient probably has nitroglycerin tablets. If the patient has not yet taken nitroglycerin, help the patient place a tablet under the tongue. (The patient must not swallow the tablet; it needs to dissolve under the tongue.) Nitroglycerin works by dilating blood vessels, thus relieving stress on the heart (Figure 10.3). If the patient does not feel relief after several minutes, he or she may be suffering an AMI. Treat any patient with angina, stable or unstable, as though he or she is having an AMI. Treatment for AMI is described in the following section.

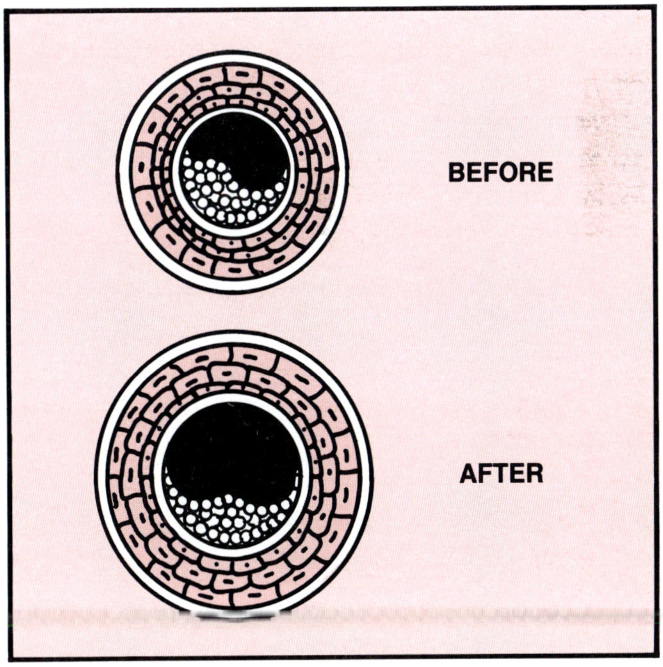


**Figure 10.3** Nitroglycerin dilates blood vessels, allowing more blood and therefore more oxygen to reach the heart.

**NOTE:** Nitroglycerin is dispensed in glass bottles and is supposed to remain potent for about one year. If the patient has transferred the tablets to another bottle, chances are good that the nitroglycerin has lost its potency. In addition, some heart patients take nitroglycerin in the form of a patch that is placed on the skin daily, usually on the upper chest or back (Figure 10.4). However, this form of nitroglycerin is not designed to provide quick relief from the pain of angina.

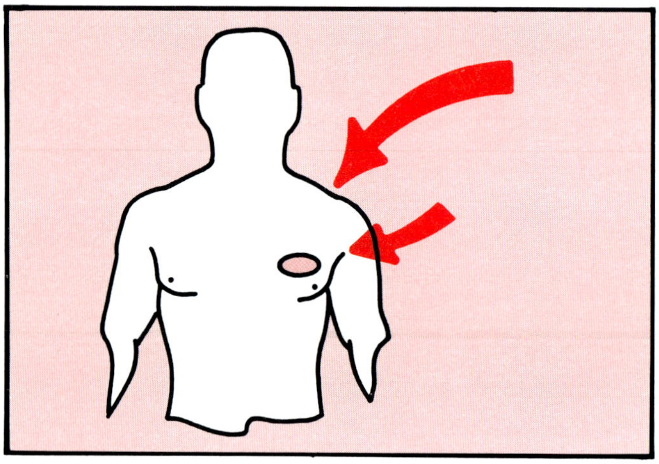

**Figure 10.4** Some heart patients take nitroglycerin continuously through patches that are placed on the skin; however, this type of nitroglycerin is not designed to provide quick relief from the pain of angina.

## AMI (Acute Myocardial Infarction)

AMI, or heart attack, occurs when the blood supply (and oxygen) to a portion of the heart is totally blocked. Blockage is usually caused by severe atherosclerosis or by a clot that forms in a coronary artery. Lack of oxygen causes a portion of the heart to die, which is referred to as an acute myocardial infarction (AMI) or heart attack.

The signs and symptoms of AMI include the following:

- Chest pain; may radiate to arms, neck, jaw, and upper back
- Profuse sweating and chills
- Pale to gray complexion
- Nausea and vomiting
- Apprehension; the patient feels as though he or she will die
- Weakness
- Difficulty or pain in breathing

The most important symptom of AMI is CHEST PAIN, which is reported by 80 to 90 percent of AMI patients. The pain of AMI is similar to that of angina, but is more intense, lasts longer (30 minutes to several hours), and is not relieved by taking nitroglycerin. Patients usually describe the pain as severe—"heavy," "squeezing," "crushing," or "tight." In approximately 25 percent of AMI patients the pain radiates to the arms, most often the left arm; the pain may also radiate to the neck, jaw, or upper back. Like angina, the pain of AMI is not influenced by coughing, deep breathing, or body movements. Table 10.1 illustrates the differences between the pain of AMI and angina.

**TABLE 10.1**
**DIFFERENCES BETWEEN ANGINA AND ACUTE MYOCARDIAL INFARCTION**

| Signs and Symptoms | Angina Pectoris | Acute Myocardial Infarction |
|---|---|---|
| Pain Intensity | Mild to moderate | Very severe, intense |
| Duration | 3 to 5 minutes | 30 minutes to several hours |
| Caused by | Stress, exertion, excitement, heavy eating | May occur during rest |
| Relieved by | Rest Nitroglycerin | Nothing brings relief |
| Associated symptoms | May be none | Profuse sweating, chills, nausea, apprehension |

The patient with AMI usually appears anxious or frightened. If the patient is also suffering from lack of oxygen, he or she may appear confused, irritable, or restless. The patient's skin may be pale, cold, or clammy. The pulse is often rapid (tachycardia), but may be slow (bradycardia). Irregularities in the pulse are common. Blood pressure is likely to be low due to reduced cardiac output.

Approximately 10 to 20 percent of patients with AMI do not experience chest pain. This is commonly known as a "silent" MI. Painless AMI is much more common in elderly people, who may exhibit sudden shortness of breath, sudden loss of consciousness, or unexplained drop in blood pressure. Treat these symptoms in elderly people as AMI.

## TREATMENT OF AMI

More than half the deaths from myocardial infarction occur within the first few hours, and many people do not call for help until several hours after pains begin. Most of these early deaths are caused by cardiac arrhythmias (irregularities in the rhythm of the heartbeat). Early treatment can mean the difference between life and death for the patient with AMI.

First of all, reassure the patient. People suffering from AMI, or who think they are suffering an AMI, are terrified. Display a calm, professional manner in order to help relieve the patient's anxiety. Explain that you are a trained first responder and that you will do all you can to make the patient more comfortable.

Chest pain is caused by lack of oxygen, and oxygen is what the AMI or angina patient needs first. Oxygen can prevent or halt the arrhythmias that kill so many AMI patients. Place the patient in the position of greatest comfort (probably sitting) and loosen any tight clothing. Administer oxygen by mask at a flow rate of six to eight liters per minute. If the patient also suffers from COPD, administer oxygen at a lower rate (about four liters per minute) and watch the patient carefully. Assist ventilations if necessary.

Do not allow the patient to move around because any activity places additional strain on the heart. When the ambulance arrives, DO NOT allow the patient to walk to the ambulance. The strain on the heart can significantly worsen the infarction. Monitor vital signs frequently, and gather up any medications so they can be transported with the patient to the medical facility.

## COMPLICATIONS OF AMI

There are three major complications of AMI: congestive heart failure (CHF), cardiogenic shock, and cardiac arrest. All are life-threatening, so monitor vital signs frequently, keeping your fingers on the patient's pulse at all times, and be alert for changes that indicate complications.

Congestive heart failure occurs when the heart is unable to pump effectively. Pump failure may be due to AMI or other illnesses. Because the heart is a two-sided pump, there are two types of heart failure: left heart failure and right heart failure.

Left heart failure occurs when the left ventricle is unable to pump out all of the blood it receives from the lungs. As a result, blood backs up behind the left ventricle and begins to accumulate in the lungs. As the pulmonary vessels fill with blood, the patient has more and more difficulty breathing.

The main signs and symptoms of left heart failure (also known as pulmonary edema) are difficulty breathing, rapid heart rate, and increased respirations. The patient may wheeze and cough up blood-tinged sputum. Left heart failure can make it so difficult to breathe that the patient suffers a lowered level of consciousness and becomes cyanotic.

Right heart failure usually occurs as a result of left heart failure. As blood backs up from the heart into the lungs, the right side of the heart must work harder to pump blood into the already engorged pulmonary vessels. Eventually, the right heart can no longer keep up with the increased work load and fails. When right heart failure occurs, blood backs up into the veins. Patients with right heart failure have distended jugular veins and develop edema (swelling caused by retention of fluid). Edema can usually be seen in the hands, feet, and abdomen (Figure 10.5).

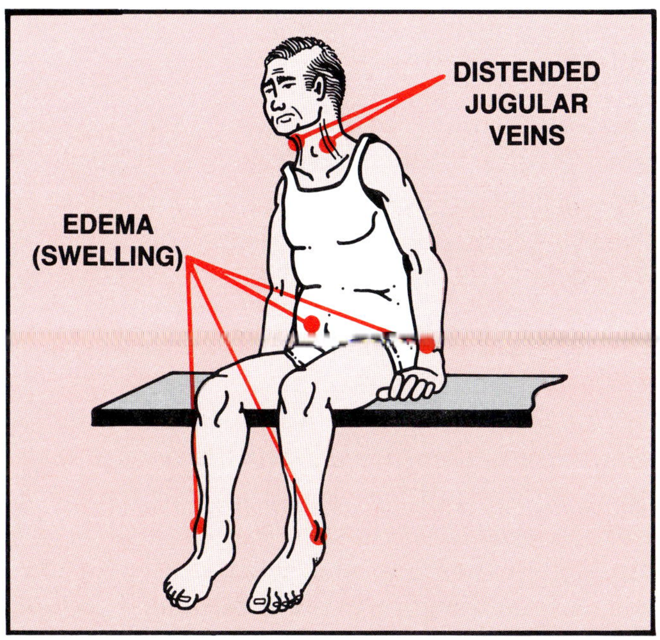


**Figure 10.5** Patients suffering from right heart failure develop swelling in the hands, feet, and abdomen.

Place a patient who is suffering heart failure in the most comfortable position, usually a sitting position with the feet dangling. Monitor the patient's vital signs and administer high-flow oxygen. Arrange for immediate transportation to a medical facility.

Cardiogenic shock occurs when the heart is damaged so badly that it cannot pump enough blood to maintain adequate tissue perfusion. Cardiogenic shock indicates extensive damage to the heart and is often fatal.

The signs and symptoms of cardiogenic shock are similar to those for other types of shock: restlessness and anxiety; pale, cool, clammy skin; cyanosis; weak, rapid pulse; rapid, shallow breathing; and falling blood pressure. (For more information on shock, see Chapter 6, Shock.)

To treat for cardiogenic shock, place the patient lying down with the legs elevated about 30 degrees. Handle the patient very gently. Administer oxygen in high concentrations. Monitor vital signs and level of consciousness frequently. Arrange for immediate transport to a medical facility.

**IF A HEART PATIENT SHOWS SIGNS OF SHOCK, GIVE OXYGEN AND ARRANGE IMMEDIATE TRANSPORT.**

Cardiac arrest, of course, presents the most immediate threat to life. Cardiac arrest occurs when the heart stops beating entirely. If this happens, begin CPR immediately. (For more information on CPR, see Chapter 5, Basic Life Support: The ABC's.)

## EMERGENCIES INVOLVING THE CENTRAL NERVOUS SYSTEM

Recall from Chapter 2 that the brain is the controlling organ of the body; furthermore, certain areas of the brain control specific body functions, such as speech, respiration, and movement. The brain is also the organ most sensitive to lack of oxygen. Any interruption in the blood (and, therefore, oxygen) supply to the brain has potentially serious consequences.

Two emergencies involving the central nervous system are strokes and seizures. Each is discussed below.

### Stroke

Stroke, also called cerebrovascular accident or CVA, occurs when blood flow to a part of the brain is interrupted. When oxygen does not reach a specific area of the brain, the functions controlled by that area of the brain are damaged or destroyed. Consequently, the symptoms of stroke vary depending upon which area of the brain has been damaged. Speech, motor functions, and sensory functions are commonly affected.

The most frequent cause of stroke is a clot, or thrombus, that forms in one of the cerebral arteries (arteries in the brain). Cerebral arteries can be damaged by atherosclerosis just as coronary arteries can, and scarred, narrowed cerebral arteries are prone to develop clots. Other common causes of stroke are cerebral embolism and cerebral hemorrhage. Cerebral embolism occurs when a blood clot formed in another part of the body breaks loose, travels through the blood, and lodges in a cerebral artery. Cerebral hemorrhage occurs when a coronary artery ruptures, usually as a result of high blood pressure or a weakened blood vessel.

Strokes can be caused by high blood pressure (hypertension), atherosclerosis, AMI, or diabetes. Most stroke victims are over 50, but young women taking oral contraceptives and blacks with sickle cell disease sometimes have strokes because they are more susceptible to cerebral embolism.

Some patients experience transient ischemic attacks (TIAs or "little strokes") from which they recover completely within 12 hours. The symptoms of TIAs — weakness, paralysis, and speech disorders — are the same as those of strokes, but they are transient, lasting from a few seconds up to 12 hours. Between attacks the patient may feel normal. Many patients who have TIAs eventually suffer complete strokes.

The signs and symptoms of stroke or TIA are as follows:

- Weakness on one side of the body (hemiparesis)

- Paralysis on one side of the body (hemiplegia)
- Speech disturbances:
  — slurred speech
  — inability to speak
  — inability to understand speech
  — difficulty in naming objects
- Staggering gait or incoordination of fine motor movements
- Visual disturbances
- Headache
- Confusion
- Seizures
- Coma (in massive stroke)

The signs and symptoms of stroke vary with each patient. Some patients have very obvious signs of stroke, such as paralysis on one side of the body, and others have very subtle signs, such as confusion. Suspect stroke in any patient, particularly an elderly patient, who suddenly exhibits confusion, altered speech, or motor disturbances.

A stroke can be a terrifying experience for an alert patient, particularly if that person is suddenly unable to move or speak. Do not assume that a stroke patient cannot hear or understand just because he or she may not be able to speak. Indicate that you understand that the patient is going through a frightening experience. Explain each step of the evaluation and treatment and try to be as reassuring as possible. However, do not give false reassurance, such as, "Don't worry, everything will be all right."

As with any other emergency situation, assess the ABC's first. Check vital signs: it is likely that the patient has an elevated blood pressure. Elevated blood pressure and a slow pulse may be a sign of swelling in the brain. Check pulses on both sides of the patient's body; note whether they are equal. Ask the patient to smile and note whether one side of the face droops. Ask several simple questions: What is your name? Can you tell me what happened? Note slurred or garbled speech. Ask the patient to squeeze your hands; one side may be markedly weaker than the other or even paralyzed.

Treat a patient with suspected stroke by

- Providing reassurance; talk as though the patient understands you, even if he or she cannot speak.
- Place the patient lying down with the head and shoulders slightly raised to relieve pressure on the brain.
- Administer oxygen.
- Monitor vital signs.

If the patient is unable to speak, you will have to obtain the patient history from relatives. Be sure to ask about any other medical problems the patient may have and any medication he or she takes. Gather any medications and arrange to have them transported with the patient to the medical facility.

## Seizures

**NOTE:** The following information on seizures was adapted with permission from "Epilepsy: Breaking Down the Walls of Understanding," published by Abbott Laboratories, Abbott Park, Illinois.

The nervous system is essentially an electrical one, with impulses constantly shuttling between the billions of neurons (nerve cells) and the parts of the body involved in activities both voluntary (such as walking) and involuntary (such as breathing). If a person's brain, with its 12 billion nerve cells, is damaged, some of these nerve cells may malfunction. The damaged cells "overload" and give off too much electricity.

The result of this temporary overload is a seizure that causes a sudden loss or disturbance of consciousness, often in association with motor activity. Although some people may have a single seizure, people who have recurrent seizures are said to have epilepsy. Medication can completely control or greatly lessen the frequency of most seizures.

Anything that can injure the brain can cause epilepsy. The more common causes of cellular damage that may ultimately result in epilepsy are birth defects and injuries; head injuries from accidents; bacterial meningitis; toxic reactions to drugs or alcohol; brain tumors, clots, and infections; poor nutrition; chemical imbalance; and poor blood circulation, particularly in the elderly. As a result of automobile accidents alone, 540,000 Americans suffer head injuries each year. These head injuries will cause almost 20,000 people to develop persistent epileptic seizures.

The form, intensity, and duration of seizures are related to the number and type of brain cells affected. There are two broad types of seizures: generalized and partial. They range from convulsions to momentary lapses of attention.

When large areas of the brain are involved, the seizures are termed "generalized." Generalized seizures affect both consciousness and motor function from the outset of the seizure. When a smaller portion of the brain is affected, the seizures are called "partial." Partial seizures have specific effects depending on the part of the brain involved.

### PARTIAL SEIZURES

The most common partial seizure is what is now termed complex-partial and formerly was known as a temporal lobe or psychomotor seizure. The complex-partial seizure consists of three brief phases: first, the person stops ongoing activity and assumes a dazed or staring expression. Then the patient may begin a pattern of repetitious, automatic, purposeless behavior that lasts for one to two minutes. Such behavior may include lip smacking, picking at clothes, or buttoning and unbuttoning clothes. As the person returns to consciousness, a short period of disorientation and confusion occurs, sometimes followed by fear, anger, or hostility. Do not restrain someone who appears to be having a complex-partial seizure unless it is necessary for safety. Provide reassurance if the patient is temporarily disoriented. Advise the patient to see a physician.

### GENERALIZED SEIZURES

There are two major types of generalized seizures: absence and tonic-clonic. Absence seizures are especially prevalent in children 4 to 14 years old. Absence (pronounced abb-sáwnce) seizures were formerly known as petit mal seizures. The absence seizure is considerably milder in form than the tonic-clonic seizure, and in fact, often passes for daydreaming.

The absence seizure is most commonly characterized by a brief (7 to 10 seconds) lapse of consciousness with staring, eyeblinking, or upward rolling of the eyes. It is not uncommon for a child to have 50 to 100 absence seizures a day. This type of seizure is almost never a medical emergency.

The most common generalized seizure is the tonic-clonic seizure, formerly known as a grand mal seizure. About 80 percent of those with epilepsy experience tonic-clonic seizures.

A tonic-clonic seizure is characterized by a convulsion in which the person's body stiffens, arms flex, legs, head, and neck extend, and the jaws clamp shut; this is the "tonic" phase. The person falls to the ground, often uttering a hoarse cry, and temporarily loses consciousness for about two to five minutes. During this time, breathing appears difficult; the body jerks; saliva may accumulate in the mouth; and the bladder or bowels may empty. During this phase of the seizure, the person may turn quite blue due to lack of oxygen. Eventually, the jerking motions cease and the person regains consciousness, somewhat disoriented and fatigued from the intense muscular activity.

The tonic-clonic seizure is the type of seizure that is most likely to result in a call for emergency help. Because a person suffering a tonic-clonic seizure loses consciousness, he or she may suffer injury while falling or during violent muscle contractions. A tonic-clonic seizure can be frightening to watch; it is most important that the first responder maintain an air of professional calm and concern for the patient. The procedure for caring for a person experiencing a tonic-clonic seizure is as follows:

- If you or the person with epilepsy senses an impending seizure early enough, you may be able to help the person lie on the ground or floor.
- Do not try to restrain the person. The seizure must run its course; it cannot be stopped once it has begun.
- Clear the area; particularly, remove hard or dangerous objects so the person ex-

periencing the seizure will not be injured by them.

- If the person is wearing glasses, remove them. Loosen clothing in the neck and head area.
- Turn the person to the side to allow saliva to drain from the mouth.
- If the patient's jaws are not already clenched shut, place a bite stick or padded tongue blade between the back teeth to prevent tongue, lip, or cheek biting. Take care not to get bitten. DO NOT try to pry the patient's mouth open or place any hard object in the mouth or between the teeth if the patient's jaws are already clenched. Jamming an object into someone's mouth may damage the mouth or teeth.

As the seizure ends and muscle spasms cease, make sure the patient has an open airway. It is not uncommon for people to vomit after they have had seizures, so be alert for possible nausea. Provide suction if necessary to clear out vomitus, saliva, and blood. As the patient regains consciousness, he or she will probably be confused and sleepy (the period immediately following a seizure is known as the postictal state). The patient may complain of a headache. Provide reassurance and begin to obtain a history from the patient, family members, or bystanders. Attempt to learn the following information:

- Does the patient have a history of seizures? Does the patient take medication for seizures? Failure to take prescribed medication is a common cause of seizures. Some common anticonvulsant medications are Dilantin, Tegretol, Mysoline, and phenobarbital. If the patient does have medication, be sure to have it transported with the patient to the medical facility.
- What did the seizure look like? How long did the seizure last? It may be necessary to obtain this information from bystanders if you do not witness the seizure.
- Has the patient suffered head trauma recently or in the past? Head trauma is a major cause of seizures.
- Does the patient abuse alcohol or drugs? If so, when was the last time alcohol or drugs were used? Seizures often occur during withdrawal from alcohol and barbiturates.
- Does the patient have a history of diabetes, heart disease, or stroke? Each of these conditions can lead to seizures.

### STATUS EPILEPTICUS: A TRUE EMERGENCY

Most seizures are single occurrences, and the patient recovers spontaneously. However, sometimes a person has several seizures without regaining consciousness. This condition is known as status epilepticus, which is defined as two or more seizures without an intervening period of consciousness. Status epilepticus is a major emergency because the patient is in danger of death due to lack of oxygen. The best treatment the first responder can administer in the field is to try to maintain an open airway and to administer oxygen if possible. Administering oxygen is very difficult under these circumstances because of the patient's convulsive movements.

---

**A PERSON SUFFERING FROM STATUS EPILEPTICUS NEEDS ANTICONVULSANT MEDICATION ADMINISTERED INTRAVENOUSLY TO HALT THE SEIZURES. ARRANGE FOR TRANSPORT TO A MEDICAL FACILITY AS RAPIDLY AS POSSIBLE.**

---

### FEBRILE SEIZURES

Children, of course, may have seizures for the same reasons as adults. In addition, children are very sensitive to rapid rises in body temperature and are prone to develop seizures when they have fevers, known as febrile seizures. Febrile seizures are most often seen in children under the age of two. Almost all febrile seizures are generalized, tonic-clonic seizures, which are naturally quite frightening to the child's parents. If the seizure has already run its course by the time you arrive, evaluate the child's ABC's and provide reassurance to the parents. Obtain a history: Has the child had seizures before? If so, have they always been associated with a fever, or have they occurred at other times? Is the child taking any medications?

If the child is still having a seizure, provide the same care as for an adult having a tonic-clonic seizure. Place the child on the floor or on a bed away from other furniture to prevent injury. Do not try to restrain the child. Do not try to jam a bite block between the child's clenched teeth. After the seizure ends, place the child on his or her side, clear the airway, and administer oxygen. Remove the child's clothing and try to reduce the fever somewhat by sponging the child with lukewarm water. DO NOT use alcohol, ice water, or cold water because they can cause chills. Advise the parents that the child should be seen by a physician.

## DIABETIC EMERGENCIES

In addition to oxygen, the cells of the body need sugar in order to survive. However, the cells cannot absorb sugar (in the form of glucose) without insulin. Insulin is a hormone secreted by the pancreas, which lies behind the stomach. Insulin helps the body use glucose efficiently, converting food into energy and maintaining blood glucose levels.

Diabetes mellitus, also known as sugar diabetes, is a disease that occurs when the pancreas cannot secrete enough insulin to control blood glucose levels. Cases of diabetes range from mild to severe. Mild diabetes, in which the pancreas produces some insulin, can often be managed by diet and medication. Severe diabetes results when the pancreas stops producing insulin entirely. Individuals with severe diabetes must give themselves insulin injections once or twice a day.

The balance of sugar and insulin is a delicate one, however, and can be upset by illness, failing to take insulin, exercising too vigorously (which burns up sugar), or by forgetting to eat. If the body winds up with too much sugar and not enough insulin, the result is hyperglycemia, also known as diabetic ketoacidosis. If the body has too much insulin and too little sugar, the patient suffers from hypoglycemia, also known as insulin shock. Both conditions can lead to coma. Table 10.2 describes diabetic ketoacidosis and insulin shock.

### Diabetic Ketoacidosis (Hyperglycemia)

Diabetic ketoacidosis occurs when the blood sugar level becomes too high, usually because the patient forgot to take insulin or took too small a dose. Infection or stress can also lead to diabetic ketoacidosis. Ketoacidosis usually progresses slowly, over 12 to 48 hours. During that time, the

**TABLE 10.2**
**Signs and Symptoms of Diabetic Emergencies**

| Characteristics | Diabetic Ketoacidosis (High Blood Sugar) | Insulin Shock (Low Blood Sugar) |
|---|---|---|
| Insulin | Inadequate | Excessive |
| Onset | Gradual | Very sudden |
| Food intake | Excessive | Inadequate |
| Patient's appearance | Violently ill | Very weak |
| Skin | Red and dry | Pale and moist |
| Thirst | Intense | Absent |
| Hunger | Absent | Intense |
| Vomiting | Common | Uncommon |
| Abdominal pain | Common | Uncommon |
| Respirations | Deep, rapid breathing | Normal or shallow |
| Breath | Ketonic (fruity odor) | Normal |
| Blood Pressure | Low | Normal |
| Pulse | Rapid | Normal |

patient gradually becomes sicker and sicker, finally lapsing into coma. The signs and symptoms of diabetic ketoacidosis are as follows:

- Excessive urination (polyuria)
- Excessive thirst (polydipsia)
- Warm, dry skin and dry mucous membranes, reflecting dehydration
- Deep, rapid respirations
- Fruity odor on the breath (ketonic breath)
- Tachycardia (rapid heartbeat)

As blood sugar levels rise, chemical changes cause the patient to eliminate large amounts of sugar and water in the form of urine. This excessive urination is called polyuria and can lead to dehydration. Dehydration causes the patient to become extremely thirsty (polydipsia); it also causes the skin and mucous membranes to appear warm and dry.

Although there is plenty of sugar in the body, cells cannot use it without insulin, so the body turns to another source of fuel: fats. Breakdown of fats produces acid waste products in the blood (acidosis), which the body tries to eliminate through deep, rapid breathing, known as Kussmaul's breathing. Fat breakdown also produces ketones, which are eliminated in the breath and in urine. Ketones cause the patient's breath to have a characteristic fruity odor, like that of ripe apples. The combination of chemical changes in the body may cause the patient to suffer abdominal pains, nausea, or vomiting. Vomiting, of course, only serves to make the patient's dehydration worse.

### Insulin Shock (Hypoglycemia)

Insulin shock, or hypoglycemia, often occurs when a diabetic takes too much insulin, too little food, or both. In contrast to ketoacidosis, hypoglycemia develops very rapidly. The signs and symptoms of insulin shock are as follows:

- Weak, rapid pulse
- Cold, clammy, pale skin
- Weakness and incoordination
- Headache
- Irritable, nervous, or bizarre behavior; may appear drunk
- Seizures and coma in severe cases

Because the brain depends on a constant supply of oxygen and glucose to function properly, the patient with hypoglycemia experiences an altered level of consciousness. Headache, dizziness, and confusion are common. The patient may become very irritable and begin to display bizarre behavior, such as hostility or aggression. The hypoglycemic patient may even appear drunk: uncoordinated, staggering, and drooling. Continued lack of sugar results in convulsions, collapse, and coma.

### Care and Treatment for Diabetic Emergencies

The patient in diabetic ketoacidosis (hyperglycemia) needs large amounts of *fluids* administered intravenously. The patient in insulin shock (hypoglycemia) needs large amounts of *sugar* administered as rapidly as possible, either orally or intravenously. Of the two conditions, hypoglycemia is the more serious because the brain suffers irreversible damage if it is not kept supplied with sugar. If there is any doubt about the cause of the patient's condition, assume hypoglycemia.

If the patient is still conscious, the answers to three key questions will give good clues to the nature of the patient's condition. They are:

- Have you taken medication or insulin today? Note what medications or insulin the patient takes and the dosages: some common medications are Diabinese, DBI, Cymelor, Orinase, and Tolinase. If the patient takes insulin, ask what type of insulin and how many units he or she takes.
- Have you eaten according to your normal schedule today?
- What has your level of physical activity been today?

There is a good chance that the patient with diabetic ketoacidosis *will not* have taken insulin, but *will* have eaten. On the other hand, the patient with hypoglycemia probably *will* have taken insulin, but *will not* have eaten.

If the patient's answers and physical and mental condition suggest insulin shock, give fruit juice sweetened with sugar, candy, sugar cubes, or a soft drink (not the diet kind). When in doubt as to what to do, give sugar. A hyperglycemic patient will not be harmed by it (the amount administered is small compared to the amount already in the blood). The hypoglycemic patient, on the other hand, can be saved from brain damage or death by receiving sugar.

**HYPOGLYCEMIA IS A DIRE EMERGENCY. ARRANGE FOR TRANSPORTATION TO A MEDICAL FACILITY AS RAPIDLY AS POSSIBLE.**

If a diabetic patient is already unconscious, it will be very difficult to distinguish between hyperglycemia and hypoglycemia. Check the patient's ABC's and look for a Medic Alert tag. Talk to relatives or passersby who may be able to give a description of the patient's condition and behavior before he or she lost consciousness. **IF A DIABETIC PATIENT IS UNCONSCIOUS, ASSUME HYPOGLYCEMIA.** However, **DO NOT** try to give anything by mouth to a patient who is unconscious because it may wind up in the patient's lungs. Some diabetics carry liquid glucose in a tube. Smear a little of the glucose under the patient's tongue and inside the cheeks. There is little else you can do for the unconscious diabetic patient except to maintain the airway and monitor vital signs. Arrange for immediate transportation to a medical facility. Table 10.3 sums up the treatment for conscious and unconscious diabetic patients.

**TABLE 10.3**
**Treating Diabetic Emergencies**

| Conscious Patient | Unconscious Patient |
|---|---|
| ABC's<br>Give sugar<br>Monitor vital signs<br>Arrange for immediate transport to a medical facility | ABC's<br>Monitor vital signs<br>Arrange for immediate transport to a medical facility |

## ACUTE ABDOMINAL PAIN

There are many disorders that can cause abdominal pain. For the most part, it is neither feasible nor useful to distinguish among the many causes of abdominal pain because, in general, field management is similar regardless of the cause. However, you should have a general idea of the types of disorders that may be present with abdominal pain and should know which of these may progress to life-threatening situations.

As discussed in Chapter 2, the abdominal cavity is contained by the diaphragm above, the pelvis below, the spine in back, and the muscular abdominal wall in front. The entire cavity is lined by a smooth membranous layer called the peritoneum. The abdominal cavity contains the major organs of digestion, excretion, and, in the female, reproduction (Figure 10.6).

The organs of the gastrointestinal system can be the site of a number of acute conditions. These acute conditions commonly result when a person has ulcers, when an organ becomes inflamed due to disease or infection, or when a hollow organ is blocked by a stone.

The stomach is subject to inflammation (gastritis), which can cause severe pain and hemorrhage. The stomach and duodenum are also common sites for ulcers, which eat away a portion of the lining of an organ. If the ulcer perforates (eats through) the organ wall, digestive juices and enzymes spill into the abdominal cavity, causing peritonitis (inflammation of the lining of the abdominal cavity). Perforating ulcers can also cause massive internal bleeding. The pancreas produces powerful digestive enzymes, and if it is inflamed (pancreatitis), these enzymes can spill into the abdominal cavity, again causing peritonitis and severe pain. The gallbladder, which lies in the right upper quadrant, stores bile produced in the liver. Inflammation of the gallbladder (cholecystitis) or obstruction of the bile ducts by gallstones can result in an acute condition. Stones can also develop in the kidneys (renal stones), producing excruciating pain when they lodge in one of the ureters.

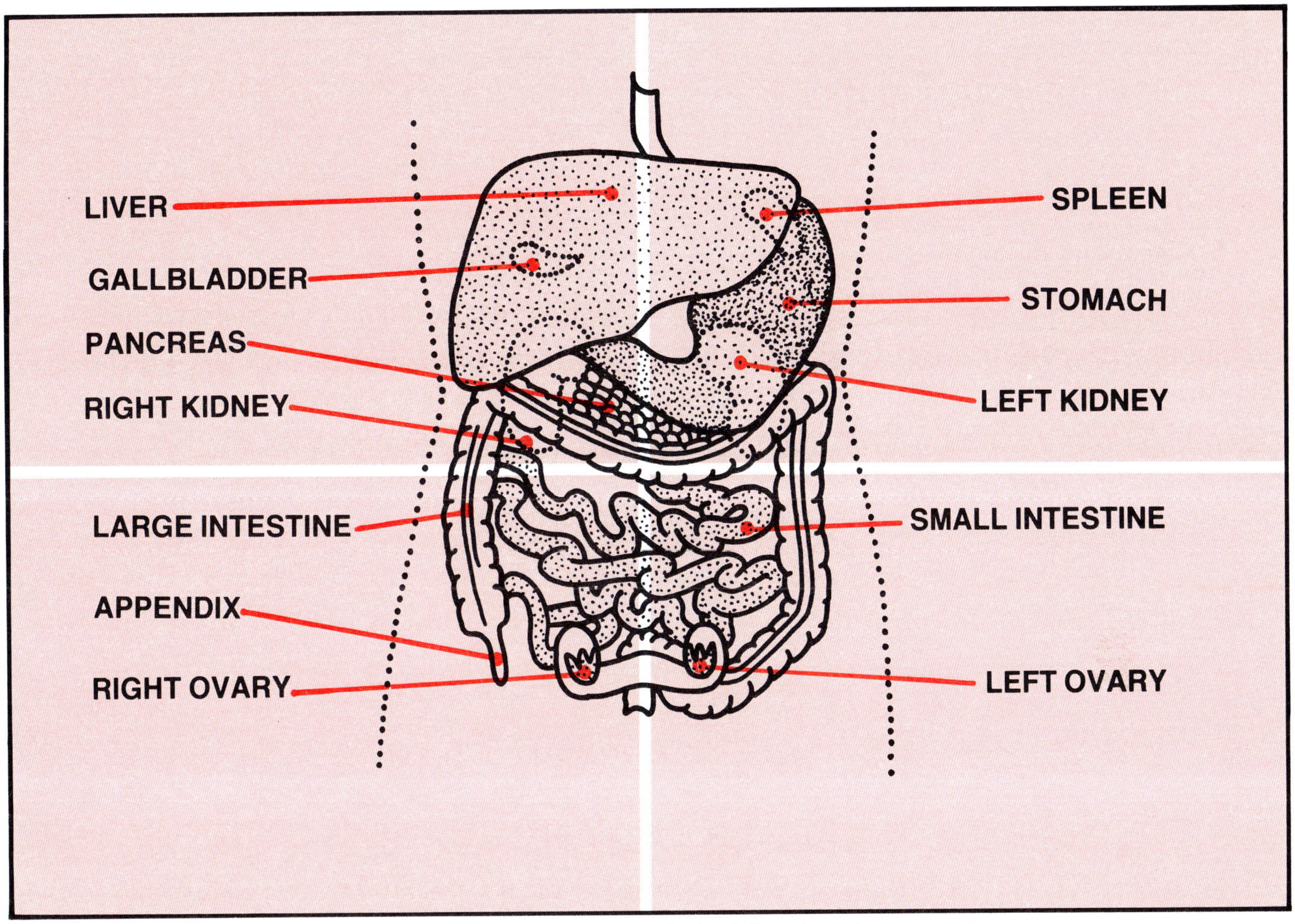


**Figure 10.6** Many organs in the abdominal cavity can become diseased, blocked, or inflamed, causing severe pain.

The large and small intestines occupy most of the abdominal cavity. Obstruction of any part of the bowels or inflammation of the colon (colitis) can cause severe pain. A small, wormlike appendage to the colon known as the appendix is susceptible to inflammation (appendicitis), which causes pain in the right lower quadrant. If an inflamed appendix ruptures, it can cause peritonitis.

The female reproductive organs are almost entirely internal. There are many conditions that can cause severe pain and/or bleeding. Some of these conditions are ectopic pregnancy (pregnancy outside the uterus), spontaneous abortion (miscarriage), pelvic inflammatory disease, and endometriosis. (For more information on ectopic pregnancy and spontaneous abortion, see Chapter 15 Emergency Childbirth.) In the urinary system, infection of the kidneys, bladder, ureters, or urethra can cause acute pain.

The most important symptom of the patient with an acute abdomen is PAIN. Try to determine the following:

- Location of the pain. Pain in the right upper quadrant, for example, suggests gallbladder or duodenal problems. Pain in the right lower quadrant often results from appendicitis.
- Radiation of the pain. Certain types of abdominal pain have typical areas of radiation. The pain of pancreatitis often radiates straight through the back, while the pain of an obstructed gallbladder may radiate around the right side to the shoulder blade. Ask if the pain has shifted since it began.
- Quality of the pain. Constant, severe pain suggests inflammation, while cramping pain often results from obstruction of a hollow organ.

- Duration of the pain. When did the pain begin? How long has it lasted? Has the patient been treated for abdominal problems, such as an ulcer, before?
- Intensity of the pain.

Besides gathering as much information as possible about the patient's pain, ask if the patient has vomited or passed bloody stools. Ask what the vomit looked like. Was it bloody? If the patient has had bowel movements, what color were they? These questions are important because a patient who is vomiting or passing blood may be bleeding internally.

When you are conducting the primary survey and taking vital signs, pay special attention to signs of impending shock: altered level of consciousness; pale, cold, clammy skin; increased heartbeat and respirations; falling blood pressure.

Do not poke at the patient's abdomen! All this does is cause the patient unnecessary pain. Touch the abdomen very gently to determine whether it is rigid or soft. Note if the abdomen seems distended.

Move the patient as little as possible. Allow the patient to lie in the position of greatest comfort. If he or she is nauseated, lying on the side is best. Be alert for vomiting. Administer oxygen and arrange for rapid transport to a medical facility.

# 11

# Behavioral Emergencies

**U.S. DEPARTMENT OF TRANSPORTATION**
**First Responder Training Course**

**Objectives:**

- Given descriptions of patients suffering from ingested poisons, inhaled poisons, bites and stings, alcohol abuse and drugs, identify the condition and describe appropriate emergency care.

**NOTE:** These objectives are covered in this chapter and in Chapter 12.

# Chapter 11
# Behavioral Emergencies

A behavioral emergency is a situation in which an individual's behavior threatens his or her own physical or psychological well being or that of others. Such behavior may be the result of a multitude of contributing factors, including diabetes, epilepsy, hypertension, drug or alcohol abuse, mental disorders, or personal injury. At the scene of an accident involving injuries, the victims and even bystanders may exhibit behavior inappropriate for the circumstances (Figure 11.1). Everyone reacts differently in emergency situations: remember that the behavior you encounter in these situations reflects an attempt to reduce anxiety. Recognizing that behavioral disturbances indicate high levels of anxiety is an essential first step in learning to deal competently and humanely with people in crisis.

While many of the behavioral problems you encounter as a first responder are temporary measures for handling stress, some may be manifestations of mental illness. Patients may exhibit depression, suicidal behavior, violent behavior, phobic behavior, or drug-induced behavior. The extreme behavior associated with each of these conditions reflects the patient's attempt to master some stress, whether internal or external, real or imagined. The stress may, in fact, be the result of any combination of these factors. As a first responder, the treatment you administer in a behavioral emergency is aimed at calming and reassuring the patient and identifying the event or events that precipitated the emergency.

When dealing with people who are in psychological crisis, remember that your own safety comes first. In many, if not most, cases involving disturbed patients, police assistance will be required. If the call for emergency assistance is dispatched as a suicidal, violent, or armed person, call for police assistance and allow the police to secure the scene before you enter. Furthermore, the police have the legal authority to search, disarm, or subdue patients who become violent. Follow the protocols for dealing with disturbed patients in your local jurisdiction.

The physical setting in which you find a patient may not reinforce your calming attitude and presence. When possible, manipulate the surroundings to create an atmosphere that is soothing to the patient and conducive to private conversation. Disperse bystanders and protect the patient from the sight of onlookers as you examine the pa-

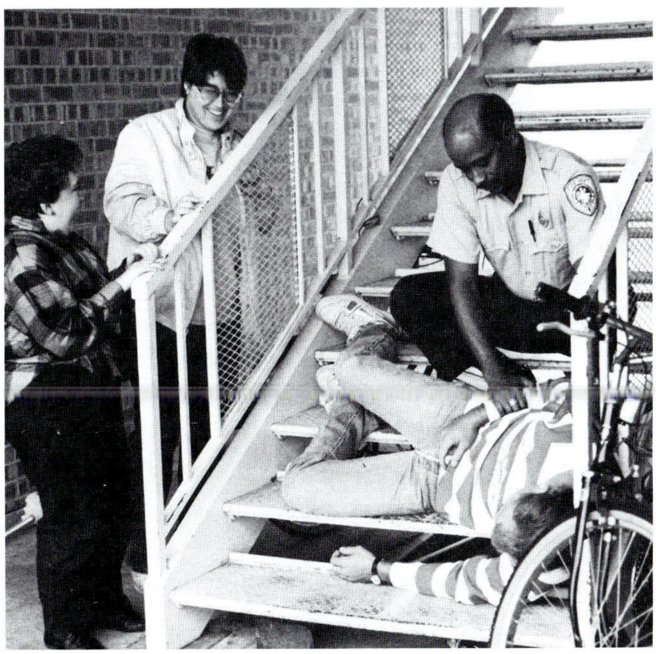

**Figure 11.1** At the scene of an accident, bystanders may behave inappropriately, for example, laughing or making jokes. Remember that these behaviors reflect an attempt to reduce anxiety.

tient. Show respect and compassion also for family and friends who may be at the scene. Assure them that you are doing all that can be done in the patient's best interests. If the words or actions of distraught family or friends seem to upset the patient, ask them to wait elsewhere until additional help arrives.

Your own behavior and manner of speaking are key factors in soothing a disturbed patient. Learn the patient's name and use it as you talk with him or her. Give the appearance of being calm and make every effort to control your own anxiety. Giving a calm appearance requires also that you be prepared to spend time with the situation. Any attempt, however subtle, to hurry the patient will more than likely heighten his or her anxiety and confusion.

The general principles for handling behavioral emergencies involve *establishing a rapport* with the disturbed patient and *encouraging the patient to talk* about his or her feelings. Place yourself at the patient's level so that you can maintain eye-to-eye contact. Do not use a patronizing tone of voice. If the patient wishes to speak only with a certain person, say a man, allow the patient to do so. Ask the patient what has contributed to the immediate emergency. Listen carefully and try to deduce the message he or she means to convey. In general, it is best not to try to direct the conversation, but articulating or rephrasing what you perceive as the cause of the patient's anxiety is often enlightening for both you and the patient. If the patient agrees with your evaluation of the situation, that information can be very helpful to those who will ultimately assume care for the patient; your grasp of the patient's dilemma may also be comforting to the patient as an indication that the situation is not hopeless. You may, in fact, articulate a problem that the patient has been unable to express, thereby relieving his or her anxiety significantly. Be honest and reassuring. In cases involving seriously disturbed patients, you can do little more than calm and reassure them and encourage them to talk until additional help arrives.

## DEPRESSION

Depression is probably the most common behavioral disturbance you will encounter as a first responder, but because it manifests itself in so many ways, you may initially mistake depression for another behavioral disturbance. Patients suffering from depression exhibit a variety of symptoms, including a very sad or listless appearance, crying spells, extreme pessimism, withdrawal, agitation, sleeplessness, and loss of appetite. Severely depressed patients express feelings of utter worthlessness or guilt, thus suicidal behavior frequently arises from cases of severe depression. Fifteen percent of patients diagnosed as clinically depressed eventually commit suicide, and depressive illness is associated with approximately fifty percent of all suicides. When dealing with depressed patients, be alert to the possibility of self-destructive impulses. NEVER leave a depressed patient unattended, not even for a very short time. Encourage the patient to talk about his or her feelings and try to identify what has precipitated the immediate emergency (Figure 11.2). Depressed patients are often withdrawn and reluctant to talk. In cases of severe depression, the patient may even be physically immobilized, incapable of movement or speech. You may find it helpful to present the patient with a simple observation, such as "You look very sad." This sympathetic overture may prompt the patient to discuss his or her feelings and circumstances. If not, maintain a

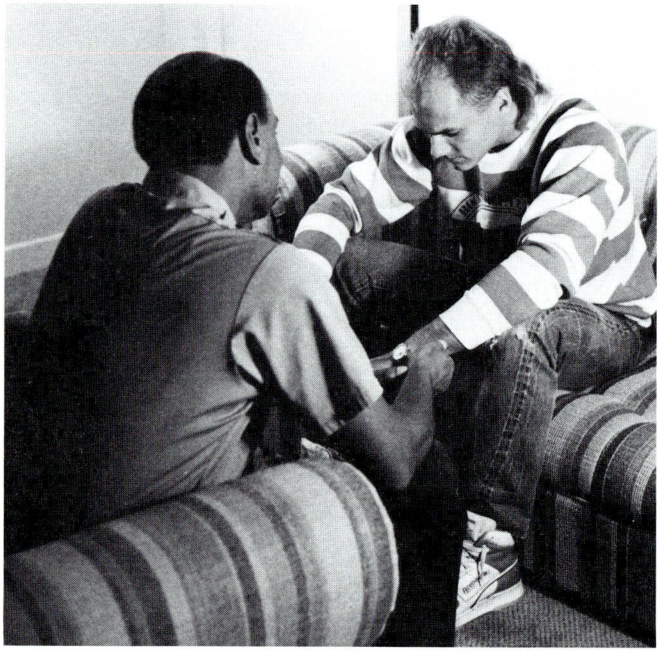

**Figure 11.2** The patient who is depressed is likely to be withdrawn. Display a sympathetic manner and encourage the patient to talk about his or her feelings.

reassuring and sympathetic attitude and continue to speak calmly whether or not the patient responds. DO NOT assume that the patient cannot hear you or that he or she is silent merely to thwart you. Keep talking and assess the patient's physical condition if he or she will allow you to do so.

Be sympathetic and understanding as patients describe their feelings and the events that have contributed to their distress, but not so sympathetic that you confirm their appraisal of the situation as hopeless. It is not unusual, of course, for depressed people to cry as they relate their circumstances; sit quietly and wait for the crying spell to pass. Expressing emotion is often therapeutic; patients usually can express themselves more easily after they have released their intense emotions. Resist the temptation to soothe these patients and to avoid what seem to be painful topics. Similarly, do not rush to finish patients sentences for them or to fill in silences. Silences and hesitations give the patient time to think.

## SUICIDAL BEHAVIOR

Suicide is an increasingly serious public health problem in the United States. In 1980 almost 27,000 people took their own lives, making suicide the tenth leading cause of death for people of all ages and the third leading cause of death for those 15 to 34 years of age. During the 11-year period from 1970 to 1980, there were 287,322 suicides in the United States, a figure representing about one suicide every 20 minutes.

While depressive illness is associated with many suicides, there are many cases in which a clear connection between the two does not exist. Suicidal behavior is linked also to violent, phobic, and addictive behavior. Suicidal individuals often report feelings of worthlessness and hopelessness, generally resulting from the loss of a loved one, whether through death or separation.

Many investigations of suicide incidents, both lethal and nonlethal, reveal conflicting feelings about life and death in suicidal individuals. In many instances, these individuals act upon their self-destructive impulses but provide for the possibility of rescue. This typically arouses feelings of hostility in rescue workers, who see such attempts as manipulative and calculated false alarms. The element of indecisiveness (ambivalence) in a suicidal individual, however, allows for successful intervention and long-range treatment aimed at averting a later attempt.

When you are called to intervene in a suicide incident, make provisions first for your own safety and that of others at the scene. A suicidal individual with a weapon must be considered potentially homicidal as well. Let the police handle the job of disarming the patient: they are trained in such procedures and you are not.

If the patient is locked into a room or building, identify yourself, explain why you are there, and ask to be let in. If the patient will not let you enter, contact the police. The patient may be armed, so do not endanger yourself unnecessarily.

As you talk with the patient, keep your voice low and calm, and make sure you keep your language at his or her level. The suicidal individual is likely to be extremely anxious or agitated, and your initial task is to alleviate the patient's anxiety as much as possible.

Successful intervention depends upon the relationship you establish with the patient, and that relationship ideally should be one of mutual trust. Remember that the potential suicide victim feels alienated and worthless and respond with the concern and attention the patient lacks (Figure 11.3).

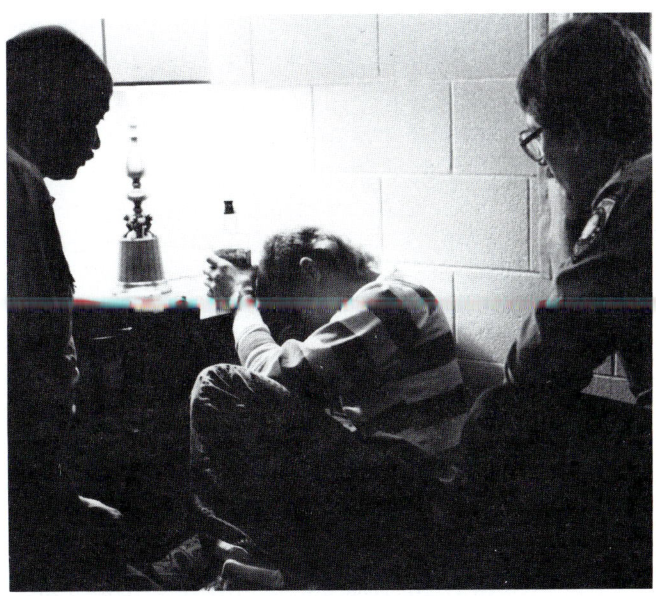

**Figure 11.3** Any suicide threat must be taken seriously. Speak to the patient in a low, calm voice and do not leave the patient alone.

Whether or not you believe the patient actually intends to commit suicide, the patient must feel that you take the threat very seriously. An individual threatening suicide is in a very precarious frame of mind and may very well carry out the threat if no one seems to appreciate its urgency.

Once you have established a viable relationship with the patient, encourage him or her to discuss the problems that have culminated in the immediate emergency. Be understanding and sympathetic, but not so sympathetic that you intensify the patient's distress. Listen quietly to whatever the patient says. It may be helpful to use noncommital words or phrases such as "Go on" or "I see." You may even say "I can understand why you're upset" if you really *can* understand, but avoid trite and empty remarks such as "I think you're being a little too hard on yourself" or "Everything is going to be all right."

A suicidal patient may take his or her own life despite your best efforts. Not all suicidal individuals are ambivalent about life and death: in some cases, the desire to die may be overwhelming. Anyone who sincerely and fervently wishes to die will find a way to do so. Under these unfortunate circumstances, you can do little or more than turn your attention to family members or friends who may be at the scene and in need of help.

If you are called to care for someone who has attempted suicide, your primary obligation is to provide basic life support. Drug overdoses must be treated for respiratory or circulatory distress. Patients with slashed wrists or other soft-tissue injuries require bleeding control. If the patient is conscious, encourage him or her to talk; never belittle or scold a patient who has unsuccessfully attempted to commit suicide. Your own behavior and management of the situation may contribute significantly to the patient's emotional recovery and avert later suicide attempts.

## VIOLENT BEHAVIOR

If the emergency is called in as a violent person, arrive with the police. When you arrive, disperse onlookers and friends or family at the scene to protect them from injury.

Competent, humane management of belligerent patients depends upon your appreciation of the fact that violent, angry behavior typically masks feelings of extreme frustration and helplessness. It is very difficult not to respond to violence in kind, but you must avoid the temptation to bait or threaten violent patients.

Because hostile patients are often frightened by their loss of control, many respond well to situations in which limits, or controls, are set. This is accomplished primarily through your own attitude and behavior. Be calm and firm and make it clear that you expect the patient to control his or her temper. Explain that you are there to help rather than punish the patient, and encourage him or her to talk about the cause of the angry display.

If the patient is unmanageable, **NEVER** attempt to restrain him or her without the authorization and help of the police (Figure 11.4). If the situation requires that the patient be overpowered and restrained, it is best to enlist the help of two or three other people so that the struggle is brief and one-sided. Not only is this technique the safest for those who must do the restraining, but it also protects the patient's ego. The patient is already suffering with the knowledge that he or she has lost control, and to be so outnumbered psychologically justifies the patient's "defeat."

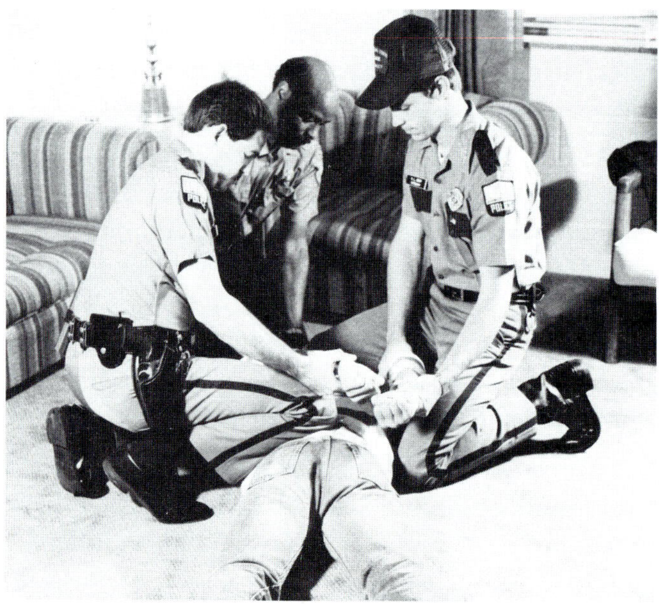

**Figure 11.4** Patients under the influence of drugs or who are under severe emotional stress may become violent. When it becomes necessary to restrain someone, do so with the help of police officers.

In some patients, violent behavior may be caused by paranoia, a psychotic condition characterized by excessive and irrational suspicion or distrust of others. Many paranoid patients are excitable and unpredictable and may have outbursts of bizarre or aggressive behavior. Treat paranoid patients as you would other violent patients. The paranoid individual will most likely be suspicious of warmth and reassurance, so maintain a friendly but somewhat distant neutrality. Do not reinforce a paranoid's delusions in an attempt to placate him or her, as this may agitate the patient even further. Remember, too, that the patient's behavior can change at a moment's notice.

## PHOBIC BEHAVIOR

A phobia is an extreme, disabling fear of a particular object, animal, or situation. Appropriately, phobic behavior is characterized by intense anxiety. Phobic individuals become highly agitated when faced with the object of their fear, and may suffer rapid or irregular heartbeat and respiration, excessive sweating, abdominal distress, and even overwhelming feelings of impending death.

A common syndrome associated with phobic behavior is caused by **hyperventilation**. Patients who are prone to hyperventilation may have a history of other symptoms that are characteristic of anxiety, such as

- Fatigue
- Nervousness
- Dizziness
- Tingling or numbness around the mouth and in the hands and feet

On physical examination, these patients show rapid respirations *(tachypnea)* and sometimes unusually deep respirations *(hyperpnea)*. These patients may also show **carpopedal spasm** — the contortion in a flexed position of the hands and feet. Patients who are predisposed to seizures are especially likely to experience them during a hyperventilation episode. Hyperventilation results in carbon dioxide depletion in the body, which can, in turn, lead to serious complications.

Your primary responsibility to phobic patients consists of protecting them from the sight of onlookers. The high anxiety associated with phobias is due in part to the fear of fainting, for example, or doing something otherwise embarrassing in public. While it is impossible to explain away the terror phobic patients experience when confronted with the object of their fear, some patients may take comfort in knowing that their phobias may subside or disappear with treatment. There are a number of effective treatment programs available through therapists and clinics that allow those with phobic conditions to overcome their fears.

Once you have dispersed bystanders or otherwise secluded yourself with the patient, assure him or her that the phobia can be treated. Be very calm and reassuring and carefully explain every step involved in the treatment you administer. If the patient is hyperventilating, for example, have him or her breathe in and out of a paper bag or similar device that will cover the nose and mouth. This causes the patient to rebreathe carbon dioxide, thus restoring the carbon dioxide level to normal. Explain to the patient the reasoning behind this treatment — your explanations and calm attitude should lessen the patient's anxiety considerably.

## ALCOHOL AND DRUG ABUSE

Alcohol and drug intoxication or overdose may induce depression, suicidal behavior, violent behavior, or phobic behavior. The specific behavior associated with drug or alcohol abuse varies from individual to individual and in accordance with the substances involved. While stimulants, depressants, and hallucinogens typically induce certain specific altered states of consciousness in users, each type of drug may be taken in combination with one or more types, thereby producing unusual behavioral and physical symptoms. Treat the behavioral symptoms of intoxicated individuals as you would those of any other patient and be alert to the possibility of physical complications. ALWAYS arrange to transport intoxicated patients to the nearest medical facility since a drug-or alcohol-induced state may mask underlying medical problems that cannot be detected in the field. The physical disorders associated with alcoholism and other forms of drug abuse can be life-threatening, so it is important to know the signs, symptoms, and treatment for intoxicated patients.

## Alcohol Abuse

Alcoholism is a major health problem in the United States today. The disease has no regard for gender, age, or social class: the "skid row bum" accounts for only a small percentage of alcoholics in this country. An estimated 6 to 10 million Americans are alcoholics, and alcohol is directly involved in 30,000 deaths and 50,000 injuries in automobile accidents annually. Because of its harmful effects on the liver, stomach, pancreas, and central nervous system, alcoholism decreases each alcoholic's life span by 10 to 20 years.

Not everyone who drinks is an alcoholic, and the signs and symptoms of uncomplicated intoxication are well known:

- Silly, giggling behavior
- Talkativeness
- Slurred speech
- Odor of alcohol on the breath

> **NOTE:** The odor of alcohol on a patient's breath does NOT indicate conclusively that his or her condition is due to alcoholic intoxication.

In cases involving severe intoxication the patient may also exhibit

- Agitated, aggressive behavior
- Mental confusion
- Extreme drowsiness
- Respiratory depression
- Loss of protective reflexes
- Coma

The alcoholic syndrome is thought to consist of two phases: problem drinking and addiction. During the first phase, the victim uses alcohol to relieve tension and to alleviate emotional distress. As the disease progresses, the victim becomes physically dependent upon alcohol and enters the second phase. In this phase, *not* drinking produces major withdrawal symptoms, such as tremors, hallucinations, seizures, and delirium tremens.

Delirium tremens is a severe, potentially fatal syndrome characterized by confusion, tremor, wakefulness, hallucinations, fever, and sweating. Hypovolemic shock is also associated with delirium tremens, and may result in cardiovascular collapse, and finally death (see Chapter 6, Shock).

Alcoholic withdrawal symptoms may last several days in the chronic alcoholic. As the victim "sobers up," he or she may complain of irritability, headache, nausea and vomiting, slowed thought, a fine tremor, and a rapid, irregular heartbeat. Hallucinations usually occur within the first 24 hours of withdrawal; withdrawal seizures may occur 12 to 48 hours after the last drink. Delirium tremens usually occurs 24 to 72 hours after the patient's last drink, but may occur up to 7 to 10 days later.

Fluid losses are likely to be high during delirium tremens. Because of increased activity, fever, and sweating, the patient may become dehydrated. Hypoglycemia and electrolyte imbalances may also complicate the patient's condition. Patients with high fevers are more likely to die from delirium tremens, which is fatal in about 15 percent of cases.

### EMERGENCY MANAGEMENT OF ALCOHOLIC WITHDRAWAL SYNDROME

Suspect delirium tremens in any patient with delirium of an unknown cause, and learn from the patient or from family members or bystanders about the patient's alcohol history. Field treatment of patients experiencing alcohol withdrawal symptoms is aimed mainly at providing basic life support and emotional reassurance. Treat alcoholic seizures, coma, and shock as you would the same symptoms in any other patient. Arrange for transportation to the nearest medical facility and be alert to the possibility of serious physical complications.

## Drug Abuse

Most drug-related calls involve overdoses, although some may involve an adverse reaction to a moderate dose, or intoxication involving a variety of drugs. Many drug users take combinations of drug types in an attempt to counteract the undesirable effects of certain drugs. This practice typically heightens the overall effect of the drugs, but often results in life-threatening physical and behavioral symptoms. Emergency intervention is more likely to be effective in cases of drugs that are taken orally because these drugs remain in the stomach for a short time before being absorbed into the bloodstream. Injected or inhaled drugs, on the other hand, are absorbed and take effect almost immediately.

Unless you are familiar with the street names for popular local drugs or have a sample of the substance(s) involved, it will be very difficult to determine exactly what the patient has taken. Table 11.1 (p. 236) lists commonly abused drugs and their street names. The street names for drugs vary locally; become familiar with those in your area.

When called to handle a situation involving drug abuse or overdose, try to learn from the patient or from bystanders

- Exactly *what* was taken
- *When* it was taken
- *How much* of it was taken
- Whether *anything else* was taken

As soon as you have gathered this essential information, call the nearest Poison Control Center or medical facility and follow the instructions you are given. If the victim is unconscious and there are no bystanders to give you information, take the time to search the patient's person and surroundings (do this in front of witnesses) before calling the Poison Control Center. If you find no clues to help identify what the patient has taken, you will probably be instructed to provide basic life support and to arrange for transportation to the nearest medical facility IMMEDIATELY. As always, pay particular attention to maintaining an open airway and be prepared to assist respirations or to perform CPR.

If you can identify the substance(s) involved, and if the patient is conscious and not convulsing, the Poison Control Center may instruct you to induce vomiting with syrup of ipecac. Ipecac is an emetic (a substance that induces vomiting). Naturally, you should follow guidelines in your area that state whether or not first responders are allowed to give this substance. Guidelines for giving ipecac are found in Chapter 12, Poisons.

Certain types of drugs, particularly stimulants and hallucinogens, may cause patients to become extremely agitated, combative, or violent. If the patient is hallucinating or suffering from a "bad trip," speak soothingly and try to reduce his or her apprehension. Some patients may become violent, attempting to harm themselves or others. These patients can be extremely difficult to subdue; call for police assistance immediately.

## TABLE 11.1 COMMONLY ABUSED DRUGS

| DRUGS | TRADE OR STREET NAMES | METHODS OF INGESTION: ORAL | INJECTED | SMOKED | SNIFFED | INHALED | COMMON EFFECTS | EFFECTS OF OVERDOSE |
|---|---|---|---|---|---|---|---|---|
| **NARCOTICS** | | | | | | | | |
| Morphine | Morphine, M, Junk, Pectoral Syrup | ✓ | ✓ | ✓ | | | Euphoria, drowsiness, constricted pupils, nausea, slow pulse, slow respirations, slurred speech | Shallow or absent respirations; cool, clammy skin; constricted pupils; cyanosis; decreased heart rate and blood pressure; seizures; possible death |
| Codeine | Robitussin A-C, Empirin with Codeine, Tylenol with Codeine | ✓ | ✓ | | | | | |
| Oxycodone | Percocet, Percodan, Tylox | ✓ | ✓ | | | | | |
| Heroin | Horse, Smack, Joy Powder | | ✓ | ✓ | ✓ | ✓ | | |
| Meperidine | Demerol, Mepergan | ✓ | ✓ | | | | | |
| Others | Darvon, Talwin, Tussionex | ✓ | ✓ | | | | | |
| **DEPRESSANTS** | | | | | | | | |
| Barbiturates | Phenobarbital, Nembutal, Amytal, Seconal, (Yellow Jackets, Downers, Goofballs, Reds, Blue Devils, Barbs) | ✓ | ✓ | | | | Slurred speech, drowsiness, drunken behavior without odor of alcohol, lowered respirations, heart rate, and blood pressure | Shallow to absent respirations; cool, clammy skin; dilated pupils; weak rapid pulse; coma; possible death |
| Benzodiazapines | Diazepam, Valium, Librium, Xanax, Serax, Tranxene, Restoril, Dalmane, Ativan | ✓ | ✓ | | | | | |
| Methaqualone | Quaalude, Parest (Ludes, Soapers) | ✓ | ✓ | | | | | |
| Chloral Hydrate | Noctec, Somnos (Knockout Drops) | ✓ | | | | | | |
| Others | Doriden, Miltown, Equanil | ✓ | ✓ | | | | | |
| **STIMULANTS** | | | | | | | | |
| Cocaine | Coke, Flake, Snow, Crack, Rock, Crystal | | ✓ | ✓ | ✓ | | Increased alertness, excitability, agitation, insomnia, loss of appetite, increased heart rate and blood pressure | Combativeness, increase in body temperature, hallucinations, increase in heart rate and blood pressure, seizures, possible death |
| Amphetamines | Dexedrine, Benzedrine (Bennies, Uppers, Speed, Crystal) | ✓ | ✓ | | | | | |
| Others | Preludin, Sanorex, Tenuate | ✓ | ✓ | | | | | |
| **HALLUCINOGENS** | | | | | | | | |
| LSD | Acid, Cubes, Sugar, Microdot | ✓ | | | | | Illusions and hallucinations, altered perception of time and distance, "faraway" appearance, increased heart rate and blood pressure | Longer, more intense "trip" episodes; possible violent behavior; psychosis, seizures, increase in pulse and blood pressure; possible death |
| Mescaline and Peyote | Mesc, Buttons, Cactus | ✓ | | | | | | |
| Amphetamine Variants | STP, MDA, TMA | ✓ | ✓ | | | | | |
| Phencyclidine | PCP, Angel Dust, Hog | ✓ | ✓ | ✓ | | | | |
| Others | Jimson Weed, Psilocyloin, DMT | ✓ | ✓ | ✓ | ✓ | | | |
| **CANNABIS** | | | | | | | | |
| Marijuana | Pot, Grass, Acapulco Gold, Thai Stick, Reefer | ✓ | | ✓ | | | | |
| Hashish | Hash | ✓ | | ✓ | | | | |
| Hashish Oil | Hash Oil | ✓ | | ✓ | | | | |
| Tetrahydrocannabinol | THC | ✓ | | ✓ | | | | |
| **INHALANTS** | | | | | | | | |
| Gases | Nitrous Oxide, Fluorocarbon | | | | | ✓ | Euphoria, slurred speech, light-headedness, incoordination, increased heart rate and blood pressure | Slow/shallow to absent respirations, dilated pupils, seizures, vomiting, coma, possible death |
| Volatile Liquids and Other Substances | Plastic Model Glue, Gasoline, Spray Paint, Paint Thinner, Typewriter Correcting Fluid | | | | | | | |
| **ANTIDEPRESSANTS** | | | | | | | | |
| Tricyclics | Elavil, Parnate, Adapin, Sinequan, Triavil, Vivactil | ✓ | ✓ | | | | General sedative effects, dry mouth, slight increase in heart rate | Rapid, irregular heart rate; hallucinations; lethargy; vomiting; dilated pupils; possible death |

# 12

# Poisons

**U.S. DEPARTMENT OF TRANSPORTATION**
**First Responder Training Course**

**Objectives:**

- Given descriptions of patients suffering from ingested poisons, inhaled poisons, bites and stings, alcohol abuse and drugs, identify the condition and describe appropriate emergency care.

# Chapter 12
# Poisons

A poison is any substance that can cause illness or death when consumed or absorbed by the body. Poisons interfere chemically with body cells by exciting or depressing their functions, or by destroying them altogether. Between 3 and 5 million poisonings occur each year, both accidental and intentional, resulting in well over 9,000 deaths. Poisoning may occur through ingestion, inhalation, injection, or absorption through the skin, eyes, or mucous membranes.

The most common type of poisoning occurs by ingestion, that is, the poison is taken by mouth and swallowed. Ninety percent of all poisonings involve children because of their natural curiosity and their tendency to ingest whatever is at hand. Everyday household materials, especially cleaning agents, prescription and nonprescription medications, insecticides, plants, and cosmetics pose a significant threat to young children. Drug ingestions in self-destructive or suicidal individuals are also examples of this type of poisoning.

Exhaust from combustion engines, gas appliances, and insecticides are common sources of poisoning by inhalation. Many people have been fatally poisoned by inhaling the combined vapors of household ammonia and chlorine bleach.

Injected poisons are introduced into the body tissues or bloodstream by agents such as insects, snakes, or animals. Accidental needle sticks and intentional injections by drug abusers are also cases of this type of poisoning.

Absorbed poisons enter the body directly through the skin or through wounds, through the eyes, and through mucous membranes. Household cleaners and insecticides are the most common materials that cause poisoning by absorption. Certain plants (such as poison ivy, poison oak, and poison sumac) may also irritate, redden, or blister the skin.

Victims of poisoning often exhibit extremely serious symptoms that present themselves very suddenly. Recognizing these symptoms and administering prompt emergency care can save the victim's life. The symptoms of poisoning vary according to the nature of the toxin and the manner in which it enters and acts upon the body. Other variables include the amount of poison involved, the time elapsed since the poison entered the body, and the size and physical condition of the victim. In general, you should suspect poisoning when an unexplained or sudden acute illness occurs, especially if the illness is characterized by gastrointestinal distress or central nervous system disorders.

## POISON CONTROL CENTERS

Poison Control Centers are located throughout the United States to provide technical assistance in cases of poisoning. These centers maintain extensive files on drugs and other potentially harmful substances, and provide emergency information on diagnosis and treatment 24 hours a day.

**IF YOU SUSPECT POISONING, CONTACT THE NEAREST POISON CONTROL CENTER.**

Poison Control Centers are often located in a local hospital. Always keep the telephone number for your regional or local Poison Control Center readily available. Naturally, the Poison Control Center can advise you more efficiently if you know the poison and the approximate quantity involved. When possible, gather information from the victim, bystanders, or evidence at the scene before calling the center.

## INGESTED POISONS

Victims of poison ingestion may exhibit a variety of symptoms, including

- Nausea and/or vomiting
- Diarrhea
- Drowsiness or unconsciousness
- Cramps or severe abdominal pain
- Abnormal breathing
- Abnormal or irregular pulse rate
- Convulsions
- Burns or stains around the victim's mouth
- Unusual breath odors or odors on the victim's clothing
- Sweating
- Dilated or constricted pupils
- Excessive salivation or foaming at the mouth

If you suspect poison ingestion, look around for a possible source, and if you find a container, be sure to have it transported with the victim to a medical facility. The labels of many containers for toxic or potentially harmful substances can be invaluable to medical personnel in diagnosing and treating the victim once he or she arrives at the emergency room. If the victim has vomited, be sure to take a sample of the vomitus as well. Try to learn either from the victim or bystanders:

- What was ingested?
- When was it ingested?
- How much was ingested?

Keep in mind that more than one substance may have been ingested. Keep in mind also that ingested poisons usually remain in the stomach for only a brief time before they are absorbed into the bloodstream, so emergency care must begin immediately.

### Emergency Treatment for Poison Ingestion

First, try to identify the substance the victim ingested. For emergency purposes there are only two classes of substances to consider:

- Those designed to be taken by mouth (such as medicines or other drugs)
- Those not intended to be taken by mouth (such as household cleaning agents, plants, and chemicals)

If the ingested substance *is* intended to be swallowed, call the Poison Control Center or nearest medical facility IMMEDIATELY and follow the instructions you are given over the telephone.

If the ingested substance *is not* intended to be swallowed, give the victim one or two glasses of milk or water to dilute the poison, *then* call the Poison Control Center or nearest medical facility and follow the instructions you are given over the telephone.

**WARNING: NEVER GIVE ANYTHING BY MOUTH TO ANYONE WHO IS UNCONSCIOUS, CONVULSING, OR HAVING DIFFICULTY SWALLOWING.** If the victim cannot swallow properly, anything given by mouth may wind up in the victim's lungs.

If the victim is conscious and not convulsing, the Poison Control Center or hospital may instruct you to induce vomiting with syrup of ipecac. Syrup of ipecac is an emetic (a substance that induces vomiting) available without prescription in one-ounce bottles. Parents or grandparents of small children should always have a bottle of ipecac on hand for each child or grandchild in the house.

Give one to two teaspoons (4 mL to 8 mL) of syrup of ipecac if the victim is under a year old. For children over a year old and adults, give three teaspoons (12 mL). The appropriate dose causes vomiting within 30 minutes in most cases; the average time is usually 20 minutes or less. Syrup of ipecac works best when the dose is followed immediately by one or two glasses of water. If the victim is a very young or frightened child, you may be more successful giving the water before you give the ipecac.

If vomiting does not occur in 20 minutes, repeat the dose once. If the victim does not vomit within 30 more minutes, the ipecac will have to be recovered from his or her stomach at the nearest medical facility.

If the Poison Control Center or hospital advises you to induce vomiting and no syrup of ipecac is available, you will probably be instructed to trigger the victim's gag reflex with your finger or some other blunt object.

When the victim vomits, hold his or her head lower than the rest of the body over a container that can be sealed and transported with the victim to the nearest medical facility. Keep in mind that an episode of vomiting does not necessarily empty the stomach completely. Arrange to transport the victim for further medical attention even after he or she has vomited.

In some cases, the Poison Control Center or hospital will instruct you NOT to induce vomiting. Depending upon the ingested substance (or substances) and the patient's condition, causing the patient to vomit may do considerably more harm than good. **DO NOT INDUCE VOMITING IF**

- The victim is semiconscious or unconscious.
- The victim has a serious heart disease or heart condition.
- The victim is having convulsions or has convulsed.
- The victim has swallowd a petroleum product (kerosene, gasoline, coal oil, fuel oil, paint thinner, cleaning fluid).
- The victim has swallowed a corrosive substance (oven cleaner, drain cleaner, toilet bowl cleaner, ammonia, bleach, lye, strong detergents).

## Food Poisoning

Food poisoning is an illness caused by the ingestion of foods that contain poisonous substances. The most common food poisoning agents are bacterial, but foods may also be contaminated with viruses, insecticides, or other toxic substances.

Insanitary food handling may result in bacterial or viral contamination, just as improper cooking practices may allow bacteria to germinate and multiply in foods. Fish and shellfish are common culprits in food poisoning cases because they sometimes feed on marine organisms that are toxic to humans. The organisms are concentrated in the flesh and internal organs of the fish, so poisoning occurs when the fish are consumed.

Some foods are more susceptible to contamination than others. The most common offending foods include meats of all sorts, eggs, dairy products, fish, and shellfish. The signs and symptoms of food poisoning may appear thirty minutes to thirty hours after the infected food is ingested, depending upon the bacteria or toxin involved. These symptoms include

- Fever
- Chills
- Severe headache
- Gastrointestinal distress, such as abdominal pain and diarrhea
- Respiratory distress
- Nausea and vomiting
- Weakness
- Irregular heartbeat
- Tingling sensations
- Numbness
- Burning sensation about the lips and mouth
- Seizures
- Hallucinations
- Shock
- Coma

If a patient has no underlying medical condition and no history of drug abuse, yet exhibits bizarre, acute symptoms, it is wise to ask what he or she has eaten within the last twenty-four hours. If a portion of the suspect food remains, seal it in a container and have it transported with the patient. If possible, take a sample of the patient's vomitus to be analyzed as well.

The treatment for victims of food poisoning is supportive. Provide basic life support and treat for shock as the patient's condition indicates (and be alert to the possibility of anaphylactic shock.) Arrange for transportation to the nearest medical facility.

## POISONING BY INHALATION

Most cases of poisoning by inhalation involve carbon monoxide gas. Because carbon monoxide is odorless, colorless, and tasteless, many victims of accidental exposure have no idea they are being poisoned. Inhaling carbon monoxide gas is also a popular means of committing suicide in the United States, accounting for about twenty percent of all adult suicide deaths.

Carbon monoxide is produced by the incomplete burning of organic materials, including wood, paper, gasoline, natural gas, coal, and charcoal. Dangerous concentrations can occur wherever heating systems are in disrepair or poorly ventilated. Carbon monoxide combines with hemoglobin in the red blood cells, which renders the blood cells incapable of carrying oxygen. When a significant number of red blood cells are affected, the victim begins to suffer the effects of insufficient oxygen in the blood and tissues and ultimately suffocates.

The symptoms of carbon monoxide poisoning vary according to the concentration of carbon monoxide at the scene, the duration of exposure, and the victim's physical condition. Mild symptoms may include difficult breathing, throbbing headache, nausea, and vomiting. As the body becomes increasingly starved for oxygen, victims may also experience impaired vision and muscular control, abnormal heartbeat, rapid breathing, seizures, respiratory failure, coma, and finally, death.

The treatment for carbon monoxide poisoning is aimed at eliminating the poison from the blood and consists simply of removing the victim from the source of exposure. Be sure to protect yourself from being overcome, and get the victim into fresh air. Assess the victim's condition and administer high-flow oxygen. Administer CPR if necessary. Arrange for rapid transportation to the nearest medical facility.

The treatment for other inhalation poisonings, such as those involving natural gas leaks in the home, pesticides, or other hazardous materials, is the same. Protect yourself from dangerous exposures and remove the victim to fresh air. Provide basic life support and arrange for transportation to the nearest medical facility.

## INJECTED POISONS

### Snakebite

More than 8,000 venomous snakebites are reported each year in the United States, yet only five to fifteen of the bites are fatal. Many victims, however, sustain serious muscle and tissue damage; some lose fingers or even portions of arms or legs. Proper emergency treatment for snakebite victims can mean the difference between a small scar and more extensive disfigurement.

Of the 2,500 species of snakes in the world, around 400 are considered poisonous. Poisonous snakes manufacture and store venom in highly developed salivary glands. When the venom is discharged, it passes into the snake's fangs by way of paired connecting ducts. The tip of each fang is a very sharp cutting edge, and just above the tip is the opening through which the snake injects its venom. For envenomation to occur, then, the snake must strike at an angle and with sufficient force to drive at least one fang into its victim to a depth exceeding the distance between the tip and the venom orifice of the fang.

Pit vipers and coral snakes are the only poisonous snakes found in the United States.

#### PIT VIPERS

Pit vipers, so called because of the paired facial depressions (loreal pits) between the nostrils and mouth, inflict by far the most serious snakebite injuries in this country. The loreal pits allow pit vipers to detect the body heat of warm-blooded prey in dim light or even in total darkness. They are muscular, heavy snakes with triangular-shaped heads and elliptical pupils (cat's eyes). A pit viper's fangs are very long with respect to the size of its mouth and must be retracted for the snake to even close its mouth. Actually, the snake "folds" its fangs so that they are parallel to the roof of its mouth when they are not needed. When the snake opens its mouth, it can erect one or both fangs. Three types of pit vipers are found in the United States: rattlesnakes, cottonmouths, and copperheads.

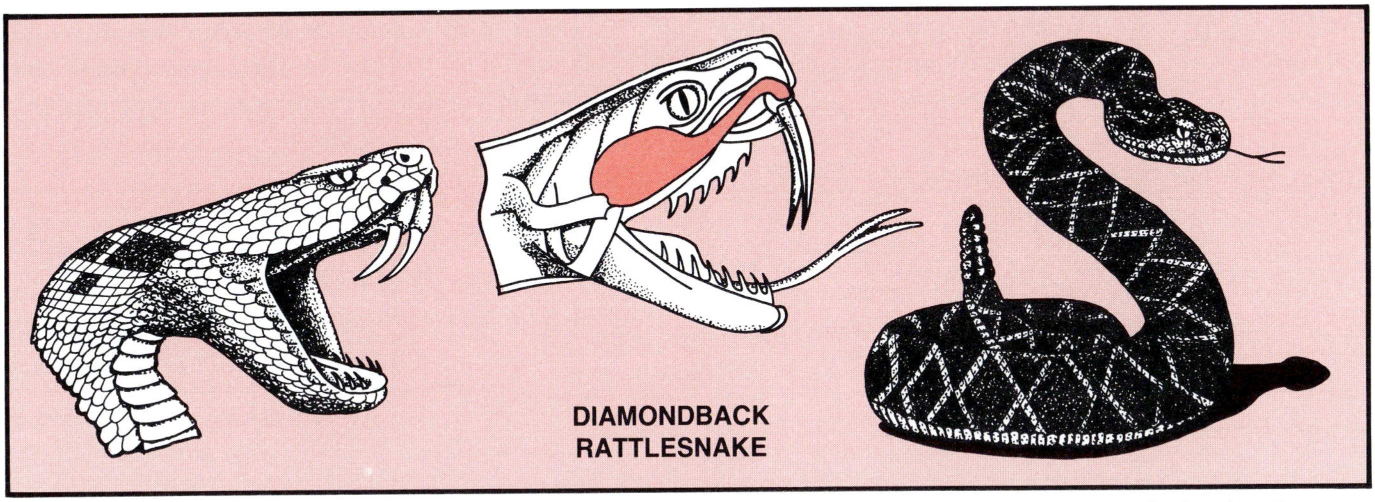


**Figure 12.1** All pit vipers have triangular heads that are wider than their necks and pits between the eye and nostril. The diamondback rattlesnake shown above is one of the largest of the pit vipers.

Most snakebite fatalities in the United States are caused by rattlesnakes. This snake's rattle, a sound-producing organ at the end of its tail, distinguishes it from other pit vipers. A diamondback rattlesnake (Figure 12.1) may grow to be eight feet (2.4 m) long and weigh as much as 30 pounds (14 kg). A large rattlesnake can inject a large quantity of venom, particularly if it has not discharged its supply recently.

Cottonmouths (also called water moccasins) are usually dark olive or brown in color. This snake is named for the cottonwhite mouth tissue it reveals when threatened (Figure 12.2).

Copperhead snakes can be distinguished from the other pit vipers by their coloring. They have a general pattern of copper-colored, chestnut, or dark brown colors on a light background (Figure 12.3).

### CORAL SNAKES

Coral snakebites are uncommon, and envenomation is even more rare. For many years, in fact, these snakes were thought to be nonpoisonous. Most bites occur when someone tries or actually handles a coral snake. The bright colors of these snakes make them especially attractive to children, who may try to play with them. The fangs of coral snakes are much shorter than those of pit vipers and cannot be moved, that is, they remain permanently erect. Coral snakes are more slender than pit vipers, and their heads are not significantly larger than their necks. Unlike pit vipers, coral snakes have round pupils. Two types of coral snakes are found in the United States: Eastern coral snakes and Sonora (Arizona) coral snakes.

Eastern coral snakes have bands of red, yellow, white, and black that encircle their entire

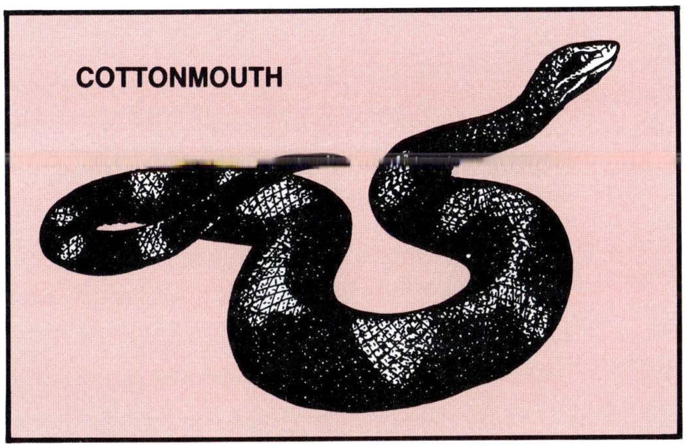


**Figure 12.2** The cottonmouth is a dark-colored pit viper that reveals a white mouth when threatened.

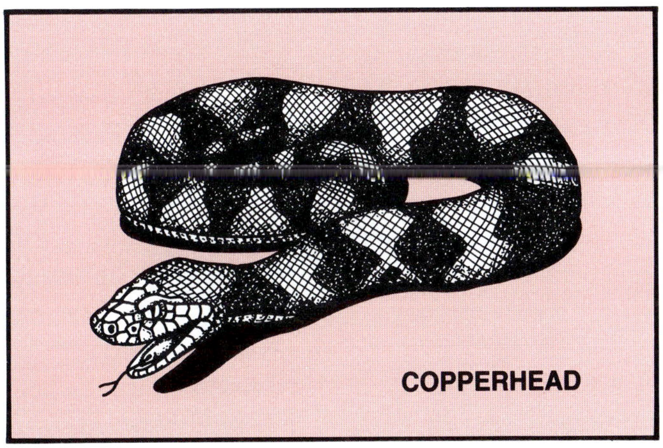


**Figure 12.3** The copperhead displays a copper or dark brown pattern on a light background.

bodies (Figure 12.4). In general, adjacent red and yellow bands distinguish coral snakes from nonpoisonous imitators. All-black specimens, however, of the Eastern coral snake have been reported in Texas. Eastern coral snakes may grow to be 2½ to 3 feet (0.7 m to 0.9 m) long.

The Sonora coral snake resembles the Eastern coral snake in every way except in size, averaging only about 15 to 18 inches (381 mm to 457 mm) in length.

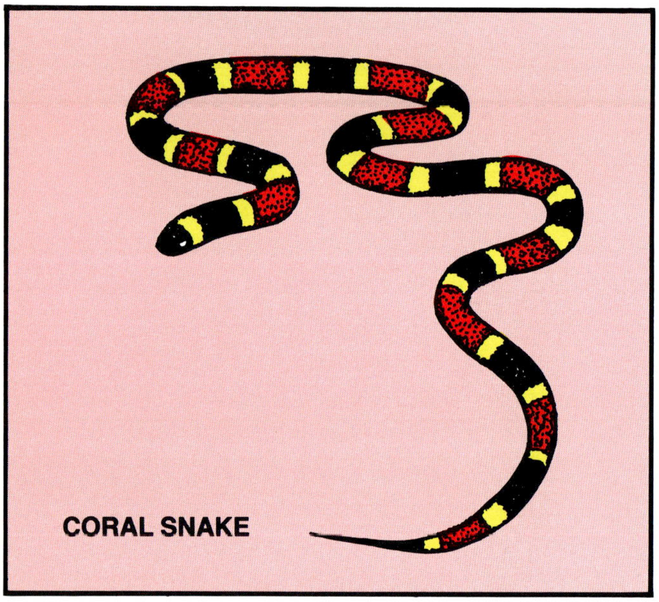


**Figure 12.4** The Eastern coral snake is distinguished by red, yellow, and black bands. Adjacent red and yellow bands indicate a poisonous snake; red and yellow bands separated by another color are found on nonpoisonous snakes.

## Caring for the Snakebite Victim

Because snakebite incidents generally elicit extreme emotional reactions, and because muscular activity hastens the absorption of snake venom, your first task upon arrival at the scene is usually to keep the victim as calm and still as possible. Many people are convinced that all bites from venomous snakes are fatal. Assure the victim that this is not the case. Next, inspect the bite. Obvious fang marks indicate a strong likelihood that the victim has been envenomated. Scratch wounds, however, do not rule out that possibility. Coral snakes, because of their size and the relative shortness of their fangs, often have an incomplete bite. Unless you can positively identify the snake that inflicted the bite, assume that a poisonous snake was responsible.

Learn from the victim whether the snake bit more than once. Ask the victim to describe the kind of pain and symptoms he or she is experiencing. Common symptoms of snake venom poisoning include

- Strange tastes (the first symptom in many cases)
- General weakness
- Blurred vision
- Tingling feeling in the lips, scalp, digits, or extremities
- Nausea
- Vomiting
- Weak, rapid pulse
- Respiratory distress
- Shock

Severe envenomations will involve several, or all, of these symptoms. Unless the venom has been injected directly into the bloodstream (a rare occurrence), the symptoms may take hours or even days to appear. The immediate evidence of envenomation may be limited to the wound itself and some swelling.

Treatment for envenomation depends upon how much time has elapsed since the victim was bitten. If the time elapsed is only two or three minutes, begin suction:

Step 1: Remove any rings and bracelets from the injured extremity.

Step 2: Apply a constricting band to the injured extremity about one or two inches (25 mm to 51 mm) above the bite. The band should be loose enough for you to slide your index finger under it with some resistance. If the bite is on a finger or toe place the band just above the wrist or foot.

Step 3: Make a longitudinal (along the long axis of the extremity) incision through each puncture wound about ¼-inch (6 mm) deep and ½ inch (12 mm) long.

Step 4: Apply suction to these incisions for at least 30 minutes, using any available means. If no other method of applying suction is available (such as that provided in a snakebite kit), suck on the wound and spit out the aspirated material. If you should accidentally swallow some of the venom, there is little cause for concern, since it will be inactivated in your stomach.

Step 5: Keep the victim still and quiet. Do not give food, drink, or allow the victim to smoke. Watch for signs of anaphylactic shock.

Step 6: Arrange for immediate transportation to the nearest medical facility where antivenin can be administered and further surgical treatment performed. Position the injured extremity so that it is slightly lower than the heart, and monitor any swelling and the speed with which it progresses. Keep the constriction band just ahead of the swelling.

Many authorities no longer advocate the suction treatment for snakebite cases. Some bites can be as deep as one inch (25 mm) or more, and when the penetration is deep enough to puncture the larger muscles, suction is ineffective. If, however, penetration is ¼ inch (6 mm) or less, and if suction is begun within the first two to three minutes after envenomation, as much as 22-50 percent of the venom can be removed. Nonetheless, muscle damage, infection, and excessive bleeding are serious risks associated with suction treatment.

If more than three minutes has elapsed since the victim was bitten or if the penetration is very deep, the recommended treatment for snakebite is very simple:

Step 1: Remove any rings and bracelets from the injured extremity.

Step 2: Apply a constricting band to the injured extremity about one or two inches (25 mm to 51 mm) above the bite. The band should be loose enough for you to slide your index finger under it with some resistance. If the bite is on a finger or toe, place the band just above the wrist or foot.

Step 3: Keep the victim still and quiet. Do not give food, drink, or allow the victim to smoke.

Step 4: Arrange for rapid transport to the nearest medical facility. Position the injured extremity so that it is slightly lower than the heart, and monitor any swelling and the speed with which it progresses. Keep the constriction band just ahead of the swelling.

If circumstances allow you to kill or capture the offending snake without risk to yourself or others at the scene, do so, and transport the snake for positive identification.

## Spider Bites

In the United States, two types of spiders inflict bites that may require emergency care: black widow spiders and brown recluse (fiddleback) spiders.

### BLACK WIDOW SPIDERS

The black widow spider is a small (about one and one-half inch [38 mm] in diameter, including its legs), glossy black spider with a red or orange hourglass-shaped marking on the underside of the female's abdomen (Figure 12.5). The male does not have the mark and is not poisonous. This spider's

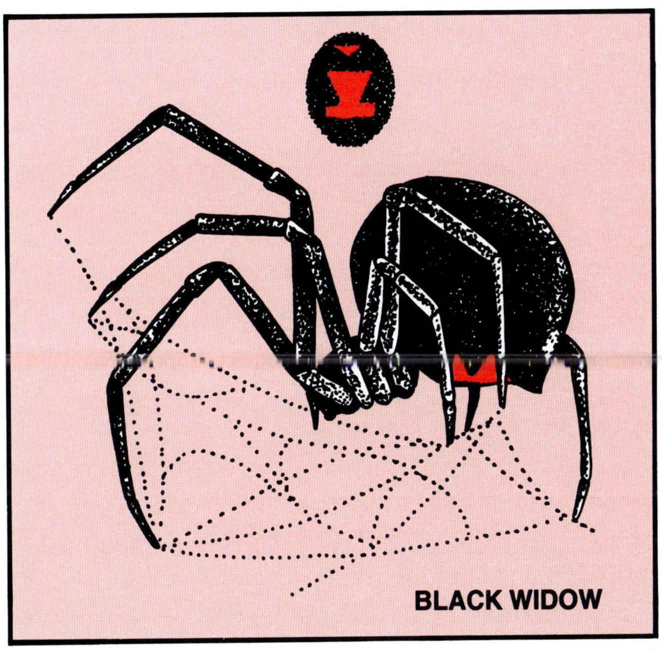


**Figure 12.5** The female black widow spider has an hourglass-shaped red mark on the abdomen; the male has no mark and is not poisonous.

bite may not be painful initially, but a dull or numbing pain usually develops around the bite within 15 to 20 minutes. If the bite is on a lower extremity, the victim will usually experience muscle spasm in the abdomen; if it is on an upper extremity, the pain and spasms will spread to the shoulders, back, and chest. Other symptoms of a black widow spider bite include nausea, vomiting, sweating, and headache.

### BROWN RECLUSE (FIDDLEBACK) SPIDERS

Smaller than the black widow, the brown recluse spider has a light brown oval-shaped body with a distinctive fiddle-shaped mark on its back (Figure 12.6). The actual bite of the brown recluse is usually painless. Blisters form at the site of the bite after several hours and the area becomes red and tender. After two or three days the bite becomes dark and ulcerated (rotted). The victim may complain of headache, general weakness, fever, joint pains, and may have a measles-like rash.

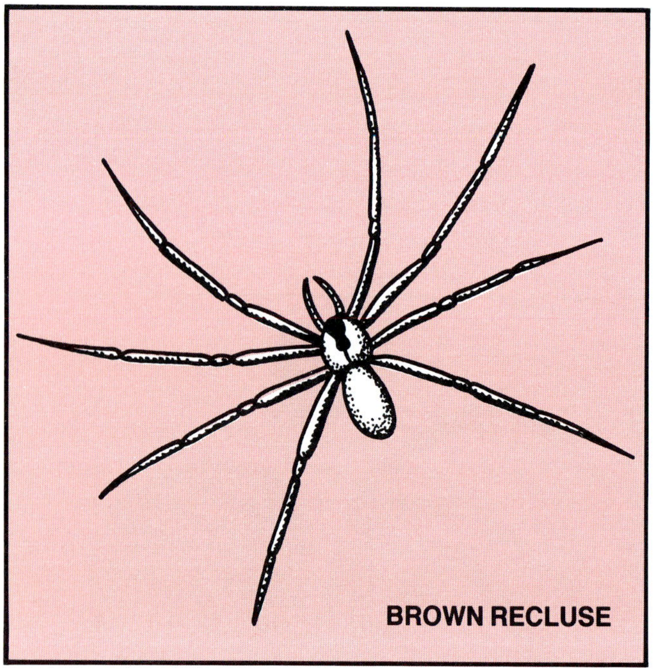


**Figure 12.6** The brown recluse spider has a dark, fiddle-shaped mark on its back.

## Emergency Treatment for Spider Bites

A bite from either of these spiders should be treated by a physician as soon as possible. Clean the wound with an antiseptic such as alcohol or hydrogen peroxide, keep the patient quiet, and arrange for transportation to a medical facility. Watch for signs of anaphylactic shock. If the offending spider is at the scene (a very rare circumstance), capture it and have it transported with the victim.

### HYMENOPTERA STINGS

The venom produced by insects of the family hymenoptera (bees, wasps, hornets, yellow jackets, and ants) is much less potent than that produced by certain snakes and spiders, yet hymenoptera stings cause ten times as many deaths annually as poisonous snakebites (Figure 12.7). The reason for this apparent paradox is the violent allergic reactions (anaphylaxis) insect bites cause in some people. (For more information on anaphylactic shock, see Chapter 10, Medical Emergencies.)

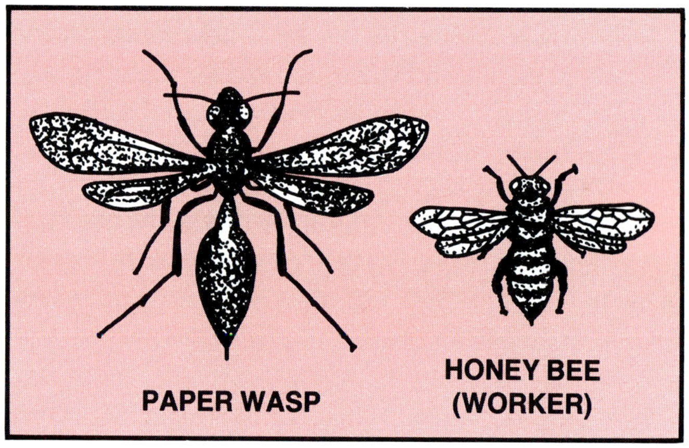


**Figure 12.7** Stings from insects of the family hymenoptera can be dangerous because some people develop severe allergic reactions. Wasps and bees are common offenders.

It is unlikely that you will be called to treat the victim of an insect bite unless he or she is exhibiting signs of an allergic reaction. Swelling in the area of the sting, even if it involves an entire extremity, is not necessarily evidence of an allergy; wheals and swelling in an area other than the location of the bite indicate that the victim is seriously allergic to the insect's venom. Other signs of allergic reaction to an insect sting include

- Itching of the hands or feet
- Headache
- Nausea
- Stomach cramps
- Rapid, weak pulse
- Labored breathing

The treatment for an uncomplicated sting consists of relieving the victim's pain and anxiety and preventing infections. First, determine whether the stinger is still attached to the victim. If so, use a knife blade or card to scrape the stinger sideways away from the wound (Figure 12.8). Never pluck a stinger from the wound: squeezing the stinger pumps more venom into the victim. Once you have removed the stinger, wash the area thoroughly with soap and water. Apply ice packs to reduce swelling. If the victim has multiple stings or has been stung around the eyes, it is best to arrange for transport to the nearest medical facility, even if there are no signs of an allergic reaction.

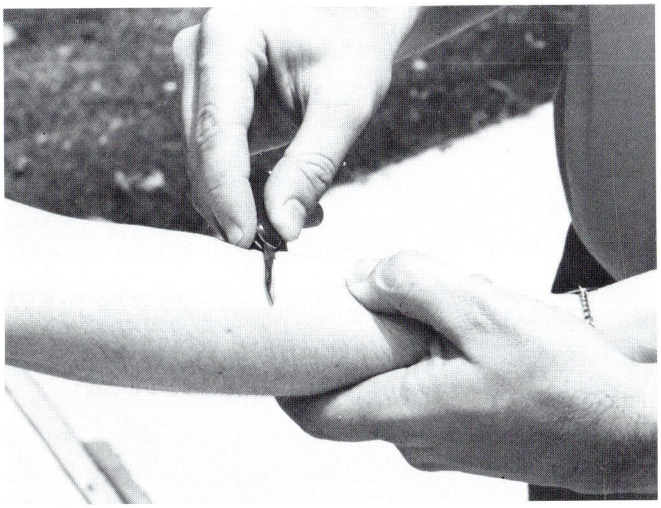

**Figure 12.8** If the stinger is still attached to the victim use a knife blade or card to scrape the stinger sideways away from the wound.

If you should treat a patient who has been stung only once (and not about the eyes) and who exhibits no signs of an allergic reaction, advise him or her of the warning symptoms of anaphylaxis before you leave the scene. Stress the importance of prompt medical care in the event that any symptoms occur. If necessary, have the patient sign a form stating that he or she refused transport.

## Animal Bites

All warm-blooded animals can transmit rabies, but some animals are much more likely to be infected with the disease than others. Carnivorous wild animals (particularly skunks, raccoons, and foxes) and bats are the animals most commonly infected. These same animals are responsible for the majority of cases of human and domestic animal rabies in the United States. Rodents (including squirrels, hamsters, guinea pigs, gerbils, chipmunks, rats, and mice) and rabbits, on the other hand, are rarely infected and have not been known to cause human rabies in this country. Although only five to six percent of all animal rabies cases involve dogs and cats, they are the offending animals in most cases that involve antirabies treatment for humans.

Two types of rabies appear in animals: "furious" and "dumb" rabies. Each type manifests itself with certain behavioral and physical symptoms. An animal with "furious" rabies initially departs from its usual temperament, becoming either excessively withdrawn or unusually affectionate. After this stage passes (in about two or three days), the animal wanders away from home and the "mad" phase of the disease sets in. During this phase the animal bites anything in its path and appears to be frothing at the mouth. The drooling is caused by difficulty in swallowing due to paralysis of the muscles surrounding the animal's throat and mouth. As the disease progresses, the paralysis gradually spreads to the limbs and vital organs and the animal dies.

An animal with "dumb" rabies does not suffer the roving, or "mad" phase. Instead, the first recognizable sign of rabies in these animals is paralysis, usually of the lower jaw. As in "furious" cases, the animal gradually lapses into a paralytic state and dies.

Rabies is a virus present in the saliva of infected animals, and can only be transmitted by introducing the virus onto the mucous membranes or into open wounds on the skin. Thus, a bite, scratch, abrasion, open wound, or mucous membrane contaminated with the saliva from a rabid animal constitutes exposure to rabies. Casual contact, such as petting an infected animal, does not constitute exposure to the disease. If the circumstances of the biting incident suggest that the victim has been exposed to rabies, he or she will receive a series of injections to combat the fatal virus.

The rabies control laws in most states dictate that any domesticated animal that bites someone must be confined and observed for ten days after the day of the attack. Learn from the victim and/or bystanders the identity of the animal's owner and, if possible, the address and phone number. If the biting animal is wild, the laws require that the animal be killed as soon as possible after the attack. The presence or absence of rabies is confirmed through a laboratory analysis of the brain tissue of the suspected carrier. In either case, contact the appropriate authorities to capture or kill the animal.

### Treatment for Animal Bites

When you are called to the scene of an animal bite incident, determine the type of animal involved. Learn from the victim and bystanders whether the attack was provoked, that is, under what circumstances the animal bit the victim. An unprovoked attack indicates a stronger likelihood that the animal is rabid than a provoked attack. In general, you should regard a bite inflicted on someone trying to feed or handle an apparently healthy animal as a provoked attack.

The most important aspect of treating the victim of an animal bite (whether you judge the animal to be rabid or not) is local cleansing of the wound. Scrub the wound vigorously with soap and running water (Figure 12.9). Use a cloth or sponge if one is available to assure a more thorough and forceful scrubbing. Arrange for transportation to the nearest medical facility.

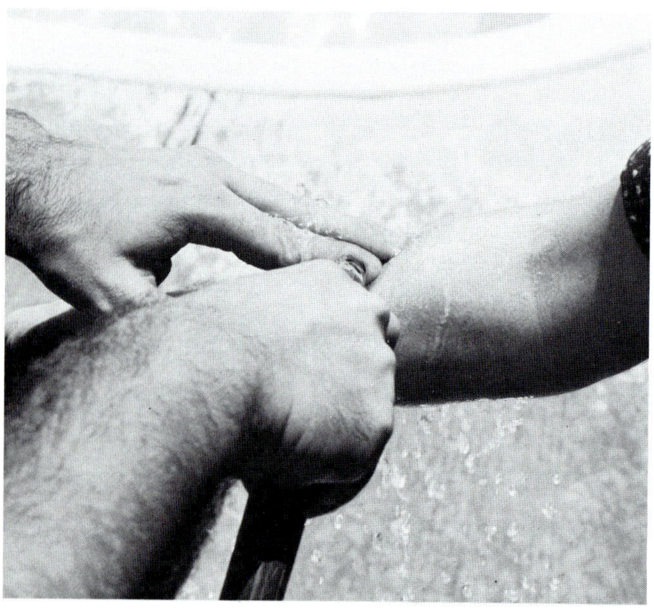

**Figure 12.9** Scrub an animal bite thoroughly with soap and water.

### Human Bites

A bite inflicted by a human being is potentially more serious than a bite inflicted by an animal because of the abundance of bacteria that live and multiply in the human mouth. A patient who has been bitten by another person, or, as generally happens, whose fist has come into contact with someone's teeth during a fight, should be evaluated at the nearest medical facility. Treat the wound as you would an animal bite: scrub it vigorously with soap and running water. Use a cloth or sponge if one is available to assure a more thorough cleansing. Arrange for transportation to the nearest medical facility.

### Marine Animal Bites and Stings

First responders in coastal areas of the United States should be familiar with the venomous or otherwise dangerous marine life inhabiting the local waters. They should also be familiar with the preferred local treatments for the injuries marine animals may cause. Wounds inflicted by marine animals may cause severe allergic reactions (anaphylaxis) in some victims, particularly those who have suffered similar injuries in the past. If the patient goes into anaphylactic shock, the best care you can provide is care for the whole patient. Monitor his or her pulse and respiration, administer oxygen, and be prepared to administer cardiopulmonary resuscitation. Transport the patient to the nearest medical facility immediately.

Most injuries inflicted by marine animals occur when the victim steps on, handles, or swims alongside a dangerous animal. Three types of wounds may be caused by marine animals: stings, punctures, bites and lacerations.

#### STINGS

Stinging marine animals, such as jellyfish, hydras, corals, and sea anemones attach nematocysts, or stinging tentacles, to their victims (Figure 12.10). The nematocysts cause intense pain that sometimes disables swimmers and causes them to drown. Some victims may experience joint and muscle pain, respiratory distress, severe rash, or swelling. The recommended treatment for a sting injury inflicted by a marine animal requires that you wear gloves. This standard treatment for un-

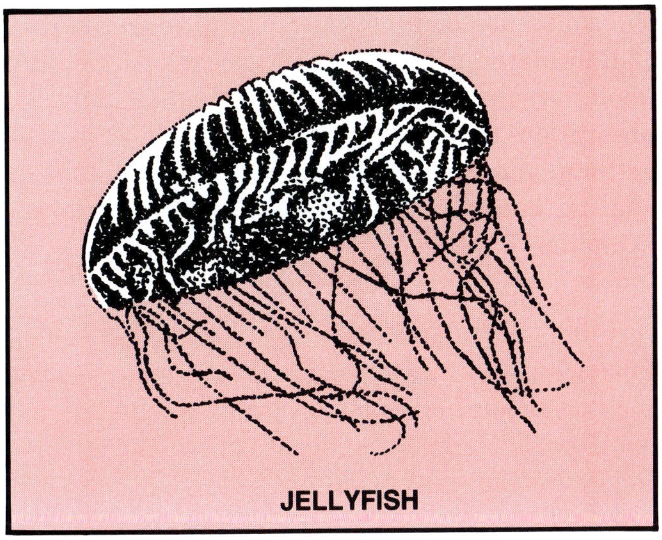


**Figure 12.10** The stinging tentacles attached to victims by jellyfish cause severe pain.

complicated stings is aimed at removing the nematocysts from the victim.

Step 1: Wash the injured part in sea water.

Step 2: Remove as many tentacles as you can with your fingers (be sure to wear gloves!).

Step 3: Pour strong alcohol over the wound.

Step 4: Sprinkle a dry powder over the wound. Flour works well, but meat tenderizer works even better because it neutralizes the proteins in the venom.

Step 5: Scrape any remaining tentacles from the wound using a knife blade or card.

Step 6: Wash the injured part in sea water once more.

Step 7: Arrange for transport to the nearest medical facility.

### PUNCTURES

Most injuries caused by puncturing marine animals occur when the spiny animals are stepped on. Coneshells, spiny starfish, stingrays, sea urchins, and sculpins produce toxic materials that enter the wound when the spine punctures the victim's skin (Figure 12.11). The resulting puncture wound is very painful and the toxin may cause nausea, vomiting, weakness, and fainting.

Because of the circumstances under which puncture injuries occur, most wounds of this type are on one of the victim's feet. The treatment for an

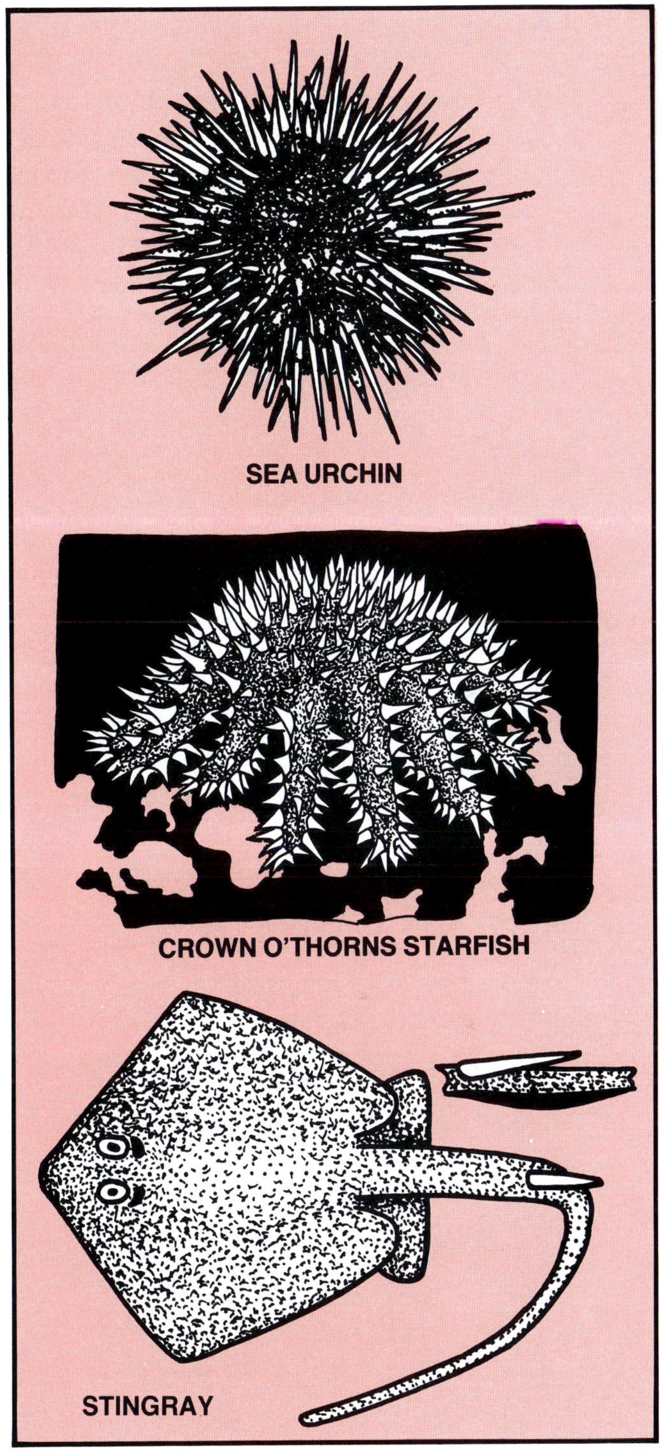


**Figure 12.11** Spiny sea animals, such as sea urchins, starfish, and stingrays, produce toxic materials that are introduced into the body when the victim's skin is punctured.

uncomplicated puncture injury inactivates the venom in the wound by using high temperatures:

Step 1: Inspect the wound and remove any spines that may have broken off in the victim's foot.

Step 2: Immerse both of the victim's feet in hot 110° to 114°F (43°C to 46°C) water for 30 to 60 minutes. Immersing the uninjured foot protects the injured foot from scalding: the injured foot may be numb, and the victim may not realize that it is burned without submerging the uninjured foot to gauge the water temperature.

Step 3: Elevate the injured limb and arrange for transport to the nearest medical facility.

### BITES AND LACERATIONS

Sea snakes, octopuses, sharks, and barracuda can inflict serious soft tissue injuries upon victims who happen to swim alongside one of the dangerous animals (Figure 12.12). If you are called to treat the victim of such an attack, provide basic life support: control bleeding and monitor the victim's pulse and respiration. Guard against shock and be prepared to administer cardiopulmonary resuscitation. Arrange for immediate transport to the nearest medical facility.

## POISONING BY ABSORPTION

Some poisons, most commonly insecticides, may enter the body through the skin, eyes, or mucous membranes. An individual working with insecticides may be poisoned by direct contact with the substance or by merely handling or wearing contaminated gloves or work clothes. Depending upon the substance, the initial symptoms of poison absorption may mimic those of heat stroke or asthma, and the victim may not realize that he or she is being poisoned even as more severe symptoms develop.

The first noticeable symptoms of poison absorption include weakness, fatigue, giddiness, headache, and nausea. Secondary symptoms may include abdominal cramps, chest pain, blurred vision, constricted pupils, sweating, difficult breathing, vomiting, and diarrhea. In severe cases, the victim becomes paralyzed and finally, comatose.

When you are called to treat a victim of poison absorption, wear protective clothing and rubber gloves to protect yourself from contamination. Remove contaminated clothing from the patient immediately, including shoes, and bathe the patient with soap and cool water for ten to fifteen minutes. Similarly, if the patient's eyes are contaminated, rinse them repeatedly with cool water. Provide basic life support and try to identify the specific poison involved, then call the nearest Poison Control Center or hospital. There are known antidotes and medical management procedures available for most insecticides, but proper treatment depends upon a knowledge of the substance(s) involved.

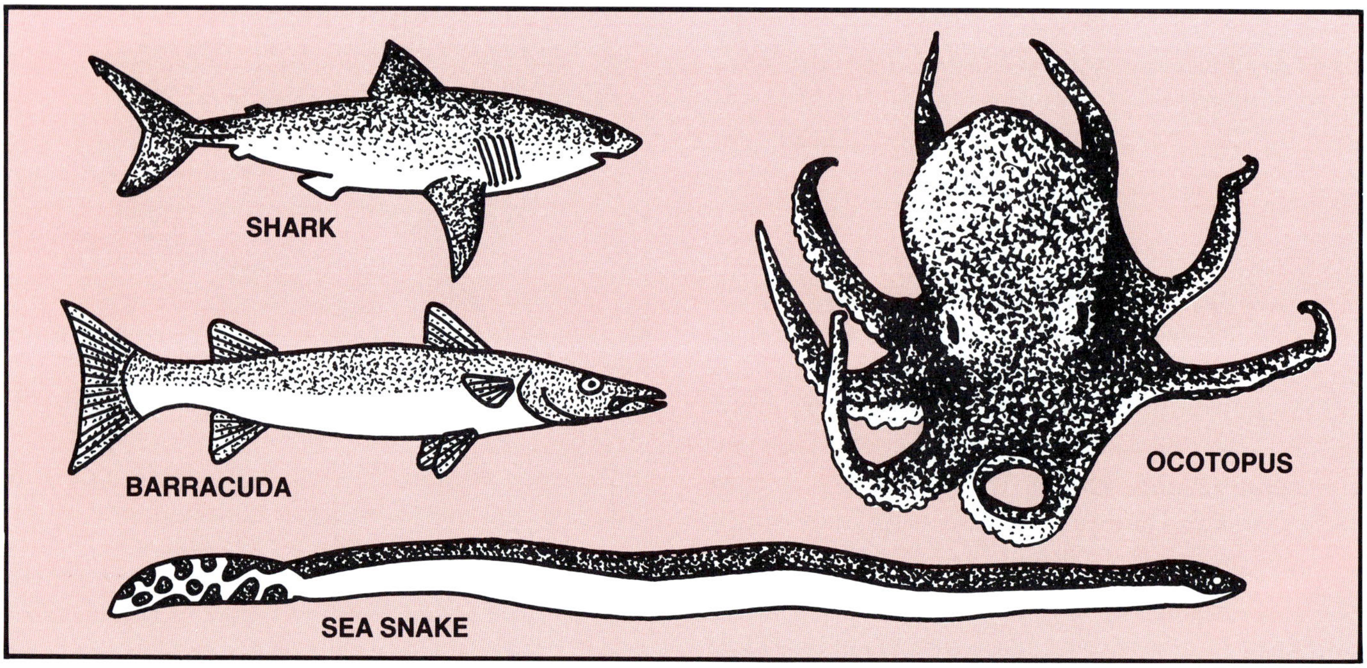


**Figure 12.12** Bites are the primary danger from such animals as sea snakes, octopuses, sharks, and barracuda.

# 13

# Burns

**NFPA STANDARD 1001**
**Emergency Medical Care**
**Fire Fighter II**

**4-4.6** The fire fighter shall identify characteristics and emergency medical care of thermal burns according to severity.

**4-4.8** The fire fighter shall identify the emergency medical care for chemical burns, including chemical burns of the eyes.



**U.S. DEPARTMENT OF TRANSPORTATION**
**First Responder Training Course**

**Objectives:**

- Given descriptions of patients burned by heat, indicate the degree and criticality of the burn and describe emergency care procedures.
- Given descriptions of patients burned by chemicals and electricity, describe emergency care procedures.

# Chapter 13
# Burns

Every year, nearly 2 million people are burned seriously enough to need medical attention. Of these burn victims, 75,000 are hospitalized, and 10,000 die. Burns are the third leading cause of accidental death in the United States, and *the* leading cause of accidental death for children 1 to 15 years old.

In addition to providing emergency burn care to the public, firefighter/first responders have a special incentive for becoming experts in emergency burn care: they also risk becoming burn victims themselves because of the nature of their job. (More than 7,000 firefighters suffered burns requiring medical treatment in 1983.)

Severe burns are considered by many to be the most serious of all injuries, and with good reason. When large amounts of skin are destroyed, body processes are upset, leaving the victim at serious risk of death from infection or other complications.

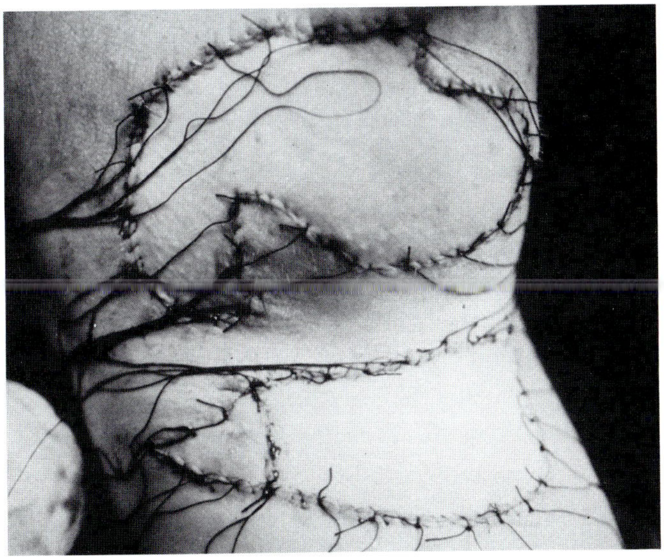

**Figure 13.1** Skin grafts, which are used to replace badly burned skin, are taken from unburned areas on the body. Here, a burn victim is receiving grafts to the lower face and neck.

Burn treatment focuses on three areas, in order of importance: survival, function, and appearance. Infection is the primary cause of death after the fifth post-burn day. Patients receive massive doses of antibiotics, and shreds of dead skin around the burn are removed to prevent bacteria from infecting the wounds further. This skin-removal process is known as debridement and is excruciatingly painful. Dressings are changed several times a day, another extremely painful process that can take hours for each dressing change. Other common complications from severe burns are pneumonia, kidney failure, heart failure, pulmonary embolism, and gastrointestinal hemorrhage.

Badly burned skin does not heal by itself and requires skin grafts, to close the wounds. Skin grafts using cadaver skin, pig skin, or synthetic skin, provide temporary coverage. But the only grafts that will not be rejected are those taken from unburned areas on the patient's own body, known as donor sites (Figure 13.1). For extensive burns, the grafting process must be repeated again and again, after the donor sites are healed and additional skin can be harvested.

Because burns tend to contract, function — the ability to move and use body parts — is threatened. To restore function, patients begin exercises to maintain muscle tone, skin elasticity, and joint movement. Splints, elastic bandages, and further surgery are employed to reduce contractures.

Only after function is restored to the greatest extent possible can surgeons turn to the final step:

cosmetic reconstruction. Skin grafts help to restore the burn patient's appearance, but scarring is inevitable, and most burn patients will never look like they did previously. Intensive psychotherapy is often needed to help patients and their families learn to deal with their appearance.

Although advances in hospital medical care, such as improved infection control, more aggressive burn treatment, and better grafting techniques, have saved the lives of many critically burned victims, burn care still begins at the scene with the arrival of first responders and EMTs. The care you provide is a critical first step in what will be a long (and painful) process of treatment and reconstructive surgery for major burns. Improper or inadequate care at the emergency scene will increase the patient's discomfort, make the job of emergency personnel in the hospital harder, and may lessen the patient's chances for survival.

By keeping in mind the functions served by the skin and by knowing the threat to life and body systems posed by serious burns, first responders can provide more effective care at the emergency scene.

## SKIN: THE BODY'S LARGEST ORGAN

The skin is the body's largest organ and serves many functions. Skin is waterproof and serves as a protective covering for the body, keeping out harmful bacteria. The skin assists in regulating body temperature, and along with the kidneys and lungs, excretes waste material from the body. It controls the flow of fluids, keeping external fluids from passing into the tissues, and prevents the loss of critical body fluids from the tissues. In addition, the skin acts as a sensory organ, detecting changes in temperature and body position, and sensations of pain. When this protective covering is damaged, the body is open to invasion by bacteria, to temperature changes, and to major disturbances in fluid balance.

Skin also plays a psychological role nearly as important as its physiological role. People's first impressions of others are often based on the appearance of the skin. If the skin is disfigured, as from a severe burn, the social impact of "looking different" can be devastating.

The skin is composed of two principal layers, the epidermis and the dermis (Figure 13.2). The epidermis, or outermost layer, is the body's first line of defense. The outer cells of the epidermis are constantly being shed. The deeper layers of the epidermis contain melanin, which is the pigment responsible for skin color.

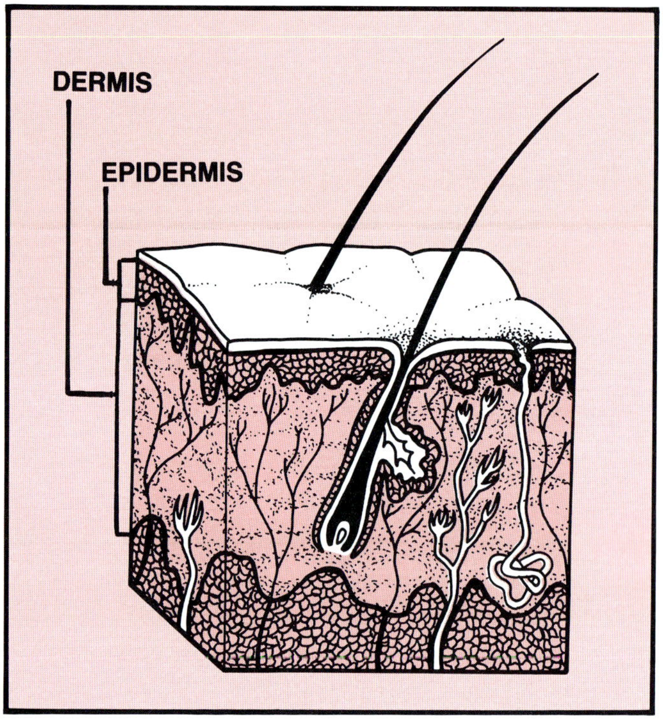


**Figure 13.2** The epidermis is the outermost layer of skin. The dermis lies below it and contains many important structures, such as hair follicles and nerves.

Below the epidermis is a tough, highly elastic layer of connective tissue called the dermis. The dermis contains many specialized skin structures, including nerve endings, blood vessels, sweat glands, sebaceous glands (oil glands), and hair follicles.

Superficial burns do only temporary damage to the epidermis, but deep burns damage the epidermis, the dermis, and may even damage the underlying muscle (Figure 13.3). Deeply or extensively damaged skin can no longer perform its functions: the body loses its ability to regulate temperature, vital fluids escape causing shock, and, most serious of all, bacteria can easily invade the body. Generally, the burns themselves do not kill; complications resulting from them do. That is why emergency treatment of burns focuses on helping to restore some of the skin's lost functions.

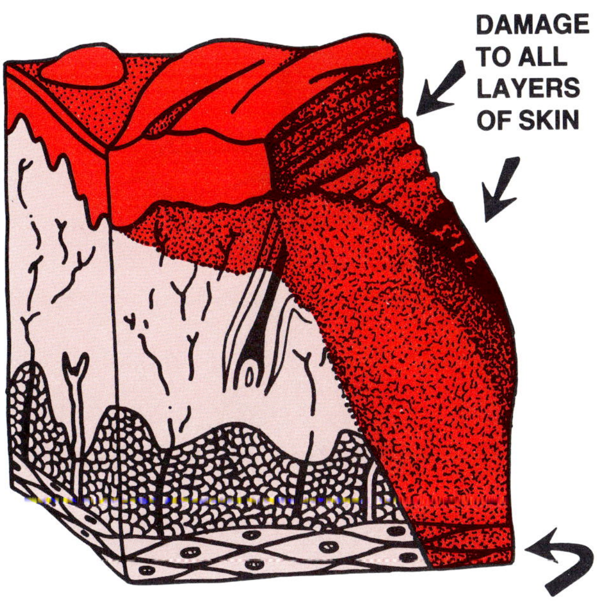


**Figure 13.3** Deep burns can damage not only all layers of skin but also the underlying fat and muscle.

## TYPES OF BURNS

Burns can be caused by exposure to heat or extreme cold, exposure to caustic chemicals, contact with sources of electrical current, or exposure to radioactive materials.

By far the largest percentage of burns (80 percent) are thermal burns. Thermal burns result from contact with fire, very hot liquids, or hot surfaces, such as hot metal. In the home, cooking accidents are common and result in scald burns that often involve children. The severity of the injury produced by a thermal burn depends on the temperature of the burning agent and the length of time it is in contact with the skin. Reduction of either of these factors will reduce the severity of injury. Causes of thermal injuries often result from faulty heating systems and open fires or fireplaces. In warm weather, outdoor activity devices such as barbeque grills or gasoline-powered engines in boats or lawn mowers are often fire hazards.

Electrical burns are caused by the heat produced when electric current passes through the body. Typically, an entrance and an exit wound are visible, with variable amounts of tissue destruction at these two sites. Initially, it is often impossible to know the extent of injury because the overlying skin may be undamaged, yet conceal dead tissue underneath. Only after careful clinical observation of the patient and diagnostic workup is the extent of the damage apparent. In some cases, especially those involving injury to the extremities, surgical exploration may be necessary to determine the extent of tissue damage. The severity of an electrical injury depends upon the surface area of the point of contact with the current, the length of time of contact, and the amperage of the current.

Chemical burns are caused by skin contact with caustic chemicals. Household chemicals that may cause injury include lye preparations, drain openers, battery acid, and other corrosive substances. Industrial accidents may also result in chemical burns. Length of exposure to the substance is the major factor determining the severity of a chemical burn. The pattern of the burn may be spotty, or it may cover a large surface, depending on how the agent came in contact with the skin. Tissue damage is often deep, especially if the substance was not immediately and completely removed. A particular hazard of chemical burns is that of swallowing some of the burning agent, resulting in death or extensive damage to the gastrointestinal system.

Radiation burns are caused by overexposure to x-rays, radioactive substances, nuclear blast, or sunlight. The most commonly seen radiation burn is a sunburn. Sunburns are not usually serious injuries; however, if large areas of the body are burned or blistered, the sunburn is more serious.

## CLASSIFICATION OF BURNS

The damage to the skin that results from a burn is classified as first, second, or third degree, depending on the depth of the burn. The severity of a burn is classified by both the *depth* of the burn and by the *amount* of tissue damaged. Therefore, a second-degree burn covering 60 percent of the body may be more serious than a third-degree burn covering 20 percent of the body.

FIRST-DEGREE BURNS. First-degree burns damage only the most superficial layers of the skin. Such burns produce redness and pain, as in a scald or moderate sunburn. First-degree burns

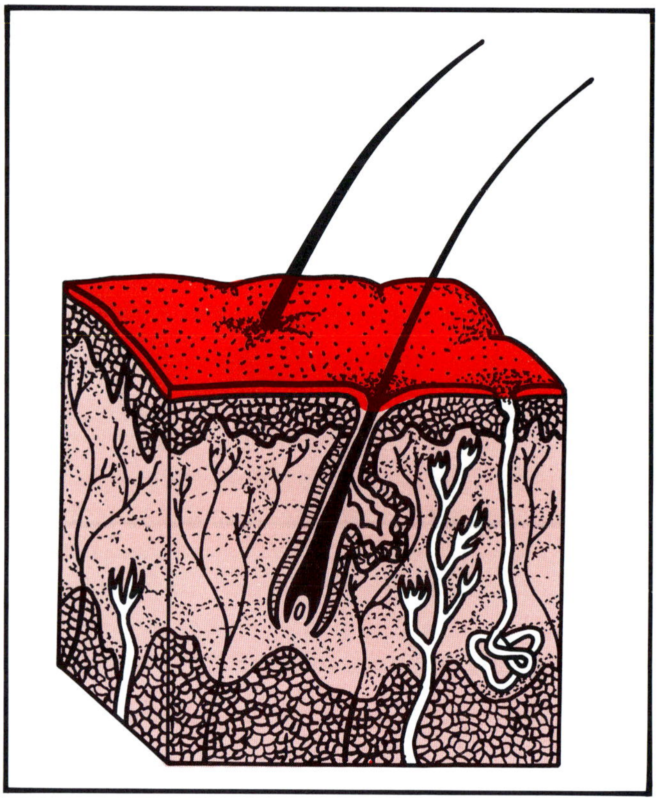

**Figure 13.4** First-degree burns involve only the top layer of skin. They are characterized by redness and pain.

usually heal in about one week, after the outer epidermal layers peel off (Figure 13.4).

SECOND-DEGREE BURNS. Second-degree burns penetrate deeper into the skin than first-degree burns. These burns are marked by blisters and swelling (edema) (Figure 13.5). Second-degree burns are often extremely painful because nerve endings become irritated and very sensitive to touch or other stimulation. Deep second-degree burns, however, may not be very painful due to nerve damage. Significant fluid loss through damaged skin can result, but if the burn is kept clean and does not become infected, it will usually heal in two to three weeks. Second-degree burns are most often caused by contact with boiling liquids. First- and second-degree burns are also known as partial thickness burns.

THIRD-DEGREE BURNS. Third-degree burns are also known as full-thickness burns because the full thickness of the skin, and perhaps even the subcutaneous fat and underlying muscle are damaged or destroyed (Figure 13.6). The skin is pale and dry; it may appear charred and leathery and smell "burned." Because nerve endings have

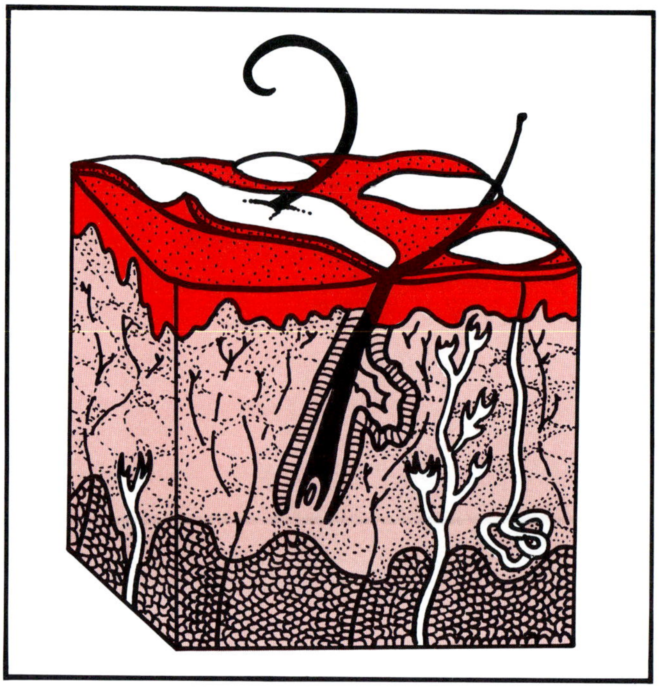

**Figure 13.5** Second-degree burns penetrate deeper into the skin and are characterized by blisters and swelling.

been destroyed, third-degree burns are usually not painful. Severely damaged skin cannot perform its protective functions, so patients with third-degree burns are likely to undergo rapid and significant fluid loss, which results in hypovolemic shock.

Full thickness burns, because of the deep destruction of tissue, cannot heal themselves by the growth of new skin. The only way for this wound to heal is by contracture, or drawing the undamaged

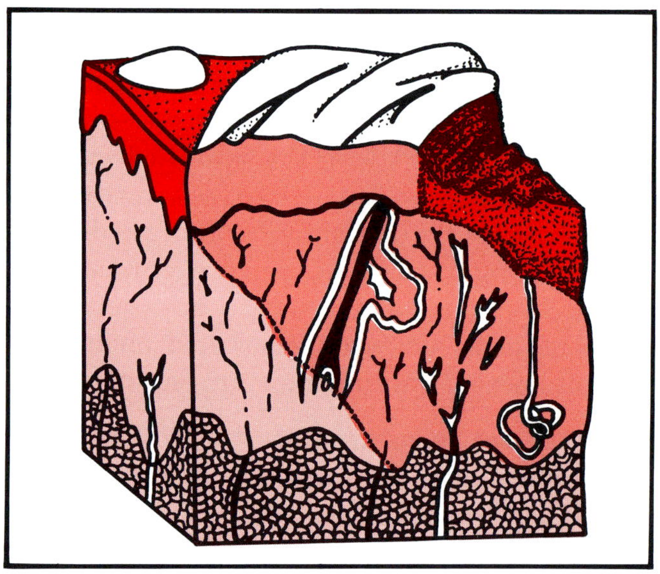

**Figure 13.6** Third-degree burns destroy the full thickness of skin. Because nerves are also destroyed, these burns are often not painful.

skin together to cover the damaged area. Skin grafting from other parts of the body is necessary to provide full function for the burned area and to prevent excessive scarring.

### Determining Severity of Burns

The severity of burns is gauged by both the depth of the burns and by the amount of tissue damaged. The "rule of nines" is used to estimate the percentage of body surface burned (Figure 13.7). This system assigns a percentage value to each part of the body; for example, an entire arm, front and back, makes up nine percent of the body. Note that the child's chart differs from an adult's; in particular, a child's head is much larger than an adult's in proportion to the rest of the body.

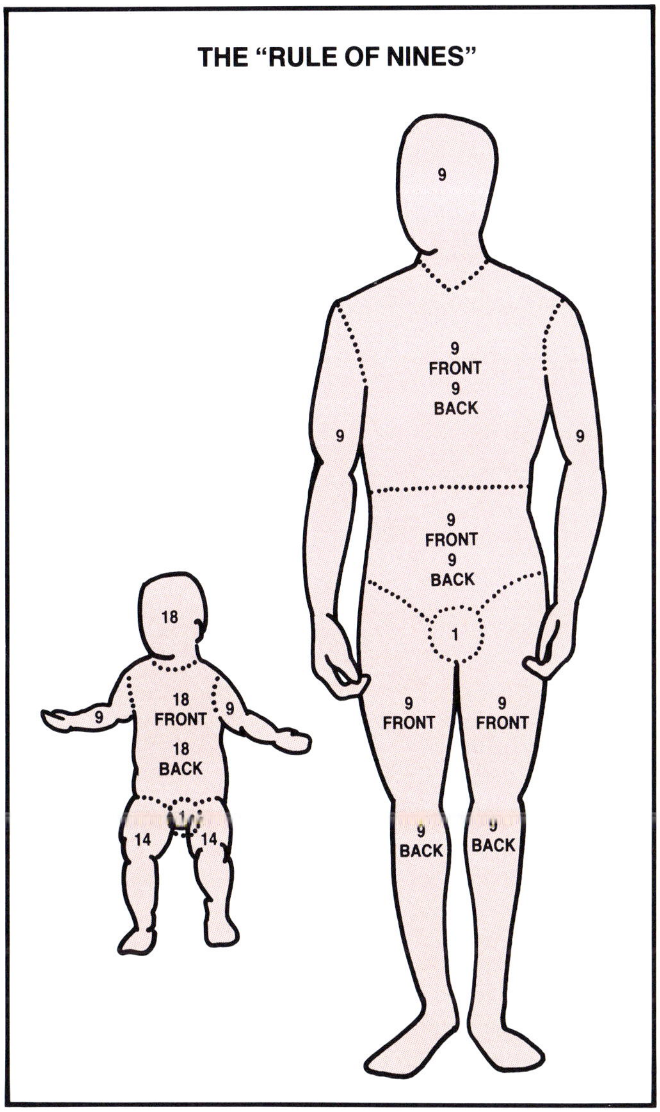


**Figure 13.7** The "rule of nines" is a helpful guide for estimating the extent of a burn.

There are several other factors that determine whether a burn is considered to be minor, moderate, or critical (severe). Critical burns are those that involve any of the following factors:

- Burns complicated by respiratory tract injuries
- Almost all burns of the face, hands, feet, genitalia, or buttocks
- Burns complicated by fractures or major soft-tissue injury
- Electrical and deep acid burns
- Burns occurring in patients with serious underlying physical problems, such as a heart condition or diabetes

Burns of the face are considered critical because of the possibility of respiratory tract involvement. In addition, burns that disfigure the face are psychologically much more damaging to the patient because they cannot be hidden. Burns of the hands and feet are serious because edema (swelling) of the hands and feet cuts off circulation to those areas and may result in loss of function. In addition, hands, like the face, cannot be hidden. Burns of the genitalia and buttocks are serious because these areas are prone to early infection.

Moderate burns include second-degree burns that involve 15 to 30 percent of the body surface and third-degree burns that involve 2 to 10 percent of the body surface, excluding burns of the face, hands, or feet.

Minor burns include first-degree burns affecting less than 20 percent of the body surface; second-degree burns that affect less than 15 percent of the body surface; third-degree burns of less than 2 percent of the body, excluding burns of the face, hands, or feet.

**NOTE:** Always consider a burn more serious if the victim is a child or an elderly person. Children under 2 and people over 60 have a higher mortality rate than other age groups with similar burn injuries. Very young children have a lower resistance to infection and older patients frequently have underlying conditions that complicate burn treatment.

The primary objectives when treating patients for burns are as follows:

- STOP THE BURNING PROCESS.
- Maintain the ABC's.
- Help to relieve pain.
- Treat for shock.
- Aid in preventing infection.

Always try to get a good history from the patient, relatives, or bystanders. Obtain the following information:

- How long ago did the burn occur?
- What, if anything, has been done by the patient or bystanders for the injury?
- Was the patient confined in a closed space with smoke, steam, or other products of combustion? If so, for how long? Did the patient lose consciousness?
- With what was the patient burned — open flame, hot liquids, or chemicals?
- Does the patient have any history of significant heart disease that might complicate fluid therapy? Is there a history of lung problems that might cause a more severe reaction to smoke inhalation? Are there any other serious underlying illnesses, such as diabetes?
- Does the patient have any allergies, including allergies to any medications?

## Thermal Burns

The first act in treating a burn victim is to EXTINGUISH ANY CLOTHING ON FIRE. Stop a person whose clothes are on fire from running; running does not put out the fire, but serves to fan the flames. Nor should the victim remain standing. A standing victim is more apt to inhale flames and to ignite the hair. Place the patient on the floor or ground and smother the flames by the fastest possible means: rolled in a blanket or doused with large quantities of water, such as from a garden hose or booster line. Once the fire is out, remove all smoldering clothing because burning can continue if the clothing is left on. Do not pull clothing or it will cause more damage to the skin; cut it off if necessary. If any clothing remains stuck to the skin, leave it there. Remove bracelets, rings, and other potentially constricting items because swelling of the hands and fingers may occur rapidly after a burn.

If the patient has suffered any injury that may cause damage to the spinal cord, such as from jumping out of a window, assume a spinal injury and treat accordingly. Immobilize the patient's head and neck before you do anything else.

LOOK TO THE PATIENT'S AIRWAY. Check for signs of respiratory involvement associated with the burn (Figure 13.8):

- Burns around the face
- Patient who has been unconscious in a burning area
- Patient who has been exposed to smoke or hot gases, especially if the burn occurred in a closed space
- Singed nasal hairs
- Sooty sputum
- Hoarseness or cyanosis

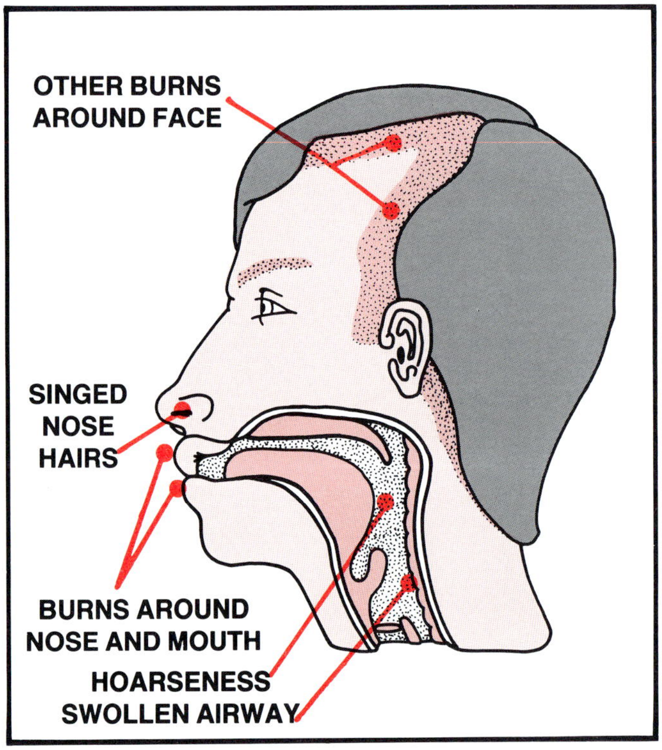


**Figure 13.8** Consider any burn critical if the patient shows signs of respiratory tract involvement.

Assume that anyone who has been in a fire or other smoky atmosphere has damage to the respiratory tract (see Inhalation Injuries below). Damage to the respiratory tract, along with shock, accounts for the majority of deaths in the first 12 hours following burns. Burns in the upper airway produce the same damage to tissues as they do anywhere else in the body; however, swelling of the larynx can rapidly seal off the airway. Administer high-flow oxygen by mask and arrange for immediate transport to a medical facility.

Take the patient's vital signs and monitor them every five minutes. Watch especially for increase in the pulse rate, which can signal impending shock. If the patient does show signs of shock, look for other injuries beside the burns that may cause shock, such as internal injuries. Keep the patient lying down with the legs elevated.

Cover the burns with a dry, sterile dressing. A commercial burn sheet or a sheet that has been sterilized and packaged is good for extensive burns. If you do not have a sterile sheet, cover the patient with a clean sheet. For burned hands and feet, insert sterile gauze pads between fingers and toes (Figure 13.9). If the eyes or eyelids are burned, cover them with sterile, moist dressings.

**NOTE:** Some burn experts prefer that burns be covered with moist dressings. Follow the guidelines in your local jurisdiction.

FIRST-DEGREE BURNS. First-degree burns can be very painful, but are usually not fatal unless they involve very large areas of the body. Within 15 to 30 minutes of the injury, immerse the burned area in cool water. Apply cool, wet towels to burns of the face and trunk. Do not cool too much of the body at once or you may cause the patient to develop chills. After cooling the burn, cover it with a dry, sterile dressing.

**CAUTION:** NEVER PUT CREAMS, OINTMENTS, PETROLEUM JELLY, BUTTER, OR ANYTHING GOOEY ON A BURN. Ointments or creams can help trap heat in the burn. Moreover, anything put on a burn will only have to be scrubbed off in the emergency room, at considerable extra pain to the patient. If someone has already put butter or petroleum jelly on the burn (many people still mistakenly believe that this treatment helps), cool the burn and cover it with a dry, sterile dressing.

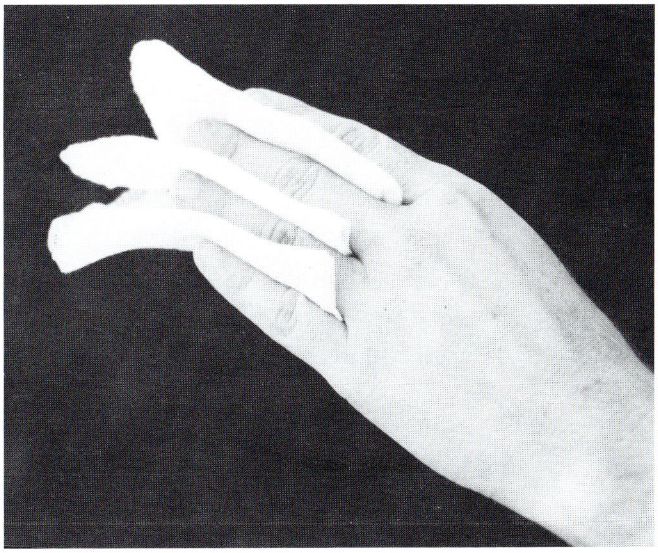

**Figure 13.9** Insert sterile gauze pads between burned fingers or toes.

SECOND-DEGREE BURNS. Second-degree burns are also very painful, unless they are deep enough to cause significant nerve damage. Treatment of second-degree burns is very similar to that of first-degree burns. Immerse the burned area in cool water or apply a cool compress. DO NOT apply ice directly to a burn; wrap the ice before applying it to the skin. Be careful not to break any blisters that may have formed; blisters form a sterile dressing. Cover the burned area with a dry, sterile dressing or a clean sheet.

THIRD-DEGREE BURNS. It is not always possible to distinguish between a deep second-degree burn and third-degree burn in the field. In addition, people usually have combination burns — some parts of the burn second degree, some parts third degree. A characteristic of third-degree burns is diminished pain or absence of pain due to destruction of nerve endings. Once again, cool the burn and cover it with a dry, sterile dressing or burn sheet. Remember that skin that has suffered extensive damage is no longer able to help regulate body temperature and protect against infection. If necessary, cover the patient with a blanket, not to add heat, but to help prevent a loss of heat. Covering the burn also helps keep air (and bacteria) away from the body.

After assessing the patient's ABC's, cooling and dressing the burns, and estimating the extent of the burns, perform a secondary survey. Tend to any associated injuries, such a fractures. DO NOT give anything by mouth.

## Inhalation Injuries

A particularly dangerous complication of thermal burns is injury to the respiratory system or airway, known as an inhalation injury. It has been estimated that up to 80 percent of fire deaths occur from smoke inhalation. The destructive agents causing these injuries are usually products of combustion rather than direct flame. Breathing smoke, toxic gases, or even very hot air can cause injury to the airway, resulting in swelling and extreme difficulty in breathing. An inhalation injury is more likely to occur if the fire is in an enclosed space, such as a house fire, because a higher concentration of toxic gases and smoke is present in the air. An inhalation injury can be very serious, and the patient may require respiratory support until swelling is reduced and he or she is able to breathe independently.

Also present at the scene of a fire are smoke, toxic gases, and superheated air. Smoke inhalation is a silent killer; many victims succumb very quickly. They are often found looking as though they are peacefully asleep.

Smoke from a fire is basically a suspension of small carbon particles and soot. Many times toxic fire gases condense on these smoke particles and enter the respiratory tract. The smaller the particle, the better the chance it will go to the alveoli, where it will do the most damage. If smoke or soot is swallowed, it will irritate the gastrointestinal tract.

Fire also brings elevated temperatures. Ceiling temperatures in a burning room can reach over 1,000°F (538°C). Inhaling superheated air, especially moist superheated air (such as happens after water is applied to a fire), can cause intense burns of the respiratory tract. Pulmonary edema (swelling), which can completely block the airways, results quickly.

Fire gases are the largest contributor to fire deaths (Figure 13.10). Most fire gases are colorless

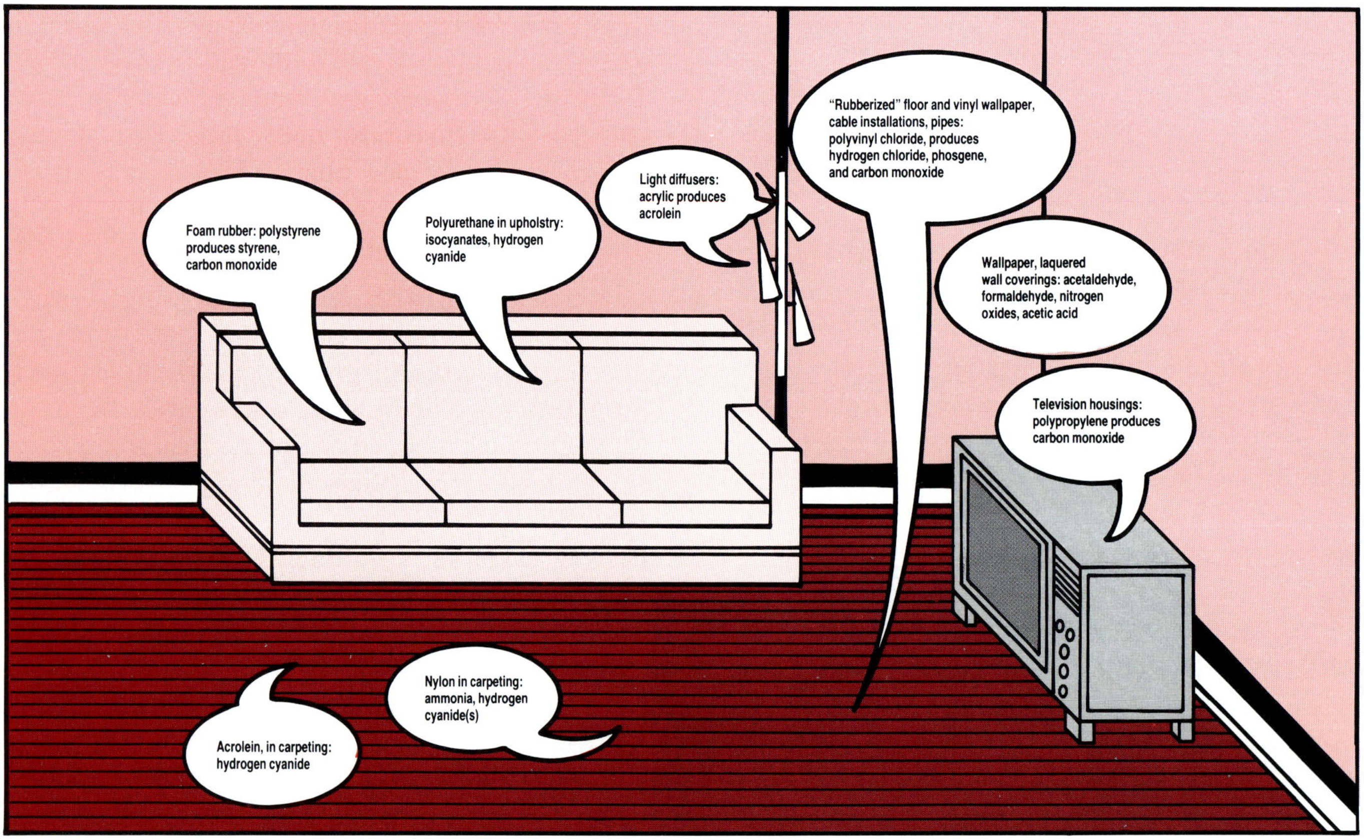


**Figure 13.10** Toxic gases released during combustion are the largest contributors to fire deaths involving inhalation injuries.

and odorless, so it is difficult to tell when the patient has been exposed. Naturally, as a firefighter/first responder, you should know better than to attempt to rescue anyone from a fiery atmosphere without wearing full protective clothing and positive pressure self-contained breathing apparatus.

Carbon monoxide (CO) is a colorless, odorless gas present at almost every fire. CO is present when incomplete combustion occurs, especially during the overhaul phase of fire fighting, when many firefighters remove their SCBA. Hemoglobin has an affinity for CO 250 times greater than for oxygen, so whenever CO is present, the blood would much rather carry it than oxygen. The first sign of exposure to CO is headache. The victim should be removed from the smoky atmosphere and given oxygen in high concentrations by mask (Table 13.1).

**TABLE 13.1**
**TOXIC EFFECTS OF CARBON MONOXIDE**

| CO (Parts per Million) | Percent CO in Air | Symptoms |
|---|---|---|
| 100 | 0.01 | No symptoms — no damage. |
| 200 | 0.02 | Mild headache; few other symptoms. |
| 400 | 0.04 | Headache after 1 to 2 hours. |
| 800 | 0.08 | Headache after 45 minutes; nausea, collapse, and unconsciousness after 2 hours. |
| 1,000 | 0.10 | Dangerous — unconsciousness after 1 hour. |
| 1,600 | 0.16 | Headache, dizziness, nausea after 20 minutes. |
| 3,200 | 0.32 | Headache, dizziness, nausea after 5 to 10 minutes; unconsciousness after 30 minutes. |
| 6,400 | 0.64 | Headache, dizziness, after 1 to 2 minutes; unconsciousness after 10 to 15 minutes. |
| 12,800 | 1.28 | Immediate unconsciousness, danger of death in 1 to 3 minutes. |

Carbon dioxide ($CO_2$) is also present at fires, but at much smaller concentrations than carbon monoxide. $CO_2$ results from complete combustion. The main symptoms of $CO_2$ exposure are dizziness and rapid breathing. (Remember, for healthy people, carbon dioxide levels in the blood provide the stimulus to breathe.)

Another major fire gas is hydrogen chloride (HCL). Any chlorine-based plastic, such as polyvinyl chloride (PVC), will liberate hydrogen chloride gas during a fire. PVC is used as electrical insulation, upholstery material, and in wall coverings. PVC does not burn with a flame as such, but smolders and releases toxic gases. When HCL is inhaled, it becomes hydrochloric acid in the respiratory tract, causing pulmonary edema (swelling) and laryngospasm. HCL not only causes acid burns but also dissolves in the blood stream, acidifying the blood and destroying the blood's ability to carry oxygen. A patient who is conscious and who does not appear to have respiratory tract burns may still have been exposed to HCL. Administer oxygen in high concentrations by mask.

Hydrogen cyanide (HCN) is another major fire gas. HCN is generated when nitrogen-containing substances burn and smolder. Substances that contain nitrogen are nylon and other plastic and synthetic fibers, and some natural fibers, such as wool. The plastic used in telephones is a common source of HCN. HCN interferes with cellular respiration. Very low concentrations can result in weakness, headache, and confusion. Higher concentrations cause collapse and cessation of breathing. Again, treatment is the administration of high-flow oxygen at high concentrations and artificial respiration if necessary.

Formaldehyde and acetaldehyde are gases that attach to carbon and soot particles. They are used as preservatives and may be part of wall coverings or lacquered wood. Exposure to formaldehyde or acetaldehyde causes eye irritation and depression of the central nervous system. Treatment includes high-flow oxygen at high concentrations and rinsing the eyes if necessary.

Formic acid is commonly encountered at fires. It is generated when dyed textiles burn. Formic acid is an eye and nose irritant. It also causes coughing, difficulty in breathing, nausea, and skin burns.

Acrolein can be encountered at plastics or petroleum fires. It is a very potent respiratory, eye, and skin irritant. Inhalation of acrolein can cause delayed pulmonary edema and chronic respiratory disease.

The fire gases mentioned here are by no means a complete list of gases that can be encountered at a fire. In addition, a number of gases are likely to be present at a fire in varying concentrations. These mixed gases result in a combined toxic effect when inhaled. As a firefighter and as a first responder, remember **ALWAYS** to wear SCBA at a fire or when rescuing someone from a fire or toxic atmosphere. The best treatment for inhalation injuries is to administer high-flow, high-concentration oxygen and arrange for rapid transport to a medical facility.

## Chemical Burns

Chemical burns occur when the skin comes in contact with strong acids, alkalies, or other corrosive materials. The burn progresses as long as the corrosive substance remains in contact with the skin. Thus, the cornerstone of therapy for these burns is removal of the chemical from contact with the patient's body.

Chemical burns can be caused by contact with wet or dry chemicals. In general, all wet chemicals should be flushed with water. Dry chemicals should be brushed away unless large quantities of water are available.

Speed is essential when dealing with a chemical burn:

- Flush the burned area with large amounts of water. If the patient is in or around the home, a shower or garden hose is ideal for this purpose. If the patient is on the job, use an industrial shower if one is available. If you use a booster line, apply water at low pressure and use a wide fog pattern.
- Quickly remove any of the patient's clothing that may be contaminated with the chemical, especially shoes, socks, and jewelry. Do not waste any time; if necessary, remove clothing while you are flushing the burned area.
- Continue flushing for at least 15 minutes.
- Prevent personal injury by avoiding skin or clothing contact with the chemical.
- When flushing is complete, cover the burned area with a dry, sterile dressing.
- Do not waste time looking for a specific antidote. Flushing with water is usually more effective, except in special cases involving chemicals that are insoluble in water.

When chemical burns are caused by substances that are not water soluble or that can cause adverse reactions when mixed with water, take the following precautions:

- DRY LIME produces a highly corrosive substance when combined with water. For this reason, remove the patient's clothing and brush the lime from the skin first. Then flush with LARGE (not forceful) amounts of water. Just a small amount of water will do more harm than good.
- Because PHENOL (carbolic acid) is not water soluble, water irrigation alone is largely ineffective. Phenol is soluble in alcohol and in oil (such as vegetable oil or castor oil). Place the patient under running water, wash the affected area with alcohol or oil, and continue flushing with large amounts of water.
- SODIUM METALS and SULFURIC ACID produce considerable heat and are potentially explosive when mixed with water. Unless a hose or shower is available, do not flush with water when dealing with these agents. Cover burns caused by sodium metals with oil; this will stop the reaction. Petroleum jelly is also useful. Wash areas exposed to sulfuric acid with a mild soap, then flush with large amounts of water.

### CHEMICAL BURNS TO THE EYES

Acids, alkalies, chemical powders, and liquid chemicals can cause permanent eye damage or even blindness after very brief contact with the eyes. DO NOT WASTE TIME TRYING TO FIND OUT WHAT CHEMICAL IS IN THE EYE. Immediately begin flushing the eyes with large amounts of gently flowing water and continue flushing for at least 20 minutes. Probably the easiest way to flush the eyes is to support the patient's head under a running faucet (Figure 13.11). You may need to help hold the patient's eyelids open, particularly if he or she is in great pain. Be

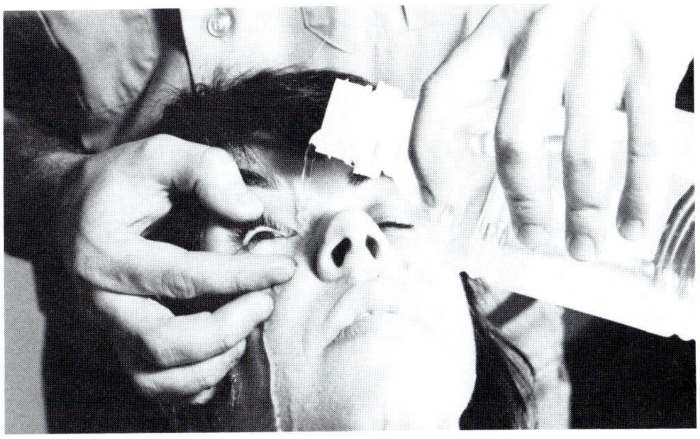

**Figure 13.11** When a chemical comes in contact with the eyes, flush the eyes with gently flowing water for at least 20 minutes.

sure to rinse under the eyelids. Do not use anything but water to flush the eyes. Any contact lenses need to come out as soon as possible, because they will prevent water from reaching the corneas. If the lenses do not come out as you begin flushing, allow the patient to remove them quickly or help the patient remove them. (For more information on removing contact lenses, see Chapter 7, Bleeding Control and Soft-Tissue Injuries.)

## Electrical Burns

Electrical burns occur when the body comes between the source of an electrical charge and the grounding site. When this happens, the body becomes a conductor for the electricity as it flows to the ground. Electrical injuries can be caused by alternating current or direct current. Alternating current is more deadly because it causes severe muscle contractions that can immobilize the victim, causing him or her to be "frozen" to the source of the current.

The skin is nonconductive to low-voltage electricity. If the skin is broken or moist, however, resistance becomes much lower. Electricity does its major damage inside the body, not to the skin itself. This is because electricity is converted into extreme heat as it travels from the point of contact through the body. Low voltage follows the path of least resistance, which is usually the blood vessels. High voltage follows the shortest path. Bones are most resistant to electricity; muscles less so; and blood vessels and nerves are very sensitive to extreme heat. Therefore, massive internal injury to muscles, nerves, tissues, blood vessels, and internal organs is common. Electrical burns commonly cause two surface injuries: an entrance wound where the current enters the body, and an exit wound where the current leaves the body.

In addition to internal damage, electricity often causes respiratory arrest and/or cardiac arrest due to ventricular fibrillation (rapid, ineffective contraction of the cardiac ventricles). For this reason, the patient's ABC's must be stabilized before burns are evaluated.

If you are called to aid someone who has come in contact with an electrical current, your first impulse may be to rush to assist the patient. BE CAUTIOUS OR YOU MAY BECOME A VICTIM YOURSELF. At the scene of the accident, keep the following points in mind:

- The patient may still be in contact with the source of the current (Figure 13.12). Do not endanger yourself by touching the patient, metal objects, water, or wet ground. Unless your department is trained in the use of hot sticks, lineman's gloves, and in moving electrical wires, do not try to provide medical assistance until all electrical hazards have been removed by the power company.

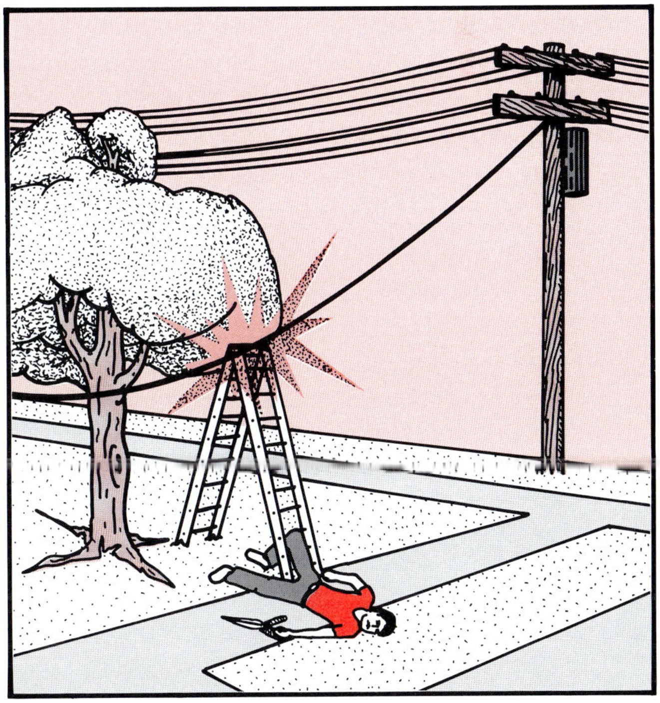

**Figure 13.12** If you have not been trained in handling electrical emergencies, do not try to provide assistance to a victim who is in contact with a source of current until the electrical hazard has been removed by trained personnel.

- Assume that all downed wires are live wires unless informed otherwise by a power company employee.

- Do not touch any wires, power lines, or other electrical sources until they have been deactivated by a power company employee.

- Instruct anyone who is trapped in an automobile by downed power lines to stay inside the car until the power company can turn off the power source and remove the lines.

As soon as the patient can be safely moved from the source of the injury, LOOK TO THE ABC's FIRST BEFORE YOU LOOK AT THE BURNS. It is more than likely that the patient has suffered respiratory or cardiac arrest from electric current passing through the body. Open the patient's airway using the modified jaw-thrust maneuver (assume a spinal cord injury), determine if the patient is breathing, and administer CPR if necessary. Often, a patient who appears dead can be revived by rapid attention to the ABC's.

Once the patient's vital signs are stabilized, examine the burns as part of the secondary survey. Always look for both an entrance wound and an exit wound on a patient with an electrical burn. Both entrance and exit wounds may resemble a bull's-eye, with a central charred zone of third-degree burns; a middle zone of cold, gray tissue; and an outer red zone. Cool the burns, then cover them with a dry, sterile dressing. Arrange for immediate transport to a medical facility. Remember, ALL electrical burns are serious and must be evaluated in a medical facility.

Two other types of electrical injuries, flash burns and flame burns, do not produce the extensive internal injuries that result when electricity passes through the body. Flash burns usually result from an arc of electricity. Although the duration of the flash may be brief, it usually causes extensive superficial injuries. Flame burns result when clothing or objects in direct contact with the skin are ignited by an electrical current. Treat these burns the same as similar thermal burns.

### LIGHTNING INJURIES

Most lightning injuries occur as a result of the "splash" of lightning from a nearby tree or other conducting object rather than as the result of a direct hit. Although the voltage from a bolt of lightning far exceeds that from a power line, the current is direct rather than alternating, and the time of exposure is very brief (less than one second).

Basically, treatment of injuries from lightning is the same as for other types of electrical burns. Again, LOOK TO THE ABC's FIRST BEFORE YOU LOOK AT THE BURNS. Open the patient's airway using the jaw-thrust maneuver (assume a spinal cord injury), determine if the patient is breathing, and administer CPR if necessary. Victims of lightning strikes often suffer temporary amnesia, so watch the patient's level of consciousness carefully. Cover any burns, which often have a zigzag pattern, with dry, sterile dressings. Arrange for immediate transport to a medical facility.

# 14

# Injuries and Illnesses From Heat and Cold

**U.S. DEPARTMENT OF TRANSPORTATION**
**First Responder Training Course**

**Objectives:**

- Given descriptions of patients exposed to heat and cold, identify the condition and describe emergency care procedures.

# Chapter 14
# Injuries and Illnesses from Heat and Cold

The body is divided into two functional areas for temperature control: a core and a shell. The core includes part of the skeletal muscle and the contents of the body cavities: the skull, vertebral column, thorax (chest), abdomen, and pelvis. The shell is the area where heat transfer between the body and the environment occurs; it includes the skin and tissues beneath the skin.

To function properly, the body must maintain its core temperature at 98.6°F (37°C). When it is hot, the body sheds excess heat by dilating blood vessels near the skin and by perspiring. When it is cold, the body conserves heat by increasing heat production and decreasing heat loss.

## HEAT ILLNESS

Exposure to excessive heat may result in heat cramps, heat exhaustion, or heat stroke. People who are most likely to be affected by excessive heat are the very young, the aged, obese people, alcoholics, and those who suffer from any disease that impairs body strength. Temperatures over 95°F (35°C) and high humidity are particularly dangerous for those vulnerable to heat illnesses. Even people who are in good physical condition can suffer heat illnesses if they overexert themselves.

A hot environment is one that is above normal room temperature 77°F (25°C). When the environmental temperature rises, heat produced through metabolism accumulates in the body. To lose this heat, the body employs several processes. First, the body sends heat to the surface by dilating blood vessels near the skin, which allows heat to dissipate in the atmosphere. When the outside temperature rises above body temperature, however, there is no longer enough temperature difference for this process to be effective. Then the body turns to another means of ridding itself of the excess heat: evaporation of water. Water evaporates from both the large airways (the breath) and the skin surface (sweat).

How much water evaporates from the airways and the skin depends upon the relative humidity, that is, the amount of water vapor in the air compared to the maximum amount that *could* be in the air. As the relative humidity rises, less water evaporates from the body. In contrast, when the relative humidity is low (and the air is dry), more water evaporates. Thus, hot, dry climates are more comfortable than hot, humid climates.

The evaporation of sweat from the skin is also affected by the amount of clothing worn and the rate of air flow past the skin surface. Wearing fewer clothes increases water evaporation from the skin; wearing more clothes decreases water evaporation. Likewise, greater air flow, such as that from a fan or breeze, increases water evaporation and less air flow decreases it.

Sweat is a diluted solution of sodium chloride (common salt). A normal adult can sweat about one liter per hour. This sweat effectively reduces body temperature but depletes the body of water and sodium.

### Heat Cramps

Heat cramps are muscle pains, usually in the legs or abdomen, that result when profuse sweating depletes the body of salt. Heat cramps usually afflict people in good physical condition who overexert themselves in sports or overwork when the heat and humidity are high. Heat cramps usually begin suddenly during vigorous activity. They may be mild, with only slight abdominal cramping and tingling in the extremities. Often, however, they produce severe and incapacitating pain in the extremities and abdomen. The patient may become hypotensive and nauseated, but the patient's mind will remain clear. The pulse is generally rapid and the skin pale and moist, but the patient's temperature is usually normal. If untreated, heat cramps may progress to heat exhaustion.

Treat heat cramps by getting the patient out of the heat and helping to restore the patient's lost salt and water.

- Move the patient to a cool place.
- If the patient is not nauseated, give one to two glasses of salt-containing solution, such as lemonade with a half teaspoon of salt added, or commercial drinks that contain sodium, such as Gatorade or Take Five. Have the patient drink slowly.
- Do not give salt tablets because they may cause or worsen nausea.
- Massage the patient's legs if it brings relief. Some patients may want to "walk it off."
- If the patient is nauseated, he or she needs replacement fluids administered intravenously.
- As salt and water are replaced, the patient's symptoms should disappear. Strongly advise the patient not to return to strenuous activity for at least 12 hours. The patient may want to resume earlier activities, but you should make it clear that further exertion may lead to heat exhaustion or heat stroke, both much more serious conditions.

## Heat Exhaustion

Heat exhaustion, also known as heat prostration, also results from excessive water and salt loss due to heavy sweating. Like heat cramps, heat exhaustion also tends to occur in persons working or exercising in hot environments. Particularly at risk are elderly, dehydrated individuals, and people who are taking diuretic medications (which eliminate fluid). The elderly are more prone to heat exhaustion because of their diminished thirst mechanism, which tends to reduce their intake of fluids even when they are dehydrated.

Because heat exhaustion is caused by loss of fluid, the signs and symptoms are those of mild hypovolemic shock. The patient is perspiring profusely, the skin is pale and clammy, the pulse is rapid and weak, and breathing is usually rapid and shallow. Blood pressure may be decreased due to peripheral pooling of the blood, and the pupils may be dilated. The patient may also be somewhat disoriented. Body temperature is either normal or decreased.

Heat exhaustion may come on suddenly, with syncope (fainting) and collapse, or may begin with such symptoms as headache, fatigue, dizziness, nausea, and sometimes, abdominal cramping. Untreated heat exhaustion may progress to heat stroke.

To treat the patient suffering from heat exhaustion

Step 1: Move the patient to a cool place, take off as much of the patient's clothing as possible, and place him or her supine, with the legs elevated.

Step 2: Sponge the patient with cold water or alcohol, and fan the patient if the humidity is not excessively high. Do not chill the patient, just make him or her comfortably cool.

Step 3: If the patient is nauseated, do not give fluids by mouth.

Step 4: Monitor vital signs every five minutes and arrange for transportation to a medical facility.

If the patient fails to recover rapidly, vomits, has diarrhea, or suffers from a medical condition (such as heart or lung disease), consider heat exhaustion an emergency. Arrange for immediate transportation to a medical facility.

## Heat Stroke

Heat stroke, also called sun stroke, is the least common but the most serious heat illness. Heat stroke is caused by a severe disturbance in the body's heat-regulating mechanism. It is a dire emergency with a mortality rate of 25 to 50 percent. The same situation that places individuals at risk of heat cramps and heat exhaustion — overexertion in a hot, humid environment — also places people at risk of heat stroke. People who are elderly, obese, alcoholic, or who suffer from chronic illnesses such as heart disease or diabetes are particularly susceptible to heat stroke. Individuals who take diuretics or tranquilizers are also vulnerable. These people, who often become ill during heat waves, at first sweat profusely to dissipate excess heat but eventually become too dehydrated to sweat any more and their core body temperature rises rapidly.

Another group of people who often suffer heat strokes are younger, athletic individuals who exercise vigorously in hot, humid weather. The humidity in the atmosphere prevents sweat from evaporating, and continued exercise produces heat faster than the body can dissipate it. Although this individual is not usually dehydrated and may even be sweating heavily, he or she collapses because the body's cooling mechanisms have become overwhelmed.

The signs and symptoms of heat stroke can develop very rapidly. As the body's sweating mechanism fails, the body's core temperature rises rapidly, reaching 105° or 106°F (40°C or 41°C). The patient becomes disoriented, confused, delirious, or lapses into coma because the brain cells cannot cope with such high temperatures. The skin is hot and dry, and may be flushed or ashen. The pulse is very rapid and bounding, but may become thready due to vasomotor collapse. Respirations are very rapid.

**HEAT STROKE IS A TRUE EMERGENCY. ACT QUICKLY OR THE PATIENT WILL SUFFER IRREVERSIBLE BRAIN DAMAGE OR DEATH.**

To treat the patient suffering from heat stroke

Step 1: COOL THE PATIENT DOWN AS RAPIDLY AS POSSIBLE. This is the most important step you can take to save the patient's life. Move the patient to a cool environment and take off as much of his or her clothing as possible. If the patient is found in the home, immediately start running cold water in the bathtub and immerse the patient up to the neck. Add as many ice cubes as you can find to the water. Send relatives and bystanders to get more ice. If the patient is outside or there is no bathtub available, use a garden hose or booster line and recruit others to bring crushed ice. Rub the ice on the patient's body and rub the extremities to stimulate blood flow to the body's surface.

Step 2: ADMINISTER OXYGEN by mask to help relieve the strain on the heart and on the brain. Remember, brain cells are those first affected by lack of oxygen, and the heart needs much more oxygen than usual when the body's temperature is high.

Step 3: If you have a thermometer, take the patient's temperature. Continue cooling efforts until the patient's temperature is below 102°F (39°C). DO NOT COOL THE PATIENT SO MUCH THAT HE OR SHE BEGINS TO SHIVER. Shivering is one way the body produces heat, which is the last thing the patient needs right now.

Step 4: Continue to monitor vital signs frequently and arrange for rapid transport to a medical facility.

Table 14.1 summarizes emergencies due to heat exposure.

## INJURIES FROM COLD

The human body can be as seriously damaged by excessive cold as it can by excessive heat. Because humans have only limited protection against cold temperatures, they must wear warm clothing, build shelters, and heat their homes. When people find themselves in cold temperatures without adequate protection, they can suffer surface damage to the skin, known as frostbite, or general cooling of the body, known as hypothermia. Frostbite, if severe, can lead to tissue death (gangrene) and necessitate amputation of the frozen tissue. Hypother-

**TABLE 14.1**
**EMERGENCIES DUE TO HEAT EXPOSURE**

| | HEAT CRAMPS | HEAT EXHAUSTION | HEAT STROKE |
|---|---|---|---|
| Cause | Salt and water loss | Salt and water loss | Failure of body's heat-regulating mechanism |
| Cramping | Yes, especially in legs and abdomen | Possibly, especially in abdomen | No |
| State of conciousness | Alert | May be disoriented | Disoriented, delirious, or unconscious |
| Skin | Cool, moist | Cool, pale, moist | Hot and dry; Flushed or may be ashen |
| Temperature | Normal | Normal or low | Very high |
| Pulse | Rapid | Rapid and weak | Rapid, bounding |
| Blood pressure | May be low | May be low | May be high |
| Treatment | Move patient to a cool place<br>Give salt and water if patient is not nauseated | Move patient to a cool place<br>Place patient lying down; remove as much clothing as possible<br>Sponge patient with cold water or alcohol<br>Do not give fluids if patient is nauseated<br>Monitor vital signs | **COOL PATIENT AS RAPIDLY AS POSSIBLE:** place patient in a cold bath or shower and rub ice on patient's body<br>Administer oxygen by mask<br>Arrange for rapid transport to a medical facility |

mia is a life-threatening condition that results when the body's core temperature cools as a result of exposure to cold.

The main factors that influence the extent of cold injuries are temperature, length of exposure, thermal conductivity of the environment, and wind. Particularly dangerous is cold, wet, windy weather (Figure 14.1).

Anything that is warm radiates heat into the surrounding air, so people lose body heat when they are in temperatures cooler than their bodies. Heat is lost rapidly from above the shoulders; it is estimated that 50 percent of the heat generated by the body can be lost if the head and neck are uncovered.

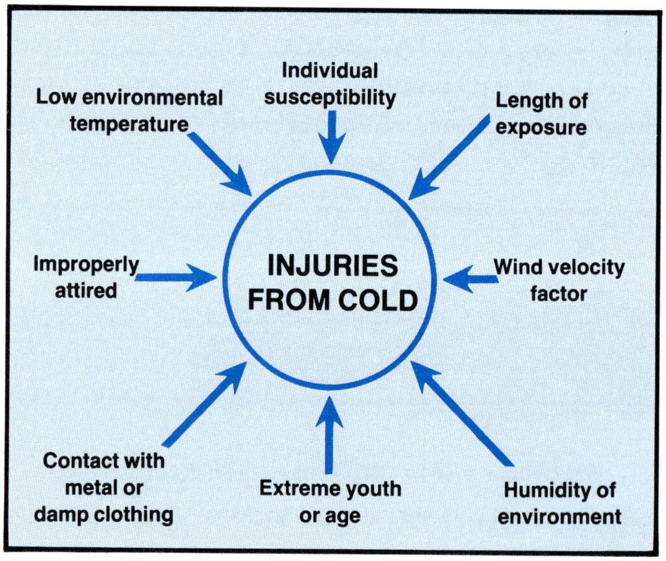


**Figure 14.1** Many factors influence the likelihood and extent of cold injuries.

Another way heat is lost is when cooler air moves over the body. Still air is a very poor conductor of heat, which is why a person in dry clothes standing in a windless area can tolerate colder temperatures better than a person in a damp atmosphere with a moderate wind. Wind, however, is much more efficient at removing heat. This is why wind chill factors are given along with temperatures when it is cold (Figure 14.2). Wind chill factors measure the cooling power of the temperature plus the wind. For example, a temperature of 15°F (-9°C) has a cooling power of 15°F (-9°C); if this same temperature is accompanied by a 10 mph (16 km/h) wind, the temperature has a cooling power of -2°F (-19°C).

**INDEX OF WIND-CHILL FACTOR**
(IN DEGREES FAHRENHEIT)

| TEMPERATURE (Degrees Fahrenheit) | WIND SPEED (MPH) | | | | | | | | |
|---|---|---|---|---|---|---|---|---|---|
| | CALM | 5 | 10 | 15 | 20 | 25 | 30 | 35 | 40 |
| 35 | 35 | 33 | 21 | 16 | 12 | 7 | 5 | 3 | 1 |
| 30 | 30 | 27 | 16 | 11 | 3 | 0 | −2 | −4 | −4 |
| 25 | 25 | 21 | 9 | 1 | −4 | −7 | −11 | −13 | −15 |
| 20 | 20 | 16 | 2 | −6 | −9 | −15 | −18 | −20 | −22 |
| 15 | 15 | 12 | −2 | −11 | −17 | −22 | −26 | −27 | −29 |
| 10 | 10 | 7 | −9 | −18 | −24 | −29 | −33 | −35 | −36 |
| 5 | 5 | 1 | −15 | −25 | −32 | −37 | −41 | −43 | −45 |
| 0 | 0 | −6 | −22 | −33 | −40 | −45 | −49 | −52 | −54 |
| −5 | −5 | −11 | −27 | −40 | −46 | −52 | −56 | −60 | −62 |
| −10 | −10 | −15 | −31 | −45 | −52 | −58 | −63 | −67 | −69 |
| −15 | −15 | −20 | −38 | −51 | −60 | −67 | −70 | −72 | −76 |
| −20 | −20 | −26 | −45 | −60 | −68 | −75 | −78 | −83 | −87 |
| −25 | −25 | −31 | −52 | −65 | −76 | −83 | −87 | −90 | −94 |
| −30 | −30 | −35 | −58 | −70 | −81 | −89 | −94 | −98 | −101 |

COLD · VERY COLD · BITTER COLD · EXTREME COLD

**Figure 14.2** The wind-chill factor measures the cooling power of the temperature plus the wind.

Finally, water conducts heat much more rapidly than air does, so heat leaves the body much faster if a person has on wet clothing or is in the water. Clothing that is damp from snow, rain, or perspiration will conduct heat away from the body rapidly.

## How the Body Conserves Heat

Remember that the body must conserve its core temperature of 98.6°F (37°C). When it is cold, the body seeks to maintain its core temperature by increasing heat production, and by decreasing heat loss.

To increase heat production, the body steps up its rate of metabolism, which is the breakdown of food to produce energy. Another way to increase heat production is by an increase in muscle activity. Walking, running, or moving about are voluntary ways to increase heat production. Shivering, which is an involuntary muscle activity, also significantly increases heat production.

The body has several ways to decrease heat loss. First, blood vessels near the skin constrict, which reduces blood flow in skin capillaries and, thus, reduces heat loss from them. In cold temperatures, the skin can become as much as 15 degrees colder than the body's core temperature. In addition, sweating is reduced or stopped altogether.

## Hypothermia

Hypothermia — an abnormally low internal body temperature caused by exposure to cold — kills thousands of people each year. Although hypothermia is most often encountered in winter, it can also be a problem anytime people fall into cold water. Remember, cold water conducts heat away from the body much faster than cold air does, so people in warmer climates can also suffer hypothermia.

Hypothermia does not result from outdoor exposure alone. It can also occur as a result of cool indoor temperatures. At greatest risk are the elderly, who probably account for nearly half of all hypothermia victims. Factors such as living alone, low income, poor diet, other illnesses, limited physical activity, and use of alcohol or certain prescription drugs place many older persons at greater risk of hypothermia. Hypothermia can also worsen preexisting conditions and diseases in older people.

Other people at increased risk of hypothermia are alcoholics who fall asleep outside; sedated by the effects of alcohol, they slip into coma and death. Mountaineers, skiers, and anyone working outdoors in the cold can suffer hypothermia if not adequately protected from the cold.

When the body core temperature falls below 93°F (34°C), the body's regulatory systems begin to fail (Table 14.2). The respiratory control center becomes depressed, oxygen consumption and carbon dioxide production slow as metabolism decreases. Because lowered metabolism produces less heat, the core temperature falls further. Progressive loss of consciousness occurs when the body's core temperature falls below 86°F (30°C). As the victim of hypothermia cools (and so do the brain cells), he or she becomes lethargic, apathetic, and profoundly sleepy. People usually lose consciousness when the body core temperature falls to 81°F (27°C). Cardiac arrhythmias (irregularities in the rhythm of the heartbeat) are also common at this stage. The lowest temperature one can survive in is usually considered to be about 73°F (23°C), although most people suffering from hypothermia die sooner. One survival has been reported, however, in a patient whose core temperature plummeted to 50°F (10°C), so victims of hypothermia merit revival attempts even if they appear to be dead. The general rule is that the patient should be considered alive until he or she has been rewarmed and is pronounced dead.

**TABLE 14.2**
**LEVELS OF HYPOTHERMIA**

| °F | °C | |
|---|---|---|
| 99.6 | 37.6 | Normal rectal temperature |
| 98.6 | 37 | Normal oral temperature |
| 96.8 | 36 | Body increases heat production through increased metabolic rate, shivering |
| 95 | 35 | Maximum shivering |
| 93 | 34 | Patients usually responsive; blood pressure normal |
| 91.4 | 33 | SEVERE HYPOTHERMIA BELOW THIS TEMPERATURE |
| 89.6 | 32 | Consciousness clouded; shivering stops; muscles rigid |
| 85.2 | 29 | Slow pulse and respirations |
| 81 | 27 | Patients usually unconscious; heartbeat may be irregular; rough handling may cause heart to fibrillate |
| 80.6 | 27 | Patients appear dead — pupils do not react to light |
| 77 | 25 | Heart may fibrillate spontaneously |
| 68 | 20 | Heartbeat stops |

The body's core temperature can drop in minutes in cold water, in hours outside in cold weather, or over several days in an underheated house or apartment. Suspect possible hypothermia in all patients, particularly elderly patients, who have altered mental states and who have been exposed to the cold. In addition, suspect hypothermia in anyone who has been accidentally submerged in water.

### CARE AND TREATMENT FOR THE PATIENT WITH HYPOTHERMIA

The patient who is still conscious is considered to be suffering from mild to moderate hypothermia. He or she may have pale, cold skin, be shivering, or act listless. First of all, **GET THE PATIENT OUT OF THE COLD IN ORDER TO PREVENT A FURTHER DROP IN THE BODY'S CORE TEMPERATURE. ARRANGE FOR IMMEDIATE TRANSPORT TO A MEDICAL FACILITY.** To prepare the patient for transport, remove all wet clothing and replace it with dry clothing. HANDLE THE PATIENT GENTLY. DO NOT rub the patient's arms or legs. Keep the patient laying down and wrapped in blankets, a sleeping bag, or any other insulating materials. Be sure to cover the head and neck because 50 percent of the body's heat can be lost through the head. Leave the face uncovered. These actions are designed not to raise the patient's body core temperature, but rather to keep the core temperature from dropping further.

If additional medical help is not immediately available, begin to add external heat. Apply hot water bottles or heating pads to the patient's head, neck, chest, and groin. DO NOT place heating devices directly on the patient's skin because they may cause burns. Wrap the bottles or pads in a towel first. DO NOT apply heat to the extremities.

The effectiveness of giving a hypothermic patient warm liquids to drink is disputed. If you do give warm liquids, do so only after the uncontrollable shivering stops, the patient has a clear level of consciousness, the ability to swallow, and evidence of rewarming. The patient can drink warm liquids that have sugar in them, such as warm apple juice. DO NOT give coffee or alcohol. DO NOT allow the patient to smoke because smoking constricts blood vessels.

Attempting to rewarm a hypothermic patient in the field can be very difficult. Follow your local guidelines for attempting to rewarm a mildly hypothermic patient. Some areas recommend placing the patient in a warm bath. If you are instructed to do so, place the patient in a warm bath of 105° to 110°F (40°C to 43°C). You will have to use a thermometer to maintain water temperature, and continue to add hot water to the bath so that the water does not cool.

When it is time to transport the patient, be sure that he or she is wrapped warmly from head to toe.

Severe hypothermia, which occurs when the patient's core temperature drops below 91°F (33°C), has a high mortality rate. If the patient is still semiconscious, he or she will likely be severely disoriented, possibly deranged. At this stage shivering has stopped, muscles are rigid, and the victim's skin feels ice cold. Unconsciousness and coma follow shortly and the victim appears dead, or nearly so.

First of all, as with mild hypothermia, get the patient out of the cold and wind and arrange for immediate transport to a medical facility. **WARNING:** HANDLE THE PATIENT VERY, VERY GENTLY, AS THOUGH EVERY BONE IN HIS OR HER BODY IS BROKEN. The heart is very irritable at this stage, and rough handling or manipulation can cause the heart to fibrillate. Very carefully cut wet clothing off and replace it with dry, warm clothing.

Begin to take the patient's vital signs. Take them for at least one to three minutes because vital signs are very difficult to obtain in the severely hypothermic patient. Pupils are often dilated and nonreactive to light. It may be impossible to obtain a blood pressure because cold tissue does not conduct sounds well. Respirations can be as slow as two or three per minute. Likewise, the heart may be beating very, very slowly. Maintain an open airway but do not use airway adjuncts; too much stimulation of the throat can cause the heart to fibrillate. If your local guidelines dictate it, assist respirations at a slow rate (about 10 per minute) using a bag-valve mask.

If the patient has any regular heartbeat, do not begin CPR. Chest compressions on a patient whose heart is still beating may cause the heart to fibrillate. If you are sure that the victim has no pulse or respirations, begin CPR and continue it, even if the patient does not respond within several minutes.

**REMEMBER THAT, EVEN THOUGH A HYPOTHERMIC PATIENT MAY APPEAR LIFELESS, THE PATIENT SHOULD NOT BE PRESUMED DEAD UNTIL HE OR SHE HAS BEEN REWARMED AND PRONOUNCED DEAD.**

If you are instructed to do so, apply external heat in the same manner as for a mildly hypothermic patient. The purpose of adding external heat is to help prevent the body's core temperature from dropping further, not to actually rewarm the patient. Rewarming should be carried out very carefully in a medical facility.

As with any other semiconscious or unconscious patient, watch what you say around the patient. People who seem to be unconscious may be able to remember conversations. Do not add to the patient's distress by making unprofessional remarks.

### IMMERSION HYPOTHERMIA

As a member of the fire department, you will likely be called to assist in removing someone who has fallen into water. While it is important that the victim be removed from the water as rapidly as possible, take precautions so that you, too, do not become a victim. First, call for extra assistance; several people may end up wet and cold. Wear a life jacket and do not venture out onto the ice or into the water without a rope around your waist that is

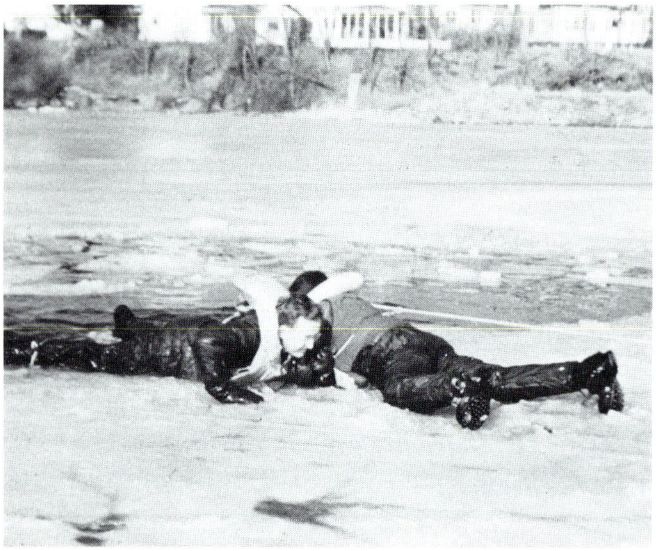

**Figure 14.3** When attempting rescue, do not venture onto the ice or into the water without a rope around the waist that is securely tied off. *Courtesy of Cranston, R.I. Fire Department.*

securely tied off (Figure 14.3). If you are making an ice rescue, only the people necessary for the rescue should be on the ice. If necessary, spread weight out by using a ladder. Keep in mind that, with cold water rescue, you have to go to the victim. Throwing ropes or flotation devices usually does not work because the victim is too cold to hold on to anything.

When water temperature is 50°F (10°C) or below, someone who accidentally becomes submerged can develop hypothermia in a very few minutes. The reason for this rapid onset of cooling is that water conducts heat away from the body much faster than air does. Moreover, temperature changes caused by submersion require that the patient be handled very carefully after being pulled out from the water.

After being removed from cold water, a victim's body core temperature continues to drop, a process known as *afterdrop*. Any exertion can increase afterdrop because it causes very cold blood in the extremities to be pumped back to the body core. Therefore, do not allow the victim to move at all if possible. As with other types of hypothermia, handle the victim very, very gently and arrange for rapid transport to a medical facility. Get the patient out of the cold and wind, and carefully remove wet clothing. Wrap the patient in warm, dry clothing and begin to apply external heat as discussed earlier. Do not give liquids if the patient is not fully conscious.

Monitor vital signs frequently, assist respirations, and add external heat as for other hypothermia victims.

## Local Injuries from Cold: Frostbite

Frostbite is the freezing or partial freezing of some part of the body due to exposure to prolonged or intense cold. Areas of the body that are unprotected or inadequately protected are most likely to develop frostbite. The nose, ears, cheeks, fingers, and toes are most often affected by the cold. Not only are these areas often uncovered or wet in the cold, they are also far from the warmer body core. Wearing too-tight gloves or shoes, which can restrict circulation, can also increase the chances of developing frostbite.

There are varying degrees of frostbite, each of which results in varying degrees of tissue injury. The mildest form of frostbite is known as frostnip, followed by superficial frostbite, and deep frostbite or freezing.

With frostnip, the skin first becomes red and inflamed, then blanches (turns gray or mottled white). Frostnip is not usually painful as it develops, and the patient is often unaware of it until someone else notices abnormally pale skin color.

To treat frostnip, get the patient out of the cold and warm the affected area by applying firm pressure with your hand. If the fingers are affected, have the patient place them into his or her armpit. As the tissue warms up, it may become red and tingle, but tissue damage is unlikely.

Actual frostbite, whether it is superficial or deep, has the potential for serious tissue damage. In fact, tissue can be damaged so badly that gangrene (tissue death) develops, necessitating amputation of the affected part.

Superficial frostbite is characterized by skin that is white, waxy, and numb. As it begins to thaw, blisters form; these blisters may be clear, red, or very dark, depending on whether or not there has been hemorrhage. If you press the affected part, it feels hard but the tissues below remain soft.

Deep frostbite is characterized by skin that is *very hard*, ice cold, and completely insensitive to the touch. If you press the affected part, the underlying tissues also feel hard. It can be very difficult to determine whether frostbite is superficial or deep. If in doubt, treat it as deep frostbite.

First, get the patient out of the cold and arrange for immediate transport to a medical facility. Handle the affected part very gently. Carefully remove any surrounding clothing and dry the tissues.

**NEVER, NEVER RUB ANY FROSTBITTEN AREA. NEVER RUB SNOW ON FROSTBITTEN TISSUES.**

The human body is 70 percent water, and when it is exposed to excessive cold, the water in the cells literally begins to freeze and form ice crystals. These ice crystals can damage or destroy cells. Rubbing or massaging the skin causes the ice crystals to do even more tissue damage.

DO NOT break any blisters that may have formed. Blisters are a type of sterile dressing, similar to the blisters from a second-degree burn. Place sterile cotton between fingers and toes, and cover the area with a dry, sterile dressing. Elevate the frostbitten part. If the patient's foot or leg is frostbitten, do not allow him or her to bear weight on it.

Some authorities advocate thawing superficial frostbite in a warm water bath; follow the guidelines in your jurisdiction. DO NOT attempt rewarming for superficial or deep frostbite if there is any chance that the tissues will be refrozen. The damage done to tissues if they are partially thawed and then refrozen is much more severe than if the tissues are left frozen. Additional damage occurs because the new ice crystals formed in the tissues during refreezing are larger than the original crystals, so more tissue is affected.

To thaw frostbitten tissue, submerge it in water that is approximately 106°F (41°C). You will have to use a thermometer and continue to add hot water so that the warming bath does not cool. Leave the part immersed for 20 to 30 minutes. Do not allow the patient to smoke because nicotine constricts the blood vessels, further reducing blood flow to the affected area. As the area thaws, the patient experiences burning, often very intense pain, and the tissues become very tender. After thawing, carefully dry the warmed area and cover it with a dry, sterile dressing. Place sterile cotton between fingers and toes.

In the case of deep frostbite, if you are less than an hour to a medical facility, leave the part frozen. Remove any wet clothing and carefully dry the affected area. Wrap it in dry, sterile dressings, and transport immediately.

If the frostbitten area has already begun to thaw, or medical help is several hours away, you may be instructed to attempt rewarming in the field. Follow the same procedures as for rewarming superficially frostbitten tissue.

# 15

# Emergency Childbirth

**U.S. DEPARTMENT OF TRANSPORTATION**
**First Responder Training Course**

**Objectives:**

- Describe procedures to follow in preparing for and assisting in normal and abnormal childbirths including caring for the mother and newborn.
- Define breech birth and prolapsed cord.
- Describe procedures to follow in the event of excessive bleeding and miscarriage.

# Chapter 15
# Emergency Childbirth

Assisting in the birth of a baby is one of the few situations in which the first responder has the opportunity to participate in a happy event, rather than one associated with illness or trauma. Childbirth is also unique in that there are two patients instead of one, each of whom requires trained care.

For the first responder, the term emergency childbirth usually refers to a normal, uncomplicated childbirth that occurs in an unexpected place. Babies are unpredictable, and do not always wait to be born until their parents have had time to reach a medical facility.

Although childbirth is an exciting event, it is also a stressful one. It is likely to become even more stressful if the mother realizes that she will not deliver her baby in the controlled surroundings of a hospital or birthing center. The mother may become even more distressed if the baby decides to arrive in a car or public place. Your job will be to reassure the mother and to provide as clean and safe an environment for childbirth as the circumstances allow.

Pregnancy and childbirth are normally pleasantly uneventful, although complications can and do occur, necessitating quick action and rapid transport to a medical facility. This chapter begins with an overview of reproduction and a brief discussion of pregnancy and complications of pregnancy that require emergency intervention. The section on childbirth covers preparation for and handling a normal delivery, followed by abnormal deliveries that usually require rapid transport to a medical facility. The chapter concludes with a discussion of possible complications after delivery that relate to both mother and baby.

## REPRODUCTION

The female reproductive system includes the ovaries, fallopian tubes, uterus, and vagina (Figure 15.1). The ovaries are two walnut-shaped organs that lie in the right and left lower quadrants. The ovaries are responsible for producing sex hormones, which not only affect the menstrual cycle,

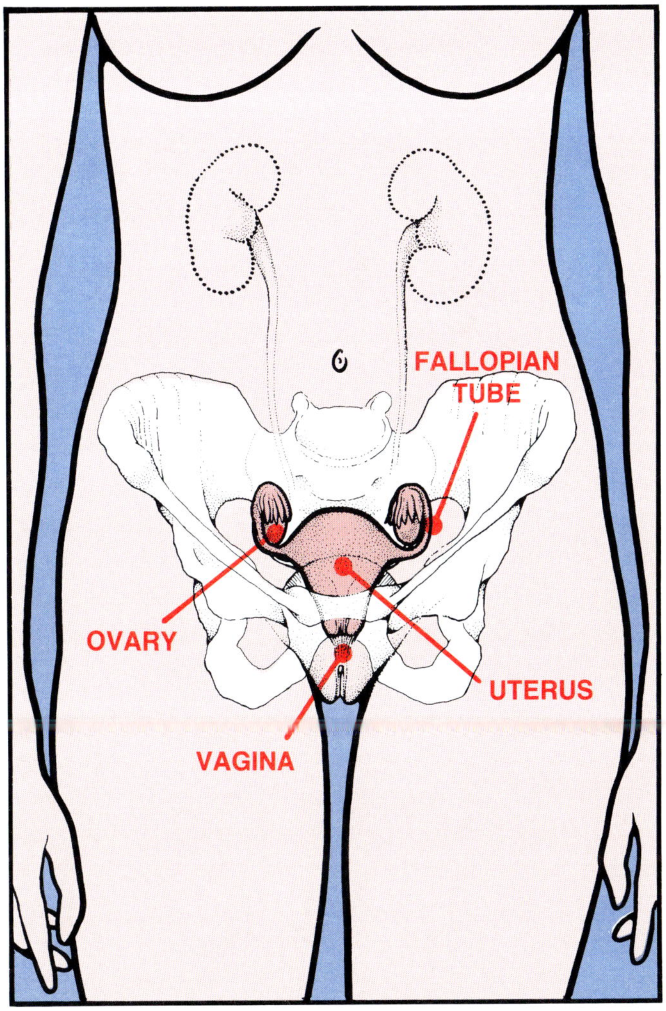


**Figure 15.1** The major organs of the female reproductive system are shown above.

but also give women their characteristic female appearance. The ovaries also produce eggs, or ova (one egg is an ovum).

After the egg is released from an ovary, it travels through the fallopian tubes, which open into the uterus. At the lower end of the uterus is the cervix, which connects the uterus with the vagina. During sexual intercourse, male sperm cells travel from the vagina through the cervix and up to the fallopian tubes, where fertilization takes place if there is an egg waiting.

The ovaries release one mature ovum, or egg, about once a month during the reproductive years. This monthly cycle of physical and hormonal changes associated with the production of eggs is known as the menstrual cycle. During the early part of the menstrual cycle, the endometrium (the inner lining of the uterus) thickens to prepare for a fertilized egg. Approximately two weeks after the last menstrual period, an ovary releases a mature egg, which travels into the fallopian tube. If the egg is not fertilized, the endometrial lining is shed. This discharge of bloody fluid is the menstrual period, which typically lasts from three to seven days. If the egg is fertilized, it continues to travel down the fallopian tube into the uterus, where it implants in the endometrium and begins to grow.

## PREGNANCY

Pregnancy begins when an egg released by the ovaries unites with a sperm cell that has been introduced into the female reproductive tract. The union of the egg and sperm cell is called fertilization, and occurs in the outer third of the fallopian tube. The fertilized egg passes into the uterus and implants in the endometrium, or inner lining of the uterus.

A pregnancy lasts approximately 280 days, or nine months, and is divided into three trimesters. During the first trimester, the fertilized egg becomes an embryo enclosed in a protective bag of waters, or amniotic sac. A special disk-shaped organ known as the placenta develops and attaches to the inner wall of the uterus. The embryo is connected to the placenta by the umbilical cord, and it is through the placenta that oxygen and nutrients pass from the mother to the embryo.

The first trimester is a critical phase of pregnancy because it is during this time that all major body systems begin to develop. Proper development can be severely affected if the mother is exposed to certain drugs, alcohol, or infectious diseases like rubella (German measles).

During the second trimester, the embryo becomes a fetus. The fetus continues to grow, developing bones and facial features. It is during this trimester that the mother first feels the fetus move inside her, usually between the 13th and 16th weeks.

During the last trimester, the fetus (and the uterus) reach their maximum sizes. The upper part of the uterus, known as the fundus, may even press up against the mother's diaphragm, making her a little short of breath. The fetal lungs mature in preparation for breathing. During the last several weeks of pregnancy, the uterus drops down as the fetus maneuvers itself into position for birth. The head, or presenting part, descends into the pelvis, and people often say that the baby has "dropped." The fetus is now at full term, 40 weeks after conception, and is ready to be born (Figure 15.2).

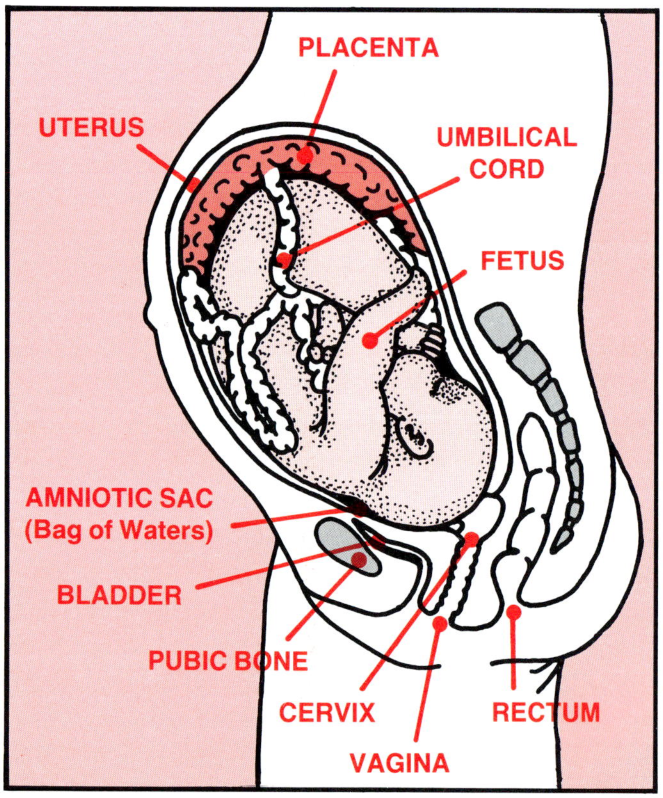


**Figure 15.2** During the last several weeks of pregnancy, the baby's head drops low into the pelvis in preparation for birth.

## Complications of Pregnancy

Although most pregnancies proceed without incident, complications can and do arise, some of them life-threatening for both mother and fetus. The complications most likely to be encountered by the first responder are sudden pain and bleeding, eclampsia (toxemia), supine hypotensive syndrome, and trauma.

Bleeding can occur at any stage of pregnancy for a variety of causes. Early in pregnancy bleeding most often results from ectopic pregnancy or spontaneous abortion (miscarriage). During the third trimester of pregnancy, bleeding may occur from placenta previa, abruptio placenta, or uterine rupture. Bleeding from any of these conditions can manifest itself vaginally, or it can be concealed inside the uterus and abdominal cavity.

### ECTOPIC PREGNANCY

Ectopic pregnancy, also known as tubal pregnancy, occurs when the fertilized egg implants itself in the fallopian tube, ovary, or abdomen (Figure 15.3). Implantation in the fallopian tube is the most common site of ectopic pregnancy. Ectopic pregnancy is more likely to occur in women who have become pregnant with an IUD in place. Tubal abnormalities or scars resulting from infections may also contribute to the occurrence of ectopic pregnancy.

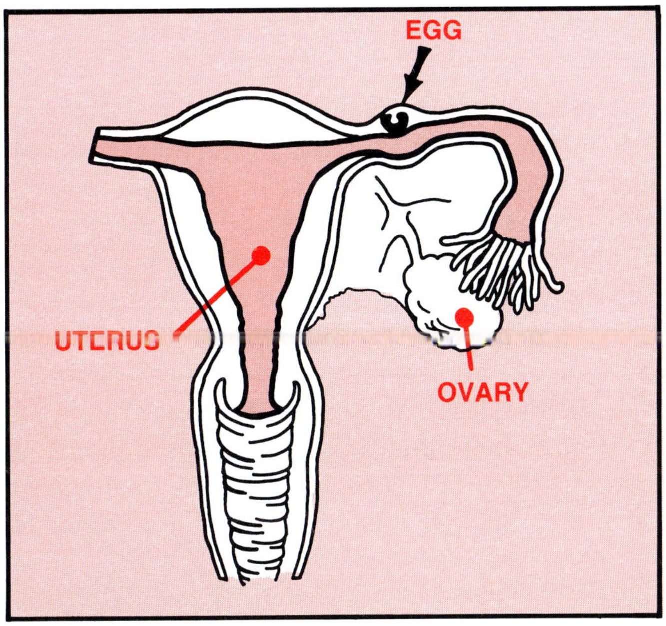


**Figure 15.3** Implantation in the fallopian tube is the most common site of ectopic pregnancy.

The fallopian tube was not designed to accommodate a fertilized egg; as the egg grows, the pressure placed on the tube causes it to rupture. The resulting blood loss causes severe pain, usually localized to one lower quadrant but sometimes radiating to the shoulders as well. Vaginal bleeding may be present or bleeding may be hidden. As blood loss continues, the classic signs and symptoms of hypovolemic shock develop: weak, rapid pulse; pale, cool, clammy skin; falling blood pressure. Place the patient supine with the legs elevated, administer oxygen, arrange for rapid transport to a medical facility, and monitor vital signs and level of consciousness frequently.

### ABORTION (MISCARRIAGE)

Abortion, or miscarriage, is the loss of a pregnancy before the fetus is capable of surviving outside the uterus. A complete abortion is one in which the entire products of conception are lost. A threatened abortion is characterized by bleeding; the bleeding may continue, resulting in a complete abortion, or it may stop, allowing the pregnancy to continue. The major signs of abortion are vaginal bleeding, which may be light or profuse, and abdominal pain similar to menstrual cramps. The woman may also pass fetal materials, which should be saved for examination by a physician. Provide emotional support for the patient, monitor her vital signs, and arrange for rapid but quiet transport to a medical facility.

### PREDELIVERY HEMORRHAGE

The three conditions described below — placenta previa, abruptio placenta, and uterine rupture — are life-threatening emergencies for both mother and fetus. Each condition occurs during the last trimester of pregnancy, and each is characterized by bleeding, pain (usually), and hypovolemic shock. Although bleeding from the vagina may not be profuse, massive amounts of blood may be concealed in the uterus and abdominal cavity. The fetus is at risk because of inadequate oxygen supply, and the mother is at risk because of hypovolemic shock. Since two lives are at stake, treat any vaginal bleeding or severe abdominal pain during the last trimester as an emergency.

Normally, the placenta implants in the upper portion of the uterus; in the case of placenta previa, however, the placenta implants low in the uterus (Figure 15.4). A placenta previa may partially or completely block the cervix. During late pregnancy, the placenta may begin to hemorrhage. Although bleeding may be profuse, it is often painless. Keep the patient lying on her left side, treat for shock, and arrange for rapid transport to a medical facility.

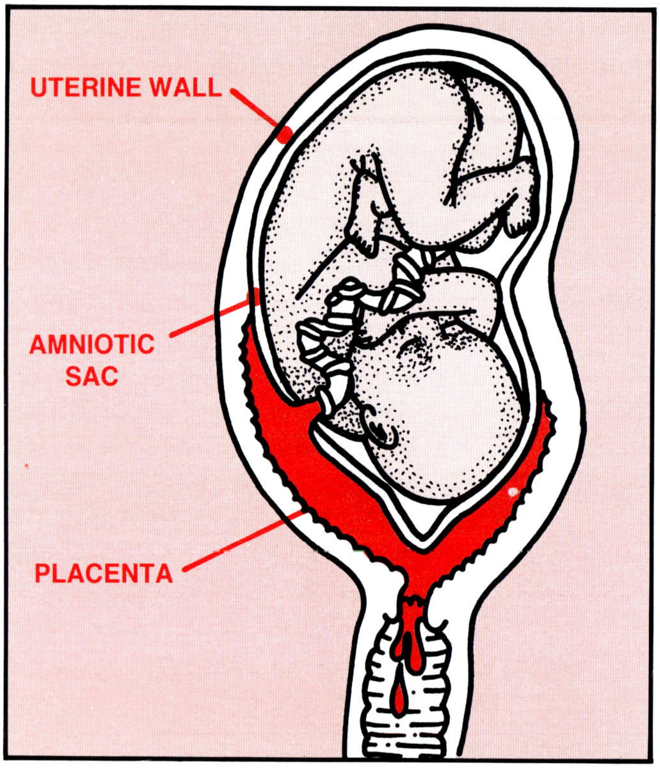


**Figure 15.4** Hemorrhage can result from placenta previa, a condition where the placenta implants itself low in the uterus.

Abruptio placenta occurs when a normally implanted placenta begins to separate from the uterine wall (Figure 15.5). The patient experiences severe abdominal pain as the uterus fills with blood. Vaginal bleeding may be light or profuse, and hypovolemic shock occurs rapidly. Keep the patient lying on her left side, treat for shock, and arrange for rapid transport to a medical facility.

Uterine rupture is rare; however, it is the most life-threatening prebirth emergency for both mother and fetus. Thinning of the uterine wall during late pregnancy and uterine scars from Cesarian deliveries are two potential causes of uterine rupture. Uterine rupture often occurs shortly after

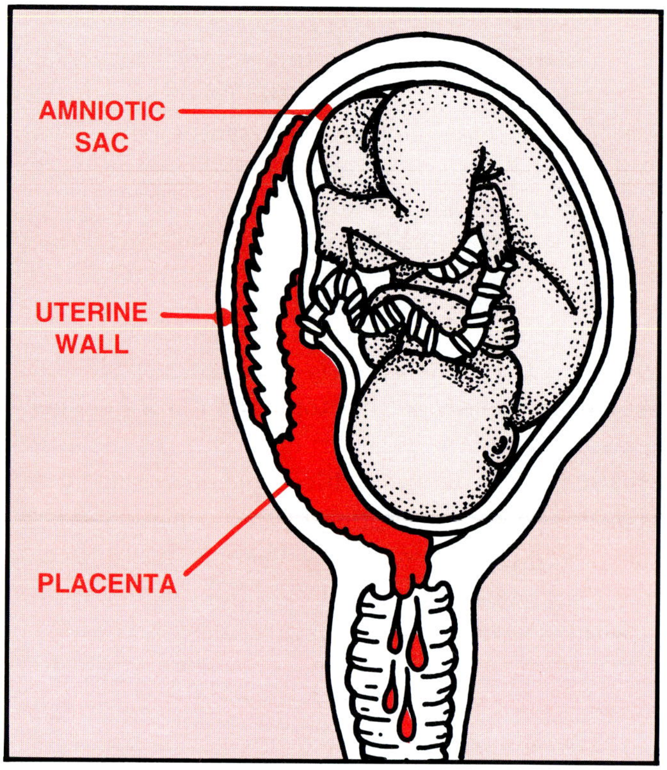


**Figure 15.5** Severe internal or external hemorrhage can result when the placenta separates prematurely from the uterine wall.

the onset of labor; the patient frequently describes a tearing sensation and sudden, severe abdominal pain. Labor contractions cease immediately. There may be very little external bleeding, but massive internal bleeding. Place the patient on her left side, administer oxygen, treat for shock, and arrange for rapid transport to a medical facility.

## ECLAMPSIA (TOXEMIA)

Eclampsia, also known as toxemia, is a serious systemic disorder that occurs during the latter part of pregnancy. It is found more frequently in women who are having their first pregnancies. Eclampsia has two stages: preeclampsia and eclampsia. The first stage, known as preeclampsia, is characterized by blood pressure greater than 140/90, protein in the urine, and edema (swelling due to retained body fluids). Edema is particularly noticeable in the face, hands, and ankles. Other symptoms of preeclampsia are headache, mid-upper abdominal pain, and blurred vision. Because preeclampsia can progress to eclampsia, any pregnant women suspected of preeclampsia should be evaluated by a physican. Prehospital treatment consists of placing the woman lying down on her left side in a quiet environment and arranging for rapid transport to a medical facility.

Eclampsia is a life-threatening emergency that is usually fatal if not treated. It can occur before, during, or after labor. Eclampsia is characterized by seizures and coma in addition to all the signs and symptoms of preeclampsia. Treat the patient by establishing and maintaining an open airway and by arranging for rapid transport to a medical facility. Keep the atmosphere as quiet as possible; bright lights, sirens, and loud noise can bring on more seizures.

#### SUPINE HYPOTENSIVE SYNDROME

The pregnant woman near delivery has a large, heavy mass in her abdomen. When she is supine (lying flat on her back), this mass, which includes the weight of the uterus, fetus, and placenta, compresses the inferior vena cava against the spinal column. The amount of blood returning to the heart is thus reduced, resulting in a drop in blood pressure. This condition is known as supine hypotensive syndrome; it is characterized by dizziness, anxiety, and low blood pressure. Treatment for supine hypotensive syndrome is quite simple: place the mother on her side, preferably her left side, which favors the return of blood to the heart. Unless injuries prevent it, the pregnant woman should always be placed on her side rather than on her back.

#### TRAUMA

The woman who suffers trauma during her pregnancy requires special attention because two lives are involved. Even if her injuries seem minor, she should be examined by a physician because there is no way to assess possible damage to the fetus outside the hospital. If injuries are more serious, be sure to establish and maintain the ABC's so that both mother and fetus are oxygenated. If the woman suffers cardiac arrest, begin CPR and continue it all the way to the hospital. If she cannot be saved, perhaps the fetus can be kept alive until it can be delivered surgically.

## LABOR AND DELIVERY

Labor is the process by which the uterus repeatedly contracts to dilate the cervix and push the baby and placenta out of the mother's body. Delivery is the actual birth of the baby. At the beginning of labor, contractions are far apart. As labor progresses, contractions become stronger and closer together. During the most active stage of labor, contractions occur every 2 to 3 minutes and last 60 seconds or longer.

There are three stages of labor: the first stage begins with the first contraction and lasts until the cervix is completely dilated (open). A completely dilated cervix is about 10 centimeters wide. The first stage lasts about 12 hours in a first-time mother, known as a primipara, and about 8 hours in a woman who has already had a child, known as a multipara. The amniotic sac frequently ruptures when the cervix is completely dilated.

The second stage of labor begins when the baby begins to descend into the birth canal (the vagina) and ends with the delivery of the baby. As the baby moves down the vagina, the head presses against the mother's rectum, making her feel as though she has to move her bowels. The mother bears down (pushes) with each contraction, and eventually the baby's head pushes against the vaginal opening, a process known as crowning. Birth of the baby follows very shortly. Pushing is very, very hard work, particularly for a primipara. The second stage of labor takes about an hour for a primipara (a first-time mother), and about 20 minutes or less for a multipara (a woman who has already had a child).

The third stage of labor lasts from the time of delivery until the placenta has been expelled and the uterus has contracted.

### Evaluating the Mother

When called to assist a woman in labor, you will first need to determine if there is time to transport the mother to a medical facility. Obtain answers to the following questions:

- When is the due date for the baby?
- Has the mother had a baby before? Labor during a first pregnancy usually lasts longer than for subsequent pregnancies; therefore, there may be time to transport during a first labor.

- How far apart are the contractions? Contractions more than five minutes apart are a good indication that there will be enough time to transport the mother. Contractions closer than two minutes apart, particularly in a woman who has already had at least one child, may indicate that birth will occur shortly. Do not base the decision whether or not to transport solely on the length of time between contractions; each labor is different, and contractions that are close together do not necessarily indicate that delivery is imminent.
- Has the amniotic sac (bag of waters) ruptured and, if so, when? If the sac ruptures more than 18 hours before birth occurs, the likelihood of fetal infection increases. If it has been many hours since the amniotic sac has ruptured, the mother may need to be transported to the medical facility for observation.
- Does the mother feel as though she has to move her bowels? This sensation, which is known as the urge to push, indicates that the baby's head has entered the vagina. Delivery is likely to occur very soon.
- Has the baby crowned? You will have to examine the mother to determine the answer to this question. Explain to the mother that you need to look to see if the baby is ready to be born. If you are a male, find a female chaperone. Have the mother remove her undergarments; look at, but do not touch, the vaginal opening. If the baby's head is bulging against the vagina, delivery is definitely going to occur very soon. (Figure 15.6).
- If there is time, ask the mother if she is under a doctor's care for any medical problems, such as heart disease, epilepsy, or diabetes. This type of information is useful for other emergency care personnel.

## Assisting With Delivery

Once it seems that birth is imminent, DO NOT allow the mother to go to the toilet. It is not her bowels that are moving, but rather the baby. In addition, DO NOT try to delay or restrain delivery in any way. Get ready to assist the mother.

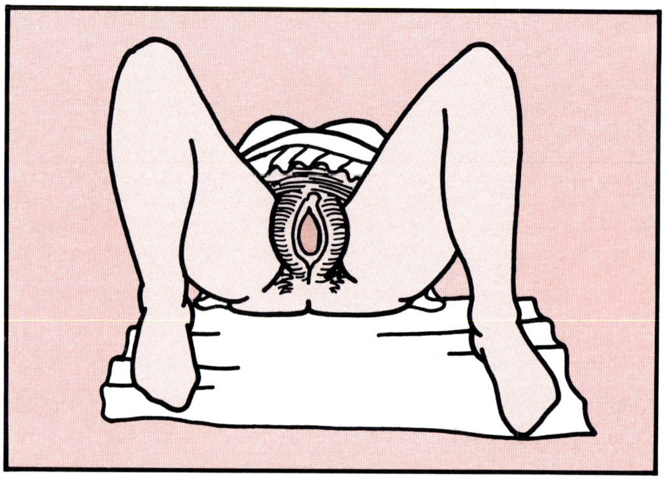

**Figure 15.6** When the baby's head bulges against the mother's vagina, a condition known as crowning, delivery will occur very soon.

The emergency vehicle should be equipped with at least one emergency obstetrics pack that includes the following: (Figure 15.7)

- Sterile drapes or towels
- Sterile 4x4 inch (102 mm x 102 mm) gauze pads
- Sterile gloves
- Small bulb syringe
- Sanitary pads
- Two or three cord clamps
- Sterile scissors
- Towel or blanket for the baby
- Several plastic bags

In addition to the sterile supplies, the following should be available:

- Aluminum foil
- Sheets or blanket for the mother
- Oxygen and suction equipment

If sterile equipment is not available, make sure everything is as clean as possible (especially your hands). If the mother is in a crowded or public place, try to find a private, clean area in which to work. This will also help lessen the mother's anxiety at having a baby in public. Allow the mother's husband or friend to remain by her side to help provide reassurance. Disperse onlookers or overex-

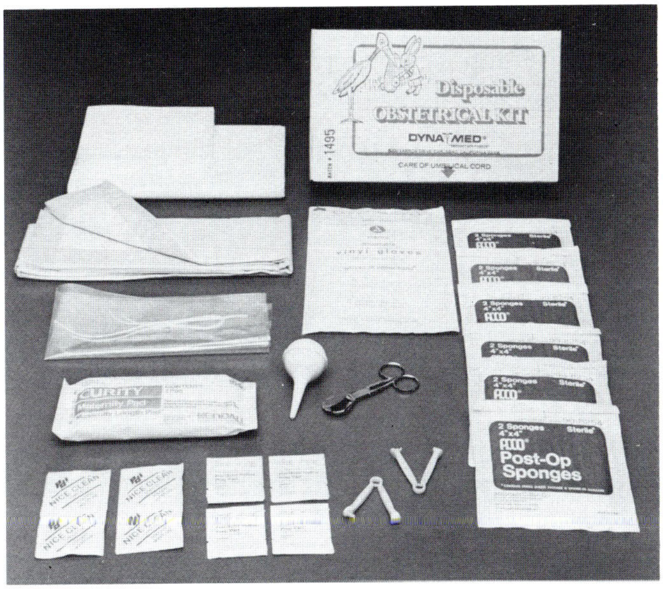


**Figure 15.7** The emergency vehicle should be equipped with an emergency obstetrics pack. *Courtesy of Dyna Med.*

cited relatives; they will only make the mother anxious. Do not coach the mother using a prepared childbirth method such as the Lamaze or Bradley methods; do allow her to use a prepared childbirth method if she wants to do so and is prepared to use it. It will help her retain some control and lessen anxiety.

Help the mother position herself for delivery. All patients should be positioned for their comfort and safety, and pregnant women are no exception. To this end, DO NOT FORCE THE MOTHER TO LIE FLAT ON HER BACK WITH HER KNEES UP. This position may give you the best view, but it makes delivery harder for the mother. The mother has a much harder time pushing when she is lying on her back. Great tension is placed on the vaginal tissues, increasing the likelihood of tearing; moreover, the weight of the baby on the mother's abdomen makes it difficult for her to breathe. Two far better positions are semisitting or side-lying, which decrease pressure on the vaginal opening and allow the mother to make better use of gravity (Figure 15.8). If the mother prefers to sit, prop her up with pillows or have someone sit behind her and support her back. If she prefers to lie on her side (place her on her left side: it favors the return of blood to the heart), have someone hold her right leg out of the way. It is not unusual for women in labor to vomit, so keep someone near the mother's head

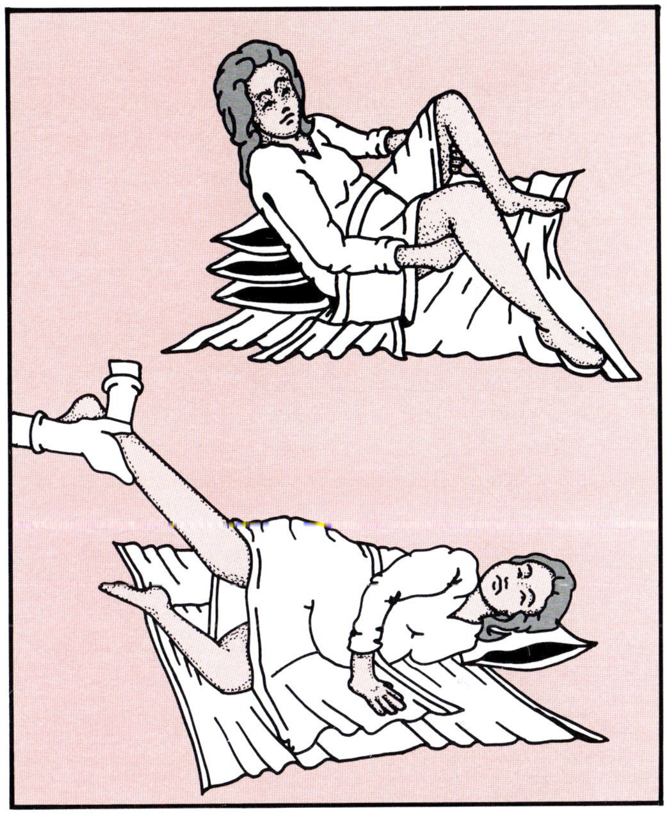

**Figure 15.8** During delivery, allow the mother to assume the position most comfortable for her. The semisitting or side-lying positions make good use of gravity and ease the weight of the baby against the abdomen.

with a container and suction equipment in case she becomes sick.

Wash your hands, then open the sterile obstetrics pack and put on gloves. Keep sterile supplies out of the way of the vaginal opening in case the amniotic sac breaks during delivery. Place a sterile drape under the mother's lower back and buttocks. Then place drapes under the vaginal opening and on the mother's abdomen and thighs. Remember your priorities: if the baby is coming fast, it is more important to assist the mother than to worry about drapes.

Reassure the mother and encourage her to relax between contractions. If the mother is pushing by grimacing, gritting her teeth, or tensing her neck muscles, you might suggest that she direct the force of her pushing *down*. When she feels that she has to push, she should clamp down hard on her diaphragm, pushing down hard and letting out her breath very slowly.

When the baby's head begins to emerge, place gentle pressure on it with the palm of your hand to prevent explosive delivery. Carefully allow the entire head to emerge and instruct the mother not to push. If she finds it difficult to resist pushing, tell her to blow short, explosive breaths through her mouth. It is impossible to blow and push at the same time.

Most babies are born face down. The head then rotates to one side almost immediately. This turning makes it easier for the shoulders to be delivered. Support the head on one hand and forearm (Figure 15.9). DO NOT PULL ON THE BABY. If the amniotic sac is still intact, tear a hole in it with scissors or your fingers and push it away from the baby's nose and mouth. Check to see if the umbilical cord is wrapped around the baby's neck (Figure 15.10). If the cord is wrapped loosely around the neck, gently slip it over the baby's head. If the cord is tight, clamp it in two places and cut it between the clamps.

Slide your hand beneath the baby's head and begin clearing the baby's nose and mouth with the bulb syringe. Clear the nose first because babies breathe through their noses, not their mouths. Squeeze the syringe first, then place the tip in the baby's nostril and release the bulb **SLOWLY** to avoid injuring the baby's fragile lungs (Figure 15.11). Remove the syringe from the baby's nose or mouth and squeeze out all mucus onto a cloth. Repeat this procedure several times.

Assist with delivery of the shoulders. The upper shoulder is usually delivered first. Gently

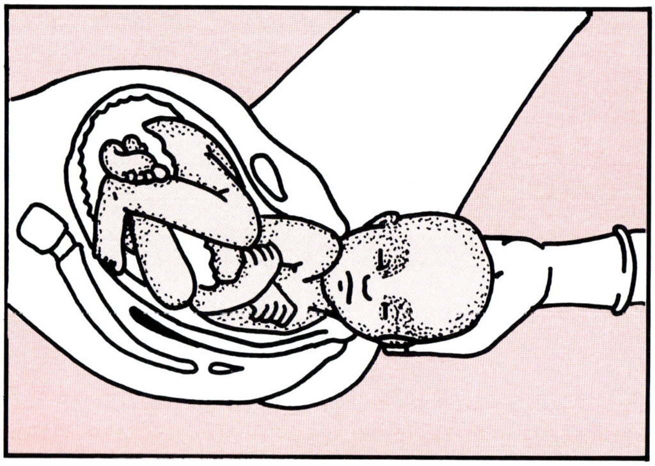

**Figure 15.9** As the baby's head emerges, support it on one hand.

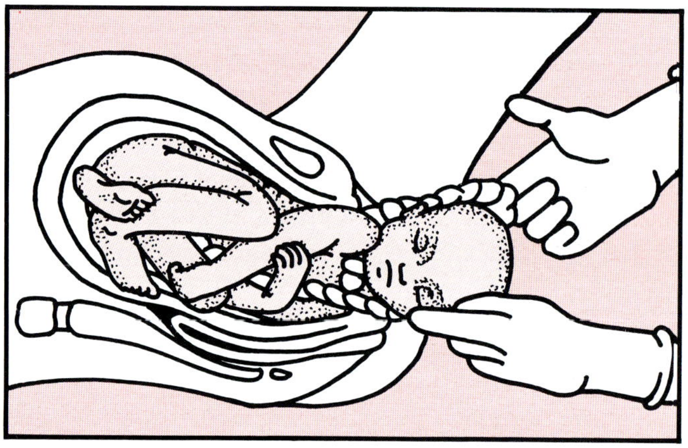

**Figure 15.10** Check to see if the umbilical cord is wrapped around the baby's neck. If this is the case, gently slip the cord over the baby's head.

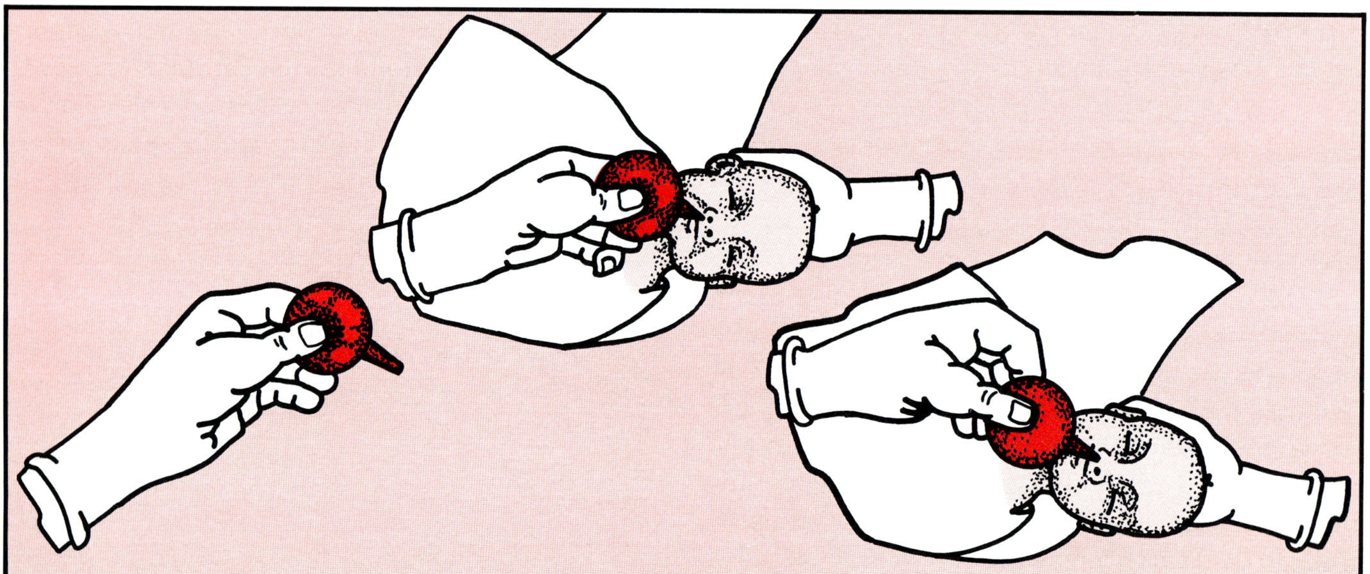

**Figure 15.11** To use a bulb syringe, squeeze the bulb, then place the tip in the baby's nostril. Release the bulb *slowly* to avoid injuring the baby's lungs. Repeat for the other nostril.

guide the baby's head down to help with delivery of the first shoulder (Figure 15.12). Then gently guide the head up to allow delivery of the second shoulder (Figure 15.13). The shoulders are the widest part of the body, so the rest of the baby is likely to deliver rapidly. **THE BABY IS SLIPPERY, SO SUPPORT HIM OR HER CAREFULLY WITH BOTH HANDS.** Note the time of birth and be sure to tell the parents whether they have a boy or a girl.

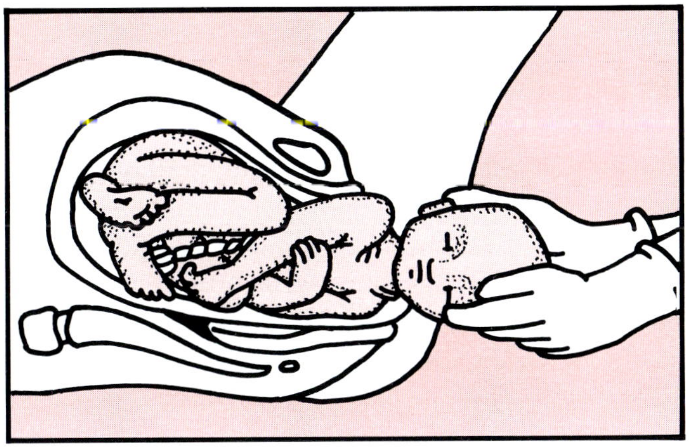

**Figure 15.12** Gently guide the head down to assist with delivery of the first shoulder.

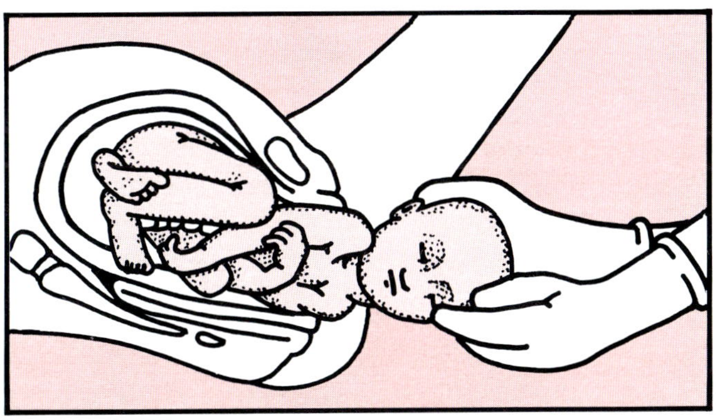

**Figure 15.13** Gently guide the head up to assist with delivery of the second shoulder.

Hold the baby at the approximate level of the placenta so that blood from the baby does not flow back into the placenta. Keep the head slightly lower than the body to aid in drainage of mucus. If necessary, suction the nose and mouth again. If the baby has not started breathing, rub the baby's back or flick your fingers against the soles of the feet. Quickly wipe off the baby and wrap it in a blanket. Newborns have difficulty maintaining their body temperatures, so do not allow the baby to become chilled. Be sure to cover the head; babies lose a great deal of body heat through their heads.

While you are waiting for the placenta to deliver, assess the baby's vital signs. The Apgar scoring system is used to evaluate newborns for heart rate, respiratory effort, muscle tone, reflex irritability, and color (Table 15.1).

**TABLE 15.1**
**APGAR SCORING CHART**

| SIGN | SCORE 0 | SCORE 1 | SCORE 2 |
|---|---|---|---|
| Heart rate | Absent | Slow (below 100) | Over 100 |
| Respiratory effort | Absent | Slow, irregular hypoventilation | Good, crying, lustily |
| Muscle tone | Flaccid | Some flexion of extremities | Active motion, well flexed |
| Reflex irritability | No response | Cry, some motion | Vigorous cry |
| Color | Blue, pale | Body pink; hands and feet blue | Completely pink |

Sixty seconds after birth of the baby, evaluate the five signs and give each sign a score of 0, 1, or 2. Then add up all 5 scores to determine the total score. Repeat the assessment at five minutes. Most newborns are vigorous and have a total score of 7 to 10; they cough or cry within seconds of delivery and require no further resuscitation. Babies with a score in the 4 to 6 range are moderately depressed. They may be pale or blue one minute after delivery, limp, and breathing weakly. These infants require some form of resuscitation.

The repeat assessment five minutes after birth is useful for noting change in the baby's vital signs. For example, at one minute a baby may have an Apgar score of 5, indicating that he or she is moderately depressed. At five minutes the baby may have an Apgar score of 8, indicating good respiration, heartbeat, and color.

Take the mother's vital signs and note her general appearance. Reassure her and have someone sponge her face if she is sweaty.

If the baby's vital signs are good and the mother is not hemorrhaging severely, prepare to clamp and cut the umbilical cord. Wait until pulses in the umbilical cord stop, then clamp it in two places. The first clamp should be at least 6 inches (152 mm) from the baby's umbilicus (belly button), and the second clamp about 2 inches (50 mm) from that. Using the sterile scissors, cut the cord between the two clamps (Figure 15.14). Handle the cord carefully because it tears easily. Examine the cut end of the cord for bleeding; if there is any bleeding, do not remove the clamp. Add another clamp about one inch (25 mm) below the first clamp. Place the baby on mother's abdomen so that she may hold her newborn. If you have orders not to cut the cord, leave it clamped and have baby and placenta delivered together to the medical facility.

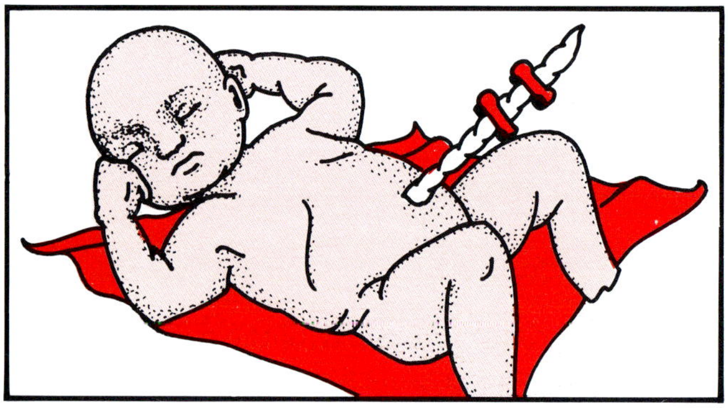

**Figure 15.14** To clamp the umbilical cord, place the first clamp about 6 inches (152 mm) from the baby's umbilicus and the second clamp about 2 inches (50 mm) from the first. Then cut the cord between the clamps.

The third stage of labor — delivery of the placenta — usually occurs spontaneously within 15 to 20 minutes after childbirth (Figure 15.15). **DO NOT PULL ON THE UMBILICAL CORD TO HASTEN DELIVERY OF THE PLACENTA.** To do so can cause severe hemorrhage in the mother. Pulling on the umbilical cord can even cause the uterus to become inverted, that is, to turn inside out. Wait for the placenta to deliver naturally, then save it in a plastic bag for examination by a physician. The physician must examine the placenta to make sure that it has been completely expelled. If pieces of the placenta are retained in the uterus, they can cause persistent bleeding and infection.

Anticipate bleeding as the placenta separates from the uterine wall. Place a sanitary napkin over

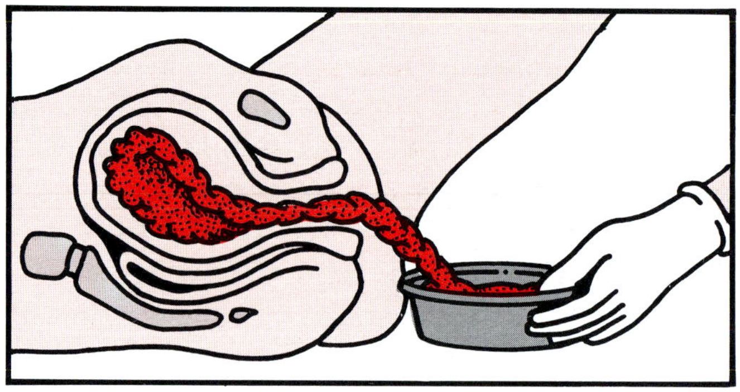

**Figure 15.15** The placenta usually delivers within 15 to 20 minutes after childbirth. DO NOT pull on the umbilical cord to speed delivery of the placenta.

the mother's vagina and allow her to put her legs together. Although some bleeding is normal, uterine contractions help close the small blood vessels in the uterus and stop bleeding before it becomes excessive. Two ways to help the uterus contract are to massage the uterus and allowing the baby to nurse. To massage the uterus, rub the mother's lower abdomen gently but firmly using circular motions (Figure 15.16). Uterine massage hurts! Explain to the mother why it is necessary. You should be able to feel the uterus harden as you massage it. Repeat the massage every five minutes until the mother arrives at the medical facility. Allowing the baby to nurse also stimulates the uterus to contract.

Help prepare mother and baby for transport. Change bloody sheets and make the mother as comfortable as possible.

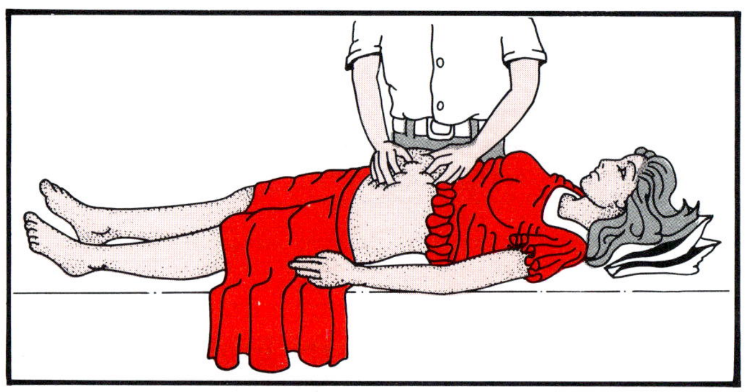

**Figure 15.16** Massage the uterus by rubbing the mother's abdomen gently but firmly using circular motions.

## Premature Babies and Multiple Births

### PREMATURE BIRTH

Any baby born before seven months of pregnancy or who weighs less than 5½ pounds (2.5 kg) is defined as premature and needs special care.

Premature babies have problems because they are so small and their organs are immature. Because they have more surface area relative to their size than full-term infants, premature babies have trouble maintaining a normal body temperature. In addition, premature babies have less subcutaneous fat to insulate them against heat loss.

Any blood loss in a premature baby is more serious because of the baby's small size. Premature babies often develop respiratory problems because their lungs are immature and they are unable to take in sufficient oxygen. Lack of oxygen due to respiratory problems leads to cardiovascular problems, bradycardia (abnormally slow heartbeat), and hypotension.

Birth weight alone is not a sure indicator of prematurity. Some low birth weight infants may be fully mature, and some premature babies may be heavier than 5½ pounds (2.5 kg). To distinguish premature from mature babies, note creases in the soles of the feet, type of scalp hair, and cartilage in the outer ears. Babies of at least 39 weeks development have creases covering the soles of their feet, coarse, silky scalp hair, and cartilage in their outer ears. Babies of less than eight months development have a single crease in the soles of their feet, fine, fuzzy scalp hair, and no external ear cartilage. In addition, premature babies are redder, skinnier, and more wrinkled than full-term babies, and their heads seem very large in comparison to their bodies.

If the mother tells you that she is not due to deliver for several months yet, or if the infant is very small, treat it as a premature delivery. To care for the premature baby, take the following extra steps:

- Premature babies are less able to tolerate lack of oxygen than mature babies. Keep the baby's nose and mouth clear of fluid with a bulb syringe.
- Keep the baby warm. Wrap the baby in a blanket and then in aluminum foil to minimize heat loss (Figure 15.17). Keep the surroundings as warm as possible and keep the baby out of any drafts.
- Prevent any bleeding from the umbilical cord because premature babies cannot tolerate the loss of even a small amount of blood.
- Make a tent above the baby with aluminum foil and administer oxygen at a low flow into the tent. Aim the oxygen at the top of the tent, not at the baby's face.
- Prevent contamination because premature infants are highly susceptible to infection. Do not breathe into the baby's face or allow anyone else to do so. Wear a disposable mask if possible.

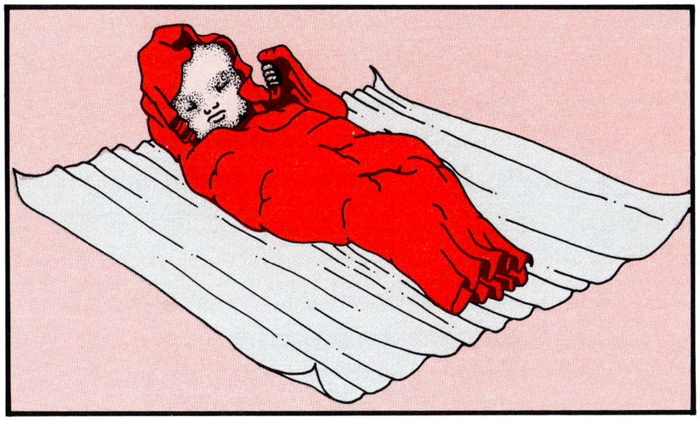

**Figure 15.17** If the baby seems premature or is very small, minimize heat loss by wrapping the baby in a blanket and then in aluminum foil.

### MULTIPLE BIRTHS

Multiple births usually do not present unique problems, except that there is more work to do, and the babies tend to be small. Suspect a multiple birth if the uterus remains unusually large after birth, or if contractions resume shortly after the birth of the first baby. Often, the mother is already aware that she is carrying more than one baby. If there is time to transport, do so; otherwise, set up for childbirth in the usual manner. After the first baby is born, clamp the cord and make sure there is no bleeding from *either* end. Delivery of the placenta(s) should occur spontaneously. Each baby may have its own placenta, or they may share one placenta. Be sure to maintain the babies' body heat. Evaluate the babies carefully because they may be small. If so, care for them in the same manner as for a premature baby.

## ABNORMAL DELIVERIES

Deliveries in which the baby's head does not present first are classified as abnormal deliveries. Three abnormal presentations are discussed in this section: breech presentation, prolapsed umbilical cord, and limb presentation. These three situations require special handling because they make delivery difficult, if not impossible, in the field, and are potentially life-threatening conditions for the baby.

## Breech Presentation

Breech presentation occurs when the buttocks, feet, or arms present first, rather than the head. If the buttocks are the presenting part and the baby has already crowned, prepare for delivery in the normal manner. Gently support the buttocks and trunk as they are delivered (Figure 15.18). Generally, the head delivers spontaneously and care for mother and infant is the same as for a standard delivery. If the head does not deliver within three minutes, however, take action to increase the amount of oxygen reaching the baby. The baby's head presses the umbilical cord against the vaginal wall, cutting off the baby's oxygen supply. Moreover, breathing is impossible if the baby's face is pressed against the vaginal wall. Insert a gloved hand into the vagina and try to place your index and middle fingers on either side of the baby's nose. Try to press your fingers back against the vagina in order to create an air space for the baby. If the head does not deliver within three minutes, arrange for immediate transport to a medical facility. Administer high-flow oxygen to the mother and put pillows and blankets under her hips. Continue to maintain the baby's airway all the way to the medical facility.

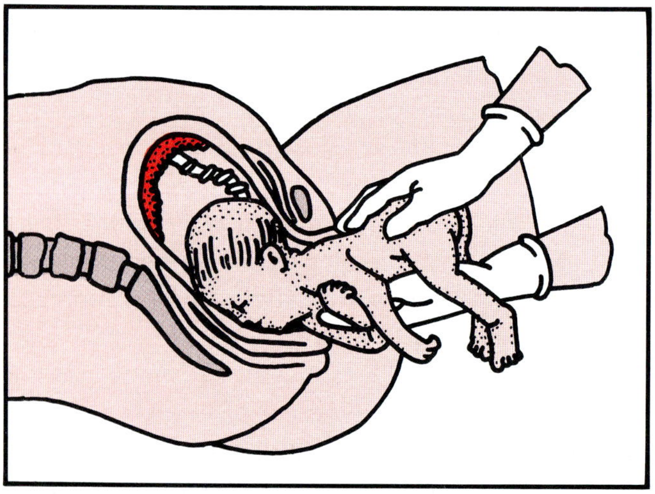

**Figure 15.18** If the baby is in a breech position, support the buttocks and trunk as they are delivered.

## Limb Presentation

If an arm or a single leg is the presenting part, support the mother's hips on pillows and arrange for immediate transport to a medical facility (Figure 15.19). A breech presentation of this type cannot be managed outside a hospital, so do not delay.

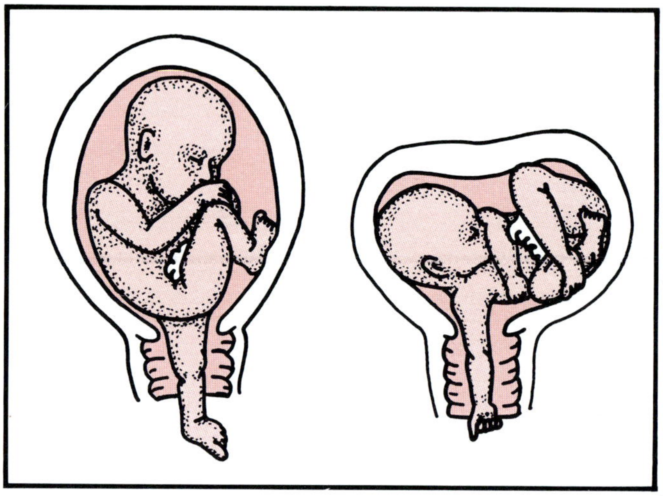

**Figure 15.19** If the breech presentation includes an arm or a single leg, support the mother's hips on pillows and arrange for immediate transport to a medical facility.

## Prolapsed Cord

Prolapsed umbilical cord occurs when the cord comes out of the vagina before the baby (Figure 15.20). Because the cord is pinched between the baby's head and the vaginal walls, the oxygen supply to the baby is drastically reduced or completely cut off. **DO NOT TRY TO PUSH THE UMBILICAL CORD BACK INTO THE VAGINA.** Place the mother in a position such that her hips are much higher than her body. Place her facing down in a knee-chest position or on her back with her hips propped up high with blankets and pillows. Both these positions make use of gravity to help keep the baby higher in the vagina. Insert a gloved hand into the vagina and gently push the baby back into the vagina several inches. Distribute your fingers evenly around the baby's head to avoid injuring the baby's soft skull. Treat the umbilical cord the same as an evisceraton: cover it lightly with a moist, sterile dressing. **GET MOTHER AND BABY TO A MEDICAL FACILITY AS RAPIDLY AS POSSIBLE.** Administer high-flow oxygen to the mother, and maintain pressure on the baby's head all the way to the medical facility.

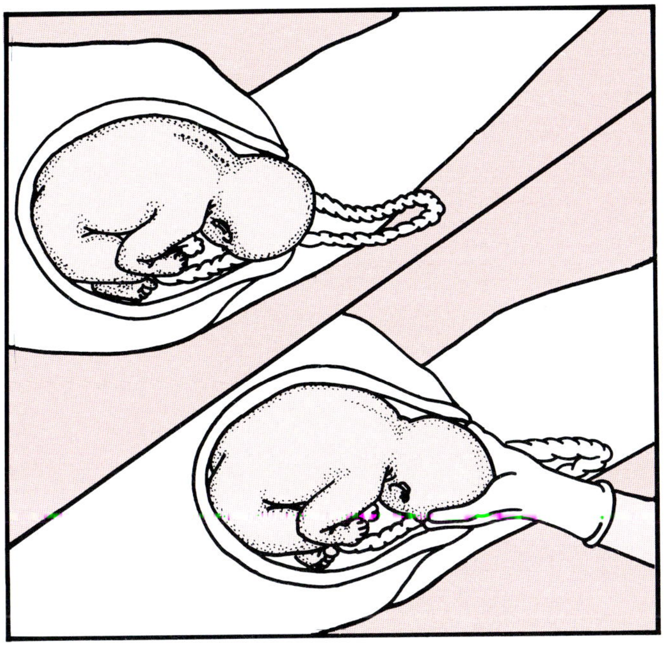

**Figure 15.20** A prolapsed umbilical cord occurs when the cord comes out of the vagina before the baby. If this happens, place the mother's hips much higher than her body and gently push the baby's head back into the vagina.

## COMPLICATIONS AFTER DELIVERY

Complications after delivery can involve the mother or baby. If the baby does not start breathing shortly after birth, resuscitative efforts must be started immediately. For the mother, possible complications of delivery include hemmorhage, uterine inversion, and pulmonary embolism.

In most cases, babies start breathing on their own. If the baby seems slow to breathe, rub the baby's back or snap your fingers against the soles of the feet. If the baby still does not breathe, you must begin mouth-to-mouth resuscitation immediately. Make sure the airway is open and that the baby's head is not hyperextended. Place your moth over the baby's nose and mouth and give very small puffs of air from your cheeks. If the baby starts breathing after several puffs, give oxygen by mask for several minutes. Hold the mask 4 or 5 inches (102 mm or 127 mm) away from the baby's face until the baby's color is normal. If the baby does not start breathing, check for a pulse. If there is no pulse, begin CPR immediately. Remember that only two fingers are needed to compress the sternum. Continue CPR until the baby arrives at a medical facility or is pronounced dead by a physician.

Occasionally, an infant is stillborn (born dead). The baby may be very small, appearing not fully developed, and very limp. If death has occurred some time before, the baby may smell bad and have a very soft head. If there is any doubt as to whether the baby is dead, start CPR and continue until the baby is pronounced dead. If the baby is obviously dead, follow the guidelines in your jurisdiction for handling stillbirth. If you are asked by the baby's parents to baptize the baby, do so by pouring a small amount of water over the baby's head and saying: "I baptize thee in the name of the Father, the Son, and the Holy Spirit. Amen."

Maternal complications of childbirth include prolonged delivery, hemorrhage, uterine inversion, and pulmonary embolism. If childbirth seems imminent but has not occurred after 20 minutes, arrange for immediate transport. There may be any number of complications that make delivery difficult, none of which can be managed outside of a medical facility.

If bleeding seems excessive after delivery of the placenta, continue uterine massage and arrange for immediate transport to a medical facility. Place the mother supine with the legs elevated. Monitor vital signs frequently and watch for signs of shock. Do not attempt to pack the vagina with dressings. Change sanitary pads as necessary and save them so that medical personnel can estimate blood loss.

Inversion, or turning inside out, of the uterus can occur as a result of excessive pressure on the uterus or from pulling on the umbilical cord in efforts to deliver the placenta. Shock commonly accompanies uterine inversion. If inversion occurs, keep the patient lying flat, and try once to replace the uterus by placing pressure on the area closest to the cervix. If the uterus cannot be replaced easily, cover all protruding tissues lightly with moist, sterile dressings. Administer oxygen and arrange for rapid transport to a medical facility.

Pulmonary embolism shortly after childbirth can be caused by a blood clot or by amniotic fluid. The mother experiences sudden, severe dyspnea (difficulty breathing), chest pain, rapid heartbeat, and falling blood pressure. Monitor vital signs frequently, administer oxygen, and arrange for rapid transport to a medical facility.

# 16

# Gaining Access and Short-Distance Transfer

## U.S DEPARTMENT OF TRANSPORTATION
### First Responder Training Course

**Objectives:**

- Given descriptions of accident scenes, describe procedures for gaining access to patients:

— In closed upright vehicles.
— In closed overturned vehicles.
— Pinned beneath vehicles.
— Pinned inside vehicles.
— In vehicles with electrical hazards.

- Given a situation, indicate:

— Whether or not a patient should be moved.
— Why the patient should or should not be moved.
— If a move is necessary, how the move should be accomplished.

- Given a "patient" and other assistants, perform:

— A direct ground lift for a patient without a spine injury.
— A direct ground lift for a patient with a spine injury.
— An extremity lift.

# Chapter 16
# Gaining Access and Short-Distance Transfer

Motor vehicle accidents often present special problems for first responders and other rescuers in terms of gaining access to patients. A damaged vehicle may have jammed doors, a crushed roof, or be twisted around the patient, preventing easy access. A combination of hand and power tools may be needed to enable rescuers to reach patients trapped inside the vehicle.

Firefighter/first responders typically are trained in extrication procedures, but on a medical call, your assignment is to provide patient care. Other firefighter/rescuers will be charged with operating power tools, rescue equipment, and keeping charged lines ready for the possibility of fire. You can and should work to stabilize any vehicles and to gain access to patients by means of hand tools. Know the limitations of your training: remember that hasty, ill-planned actions can worsen the patient's injuries and harm rescuers as well.

The sections that follow describe methods for stabilizing vehicles, ways to gain access to patients who are trapped inside vehicles, and emergency and nonemergency methods for moving patients short distances. Some of the techniques for moving patients may apply to patients found at the scene of an accident, while others are more appropriate for the patient who is encountered in a home or similar situation.

## SIZE-UP

Careful size-up and coordination of rescue efforts are a must in order to avoid further injuries to patients and to provide proper patient care. Quickly size up the scene: Note the number of vehicles and passengers, as well as how badly injured the passengers seem to be. Remember the rule when calling for ambulances — one ambulance can handle one patient requiring advanced life support or two patients requiring basic life support. If it looks as though power tools will be needed for extrication, have them dispatched immediately. It is better to have tools on the scene that are not needed than to spend valuable time with hand tools and *then* decide that power tools are needed. Have a wrecker or truck with a winch dispatched as well. Their cables are useful for stabilizing vehicles. Call for police assistance with traffic control. Note the presence of hazards, such as downed electrical lines, leaking gasoline, or fire. Rain or wet ground conditions will make the scene itself more hazardous, making it more difficult to stabilize vehicles and increasing any electrical hazards. (Refer back to Chapter 3 for further discussion of scene assessment.)

All personnel should be in full protective gear, including gloves and face protection, before stabilizing any vehicle or attempting to gain access. Other firefighters should be standing by with charged hoselines and extinguishers in case of fire. If fuel is spilled on the ground, use foam to keep the fuel's vapors from spreading and finding an ignition source. Remove the vehicle's battery cables to lessen the chances of ignition. Finally, no one in the immediate vicinity should be smoking. If enough personnel are on the scene, designate one firefighter as safety officer. The safety officer can patrol the entire accident scene, watching for and reporting hazards.

## EFFECT OF RESCUE WORK ON VICTIMS

First responders must take special care to reduce the psychological effect that some undesired, but necessary, noise, vibration, movement, and conversation have on the victim. A certain amount of noise during a rescue operation is necessary, but it should be kept to a minimum and the victim advised and prepared to lessen anxiety and fear. Avoid sudden movements, which can further injure as well as terrify the victim. Limit conversations to necessary communication: Avoid colorful descriptions of the victim's condition, the extent of damage to the vehicle, and loud and abusive language. Limit access to the scene to trained personnel.

## STABILIZING A VEHICLE

The pressure exerted on a vehicle as rescuers attempt to gain entry can cause a vehicle to roll or tip. Obviously, this situation is a serious hazard to rescuers and passengers alike. Therefore, STABILIZE ALL VEHICLES BEFORE ATTEMPTING TO GAIN ACCESS TO PASSENGERS. All vehicles should be considered unstable; even an upright, closed vehicle should have the wheels chocked to prevent it from rolling. Do not allow anyone to climb on a vehicle, to stand below a vehicle that is resting on a hill, or to get under a vehicle that has not been stabilized first. While stabilizing the vehicle, talk to the patients, reassuring them, and tell them not to move around too much.

The following items are commonly used for stabilizing vehicles:

- Cribbing
- Tires
- Air bags
- Chains and ropes (**NOTE:** Chains are preferred; ropes tend to stretch.)
- Tow truck
- High-lift jacks
- Winches

Cribbing is made from 2 x 4's or 4 x 4's and usually has rope handles to facilitate carrying. To stabilize a vehicle, cribbing is stacked one tier at a time, with each row stacked in the opposite direction (Figure 16.1). Tires are also used for cribbing, as are wooden wedges. Tires can be found in the trunk of the accident vehicle or spare tires can be used from police vehicles or ambulances.

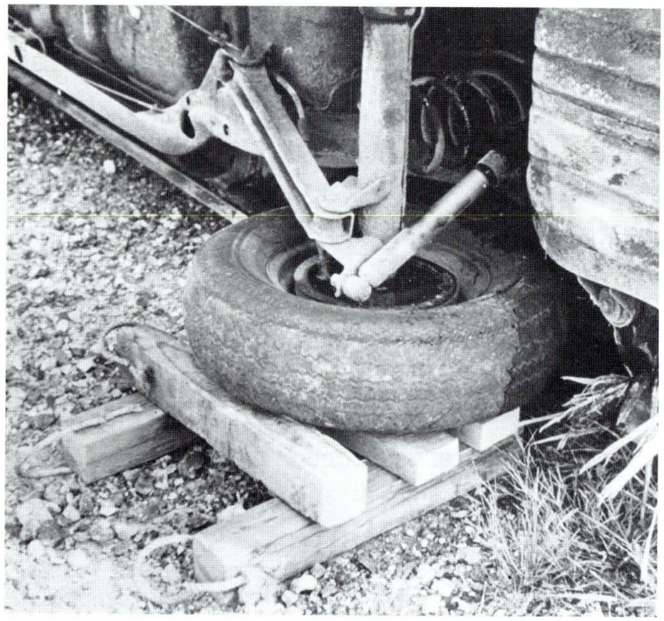

**Figure 16.1** To stabilize a vehicle, each row of cribbing should be stacked in the opposite direction. *Courtesy of Joel Woods, Maryland Fire and Rescue Institute.*

Air bags are an excellent stabilizing device. They require an air supply for inflation, such as an SCBA bottle. Air bags are rated to be inflated to a particular psi (kPa) or pressure. They are also rated to lift a certain amount of weight when inflated to their correct pressure. Do not inflate them beyond their rated capacity or try to lift an object too heavy for the bag.

If a tow truck arrives on the scene, its cable can be used to help stabilize the vehicle. Ropes can be used in the same manner, but exercise caution: ropes tend to stretch, and sharp bends produced by knots reduce a rope's strength. Rope should be at least one-half inch (13 mm) in diameter and must be tied so that it does not slip. Finish knots with one or two overhand safeties so that knots do not come loose (Figure 16.2). When you tie off a vehicle, make sure that it is tied to a stable object, such as a tree or heavy post. Tying the accident vehicle to another vehicle's front bumper may cause the car to pull. If you have to tie the accident vehicle to another vehicle, tie it to the side; it is much harder to pull a vehicle sideways.

High-lift jacks can be used to lift or brace a vehicle. Never use a jack by itself; use it with cribbing

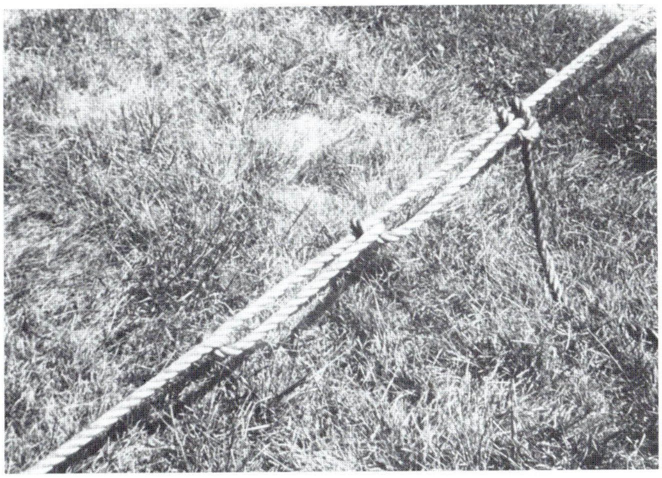

**Figure 16.2** Keep knots from coming loose by tying one or two overhand safeties. *Courtesy of Joel Woods, Maryland Fire and Rescue Institute.*

to provide additional stability. If you are using the jack for lifting, add cribbing as you jack. Do not use a bumper jack; it is too flimsy to provide any real stability.

## Closed Upright Vehicle

Even though a closed, upright vehicle may look stable, forces exerted by the use of hand or power tools can cause the car to move. Stabilize it first by chocking the wheels with wooden wedges or by letting the air out of the tires.

## Closed Vehicle on its Side

A closed vehicle on its side should be stabilized on its side before first responders attempt any entry. DO NOT attempt to right the vehicle by rocking or pushing it. Such action can easily cause the vehicle to roll over, injuring rescuers and further injuring passengers. Under no circumstances should a vehicle be tipped over with victims still inside. Tie the vehicle off with ropes or chains (Figure 16.3). If possible, use the spare tire, hood, and trunk to provide further stability. The hood and trunk lids can be opened if they can rest on the ground.

## Overturned Closed Vehicle

An overturned vehicle should be stabilized in the position in which it is found. DO NOT attempt to right the vehicle. Stabilization may be accomplished by several means — cribbing or wedges, jacks, come-alongs, air bags, or ropes (Figure 16.4).

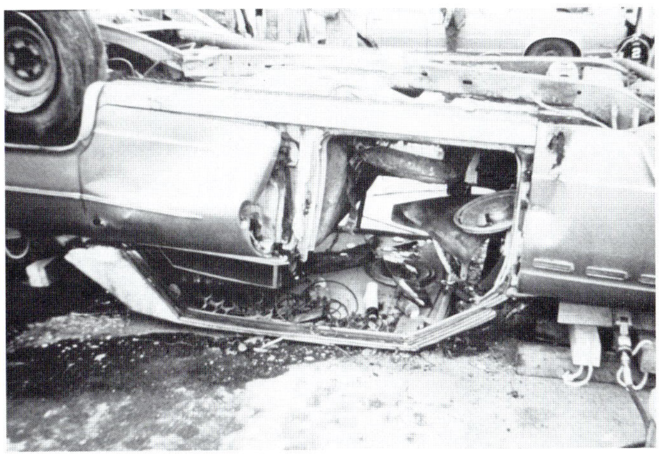

**Figure 16.4** Do not attempt to right an overturned vehicle. Rather, stabilize it with cribbing, jacks, wedges, or ropes. *Courtesy of Joel Woods, Maryland Fire and Rescue Institute.*

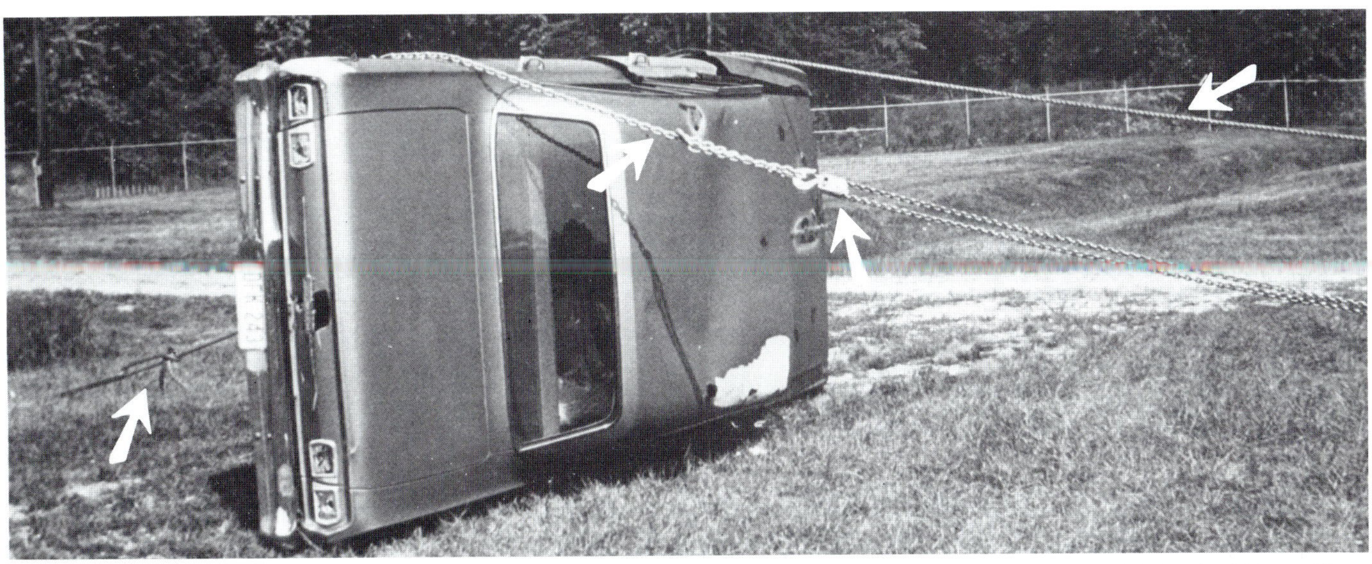

**Figure 16.3** DO NOT tip over a vehicle that has victims inside it. Tie the vehicle off with ropes or chains. *Courtesy of Joel Woods, Maryland Fire and Rescue Institute.*

## Pinned Patients

To stabilize a vehicle so that a patient pinned beneath it can be removed safely, use air bags or a hydraulic jack and cribbing. The vehicle must be shored up as it is raised so that it does not fall back down on the patient or rescuers. Do not use a car jack unless it is absolutely necessary; even then, be sure to use cribbing.

Being pinned by a vehicle may close off arteries, temporarily stopping severe bleeding. Be aware that as the vehicle is lifted from the patient, he or she may suffer a rapid onset of hypovolemic shock. Be prepared to treat the patient accordingly.

## GAINING ACCESS

The purpose for entering a vehicle is to begin assessing and treating patients. It is not necessary to immediately remove patients from vehicles unless circumstances demand it, as, for example, a fire or a patient in cardiac arrest. In such cases, the patient's injuries become secondary to preservation of life and he or she must be pulled from the vehicle as rapidly as possible.

If there are no immediate threats to life, it may take considerable effort, power tools, and time before the patient can be carefully and safely extricated (disentangled) from the vehicle. During extrication, the vehicle is removed from the patient, rather than the patient from the vehicle. This portion of the chapter concentrates on the hand tools first responders are likely to have available.

The following hand tools are commonly used for gaining access to patients in vehicles:

- Cribbing
- Pry axe, crash axe, or Halligan bar
- Hacksaw
- Baling hooks
- Air chisel
- Spring-loaded center punch
- Come-along
- Lawn mower blade and hammer
- Linoleum knife

The most efficient way to gain access to a vehicle depends upon the damage to the vehicle and the way in which the vehicle has come to rest. As with forcible entry, the rule for gaining access is "try before you pry." Often, the easiest way to gain access to a vehicle is the normal way: by opening one of the doors. Try all the doors first: one may still open. (It is foolish to begin hacking at a vehicle with an axe only to have someone else discover that one of the doors opens.) If the door is locked, someone who is skilled with a lockout tool may be able to release the locking mechanism. If the doors are jammed, dented, or otherwise inaccessible, you will have to break windows, pry the doors, cut around the door lock, or cut through the roof.

Side windows probably represent the quickest means of gaining access to a closed vehicle with jammed or inaccessible doors. Side windows are usually made of tempered glass. Tempered glass shatters when struck but does not break into big shards; rather, it breaks into very small pieces. If possible, break a window on the opposite side of the patient. If you have the equipment there, tape the window with adhesive paper or duct tape. Then place a pointed tool, such as the point of a pick-head axe, a center punch, or a screwdriver in the lower corner of the window (Figure 16.5). Strike the handle of the tool firmly with another tool but do not follow through on the stroke. Strike the glass firmly enough that the glass shatters in place but not so hard that the glass is knocked inward. Then

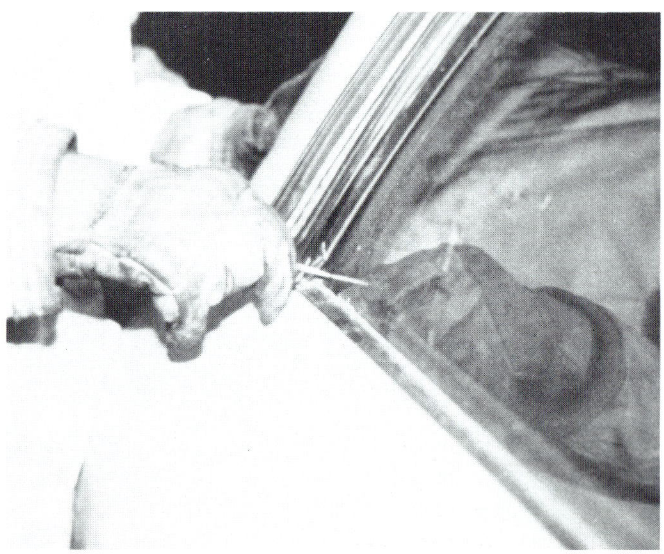

**Figure 16.5** Place a pointed tool in the lower corner of the window. *Courtesy of Joel Woods, Maryland Fire and Rescue Institute.*

reach in and open the door or pull out some of the glass to reach the door lock.

Another way to gain access is to begin prying the door with hand tools. Concentrate on the area around the door lock where all the door and lock strength is. Use a pry bar, Halligan bar, crash axe, or similar tool and begin prying. Use wedges and/or cribbing to increase the distance the tool will spread on one try. Insert the prying tool between the window and the door next to the door lock, apply leverage, and spread the metal slightly. Then, reposition the tool deeper into the objective and repeat the process. Once the door lock is exposed, the task of opening the door is easier. At the very least, prying with hand tools will provide a better surface for power tools.

Cutting around doors to bypass the lock entirely is another method of gaining entry. Use a large hand tool designed for cutting metal or a hammer and screwdriver (Figure 16.6). An air chisel also offers a fast and efficient way to cut around the lock.

Entering through the roof is often the most feasible way to gain access when a vehicle is on its side. Make a three-cornered cut using a flat-head axe and a hammer or hand cutting tool (Figure 16.7). A lawn mower blade used with a hammer makes an excellent metal cutter. When it arrives, an air chisel is a fast and efficient way to gain access through the roof. If rescuers cannot gain access through the roof, the next points of entry are the front and rear windshields.

If you are unable to gain access through the door or side windows, consider removing the windshield or taking the roof off. Both these procedures are difficult and time consuming with hand tools, so they should be tried only when other attempts at entry have failed.

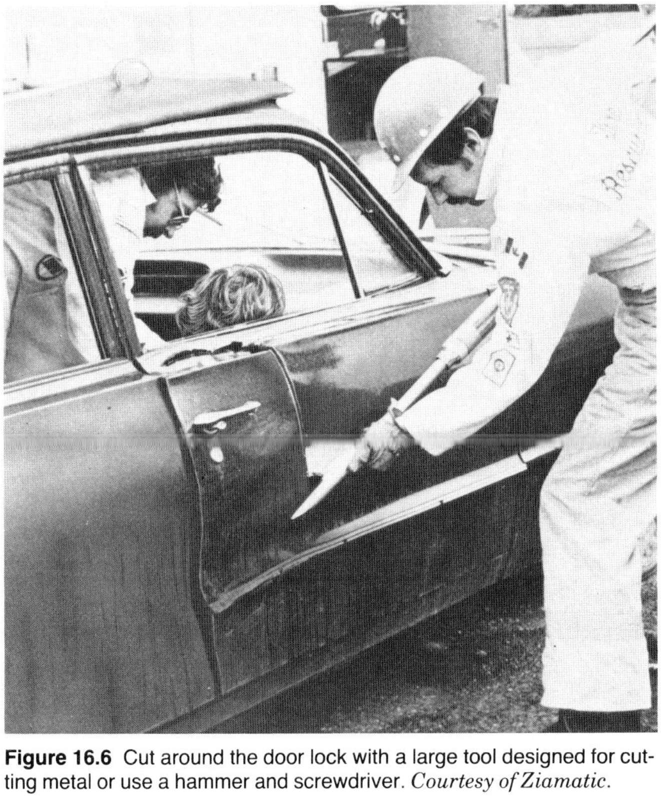

**Figure 16.6** Cut around the door lock with a large tool designed for cutting metal or use a hammer and screwdriver. *Courtesy of Ziamatic.*

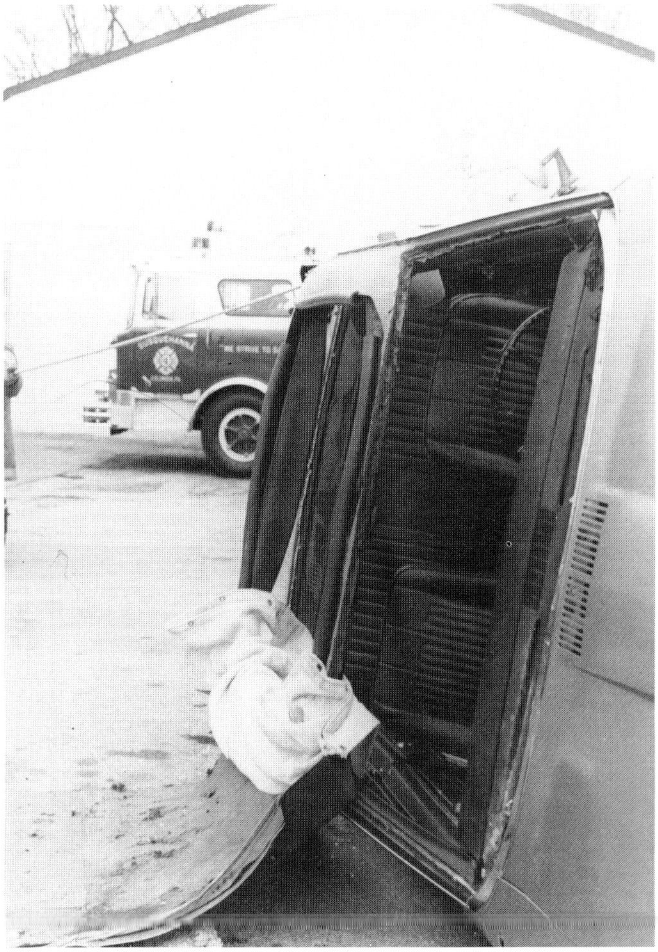

**Figure 16.7** To gain access through the roof of a vehicle, make a three-cornered cut using a hand cutting tool or a lawn mower blade and a hammer. *Courtesy of Elmer Reese.*

Windshields are made of laminated glass, which is two layers of glass glued to a layer of plastic. Laminated glass does not shatter like tempered glass does; furthermore, laminated glass is very difficult to cut. The preferred method is to remove the entire windshield. One method for removing a windshield is to pull off the molding around the windshield with a baling hook (Figure 16.8). In some newer model cars (1970s and later), windshields are set in mastic and a linoleum knife is required to cut through the glue. If there is chrome attached to glass, mastic has been used. If there is chrome plus rubber plus glass, the chrome can be peeled off from the top and sides and the windshield can be pried off with a screwdriver or other similar tool (Figure 16.9). To break laminated glass, you will have to chop through it with an axe or baling hook. Again, when breaking glass, try to break glass in an area away from the patient in order to keep as little glass as possible from falling on the patient.

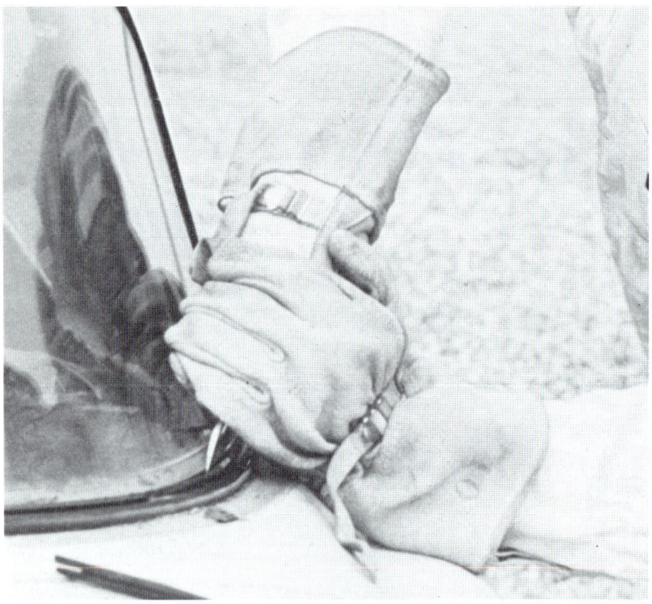

**Figure 16.8** Using a baling hook to pull off molding. *Courtesy of Joel Woods, Maryland Fire and Rescue Institute.*

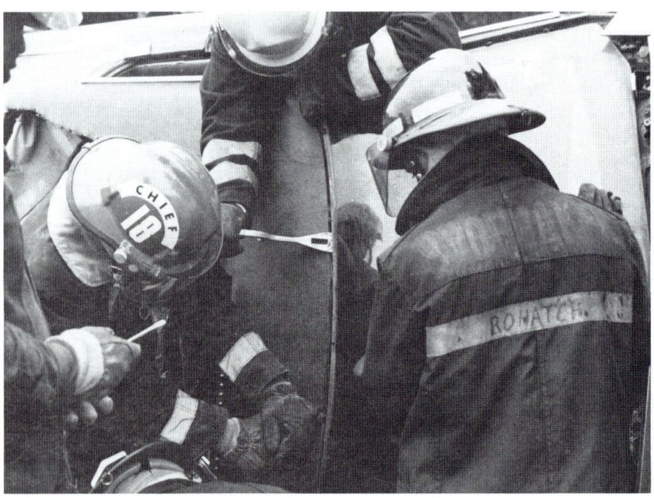

**Figure 16.9** Pry the windshield off with a screwdriver or other flat-edged tool. *Courtesy of Gary Courtney.*

Depending upon damage to the vehicle, it may be necessary to take off the roof. This is a very difficult procedure with hand tools. You may be able to use a hacksaw or axe and cut through all the door posts, then lift off the roof. An air chisel can also be used to cut the door posts.

If the vehicle is overturned or on its side, entry through the floor offers a way into the passenger area. Again, this is a difficult and time-consuming procedure with hand tools. The front and rear passenger floor boards are the best points of entry. Avoid cutting under seats, and watch for fuel lines. Remember, too, that passengers on the floor of the vehicle may be further injured when tools penetrate into the passenger area, so exercise caution.

## PATIENT ASSESSMENT

As you enter the vehicle, take in a cervical collar, blanket, flashlight, and a pad and pencil. You should be wearing full protective clothing. TURN OFF THE IGNITION FIRST. If it is impossible to turn off the ignition from inside the vehicle, have other rescuers remove the battery cables. Again, all rescuers should be wearing full protective clothing, including eye and hand protection. Battery cables must be removed with care because they may spark; they should be carefully worked off the terminal posts or cut with long bolt cutters. Firefighters should be ready with a charged line in case of fire.

As always, assess and correct the patient's ABC's first. CAREFULLY loosen clothing in the neck area and apply a cervical collar, then bandage any open wounds (Figure 16.10). If the patient needs CPR, he or she will have to be removed from the vehicle as rapidly as possible; in this case, all other injuries are secondary.

Cover the patient with a blanket to conserve body heat and to protect the patient from breaking glass. Stay with the patient and provide reassurance, particularly when power tools are started. THE RESCUER IN THE VEHICLE SHOULD STAY WITH THE PATIENT UNTIL ANOTHER MEMBER OF THE EMS SYSTEM TAKES OVER OR UNTIL EXTRICATION IS COMPLETED. In

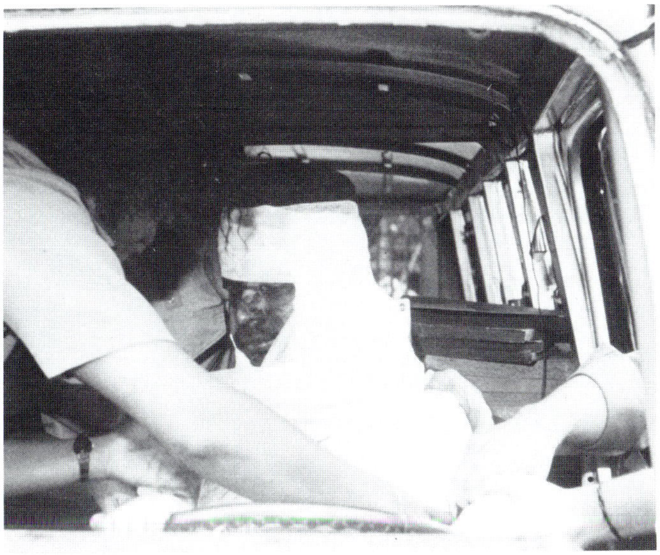

**Figure 16.10** After assessing the ABC's and applying a cervical collar, bandage open wounds. *Courtesy of Joel Woods, Maryland Fire and Rescue Institute.*

the excitement, confusion, and noise of an accident scene it is easy to get distracted by other people or extrication procedures and neglect the patient.

Look to see if interior parts of the car will have to be moved in order to free the patient. The patient may be trapped by the pedals, the steering wheel, a shifted seat, or any other mechanism. The rescuer may need to help wrap a chain around the streering column so that other rescuers can pull the steering column off the patient with a power tool (Figure 16.11). If the patient's feet are entangled in the pedals, it may be necessary to use a small power tool or hand tools to free the feet. Be sure to pad or stabilize the patient's feet first for safety.

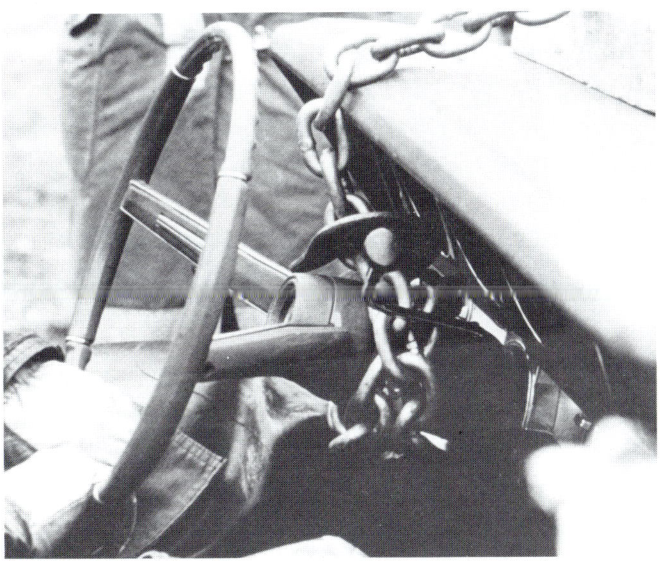

**Figure 16.11** The rescuer inside the vehicle may need to help by wrapping a chain around the steering column. *Courtesy of Joel Woods, Maryland Fire and Rescue Institute.*

If a patient is caught between the seat and the dash, it may be possible to achieve more working room by operating the seat lever and moving the seat back on its track.

Patients whose heads, arms, or other body parts have been thrown through a windshield require special attention. After stabilizing the vehicle, protect the patient from further injury by padding and stabilizing the protruding body part. Work a towel, blanket, or sheet between the body part and the windshield (Figure 16.12). Next, start pulling the glass from around the body part by using a knife or pliers. When enough glass has been removed, move the body part back through the windshield.

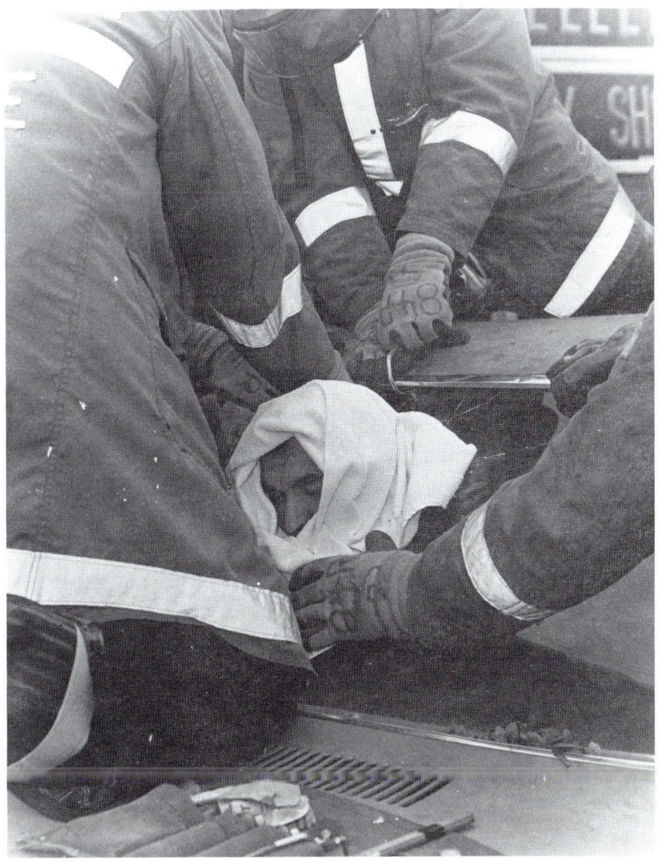

**Figure 16.12** If a body part is protruding through a windshield, pad it with a blanket or towel. *Courtesy of Elmer Reese.*

Naturally, vehicle accidents do not conveniently occur with only one car and one patient. While you are inside the vehicle, check the floor and under the seats in case a small child or infant is pinned in the vehicle. Look for dolls or toys that might indicate a young passenger. Rescuers outside the vehicle should open the trunk and check under the vehicle, again to make sure that no one — adult, child, or animal — is trapped.

## SHORT-DISTANCE TRANSFER

In general, a patient should not be moved until he or she is ready for transportation to a medical facility. All necessary emergency care should be provided first. Furthermore, a patient who has suffered trauma or who is unconscious must be assumed to have a spinal cord injury. The methods for immobilizing a patient with a spinal injury on a backboard or a scoop stretcher are described in Chapter 8, Injuries to the Skull, Spine, and Chest. The lifts, carries, and drags described in this chapter are intended for the patient who is ill or who must be moved rapidly to a place of safety.

Only if there is an immediate danger to the patient or to rescue workers should the patient be moved before treatment is provided. Emergency moves are necessary if

- There is a fire or danger of fire.
- Explosives or other hazardous materials are involved.
- It is impossible to protect the accident scene.
- It is impossible to gain access to other victims who need immediate life-saving care.
- The patient is in cardiac arrest and must be moved to a different area (and a firm surface) so that rescuers can administer CPR.

The major danger in moving a patient quickly is the possibility of aggravating a spinal injury; for example, it is impossible to quickly remove a patient from a vehicle and at the same time protect the patient's spine. In an extreme emergency, however, the patient's spinal injuries become secondary to the goal of preserving life.

If it does become necessary to perform an emergency move, make every effort to pull the patient in the direction of the long axis of the body, not sideways (Figure 16.13). Avoid jackknifing the patient. If the patient is on the floor or ground, pull

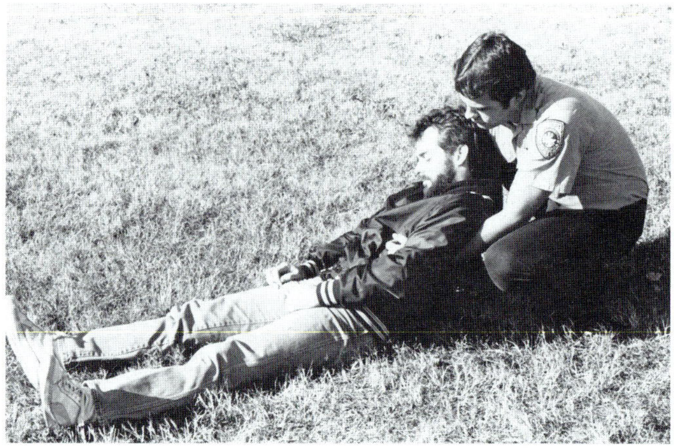

**Figure 16.13** If it does become necessary to perform an emergency move, try to pull the patient in the direction of the long axis of the body, not sideways.

on his or her clothing in the neck or shoulder area. It may be easier to pull the patient onto a blanket and then to drag the blanket. There are a number of carries and drags that may be used to move a patient from an area quickly; these are described later in the chapter.

It is always better to have two or more rescuers when attempting to lift or carry an adult. One rescuer can safely carry a child or small adult, but two, three, or four rescuers may be needed to safely lift and carry a larger adult. An unconscious individual is always more difficult to lift: this person is unable to assist in any way and a relaxed body becomes "dead weight."

It is not easy for inexperienced people to lift and carry a person correctly. Their efforts may not be well-coordinated, and they will need careful direction to avoid further injury to the patient. Anyone who helps carry a patient should guard against losing his or her balance. The carriers should lift gradually and with proper technique, so that the patient is not injured further. In addition, lifting incorrectly is one of the most common causes of injury to rescuers (Figure 16.14). Do not attempt to lift anything — person or object — while you are bent over. Rather, position yourself by kneeling close to the patient and keeping your back as straight as possible. When you lift, use the lifting power of your legs, not your arms and back.

If immobilization of an injured part is not feasible until the patient has been moved a short distance, one rescuer should place one hand under the injured part and the other hand just above or below

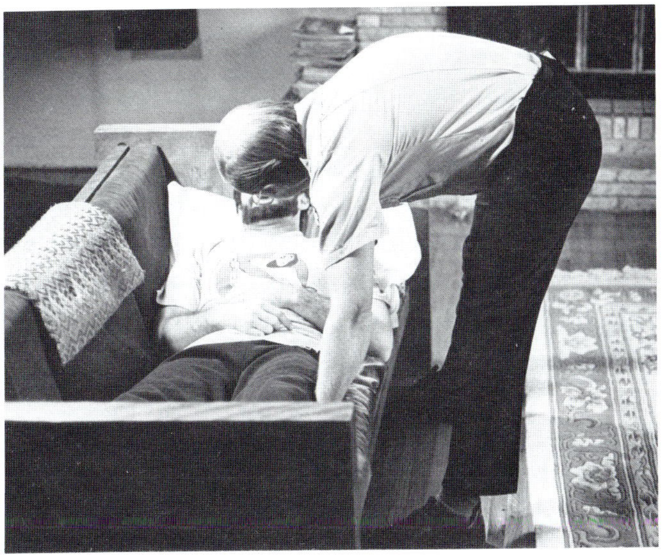

**Figure 16.14** Trying to lift while you are bent over places severe strain on the back.

the injured part. While several rescuers lift the patient, one rescuer lifts the main weight of the injured extremity, and another rescuer keeps the immediate area of the injury from bending or twisting.

## Cradle-In-Arms Carry

This carry is effective for children and small adults, but is not practical for unconscious adults due to the weight and relaxed condition of the body.

Step 1: Place one arm under the patient's arm and across the back and the other arm under the patient's knees (Figure 16.15).

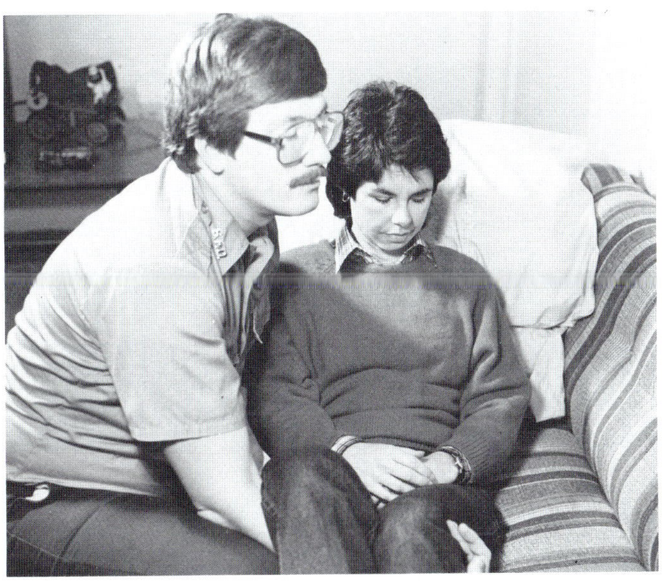

**Figure 16.15** Reach across the patient's back with one hand and under the knees with the other.

Step 2: Keeping your back straight, lift the patient to about waist height and carry the patient to safety (Figure 16.16).

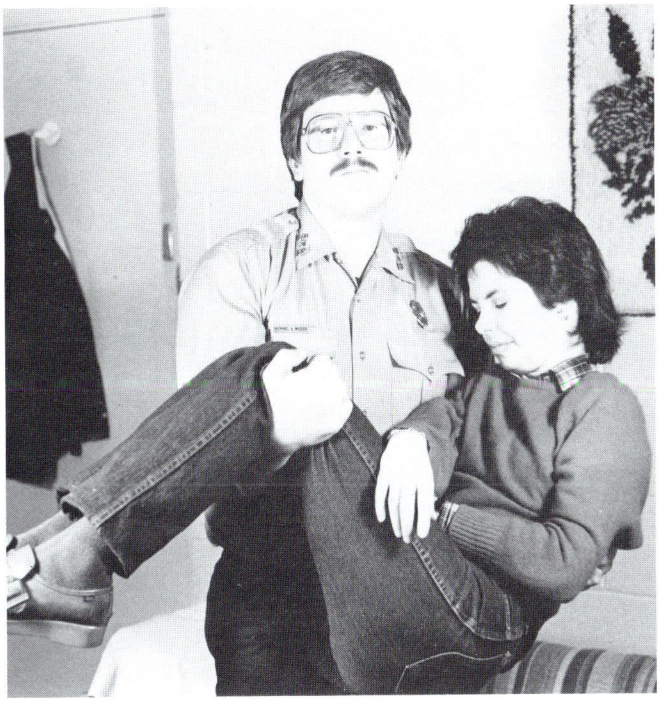

**Figure 16.16** Keep your back straight and lift the patient to about waist height.

## Seat Carry

This carry may be used on a conscious or unconscious person.

Step 1: Both rescuers link arms across the patient's back and raise the patient to a sitting position (Figure 16.17).

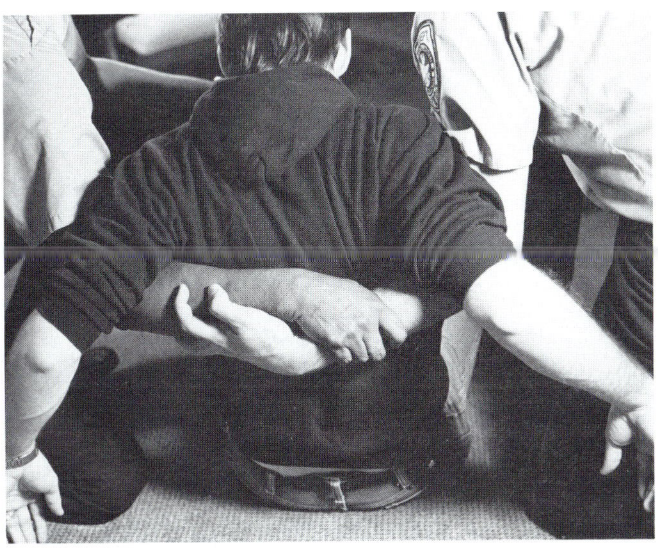

**Figure 16.17** Both rescuers link arms across the patient's back, then raise the patient to a sitting position.

Step 2: Both rescuers then reach under the patient's knees, again linking arms (Figure 16.18). The arms linked at the patient's back and legs form a seat.

Step 3: Both rescuers then stand, using the correct technique, and move the patient to safety (Figure 16.19).

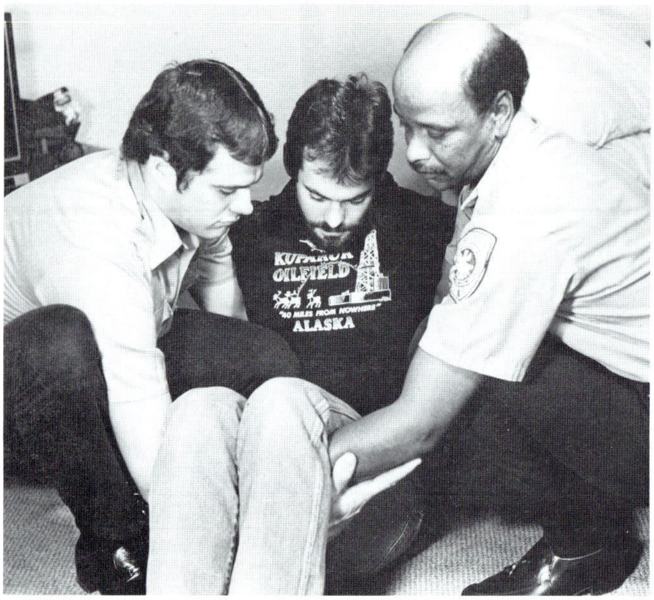


**Figure 16.18** By linking their other arms under the patient's knees, the rescuers form a seat.

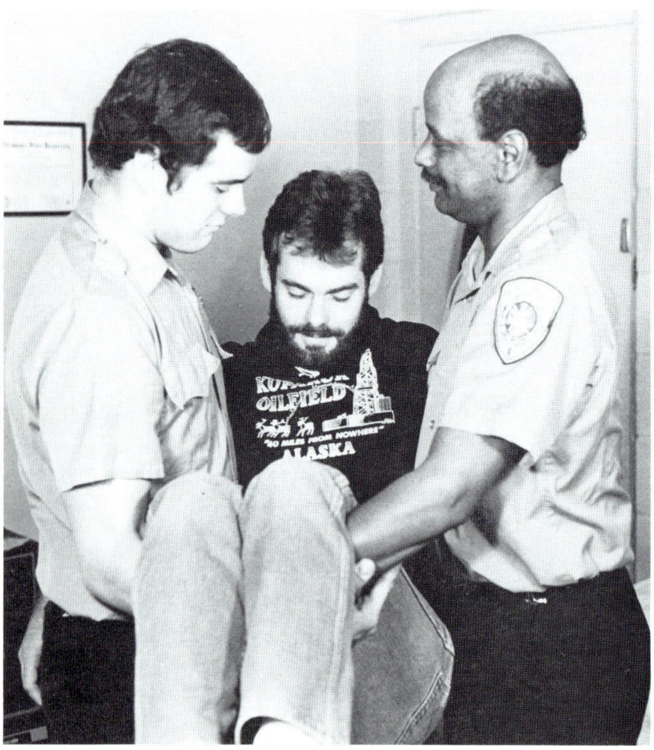


**Figure 16.19** Using the correct technique, both rescuers stand and move the patient.

## Two- or Three-Person Carry

This carry is a very common and useful way to lift a patient who is lying down. Many patients, such as geriatric patients and cancer patients, are far more comfortable when left in a lying or extended position. The two- or three-person carry is useful for moving a patient from a bed to a stretcher and is especially useful when the patient is in cramped quarters, such as a mobile home or recreational vehicle. If the patient is small, two rescuers may be sufficient; if the patient is large, four rescuers may be necessary.

Step 1: Position the stretcher so that the patient can be carried to it and placed on it without difficulty. This may require leaving the stretcher in the up or medium position.

Step 2: The rescuers should position themselves on the side of the patient that is easiest to reach and/or that will facilitate placing the patient on the stretcher. For example, picking up the patient from the right side will mean placing the patient on the stretcher from the right side. One rescuer should be positioned at the head and upper torso of the patient, one at the waist and legs, and, if necessary, one at the lower legs. If the patient is in a bed, it may be necessary to move the patient to the closest side of the bed in order to facilitate the lift.

Step 3: The rescuers should crouch or kneel as close to the patient as possible, keeping their backs straight. The rescuer at the head places one hand slightly under the patient's head and the other hand and arm under the patient's upper body. The other rescuers place their arms under the patient's torso and legs (Figure 16.20).

Step 4: On the signal from the rescuer at the head, all rescuers carefully roll the patient toward their chests (Figure 16.21).

Step 5: Again, on the signal from the rescuer at the head, all rescuers stand while keeping the patient held against their chests (Figure 16.22). The patient may now be moved to the desired location.

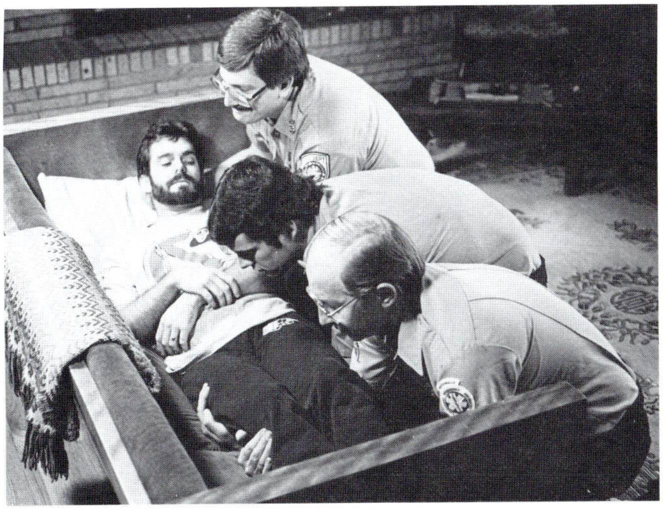

**Figure 16.20** The rescuer at the head supports the patient's head and upper body. The other rescuers support the patient's torso and legs.

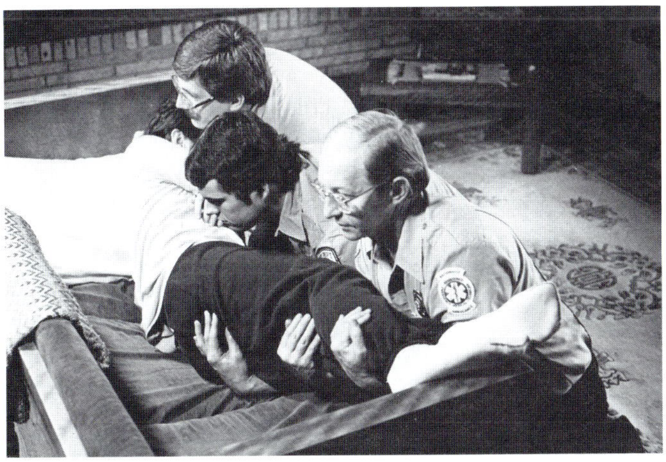

**Figure 16.21** On signal, all three rescuers roll the patient toward their chests.

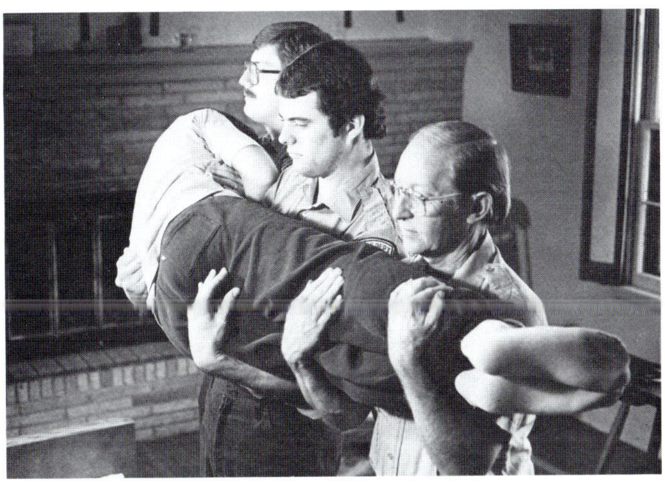

**Figure 16.22** On signal, the rescuers stand with the patient.

Step 6: Reverse the above procedures, again on the signal of the rescuer at the patient's head, to place the patient on the stretcher.

**NOTE:** With a smaller patient, two rescuers can perform this lift. One rescuer supports the patient's head and upper back and the other rescuer supports the patient's torso and legs (Figure 16.23).

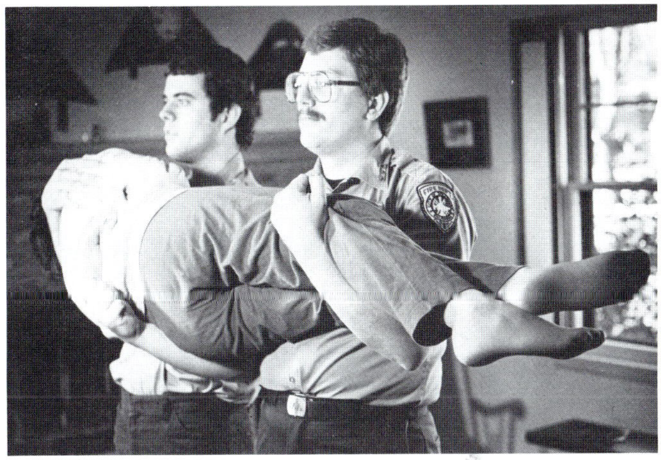

**Figure 16.23** A smaller patient may be lifted by two rescuers.

## Incline Drag

This drag can be used to move a patient down a stairway or incline, and is very useful for a unconscious patient.

Step 1: Turn the patient so that he or she is supine (lying on the back).

Step 2: The rescuer kneels at the head of the patient, reaches under the patient's arms, and hold the patient's wrists (Figure 16.24). If the patient is unconscious, it may be helpful to tie the patient's hands together.

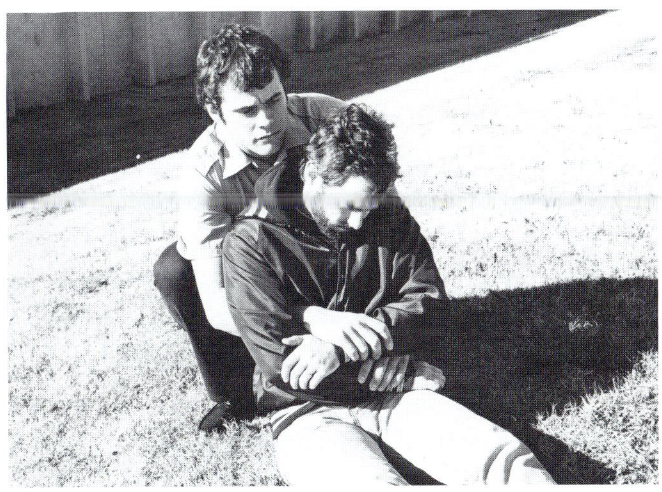

**Figure 16.24** Kneeling behind the patient, the rescuer reaches under the patient's arms and grasps the patient's wrists.

Step 3: The rescuer comes to a standing position (Figure 16.25). The patient can now be eased down a staircase to safety.

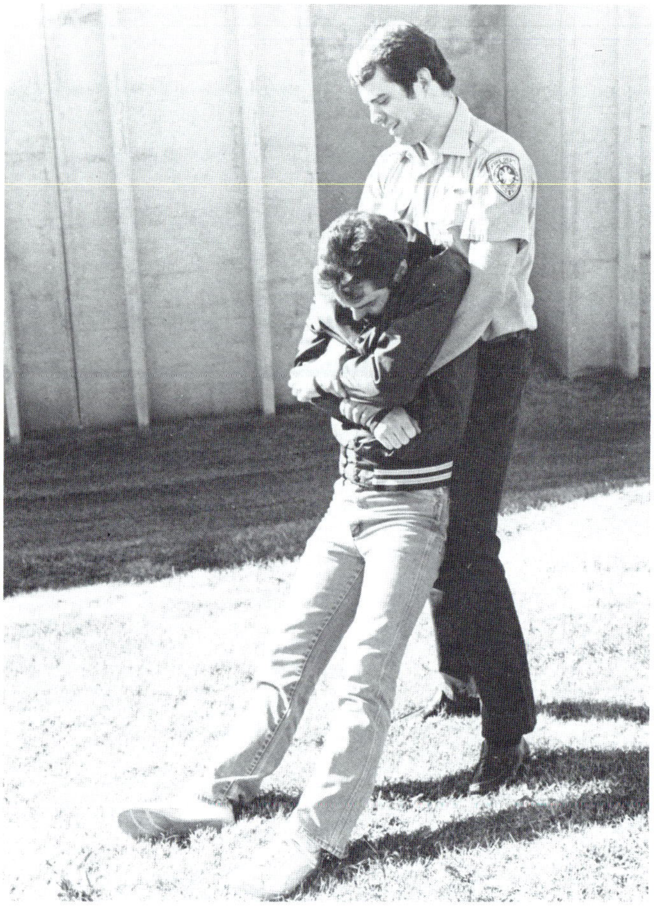

Figure 16.25 The rescuer stands with the patient.

## Blanket Drag

This drag may be executed with a blanket, rug, or sheet and can be employed by one person. The steps are as follows:

Step 1: Turn the patient so that he or she is lying face up. Place a blanket next to the patient (Figure 16.26).

Step 2: Kneel on both knees at the patient's side. Reach across the patient and grasp the patient's shoulder and hip. Roll the patient up against your knees and hold securely (Figure 16.27).

Step 3: With one hand, slide the blanket against the patient, gathering it slightly against the patient's back (Figure 16.28).

Step 4: Gently allow the patient to roll onto the blanket, then straighten the blanket out on both sides. Tuck the lower ends of the blanket around the patient's feet and drag the patient to safety (Figure 16.29).

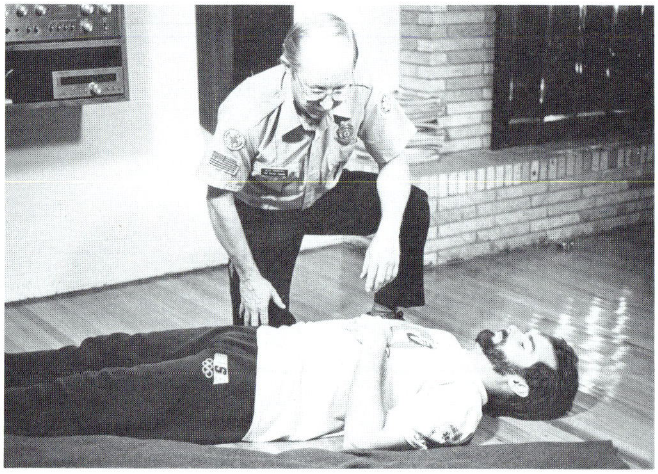

Figure 16.26 Turn the patient so that he or she is lying face up. Then place a blanket next to the patient.

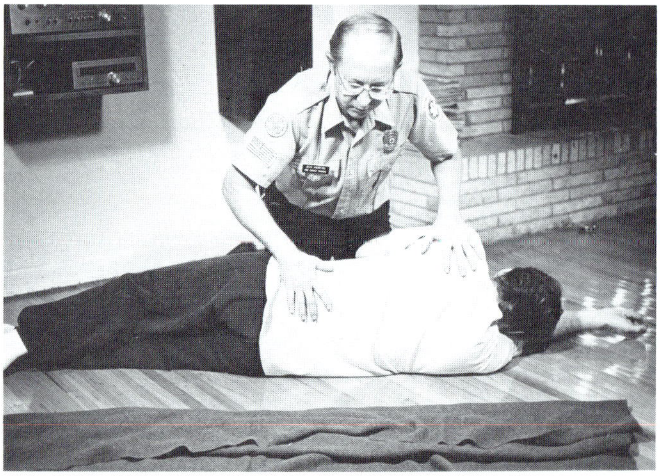

Figure 16.27 Grasp the patient's shoulder and hip and roll the patient against your knees.

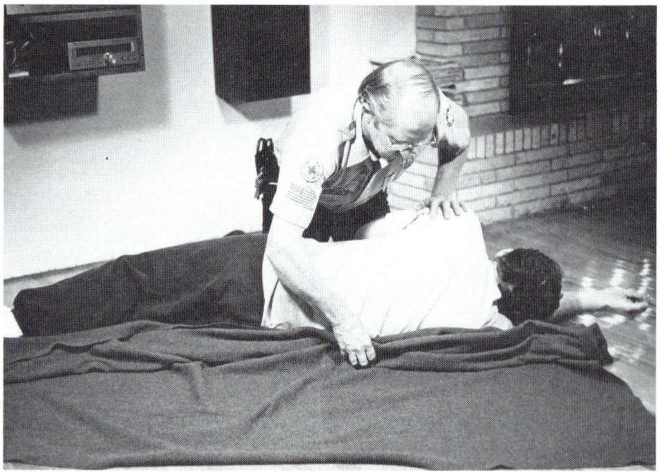

Figure 16.28 Slide the blanket against the patient, gathering it slightly against the patient's back.

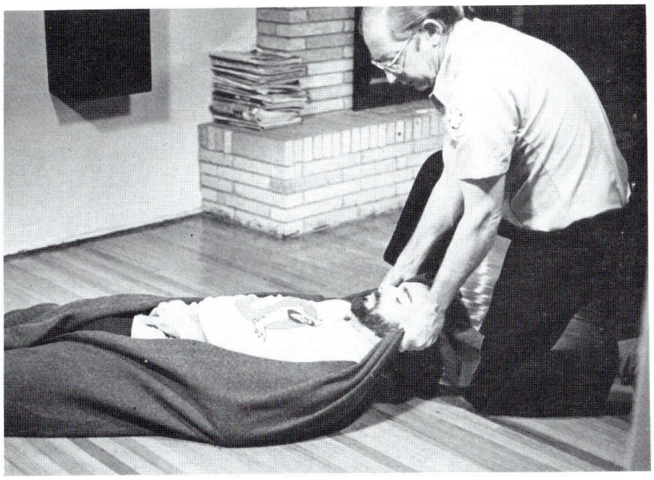

**Figure 16.29** Gently roll the patient onto the blanket and tuck the ends of the blanket around the patient's feet.

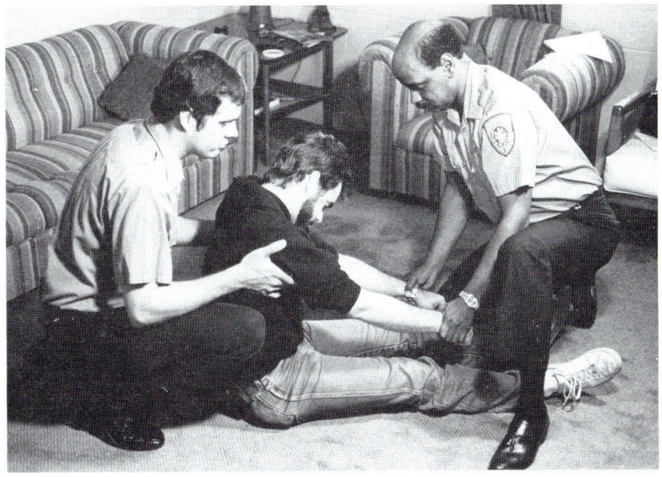

**Figure 16.31** One rescuer pulls the patient to a sitting position while the other rescuer supports the patient's back.

## Extremities Lift

The extremities lift may be used on a conscious or unconscious patient. This lift, which requires two persons, should be performed in the following manner:

Step 1: One rescuer kneels at the head of the patient, and the second rescuer kneels by the patient's knees.

Step 2: The rescuer at the head places one hand under each of the patient's shoulders while the second rescuer grasps the patient's wrists (Figure 16.30).

Step 3: The rescuer holding the patient's wrists pulls the patient to a sitting position; the other rescuer assists by supporting the patient's back (Figure 16.31).

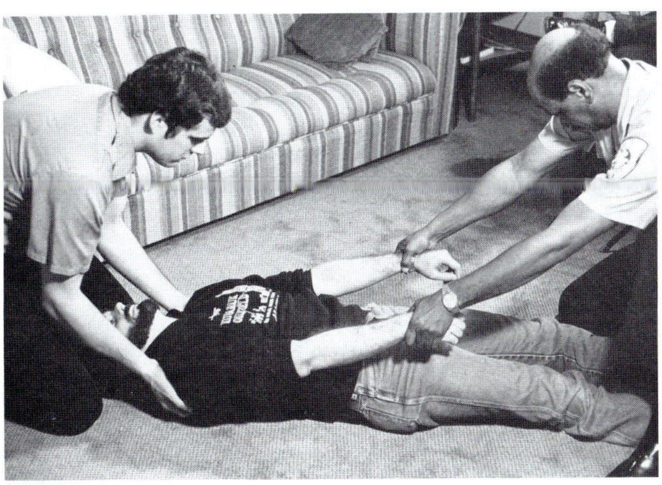

**Figure 16.30** One rescuer supports the patient's shoulders and the other grasps the patient's wrists.

Step 4: The rescuer at the patient's head reaches under the patient's arms and grasps the patient's wrists. The rescuer at the patient's feet turns around, facing away from the patient, and slips his or her hands under the patient's knees (Figure 16.32).

Step 5: Both rescuers crouch on their feet.

Step 6: On the signal of the rescuer at the patient's head, both rescuers stand and move with the patient.

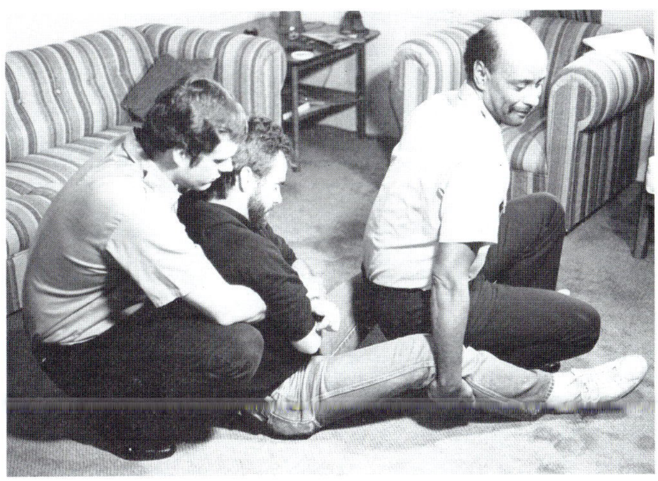

**Figure 16.32** The rescuer kneeling behind the patient reaches under the patient's arms and grasps the patient's wrists. The second rescuer turns around and slips his or her hands under the patient's knees.

## Chair Carry

The chair carry can be used for a conscious or unconscious person. Be sure that the chair you use is sturdy; do not attempt this carry using a folding chair. The steps for executing the chair carry are as follows:

METHOD 1

Step 1: Turn the patient onto his or her back.

Step 2: One rescuer raises the patient's knees until the knees, buttocks, and lower back are high enough for the second rescuer to slip the chair under the patient (Figure 16.33).

Step 3: Raise the chair to a 45-degree angle. One rescuer then carries the back of the chair and the other rescuer carries the legs of the chair (Figure 16.34).

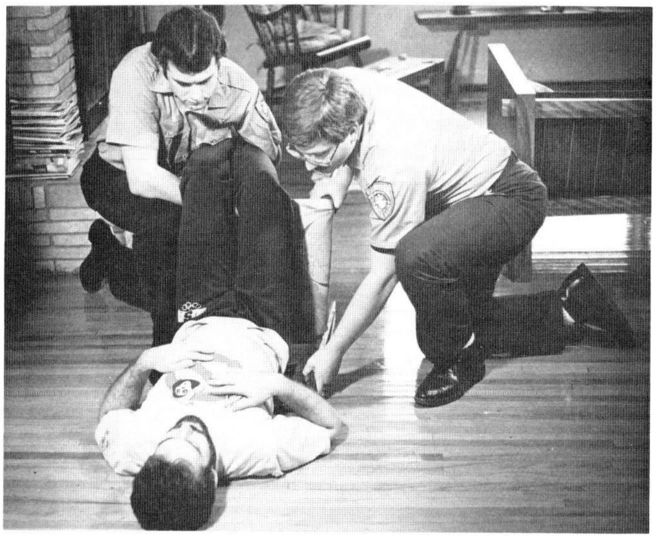

**Figure 16.33** One rescuer lifts the patient's legs and buttocks enough that the second rescuer can slide a chair under the patient.

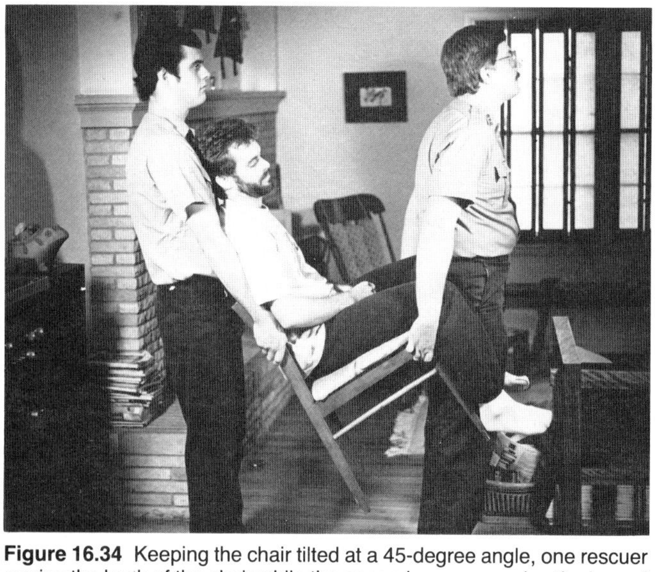

**Figure 16.34** Keeping the chair tilted at a 45-degree angle, one rescuer carries the back of the chair while the second rescuer carries the legs of the chair.

METHOD 2

Step 1: Turn the patient onto his or her back.

Step 2: The rescuer at the patient's head reaches under the patient's arms and holds the patient's wrists. The rescuer at the feet holds the patient's legs under the knees (Figure 16.35).

Step 3: Both rescuers gently lift or swing the patient onto the chair (Figure 16.36).

Step 4: Both rescuers then position themselves as in Method 1, raising the chair to a 45-degree angle. One rescuer carries the back of the chair and the other rescuer carries the legs of the chair.

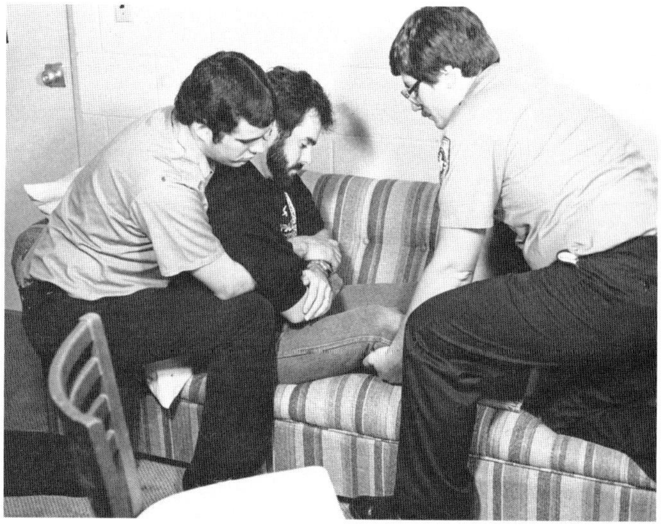

**Figure 16.35** One rescuer grasps the patient's arms, supporting the wrists, while the other rescuer slips his or her hands under the patient's knees.

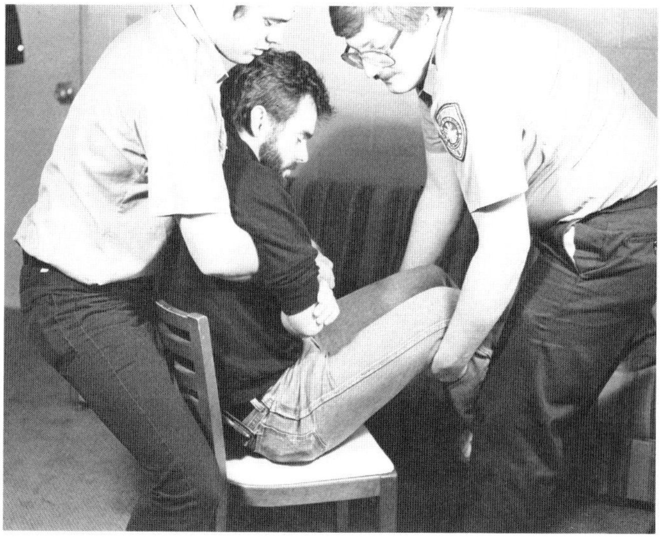

**Figure 16.36** Both rescuers gently lift the patient onto the chair.

## Stokes Basket

The Stokes basket is especially useful for moving patients from heights or over rough terrain or rubble. A Stokes basket is constructed of molded plastic attached to an aluminum frame or woven mesh covering a metal frame. Plastic Stokes baskets are rapidly becoming more popular than wire baskets because they are stronger, easier to handle, and more comfortable for the patient. In addition, many plastic Stokes baskets are molded to allow a long backboard to be placed inside; this feature is especially useful for the patient with a suspected spinal injury. To place a patient in a Stokes basket, two blankets and 50 feet (15 m) of rope are needed.

Step 1: Prepare the Stokes basket for the patient by placing one blanket lengthwise across the head of the basket, allowing one-third of the long edge to extend past the end of the basket. Place a second blanket lengthwise in the basket, allowing about one-fourth of the blanket to extend past the foot area of the basket (Figure 16.37).

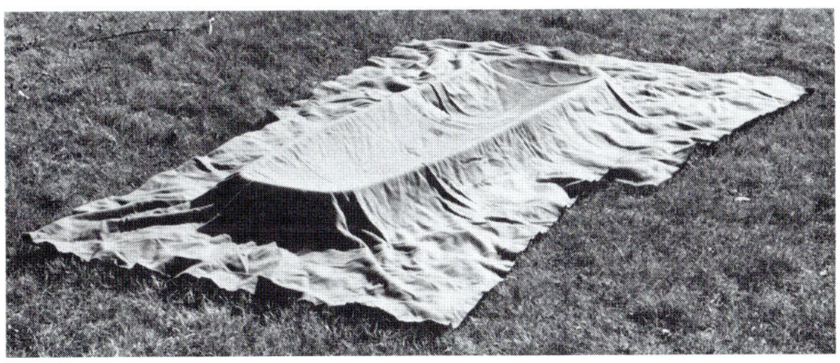

**Figure 16.37** Prepare the Stokes basket by placing one blanket lengthwise across the head of the basket and another blanket lengthwise in the basket.

Step 2: Fold the overhanging portion of the blanket at the head onto itself and place the patient in the basket (Figure 16.38).

Step 3: Fold the lengthwise blanket around the patient, then fold the blanket at the patient's head around the patient by forming folded corners and wrapping the ends across the chest (Figure 16.39). **NOTE:** If the Stokes basket has straps, fasten them at this point.

Step 4: Place the lashing rope through the openings at the foot of the stretcher, starting inside and passing the rope to the outside. Adjust the rope until an equal amount is on each side of the stretcher.

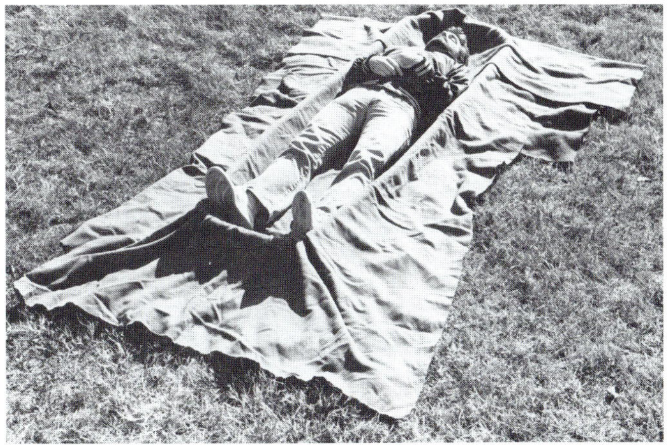

**Figure 16.38** Fold the blanket at the head of the basket onto itself and place the patient in the basket.

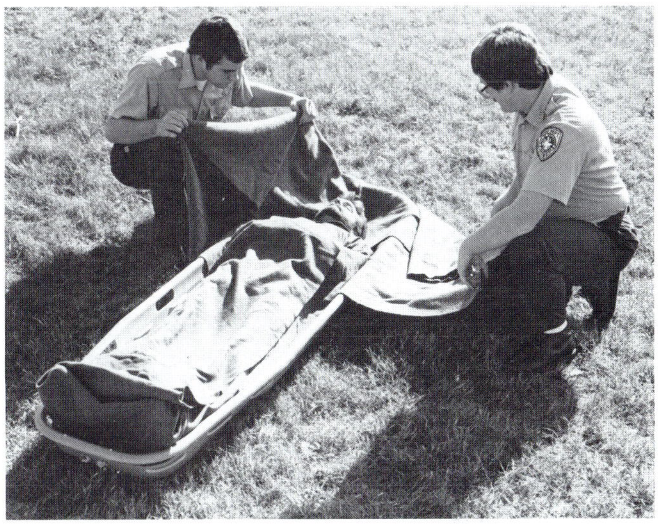

**Figure 16.39** Fold the blankets around the patient's head and body as shown.

Step 5: Secure the patient's feet. Two methods are described below.

METHOD 1: Grasp the rope at the right rail inside the basket and form a half-hitch over the patient's foot at the instep. At the left side, form another half-hitch over the patient's feet at the instep. The patient now has two half-hitches around the feet (Figure 16.40). Dress these half-hitches until they are snug. (**NOTE:** The cross-arm technique is a quick way to form two half-hitches. These can be slipped over the patient's feet and dressed until they are snug.

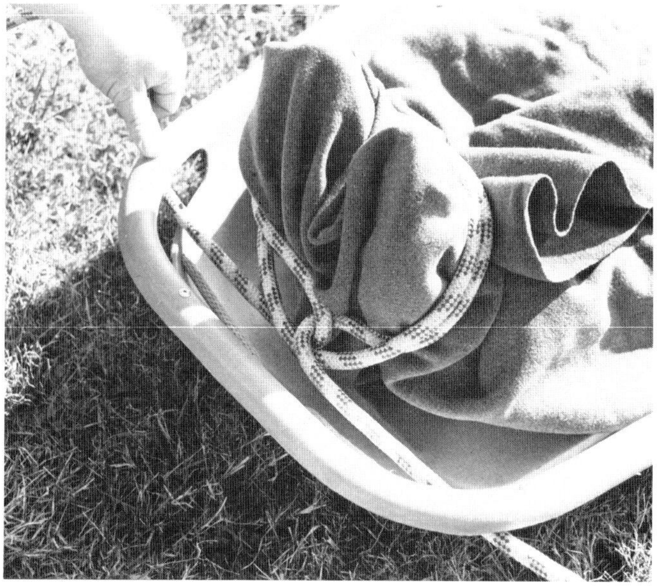

Figure 16.40 Form two half-hitches and slip them over the patient's feet.

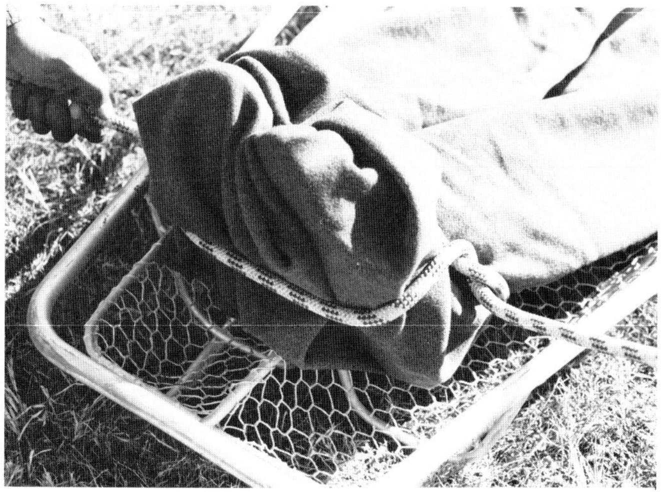

Figure 16.41b The rope should be snug around the patient's feet and ankles.

METHOD 2: (shown with a patient in a wire Stokes basket) Locate the center of the lashing rope. Place the center of the rope under the patient's feet and cross the rope over the top of the patient's feet. Holding the lower section of rope, bring it over the upper section of rope and place it around the patient's feet (Figure 16.41a, b).

Step 6: Take the right side of the rope and pass it over the rail, across the stretcher, and through the closest opening on the left side. Repeat this procedure with the left side of the rope, lacing it inside to outside. (If you are using a wire Stokes basket, thread the rope through the "D" openings.) Continue lacing right to left across the stretcher up to the patient's shoulders. With two rescuers, it is easier to lace if each rescuer passes the rope through the opening, gathers the excess rope, and hands the rope to the other rescuer to lace on the opposite side (Figure 16.42).

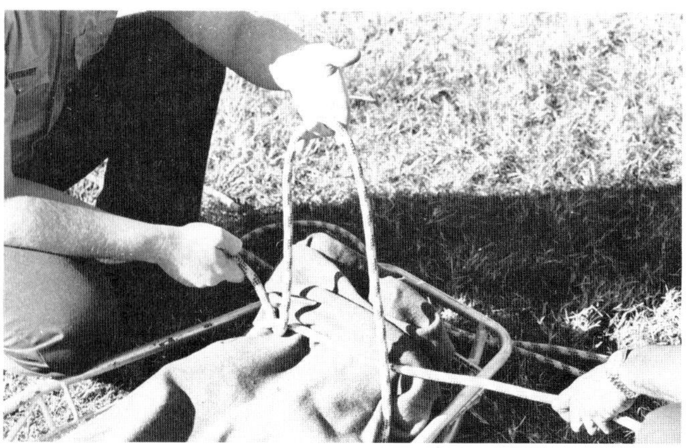

Figure 16.41a Hold the lower section of rope, bring it over the upper section of rope, and place it around the patient's feet.

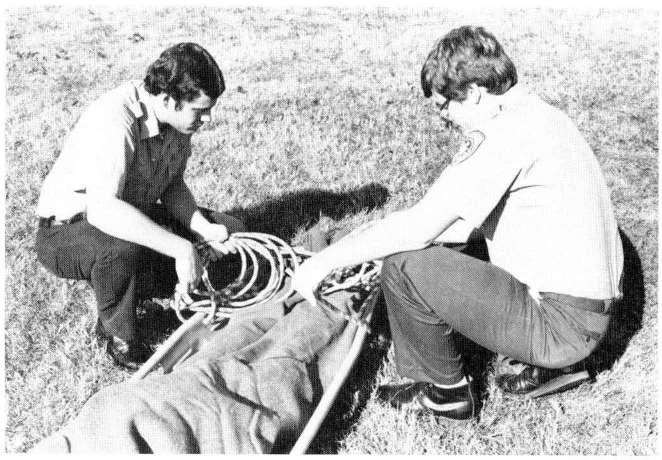

Figure 16.42 Gather excess rope and pass it across to the rescuer on the opposite side.

Step 7: At the patient's shoulders, secure the rope on each side with a clove hitch and a safety (Figure 16.43). It may be easier to tie a clove hitch on the opposite side of the stretcher. Protect the patient's face with a helmet while you are securing the rope.

Step 8: Starting back at the patient's feet, tighten the lashing by pulling up on the

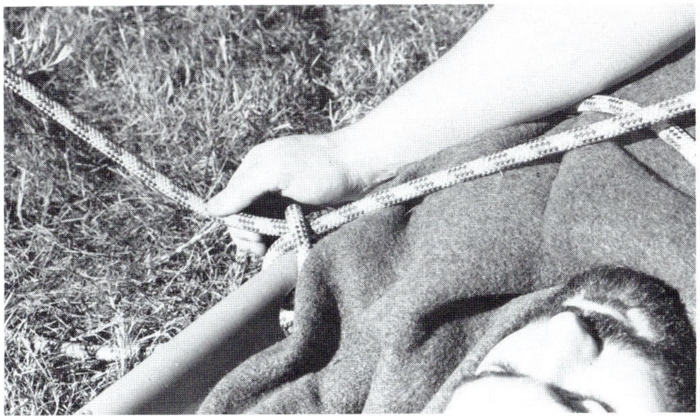

**Figure 16.43** At the patient's shoulders, tie a clove hitch and finish it with a safety.

X's, as shown, working up to the clove hitches and safeties (Figure 16.44). Dress all knots until they are snug.

Step 9: Tuck the excess rope under the lashing to secure it (Figure 16.45).

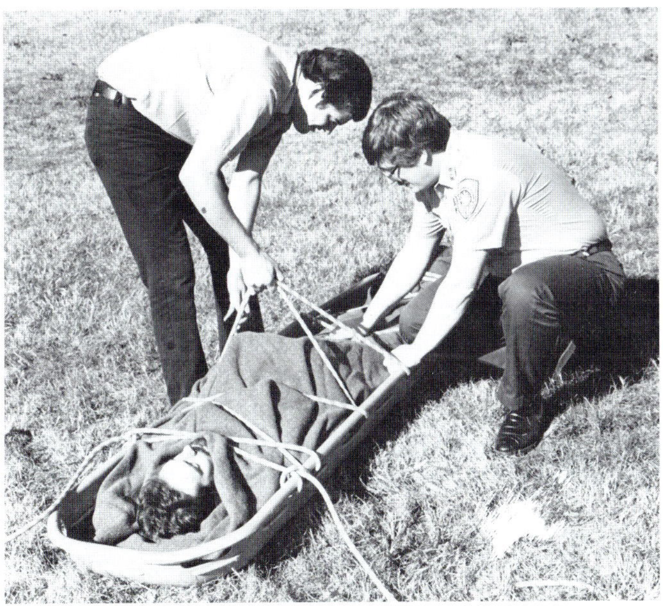

**Figure 16.44** Starting at the feet, tighten the lashing by pulling up on the X's, then dress the clove hitches and safeties until they are snug.

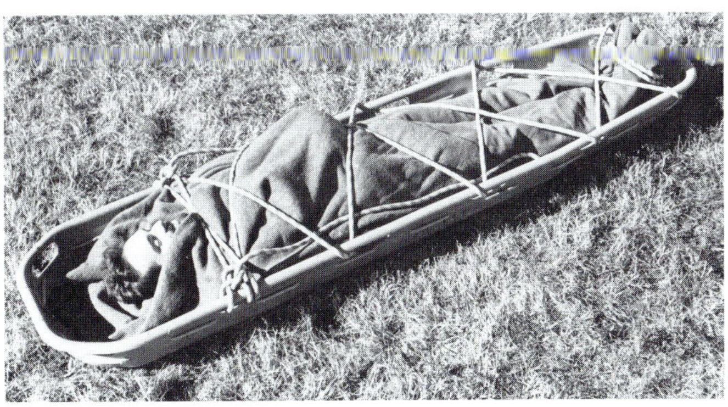

**Figure 16.45** Secure excess rope by tucking it under the lashing.

Step 10: To attach a suspension line for raising or lowering the Stokes basket, pass several feet (meters) of another 50-foot (15 m) length of rope through the openings at the head of the stretcher, then tie a bowline. For more information about Stokes baskets, see IFSTA **Rescue Practices**.

## Litters

Stretchers or litters can be improvised with bunker coats, blankets, and pike poles. A good litter may be made from two bunker coats and two pike poles. The coats can easily be slipped onto the poles by turning them inside out over the head of a rescuer while he or she holds the two poles, as illustrated in (Figure 16.46). The flaps can then be turned down around the poles and buttoned or snapped underneath.

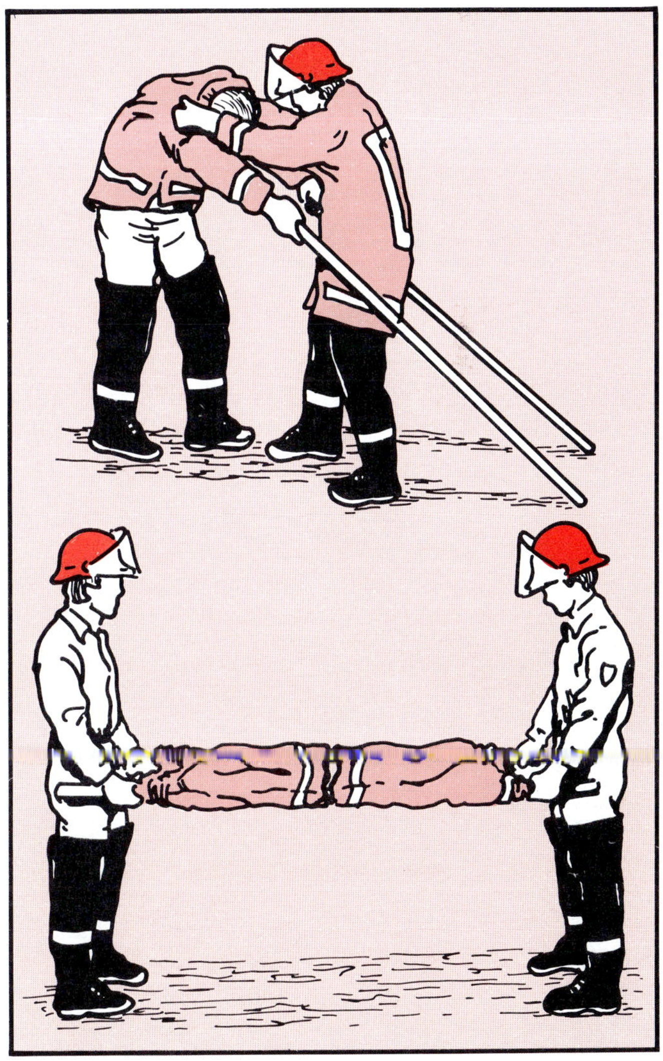

**Figure 16.46** An improvised litter can be made with bunker coats and pike poles, as shown.

Another satisfactory litter can be made from a blanket and two pike poles. Place one pole on the unfolded blanket about 1 foot (0.3 m) from its center and fold the short side of the blanket over the pole toward the other side. Place a second pole on the two thicknesses about 20 inches (508 mm) from the other pole. Then fold the remaining side of the blanket over the second pole toward the first pole, When a patient is placed upon the blanket, his or her body weight will hold the blanket securely. The procedure is shown in Figure 16.47.

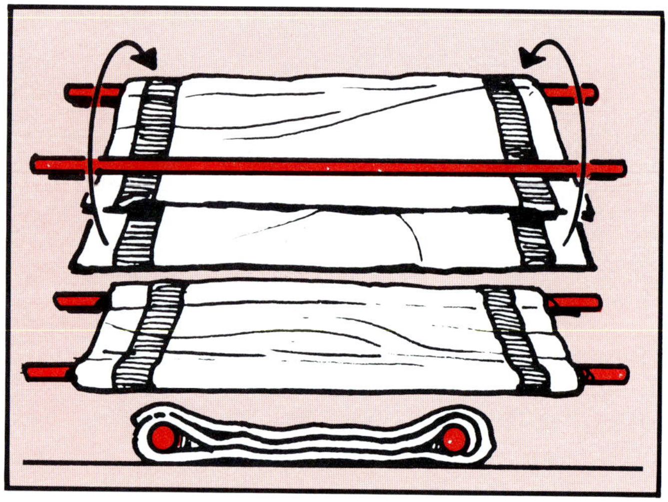

**Figure 16.47** A blanket or salvage cover can be folded around two pike poles to make an improvised litter.

17

# Emergency Vehicles and Ambulance Equipment

# Chapter 17
# Emergency Vehicles and Ambulance Equipment

First responders typically travel to the emergency scene in an engine and do not transport patients to a hospital or other emergency facility; this phase of EMS is usually handled by a public or private ambulance staffed by EMTs or paramedics. Some areas operate paramedic engines, which are fire department engines that carry a full complement of ambulance equipment. The paramedics who staff these engines are capable of providing advanced life support but do not transport the patient to a medical facility. Occasionally, an emergency in a remote location or the need to transport a patient to a specialized facility demands other emergency vehicles. In these cases, helicopters and fixed-wing aircraft can provide accessibility and rapid transportation.

This chapter begins with a brief overview of different types of ambulances, then describes ambulance equipment, its uses, and likely storage places. Emergency Driving Practices is discussed next, followed by Communications and its importance in emergency medical care. A discussion of Records and Reports follows, with emphasis on the need for complete and accurate records. The final section, Air Ambulances, describes the special uses of helicopters and fixed-wing aircraft for emergency patient transport.

Since first responders provide assistance to other members of the EMS team, efficient teamwork requires that they be familiar with other types of emergency vehicles and their equipment. The assistance you provide to EMTs and paramedics will depend upon the nature of the emergency call and upon your local guidelines. Follow these guidelines carefully; attempting to provide care above your level of training can place you at risk of a lawsuit (see Chapter 1, Introduction).

Naturally, first responders work most often with ambulance crews, which are staffed by EMTs and/or paramedics, depending upon the level of emergency care offered in your area. To qualify as an ambulance, a vehicle must meet certain standard requirements. Ambulances meeting these requirements may be manufactured as "stock" vehicles or custom built.

Four standard requirements of ambulances are as follows:

- All certified ambulances must provide space for at least one patient in need of advanced life support or two patients in need of basic life support, two attendants, and a driver.
- The ambulance must be equipped with a radio communications system.
- The ambulance must carry sufficient equipment and supplies to care for patients.
- The ambulance should be equipped for light rescue work.

Federal specifications for ambulances classify three main types of emergency medical care surface vehicles:

- The Type I ambulance has a conventional cab-chassis with a modular ambulance body (Figure 17.1). This type of ambulance has no walk-through and large equipment is stored in outside compartments.
- The Type II ambulance is a standard van and features a walk-through (Figure 17.2).

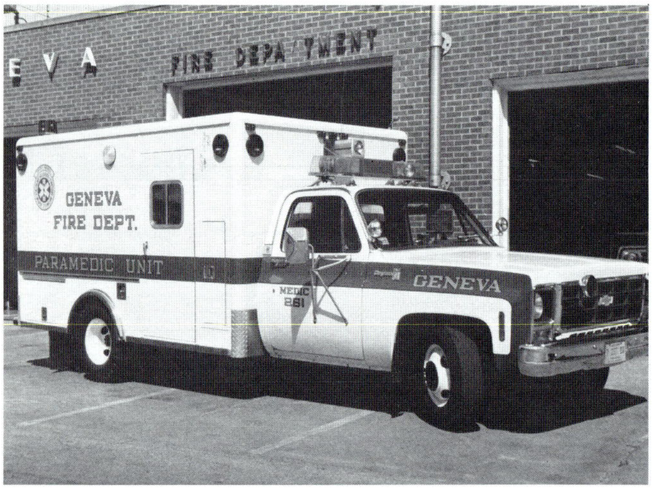


**Figure 17.1** The Type I ambulance has a conventional cab-chassis with a modular body. *Courtesy of Geneva Fire Department.*

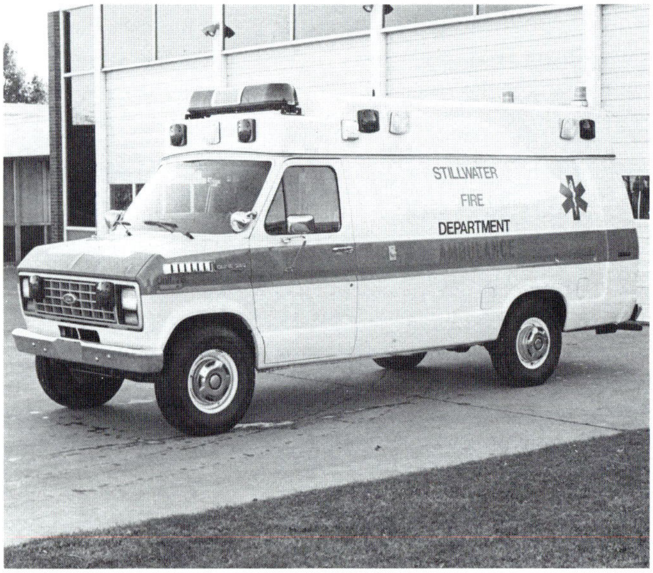


**Figure 17.2** The Type II ambulance is a standard van type. *Courtesy of Stillwater Fire Department.*

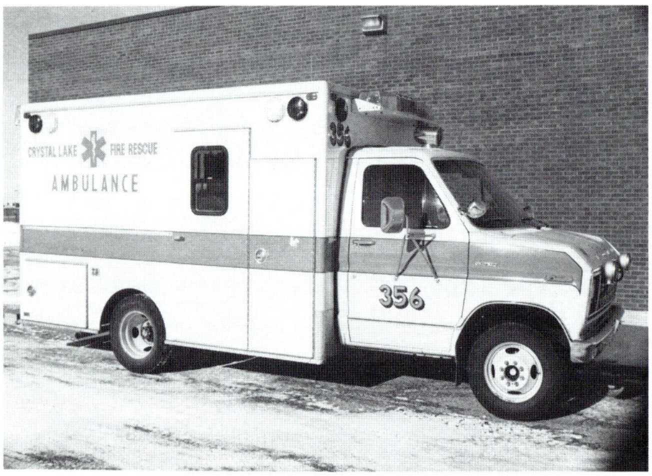


**Figure 17.3** The Type III ambulance is a van chassis with a modular body. *Courtesy of Crystal Lake Fire Department.*

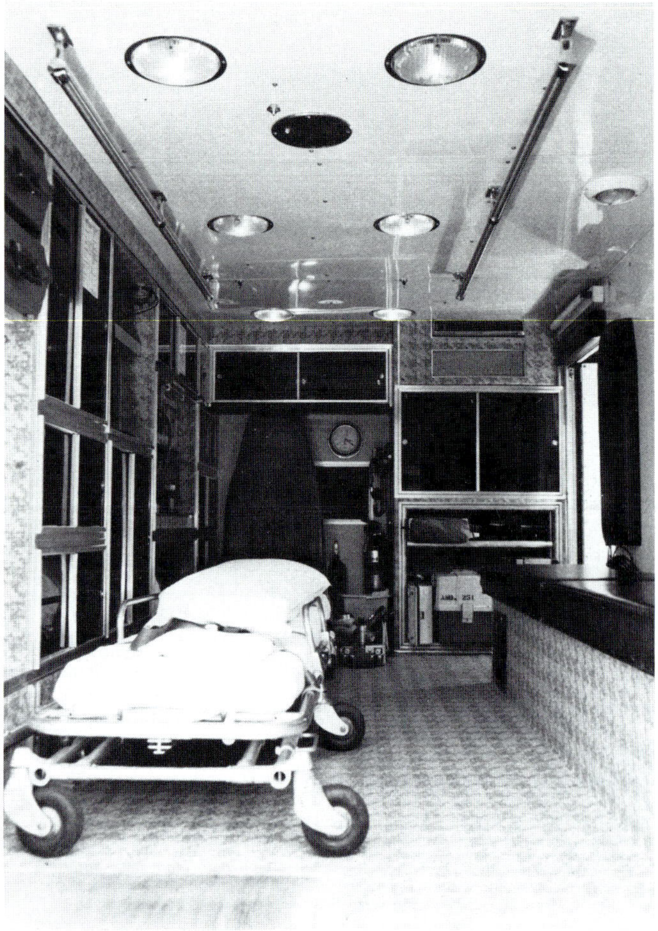

**Figure 17.4** The storage compartments of an ambulance will vary with the ambulance design. Shown above is a typical interior of a Type I or Type III ambulance. *Courtesy of Geneva Fire Department.*

This type of van has no outside storage compartments, so all equipment is stored in inside compartments or under the squad benches.

- The Type III ambulance is a van chassis with a modular body (Figure 17.3). It has a walk-through plus outside storage compartments.

The specific design details of the ambulance and the location of equipment and supplies in an ambulance are basically determined by the manufacturer of the vehicle. Consideration is given to the relative importance of each item and the user's recommendations. The interior of an ambulance is shown in Figure 17.4.

## AMBULANCE EQUIPMENT

Ambulances carry a great deal of patient care equipment and supplies. Nearly all this equipment must be stored inside the ambulance. (If the ambulance has outside storage compartments, larger equipment, such as traction splints and rescue tools, may be stored there.) All equipment must be stored so that it is readily accessible. At the same time, equipment must be secured so that it does not create a hazard while the ambulance is in motion.

On an emergency call, you may be asked to get patient care items from the ambulance. The discussion of ambulance equipment that follows briefly describes the most common types of equipment and their uses. Naturally, it will be more efficient if you have already familiarized yourself with the ambulance(s) in your area so that you know where supplies are likely to be stored. Remember, provide assistance in accordance with your local regulations. Never attempt to use any equipment that you have not been trained in or authorized to use.

## Airway Equipment

For airway care, EMTs and paramedics use much of the same airway equipment that you are already familiar with, such as oral airways and suction equipment. Oral airways are likely to be in an airway bag or box that is stored near the patient's head. First responders carry only portable suction equipment, but an ambulance carries both portable and fixed suction equipment. In some ambulances, fixed suction equipment runs off a vacuum from the engine, so the engine has to be on for the equipment to work. More commonly, fixed units run off a separate pump, so do not require engine power.

EMTs and paramedics are trained in the use of several airway devices that provide better airway management and help prevent regurgitation: the esophageal obturator airway (EOA) and the endotracheal tube. The EOA is inserted into the patient's esophagus; the endotracheal tube is inserted into the patient's trachea (Figure 17.5). The EOA is used for what is called a "blind" intubation, that is, it is slid through the mouth and placed in the esophagus. The EOA is usually a long, clear tube with a bulb on the end that comes with a mask and syringe. The syringe is used to inject a small amount of air into the mask so that it seals tightly against the patient's face. The syringe is also used

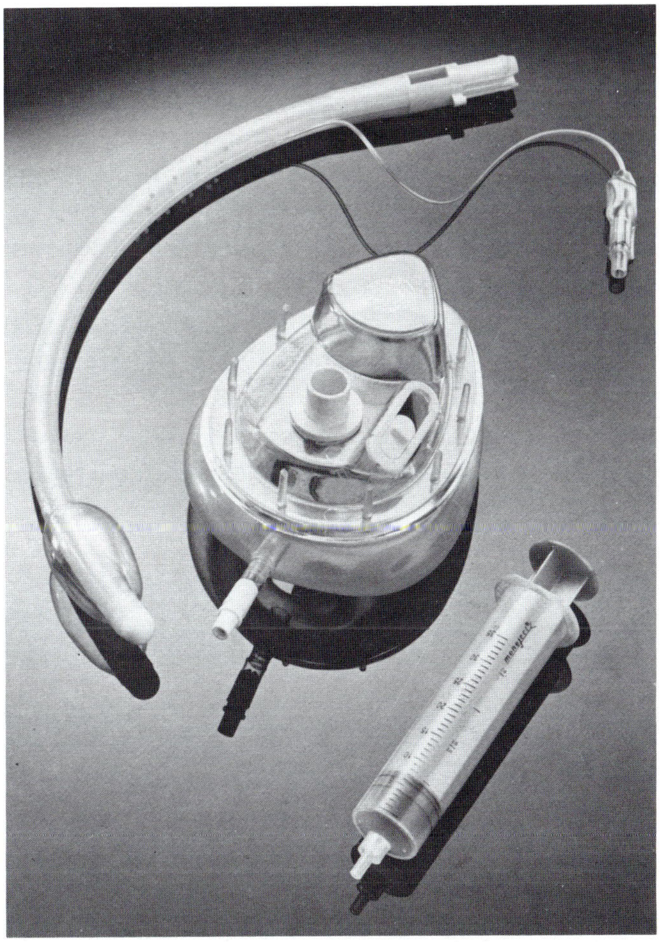

**Figure 17.5** The EOA is placed in the patient's esophagus to help prevent regurgitation. *Courtesy of Dyna Med.*

to inflate the small bulb on the end of the EOA after it is inserted. This procedure seals the esophagus, preventing air from reaching the stomach and lessening the chances of regurgitation. Once the EOA is in place, you may be asked to assist ventilations with a bag-valve mask.

**NOTE:** Sometimes an EOA must be removed because it has been inserted incorrectly or because the patient has regained consciousness. If you are assisting, be ready with suction as the EOA is removed; this action causes regurgitation.

Intubation using an endotracheal tube (also known as an ET tube) and laryngoscope is performed by paramedics. In this procedure, the paramedic uses a laryngoscope, which is a blade with a light on it, to see the patient's trachea. Then the paramedic inserts the endotracheal tube into the patient's trachea. This procedure maintains an open airway. Laryngoscopes have either straight or curved blades and are available in adult and pediatric sizes (Figure 17.6). Laryngoscopes can be sterilized and reused, but endotracheal tubes are used only once. Endotracheal tubes are available in different sizes in sterile packages. If you open a package, keep your face away from the package contents and do not touch the ET tube. Once the tube is inserted it should be taped down as soon as possible. If you are asked to assist with ventilations, be careful not to push or pull on the tube. If you push on it, you may inadvertently pull the tube out. Do not use a demand valve on a patient who has an ET tube inserted; it puts too much pressure on the lungs. Use a bag-valve mask instead. Since laryngoscopes have lights, bulbs or batteries have to be changed periodically. These should be stored in the airway kit.

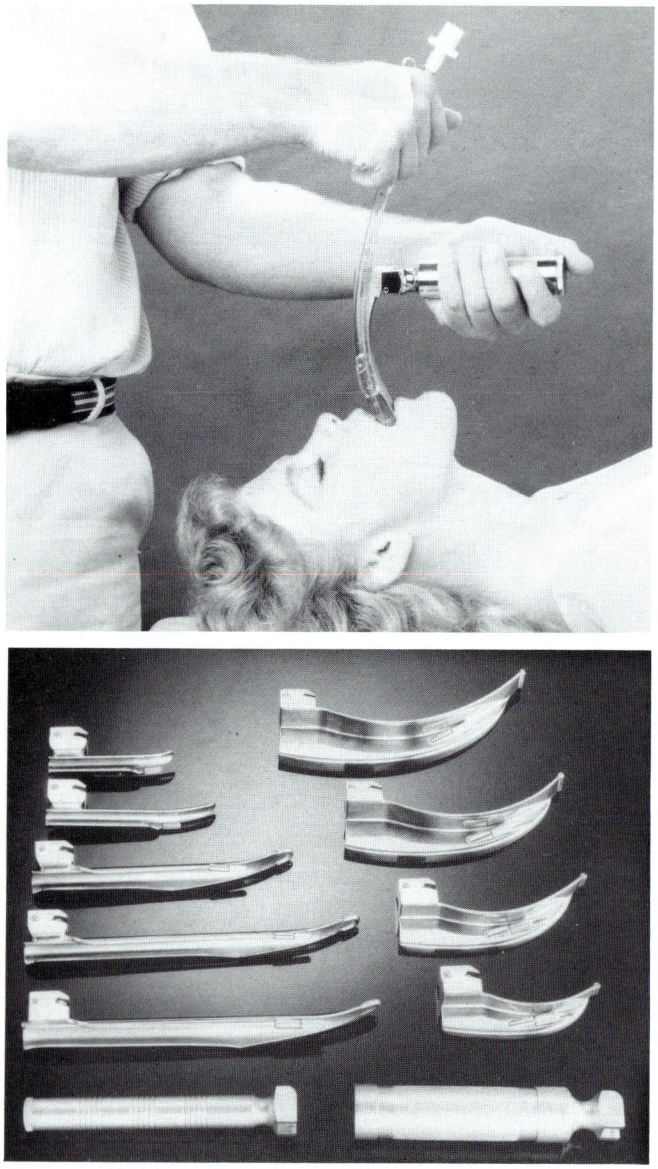

**Figure 17.6** A laryngoscope is used to help place an endotracheal tube in the patient's trachea. Laryngoscopes are available with straight or curved blades, as pictured above. *Courtesy of Dyna Med.*

Certain drugs are given down the ET tube. If the paramedic decides to do this and you are assisting with ventilations, you will have to increase the rate a little to compensate for the time lag in respirations and to help the drug dissolve.

## Breathing Equipment

An ambulance will be stocked with both portable and fixed oxygen equipment. Portable oxygen is dry oxygen, while the fixed oxygen may be humidified. Fixed oxygen is stored in large oxygen cylinders and the oxygen tubing is usually built into the ambulance. To turn on the large $0_2$ cylinder, either reach through a small port and turn the cylinder valve and/or press the switch on the wall marked *Oxygen*.

## Circulation Equipment

A heart monitor is used to detect irregularities in the function of the heart. Electrodes from the heart monitor are attached to the patient's chest and a monitoring scope or strip of paper displays the patient's heart activity. This reading is known as an electrocardiogram, or EKG. With telemetry, the EKG can also be transmitted to a hospital (Figure 17.7). Qualified personnel there can also interpret the EKG and assist with emergency care. Know where the heart monitor is mounted in the ambulance; if you are asked to get it, remember that it may be charging or hooked into the telemetry. Do not pull a monitor from the wall; disconnect all cords carefully. It may be necessary to change batteries in the monitor, so it is useful to

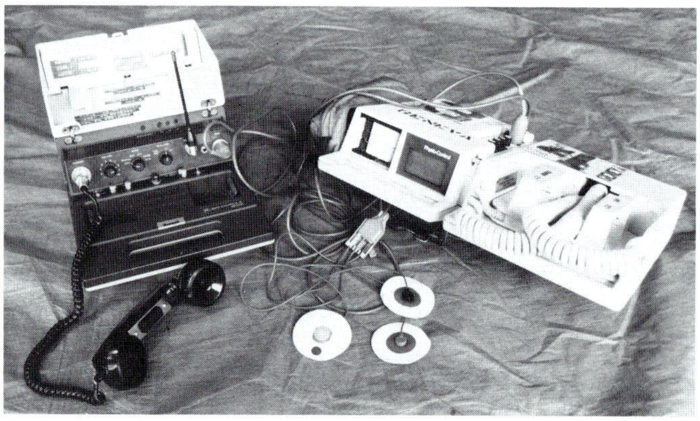

**Figure 17.7** With telemetry, information about a patient's heart activity can be transmitted to a hospital. *Courtesy of Geneva Fire Department.*

know where the batteries are kept and how to change them.

During an emergency call, the patient's heart may begin to fibrillate. Fibrillation is a type of cardiac arrest characterized by spasmodic, ineffective contraction of the heart. Heart monitoring equipment can also be used to defibrillate the patient's heart. Defibrillation is accomplished by shocking the heart with an electrical current. This procedure can be hazardous: when the "clear" signal is given, do not touch anything connected to the patient, such as IV bags, oxygen equipment, or patient monitoring equipment. Remember also that people who are in cardiac arrest frequently lose bladder control. Naturally, urine conducts electricity, so be sure to avoid contact with it during a defibrillation procedure.

Telemetry can be sent to a remote location by various means. A common method is through the unit radio or through the portable medical radio, which is often referred to as the "core unit" or "white box." The heart monitor is connected to the radio by means of a patch cord. Electrical signals generated in the monitor are then sent through the radio to the receiving location. Voice conversation near the monitor can be transmitted along with the monitor's signal or just the monitor's signal can be transmitted. A small portable antenna can be connected to the radio to improve radio operation in areas that do not have good radio reception or transmission. In areas where radio transmission is impossible, a phone coupler may be used to transmit telemetry. Some telemetry units even have recorders that use standard cassette tapes. Heart monitoring equipment and telemetry are used to monitor and evaluate actions performed at the emergency scene; when these devices are being used, remember to watch your language because it may become a permanent record.

## Intravenous Solutions (IVs) and Drugs

Most ambulances carry at least two different IV solutions: D5W and Lactated Ringers. D5W is used for patients with medical problems, such as heart patients. It is given to keep veins open so that drugs can be administered intravenously (Figure 17.8). D5W is commonly used in 250 cc and 500 cc bags. Lactated Ringers is used for fluid replacement; therefore, it is given primarily to people in shock. Lactated Ringers for emergency use is commonly stored in 1 000 cc bags.

You may be asked to hand a sterile alcohol wipe or a needle. There are two basic types of needles used to start IVs. Butterfly needles are used for infants and children and over-the-needle catheters (onc) are used for adults. Needles are referred to by size: the larger the number, the smaller the needle. After an IV is started, it is taped down so that it will not accidentally come loose. You may be asked to cut tape or to record the time the IV was started.

If it is necessary to draw blood, the paramedic or EMT may do it as soon as the over-the-needle catheter is inserted (Figure 17.9). You may be han-

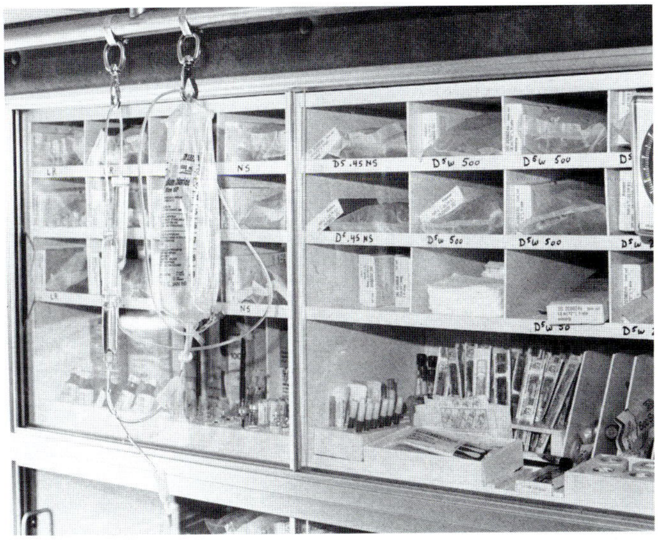

**Figure 17.8** Intravenous solutions are used to replace lost fluids or to keep veins open for the administration of drugs. *Courtesy of Albuquerque Ambulance Service.*

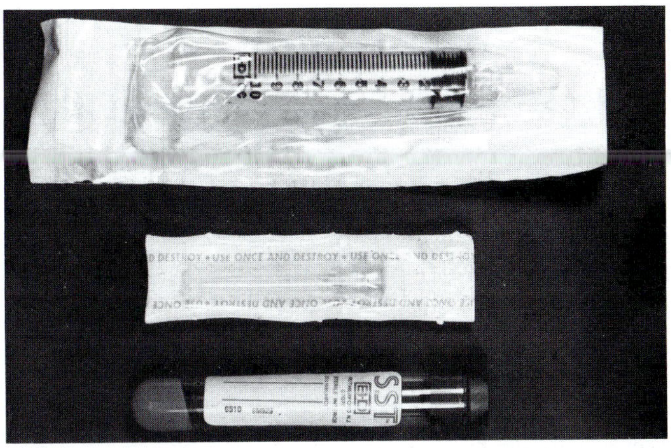

**Figure 17.9** A packaged blood draw set and its components — syringe, needle, and blood tube — are shown above.

ded a syringe containing blood; if you are permitted to do so, put a needle on the syringe and insert it into the top of the blood tube. After the syringe is emptied, carefully dispose of both needle and syringe in the appropriate container. Write the date, time, and the patient's name on the tube. **CAUTION:** If you handle any needles, be very careful not to stick yourself or others. If you do accidentally stick yourself, you will have to make a trip to the hospital for further evaluation.

Most drugs carried by EMTs and paramedics are used for cardiac patients. Some drugs are given by injection, some are mixed in IV bags, and some come already mixed. These drugs are kept in a drug box, which will be stored in an out-of-the-way place (Figure 17.10). The drug box may be locked to deter theft. A number of drugs may be administered to a patient during a cardiac emergency; it is important that the drugs and times of administration be recorded. If other personnel are very busy, you may be asked to fill out a medication added sticker.

## Other Equipment

MAST suits, spinal immobilization equipment, and splints are standard ambulance equipment. MAST suits are available in adult and pediatric sizes and are usually kept in a plastic case. Traction splints and spinal immobilization equipment, such as KED-type devices and long and short backboards, will be stored in the larger compartments (Figure 17.11). If the ambulance has outside storage compartments, these devices may be stored outside. Other splints may be stored with them or may be stored anywhere they will fit. (**NOTE:** Extrication or rescue equipment, if it is

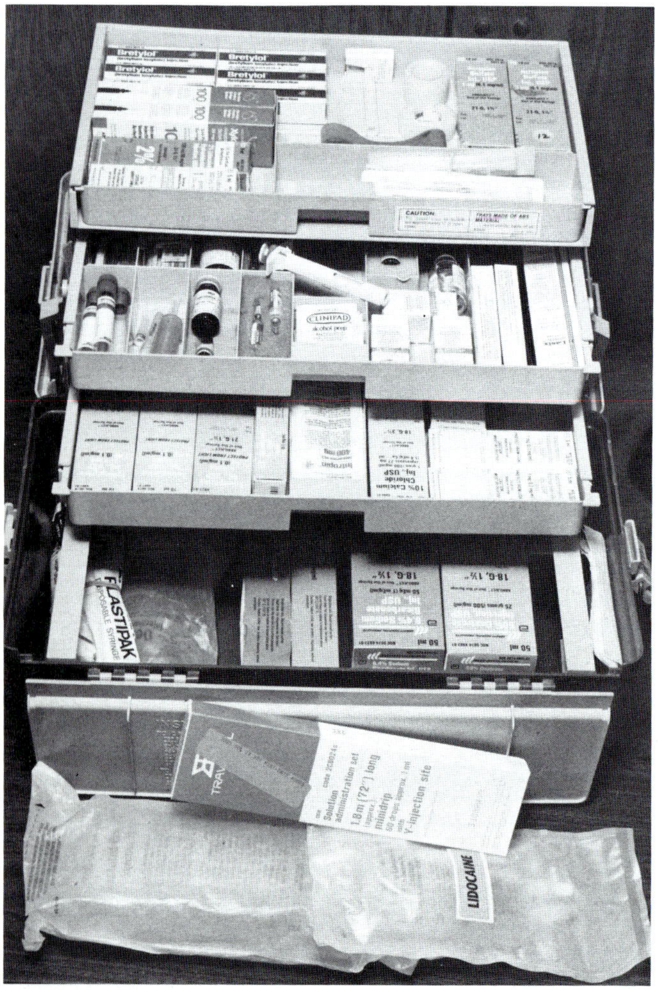


**Figure 17.10** The many different types of drugs used by EMTs and paramedics are stored in a drug box. *Courtesy of Crystal Lake Fire Department.*

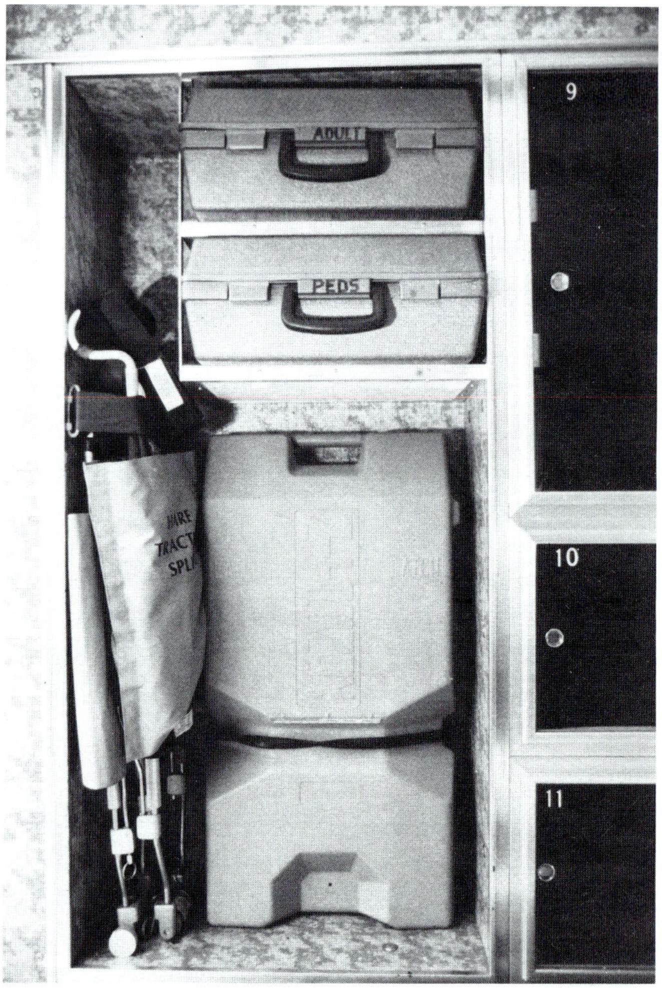


**Figure 17.11** Splints and MAST suits are usually kept in a plastic case. These cases will probably be stored in the larger compartments. *Courtesy of Geneva Fire Department.*

carried, will likely be stored in outside compartments.)

Cervical collars come in large, medium, small, and pediatric sizes. If the cervical collar has two parts, remember to get both of them. Sandbags are usually stored by the cervical collars. Large IV bags can also be used to help immobilize a patient's head.

Different kits — boxes that contain specialized patient care items — will also be stored in the ambulance. Extra jump kits, which contain a wide variety of patient care items, are likely to be kept near the attendant for quick access. A trauma kit may be stored any place that is reasonably accessible.

## Ambulance Cots

Manufacturers will specify the correct way to use their brand and style of cot; however, this section includes some basic cot handling techniques for the most common styles of cots. Cots are side mounted or center mounted, depending upon the type of ambulance. Side-mount cots are more common in vans. To release a side-mount cot, push the release mechanism on the lower left and at the same time pull the cot out and to the right. To lock a side-mount cot back into place, move it back in its holder while pushing the release mechanism. Then pull on the cot to make sure that it is securely in place. To remove a center-mount cot, push the release mechanism and pull it straight out. Reverse the procedure to put the cot back in; it will automatically lock in place. For the roll-in cot, hold the lever and the wheels will automatically drop as the cot is pulled out and collapse as the cot is pushed in (Figure 17.12).

Two people are needed to lift a cot, one positioned on each side. The proper location to hold the cot when loading or unloading is generally on the lowest bar running lengthwise along the stretcher. REMEMBER TO LIFT WITH THE PROPER TECHNIQUE: USE YOUR LEGS, NOT YOUR BACK.

When it is necessary to raise or lower a cot, only one person should work the mechanism, which is on the side and/or end of the cot. Remember to keep your foot on the bottom of the cot to steady it as you raise or lower it. Naturally, if a patient is on the cot, make sure that he or she is securely strapped in before you move it.

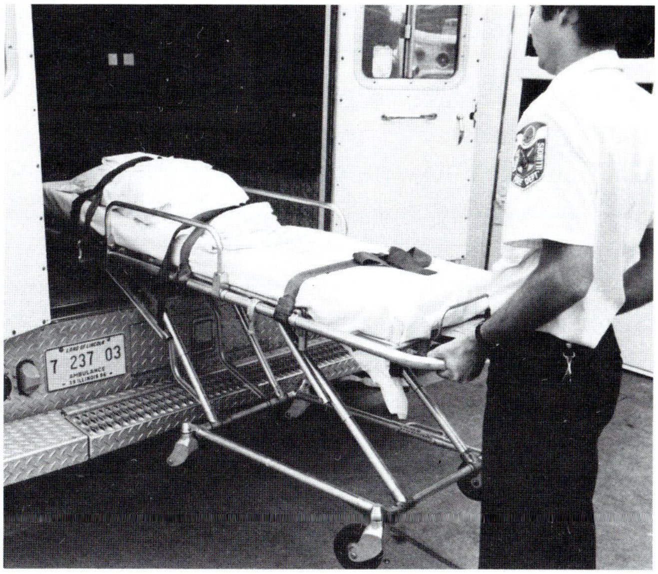


**Figure 17.12** The wheels of the roll-in cot automatically collapse as the cot is rolled in. *Courtesy of Geneva Fire Department.*

## EMERGENCY DRIVING PRACTICES

State, county, and municipal laws usually take into consideration that an emergency vehicle has certain privileges other vehicles do not have. These privileges include speed, right-of-way, parking, progressing through traffic signals, and direction of travel. These privileges are, however, not always spelled out in the law, nor are they automatic. There is no guarantee that other drivers will grant the right-of-way simply because there is an approaching ambulance. For example, an ambulance approaching an intersection with sirens wailing is *requesting* the right-of-way, not *demanding* it. The most important safety point to remember is this: **THE LAWS CONCERNING EMERGENCY VEHICLES DO NOT GIVE THE DRIVER OF AN AUTHORIZED EMERGENCY VEHICLE THE RIGHT TO DRIVE RECKLESSLY OR TO DISREGARD SAFETY PRECAUTIONS.** Driving recklessly endangers the occupants of the ambulance as well as those in the streets.

Driving at high speed is not only dangerous, it can seriously aggravate an injury or illness, particularly if the patient has a heart problem, a spinal injury, or is in shock. A good policy for an ambulance driver to follow is to drive as though a family member is on the ambulance cot and friends are in the other cars on the road.

The ambulance driver (who may be a first responder assisting on a special call) must realize that his or her primary purpose is to provide a safe and comfortable ride for the patient. The driver must keep the emergency vehicle under control at all times by considering other traffic, weather conditions, time of day, and the type of road.

If extra passengers are permitted in the ambulance, they and the driver must wear seat belts. Remember that EMTs or paramedics are attending to the patient and will go flying if the ambulance makes sudden stops or turns corners sharply. Call out a warning when stopping or turning corners, and take them slowly. STOP at intersections if the light is red. Once you can see that traffic in all directions has stopped, proceed through the intersection SLOWLY. Even if the light is green, proceed through the intersection cautiously.

The use of a siren or electronic warning signal should be limited to true emergencies. Remember that, even if it is necessary, a siren may have an adverse effect on the patient. The siren pitch may have to be varied because it is sometimes difficult for a driver in a closed car to detect one continuous tone. (The wail is considered to be the most effective warning sound. Do not fiddle with the buttons to produce unusual tones. This action reduces the decibel level of the siren considerably and wears out the siren.)

Rapid alternation of the headlights between high and low beams is effective even during the daytime. If high-beams are used, take care not to blind drivers in oncoming cars. Red or other color rotating beams of light are also very effective warning signals.

The basic rules for emergency driving can be summed up as follows:

- Use audible warning signals only for a true emergency.
- Approach an accident scene carefully and cautiously — watch for pedestrians and park in a safe place.
- Except for extreme emergencies, operate within the speed limits.
- Reduce speed through traffic lights or stop signs and use audible warning signals at these points.
- Avoid sudden stops and sharp turns.
- Remember the other person — drive defensively.
- Treat the occupants of the ambulance, particularly the patient, as you would wish to be treated.

## COMMUNICATIONS

A well-equipped ambulance should have an intercom system between driver and attendant, two-way radio, public address system, both audible and visible warning devices, and portable radios (Figure 17.13). Contact should be made with the dispatcher as soon as the emergency unit is en route. The dispatcher should be told the exact location of the incident, the time of arrival, time of departure, and time of arrival at a medical facility. The medical facility should also have direct radio communication with the ambulance so that advice and assistance from a physician can be obtained in case of cardiac arrest or similar emergency.

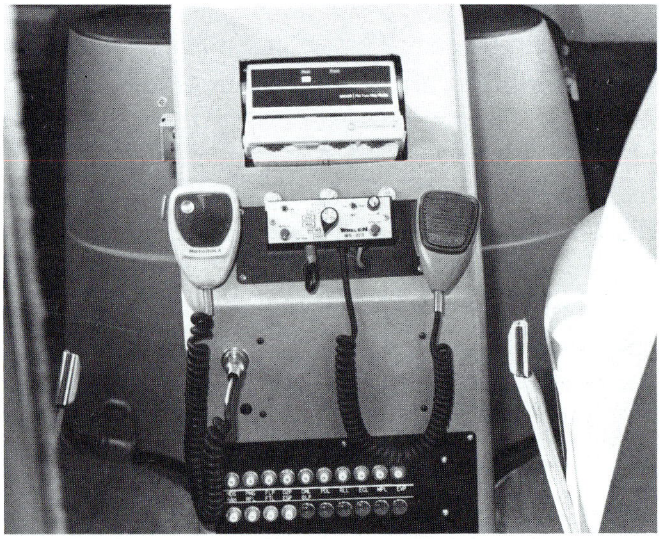

**Figure 17.13** Different types of communications equipment are needed to enable dispatchers, ambulance attendants, and hospitals to exchange information. *Courtesy of Albuquerque Ambulance Service.*

In the ambulance, the intercom system enables the driver and ambulance attendant to communicate. In this way, the attendant with the patient may request an increase or reduction in speed or direct the driver in any other respect.

Portable radio units, also known as "walkie-talkies," "mini-paks," and "handi-talkies," are most useful at the scene of an accident. These units can operate on the same frequency as a base station or can operate on a separate frequency. Portable radios do not have as much transmitting power as does the ambulance or dispatch radios. This is an important point to remember, especially if you are working in an area that is isolated or that does not have good radio transmission. It is also important to be familiar with proper radio operation since several misused portable units can interfere with essential radio traffic.

One of the most commonly used radio systems for EMS work today is the UHF duplex system. This system utilizes a series of radio repeaters that receive radio transmissions and relay them to more distant locations. An important aspect of this system is that one frequency is used for transmitting information and another frequency is used for receiving information. This allows the hospital to receive telemetry and to send instructions at the same time (Figure 17.14). In most areas, a hospital uses a designated radio channel just as an individual would a phone number. If a unit wishes to talk to a particular hospital, it will ask central dispatch for confirmation that the hospital channel is clear and available for use. They may then contact the hospital on that particular channel. Generally, each hospital also has a second radio channel to use as a backup in the event that more than one patient is being brought in at the same time. This backup channel is commonly assigned to several hospitals as their backup, which facilitates information relay in large casualty situations.

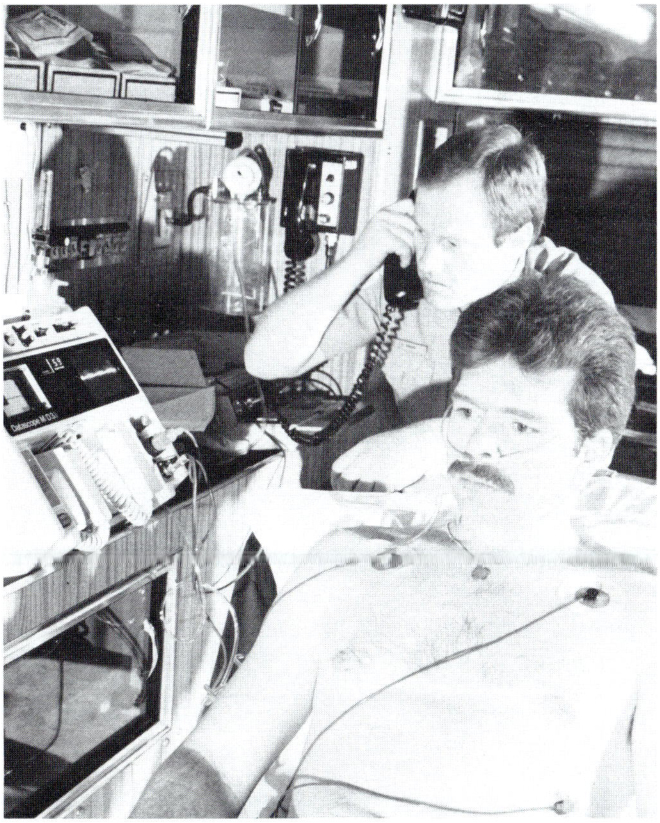

**Figure 17.14** The UHF duplex radio system allows a hospital to receive telemetry on one frequency and at the same time send instructions on another frequency. *Courtesy of Crystal Lake Fire Department.*

## RECORDS AND REPORTS

Records and reports are a vital part of emergency medical services. Complete and accurate reports enable first responders to transmit vital patient information to EMTs and paramedics, thus helping to ensure high-quality patient care. In turn, the reports filled out by EMTs and paramedics give additional information to doctors and nurses. Records and reports also serve as legal documents, another reason why they must be as complete and as accurate as possible. Finally, accurate records are necessary for evaluation purposes. A well-maintained system of records and reports enables fire department officers to evaluate personnel and training needs and to inventory equipment and supplies.

At the emergency scene, the first responder will probably fill out a simplified patient care form that includes the patient's name, chief complaint, vital signs, and treatment initiated. This information is then given to EMTs or paramedics. If you have a separate fire department form to fill out, make sure the information matches the patient care form. A Mobile Intensive Care Unit (MICU) form or run sheet form will usually be filled out by EMTs or paramedics, although you may be asked to help if there are a number of patients. Be sure to write legibly and press hard enough to transfer your writing through all copies of the forms.

All patients at the emergency scene must be accounted for, either on a run sheet or a release form. If there are several patients at the scene who will not be transported, they need to sign a release form. Be sure to have a witness sign the release form as well; preferably this person should be someone other than another firefighter. A police officer is often an excellent person to use as a witness since a police officer's presence can persuade an individual to consent to needed treatment. Make sure that EMTs or paramedics see the forms because they may want to call the hospital for further advice.

## AIR AMBULANCES

Aircraft can be invaluable for patient transportation when accessibility, time, and distance are critical factors. Sometimes land travel will be very slow due to heavy traffic, poor road conditions, or difficulty reaching the accident scene. Sometimes a patient in an outlying area requires rapid transport to a specialized facility, such as a trauma center, burn center, or neonatal center. Sometimes the geographic area covered by an ambulance service is too large or the terrain too rugged for surface vehicles to reach quickly. Under these circumstances, aircraft are often the best means of patient transport.

A specially equipped helicopter may be able to transport twice as many patients as an ambulance (Figure 17.15). A helicopter can operate at speeds approximately twice as fast as conventional surface vehicles. This ability makes it ideal for rapid transport around large metropolitan areas where specialized facilities are located. A helicopter cannot operate in heavy winds or when visibility is poor; a helicopter pilot *must* be able to see in order to land and take off.

In order to land, a helicopter requires an open, unobstructed area about 150 feet (46 m) in diameter and a reasonably clear approach for several hundred feet (30 m or more). Roadside utility poles, traffic, and uncontrolled crowds are the principal obstacles. The main safety considerations to keep in mind if you assist with a helicopter transfer are as follows:

- Clear the landing area of all debris and loose objects.
- After dark, mark the corners of the landing site with flares. DO NOT shine flashlights up at the pilot, as he or she will not be able to see.
- Approach a helicopter only from the front and in a crouched position. Move away from the helicopter in the same direction (Figure 17.16). **NEVER WALK AROUND THE TAIL ROTOR AREA.**
- If the helicopter lands on a slope, approach from the downslope side; clearance from the main rotor blade to the ground is greatly reduced on the upslope side.
- If you carry equipment near the helicopter, carry it waist high or lower, and parallel to the ground.

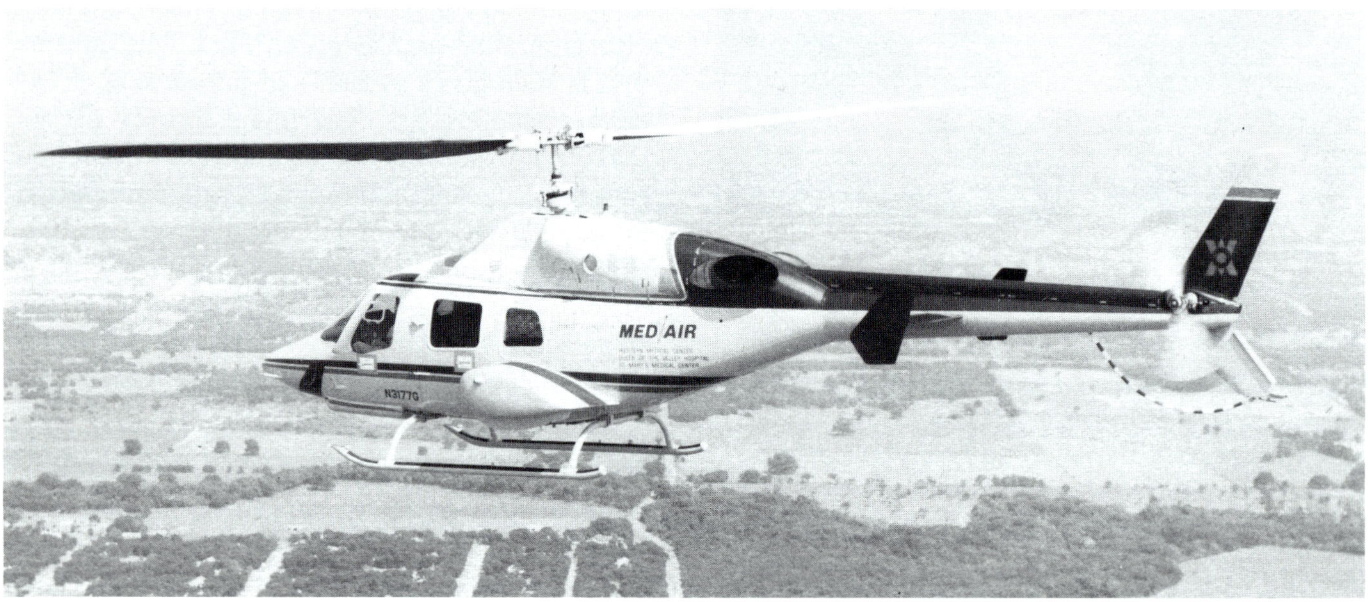


**Figure 17.15** Helicopters are an excellent way to rapidly transport patients to specialized medical facilities. *Courtesy of Bell Helicopter Textron, Inc.*

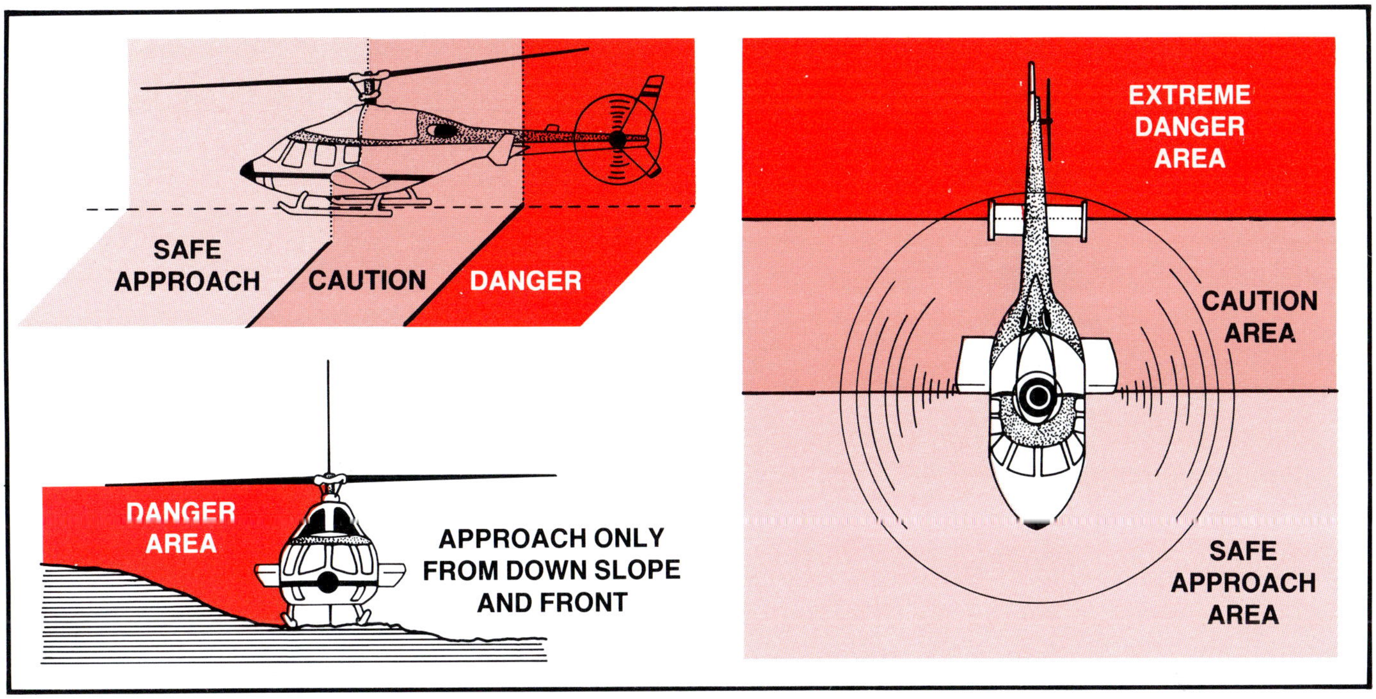


**Figure 17.16** Approach a helicopter ONLY from the front. NEVER walk near the tail rotor area.

- Keep emergency vehicles at least 50 feet (15 m) from the helicopter.
- No smoking within 100 feet (30 m) of the aircraft.

Airplanes (fixed-wing aircraft) are also used for patient transportation. They are especially useful for transfers involving great distances. Depending upon the size of the aircraft, anywhere from one to several patients may be transported at one time. The military uses large transport planes to carry many patients; however, it is more practical in the civilian setting to use smaller aircraft. A common type and size airplane used for emergency transport is pictured in Figure 17.17. A small airplane has several advantages over a helicopter:

- An airplane can transport patients approximately twice as fast as a helicopter.
- An airplane can fly in heavy winds and when visibility is poor. It can also fly above many storms that helicopters cannot. Airplanes *are* affected by bad weather, but not to the extent that helicopters are.
- An airplane is more comfortable for patient and crew because it has a pressurized cabin.
- An airplane ride is smoother and has less vibration than a helicopter ride.

The biggest disadvantage of an airplane is that it requires adequate space to take off and land. Helicopters require comparatively little landing space, but airplanes require a significant length of runway. A preselected site, such as an abandoned airstrip or a crop dusting airfield can be used, but it must be adequately lighted and agreed upon by the pilots. Law enforcement agencies can be used to block a highway if it is needed as a landing strip.

Special safety precautions also apply around an airplane. Most important, **DO NOT** approach an airplane until the propellers have stopped turning completely and the pilot or crew has motioned for you to approach. Generally, the crew will open the side door as soon as it is safe. Unlike a helicopter, the approach to a plane is from the rear.

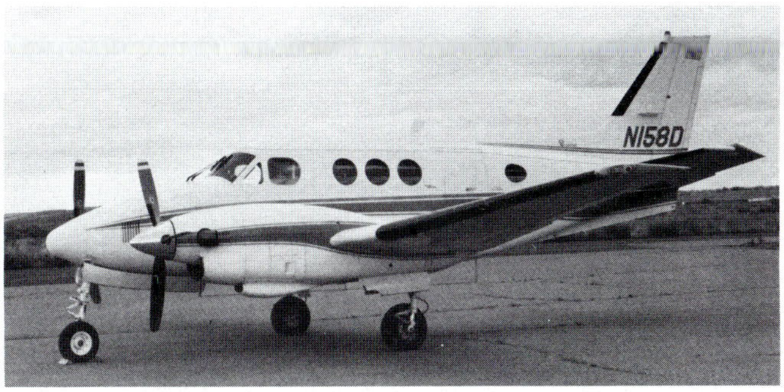


**Figure 17.17** Fixed-wing aircraft are especially useful for transporting patients over long distances. *Courtesy of Presbyterian Air Ambulance.*

# Bibliography


**Chapter 1**

1. American Academy of Orthopaedic Surgeons. *Emergency Care and Transportation of the Sick and Injured.* 2nd ed. Chicago: 1977.
2. Caroline, Nancy L., M.D. *Emergency Medical Treatment: A Text for EMT-As and EMT-Intermediates.* 1st ed. Boston: Little, Brown, and Company, 1982.
3. Holt, Francis C. "Post Traumatic Stress Disorder and the Firefighter." *Fire Engineering.* November 1985, 24-27.
4. U.S. Department of Transportation. National Highway Traffic Safety Administration. *Emergency Medical Care: A Manual for the Paramedic in the Field.* Washington, D.C.: U.S. Government Printing Office, 1983.
5. U.S. Department of Transportation, National Highway Traffic Safety Administration. *Emergency Medical Services: First Responder Training Course. Lesson 1.* Washington, D.C.: U.S. Government Printing Office, 1979.

**Chapter 2**

1. American Academy of Orthopaedic Surgeons. *Emergency Care and Transportation of the Sick and Injured.* 2nd ed. Chicago: 1977.
2. U.S. Department of Transportation. National Highway Traffic Safety Administration. *Emergency Medical Care: A Manual for the Paramedic in the Field.* Washington, D.C.: U.S. Government Printing Office, 1983.
3. U.S. Department of Transportation. National Highway Traffic Safety Administration. *Emergency Medical Services: First Responder Training Course. Lesson 2.* Washington, D.C.: U.S. Government Printing Office, 1979.
4. Vannini, Vanio, and Giuliano Pogliani, eds., and Dr. Richard T. Jolly, trans. *The Color Atlas of Human Anatomy.* New York: Beekman House, 1980.

**Chapter 3**

1. Adams, Richard. "Aiding the AIDS Victim." *Firehouse.* January 1984, 22/81.
2. Adams, Richard. "Basic Precautions Against AIDS." *Firehouse.* February 1986, 18.
3. Antoline, Michael. "Mass-Disaster Triage." *Jems.* Vol. 6, No. 11, November 1981, 46-48.
4. Antoline, Michael. "Communicable Diseases." *Jems.* Vol. 6, No. 13, December 1981, 38-40.
5. Caroline, Nancy L., M.D. *Emergency Care in the Streets.* Boston: Little, Brown, and Company, 1985.
6. Carlson, Gene P. "Don't Take Another Step." *Fire Command.* March 1984, 18-20.
7. "Communicable Disease Notice: Aids-Hepatitis B." *EMS News - Special Edition.* July 1985.
8. Dernocoeur, Jim. "Electrical Injuries." *Jems.* May 1983, 60-61.
9. "Hazardous Materials Incident Plan-Radiological Response." Phoenix Fire Department Standard Operating Procedures. November 1983.
10. Hoover, Deborah A. "Hazardous Materials and Pre-Hospital Care." Illinois State Department of Public Health, June 1985.
11. Judd, Richard L. and Dwight D. Ponsell. *"The First Responder: the critical first minutes!"* St. Louis: C.V. Mosby Co., 1982.
12. Meade, Jeff. "What You Can and Cannot Catch (From Who and What)." *Prevention.* Vol. 37, No. 11, November 1985, 52-58.
13. Moore, Kim (Lt.) "Developing Street Smarts." *Emergency Medical Services.* Vol. 15, No. 1, January/February 1986, 36-42.
14. "Q & A About AIDS." Aurora, IL: Aurora Area Blood Bank.
15. Seaver, Jon F. "The Disturbed and Unruly City." *Jems.* June 1984, 82-83.
16. "Tactical Plans - Hazardous Materials - Flammable Liquid Incidents." Phoenix Fire Department Standard Operating Procedures, January 1984.
17. "Tactical Plans - Hazardous Materials-Natural Gas Incidents." Phoenix Fire Department Standard Operating Procedures, October 1984.
18. West, Katherine H. "Chickenpox, Shingles, and EMS." *Emergency Medical Services.* Vol. 14, No. 2, March/April 1985, 48.
19. West, Katherine H. "Emergency Concepts - Infection Control." Copyright 1982. Revised 1984.

**Chapter 4**

1. Cleary, Victoria, R.N., Mary Hewett, R.N., and Alan Schemehl. *Start: A Triage Training Module.* Newport Beach, CA: Hoag Memorial Hospital, 1984.
2. Cowley, R. Adams, M.D. "Managing Steering Wheel Injuries." *Emergency.* November 1979, 65-67.
3. Dick, Thom. "Tricks of the Trade: Getting Started." *Jems.* September 1983, 24-25.
4. Dick, Thom and Glenda Jenkins. "Looking at Little People - Tips on Assessing Young Children in the Field." *Jems.* July 1981, 24-32.
5. Gille, Greg. "Patient Care - Not Injury Care." *Emergency.* March 1985, 36-37.
6. Hooper, H. Allen, M.D. "Deceleration Injuries." *Emergency.* September 1979, 59-61.
7. Jarvis, Carolyn Mueller, R.N., M.S.N. "Vital Signs." *American Journal of Nursing.* April 1976, 31-37.

8. McMahan, Frank J. "What Special Problems do Geriatric Patients Present?" *Emergency Medical Services.* March/April 1985, 19-25.

9. Neely, Keith. "The Trauma Rush." *Emergency.* March 1985, 31-34.

10. Robbins, Vincent de Paul. "Patterns of Trauma - The Forgotten Element of Assessment." *Jems.* November 1983, 46-49.

11. Spoor, John E., M.D. "Trauma Response - Beyond the ABC's." *Emergency.* February 1980, 33-35.

12. Taylor, Bruce W., R.N., C.E.N., M.I.C.N., "Altered Factors in the Assessment of the Geriatric Patient." *Emergency Medical Services.* Vol. 14, No. 2, March/April 1985, 26-30.

13. U.S. Department of Transportation. National Highway Traffic Safety Administration. *Emergency Medical Care: A Manual for the Paramedic in the Field.* Washington, D.C.: U.S. Government Printing Office, 1983.

14. U.S. Department of Transportation. National Highway Traffic Safety Administration. *Emergency Medical Services: First Responder Training Course. Lesson 3.* Washington, D.C.: U.S. Government Printing Office, 1979.

**Chapter 5**

1. American Academy of Orthopaedic Surgeons. *Emergency Care and Transportation of the Sick and Injured.* 3rd ed. Chicago: American Academy of Orthopaedic Surgeons, 1981.

2. Caroline, Nancy L., M.D. *Emergency Medical Treatment: A Text for EMTS-As and EMT-Intermediates.* 1st ed. Boston: Little, Brown and Company, 1982.

3. "First Responder SIDS Management." S.I.D.S. Regional Center, Loyola University Medical Center, Maywood, IL.

4. "Standards and Guidelines for Cardiopulmonary Resuscitation (CPR) and Emergency Cardiac Care (ECC)." *JAMA.* Vol. 255, No. 21, June 6, 1986.

5. *Student Manual for Basic Life Support.* American Heart Association, 1981.

6. "Sudden Infant Death Syndrome (SIDS) Information for Emergency Medical Technicians." S.I.D.S. Regional Center, Loyola University Medical Center, Maywood, IL.

7. U.S. Department of Transportation. National Highway Traffic Safety Administration. *Emergency Medical Care: A Manual for the Paramedic in the Field.* Washington, D.C.: U.S. Government Printing Office, 1983.

8. U.S. Department of Transportation. National Highway Traffic Safety Administration. *Emergency Medical Services: First Responder Training Course. Lessons 4 and 5.* Washington, D.C.: U.S. Government Printing Office, 1979.

**Chapter 6**

1. American Academy of Orthopaedic Surgeons. *Emergency Care and Transportation of the Sick and Injured.* 3rd ed. Chicago: American Academy of Orthopaedic Surgeons, 1981.

2. Caroline, Nancy L., M.D. *Emergency Medical Treatment: A Text for EMT-As and EMT-Intermediates.* 1st ed. Boston: Little, Brown and Company, 1982.

3. U.S. Department of Transportation. National Highway Traffic Safety Administration. *Emergency Medical Care: A Manual for the Paramedic in the Field.* Washington, D.C.: U.S. Government Printing Office, 1983.

4. U.S. Department of Transportation. National Highway Traffic Safety Administration. *Emergency Medical Services: First Responder Training Course. Lesson 8.* Washington, D.C.: U.S. Government Printing Office, 1979.

**Chapter 7**

1. Barber, Janet M. and Peter A. Dillman. *Emergency Patient Care for the EMT-A.* Reston, VA: Reston Publishing Co., 1981.

2. Bergeron, J. David. *First Responder.* Bowie, MD: Robert J. Brady Co., 1982.

3. Caroline, Nancy L., M.D. *Emergency Medical Treatment: A Text for EMT-As and EMT-Intermediates.* 1st ed. Boston: Little, Brown and Company, 1982.

4. *Emergency Victim Care.* Ohio Trade and Industrial Education Service. Ohio State University, Columbus, Ohio, 1972.

5. Gross, Gary. "After the Accident . . . Can Contact Lenses Be Removed Safely?" *Traffic Safety.* January/February 1981, 10-11, 30-31.

6. Judd, Richard L. and Dwight D. Ponsell. *"The First Responder: the critical first minutes!"* St. Louis: The C.V. Mosby Company, 1982.

7. Karren, Keith J. and Brent Q. Hafen. *First Responder: A Skills Approach.* Englewood, CO: Morton Publishing Company, 1982.

8. "Managing Contact Lens Removal." *Emergency.* Vol. 12, No. 10, October 1980, 60.

9. Scarano, Steve. "Re-Using Body Parts." *Jems.* Vol. 9, No. 6, June 1984, 81.

10. U.S. Department of Transportation. National Highway Traffic Safety Administration. *Emergency Medical Care: A Manual for the Paramedic in the Field.* Washington, D.C.: U.S. Government Printing Office, 1983.

11. U.S. Department of Transportation. National Highway Traffic Safety Administration. *Emergency Medical Services: First Responder Training Course. Lesson 9.* Washington, D.C.: U.S. Government Printing Office, 1979.

**Chapter 8**

1. American Academy of Orthopaedic Surgeons. *Emergency Care and Transportation of the Sick and Injured.* 3rd ed. Chicago: American Academy of Orthopaedic Surgeons, 1981.

2. Caroline, Nancy L., M.D. *Emergency Medical Treatment: A Text for EMT-As and EMT-Intermediates.* 1st ed. Boston: Little, Brown and Company, 1982.

3. Grant, Harvey D., Robert H. Murray, Jr., and J. David Bergeron. *Emergency Care.* 3rd. ed. Bowie, MD: Robert J. Brady Company, 1982.

4. Kelley, Thomas A. "PFRH: Proper First-Aid Reduces Handicaps. A Simple Method for Recognizing Spinal Cord Injuries." *Jems.* August 1981, 26-29.

5. Marley, Charlie. "Critical Trauma. When Time is of the Essence." *Emergency.* November 1984, 45-56.

6. Robbins, Vincent de Paul. "Patterns of Trauma: The Forgotten Element of Assessment." *Jems.* November 1983, 46-49.

7. "Techniques of Helmet Removal from Injured Patients." American College of Surgeons, Committee on Trauma. July 1980.

8. Thomas, Clayton L., M.D., M.P.H. *Taber's Cyclopedic Medical Dictionary.* Philadelphia: Davis Company, 1981.

9. Thygerson, Alton, Ed.D. "Motor Vehicle Accidents." *Emergency.* November 1984, 66-71.

10. U.S. Department of Transportion. National Highway Traffic Safety Administration. *Emergency Medical Care: A Manual for the Paramedic in the Field.* Washington, D.C.: U.S. Government Printing Office, 1983.

11. U.S. Department of Transportation. National Highway Traffic Safety Administration. *Emergency Medical Services: First Responder Training Course. Lesson 13.* Washington, D.C.: U.S. Government Printing Office, 1979.

**Chapter 9**

1. American Academy of Orthopaedic Surgeons. *Emergency Care and Transportation of the Sick and Injured.* 3rd ed. Chicago: American Academy of Orthopaedic Surgeons, 1981.

2. Caroline, Nancy L., M.D. *Emergency Medical Treatment: A Text for EMT-As and EMTS-Intermediates.* 1st ed. Boston: Little, Brown and Company, 1982.

3. U.S. Department of Transportation. National Highway Traffic Safety Administration. *Emergency Medical Care: A Manual for the Paramedic in the Field.* Washington, D.C.: U.S. Government Printing Office, 1983.

4. U.S. Department of Transportation. National Highway Traffic Safety Administration. *Emergency Medical Services: First Responder Training Course. Lesson 12.* Washington, D.C.: U.S. Government Printing Office, 1979.

**Chapter 10**

1. Abbott Laboratories. *EPILEPSY: Breaking Down the Walls of Misunderstanding.* Abbott Laboratories: Abbott Park, IL.

2. "Acute Abdominal Disorders." *Rekindle.* Vol. 14, No. 4, April 1985, 5.

3. Jacobs, Fred L. "Stroke: Emergency Assessment and Management." *Emergency Medical Services,* Vol. 14, No. 2, March/April 1985, 41-46.

4. Kunz, Jeffrey. *American Medical Association Family Medical Guide.* New York: Random House, 1982.

5. Sherman, Carla Pissarro. "Stroke: The First Minutes." *The Journal of Pre-Hospital Care.* May/June 1985, 20-25.

6. Wentz, Richard. "Oxygen Therapy and COPD." *Emergency.* January 1984, 32-33.

7. U.S. Department of Transportation. National Highway Traffic Safety Administration. *Emergency Medical Care: A Manual for the Paramedic in the Field.* Washington D.C.: U.S. Government Printing Office, 1983.

8. U.S. Department of Transportation. National Highway Traffic Safety Administration. *Emergency Medical Services: First Responder Training Course, Lesson 14.* Washington D.C.: U.S. Government Printing Office, March 1979.

**Chapter 11**

1. Adams, Rich. "Suicide Intervention." *Firehouse.* August 1985, 16.

2. Albarino, John E. "Crisis Intervention: Can It Be Managed in the Field?" *Emergency Medical Services.* January/February 1985, 46-47.

3. Brody, Jane. *Guide to Personal Health.* 199-213. New York: Avon, 1983.

4. Caroline, Nancy L., M.D. *Emergency Care in the Streets.* Boston: Little, Brown and Company, 1983.

5. *Centers For Disease Control: Suicide Surveillance, 1970-1980.* Issued April 1985. Atlanta, GA: U.S. Department of Health and Human Services.

6. Edwards, Frank J. "Psychiatric Emergencies, Part 1." *Emergency Medical Services.* Vol. 14, No. 3, May/June 1985, 46-51.

7. Edwards, Frank J. "Psychiatric Emergencies, Part 2." *Emergency Medical Services.* Vol. 14, No. 4, July/August 1985, 45-50.

8. Gorski, Terrence T. "Managing the Violent Patient." *Fire Command.* August 1981, 40-41.

9. Neely, Keith. "The Holiday Depression Syndrome." *Jems.* December 1983, 50-51.

10. Rawlins, Gary and Phillip Haile. "Handling the Suicide Call." *Jems.* June 1982, 34-36.

11. Shybut, John and Ron Carter. "An Ounce of Intervention." *Jems.* August 1981, 40-41.

**Chapter 12**

1. Antoline, Michael L. "Child Poisoning." *Jems.* March 1982, 45-48.

2. Barber, Janet M. and Peter A. Dillman. *Emergency Patient Care.* Reston, VA: Reston Publishing Co., 1981.

3. Brody, Jane. *Guide to Personal Health*. New York: Avon, 1983, 392-99.

4. Carlson, Richard W. "Envenomation Due to Snake, Arthropod, and Fish Venoms." *Emergency Management of Poisonous Reptile and Insect Bites*. University of Southern California Medical School, n.d.

5. Caroline, Nancy L., M.D. *Emergency Medical Treatment: A Text for EMT-As and EMT-Intermediates*. 1st ed. Boston: Little, Brown and Company, 1982, 374-397.

6. Hammessley, Mary Lou. "Stings With Wings and Other Nasty Things." *Emergency Product News*. July 1977, 23-31.

7. Knefler, F. Thomas. "A Practical Guide to Poisonous Snakebite." *Jems*. October 1981, 41-47.

8. "1983 Rabies Prevention." Oklahoma State Department of Health, January 1983.

9. "Plant Poisoning — It Can Happen in Your Home!" *Booster Line*. Vol. 2, No. 5, Ft. Worth: Tarrant County Fire Service Instructor's Society, May 1977.

10. "Rabies Surveillance." (Summary 1980-82) U.S. Department of Health and Human Services, August 1983.

11. Schultz, Kenneth E. "Hazardous Marine Life." *Emergency Medical Services*. Vol. 14, No. 3, May/June 1985, 62-75.

12. U.S. Department of Transportation. National Highway Traffic Safety Administration. *Emergency Medical Care: A Manual for the Paramedic in the Field*. Washington D.C.: U.S. Government Printing Office, 1983.

13. "What You Should Know About Rabies." American Veterinary Medical Association, Schaumburg, IL.

**Chapter 13**

1. American Academy of Orthopaedic Surgeons. *Emergency Care and Transportation of the Sick and Injured*. 3rd ed. Chicago: American Academy of Orthopaedic Surgeons, 1981.

2. Caroline, Nancy L., M.D. *Emergency Medical Treatment: A Text for EMT-As and EMT-Intermediates*. 1st ed. Boston: Little, Brown and Company, 1982.

3. Dernocoeur, Jim. "Electrical Injuries. Part 1: Understanding the Source." *Jems*. May 1983, 60-61.

4. Dernocoeur, Jim. "Electrical Injuries. Part 2." *Jems*. June 1983, 60-61.

5. "Emergency Care of a Burn Patient." Baptist Medical Burn Center, Oklahoma City, OK.

6. Module III, Field Training. (Emergency first aid for burns) Baptist Medical Burn Center, Oklahoma City, OK.

7. U.S. Department of Transportation. National Highway Traffic Safety Administration. *Emergency Medical Care: A Manual for the Paramedic in the Field*. Washington D.C.: U.S. Government Printing Office, 1983.

8. U.S. Department of Transportation. National Highway Traffic Safety Administration. *Emergency Medical Services: First Responder Training Course. Lesson 19*. Washington D.C.: U.S. Government Printing Office, 1979.

**Chapter 14**

1. American Academy of Orthopaedic Surgeons. *Emergency Care and Transportation of the Sick and Injured*. 3rd ed. Chicago: American Academy of Orthopaedic Surgeons, 1981.

2. Caroline, Nancy L., M.D. *Emergency Medical Treatment: A Text for EMT-As and EMT-Intermediates*. 1st ed. Boston: Little, Brown and Company, 1982.

3. Scarano, Steve. "Heat Emergencies." *Emergency*. June 1979, 51-54.

4. Sornberger, Jane. "Hypothermia — The Winter Killer." *FEMA Newsletter*. Washington, D.C.: Federal Emergency Management Agency, September/October, 1985.

5. "State of Alaska Hypothermia & Cold Water Near Drowning Guidelines." Juneau: Alaska Department of Health & Social Services, April 1982.

6. U.S. Department of Transportation. National Highway Traffic Safety Administration. *Emergency Medical Care: A Manual for the Paramedic in the Field*. Washington D.C.: U.S. Government Printing Office, 1983.

7. U.S. Department of Transportation. National Highway Traffic Safety Administration. *Emergency Medical Services: First Responder Training Course. Lesson 19*. Washington D.C.: U.S. Government Printing Office, 1979.

**Chapter 15**

1. Celebreeze, Ellen M. "Third Trimester Pre-Delivery Hemorrhage." *Emergency*. October 1981, 48-51.

2. U.S. Department of Transportation. National Highway Traffic Safety Administration. *Emergency Medical Care: A Manual for the Paramedic in the Field*. Washington D.C.: U.S. Government Printing Office, 1983.

3. U.S. Department of Transportation. National Highway Traffic Safety Administration. *Emergency Medical Services: First Responder Training Course. Lesson 16*. Washington D.C.: U.S. Government Printing Office, 1979.

4. Williams, Casie, R.N. "Emergency Childbirth." *Emergency Medical Services*. May/June 1985, 100-104.

**Chapter 16**

1. U.S. Department of Transportation. National Highway Traffic Safety Administration. *Emergency Medical Services: First Responder Training Course. Lessons 17 and 21*. Washington D.C.: U.S. Government Printing Office, 1979.

# Index

## A



## B

## C

## D

## G



## H

## I



## J



## K



## L



## M



## N

## U



## V



## W



## X



## Y

# IFSTA MANUALS

**FIRE SERVICE ORIENTATION & INDOCTRINATION**
History, traditions, and organization of the fire service; operation of the fire department and responsibilities and duties of firefighters; fire department companies and their functions; glossary of fire service terms.

**FIRE SERVICE FIRST RESPONDER**
Covers all objectives for U.S. DOT First Responder Training Course as well as NFPA 1001 Emergency Medical Care sections. The special emphasis on maintenance of the ABC's features updated CPR techniques. Also included are scenen assessment and safety, patient assessment, shock, bleeding control, spinal injuries, burns, heat and cold emergencies, medical emergencies, poisons, behavioral emergencies, emergency childbirth, short-distance transfer, and emergency vehicles and their equipment.

**FIRE SERVICE FIRST AID PRACTICES**
Brief explanations of the nervous, skeletal, muscular, abdominal, digestive, and genitourinary systems; injuries and treatment relating to each system; bleeding control and bandaging; artificial respiration, cardiopulmonary resuscitation (CPR), shock, poisoning, and emergencies caused by heat and cold; fractures, sprains, and dislocations; emergency childbirth; short-distance transfer of patients; ambulances; conducting a primary and secondary survey.

**ESSENTIALS OF FIRE FIGHTING**
This manual was prepared to meet the objectives set forth in levels I and II of NFPA, *Fire Fighter Professional Qualifications, 1981.* Included in the manual are the basics of fire behavior, extinguishers, ropes and knots, self-contained breathing apparatus, ladders, forcible entry, rescue, water supply, fire streams, hose, ventilation, salvage and overhaul, fire cause determination, fire suppression techniques, communications, sprinkler systems, and fire inspection.

**IFSTA'S 500 COMPETENCIES FOR FIREFIGHTER CERTIFICATION**
This manual identifies the competencies that must be achieved for certification as a firefighter for levels I and II. The text also identifies what the instructor needs to give the student, NFPA standards, and has space to record the student's score, local standards, and the instructor's initials.

**FIRE SERVICE GROUND LADDER PRACTICES**
Various terms applied to ladders; types, construction, maintenance, and testing of fire service ground ladders; detailed information on handling ground ladders and special tasks related to them.

**SALVAGE AND OVERHAUL PRACTICES**
Planning and preparing for salvage operations, care and preparation of equipment, methods of spreading and folding salvage covers, most effective way to handle water runoff, value of proper overhaul and equipment needed, and recognizing and preserving arson evidence.

**FORCIBLE ENTRY**
This comprehensive manual contains technical information about forcible entry tactics; tools; and door, window, and wall construction. Forcible entry methods are described for door, window, and wall entry. A new section on locks and through-the-lock entry makes this the most up-to-date manual available for forcible entry training.

**SELF-CONTAINED BREATHING APPARATUS**
Beginning with the history of breathing apparatus and the reasons they are needed, to how to use them, including maintenance and care, the firefighter is taken step by step with the aid of programmed-learning questions and answers throughout to complete knowledge of the subject. The donning, operation, and care of all types of breathing apparatus are covered in depth, as are training in SCBA use, breathing-air purification, and recharging cylinders. There are also special chapters on emergency escape procedures and interior search and rescue.

**FIRE VENTILATION PRACTICES**
Objectives and advantages of ventilation; requirements for burning, flammable liquid characteristics and products of combustion; phases of burning, backdrafts, and the transmission of heat; construction features to be considered; the ventilation process including evaluating and size up is discussed at length.

**FIRE SERVICE RESCUE PRACTICES**
Sections include water and ice rescue, trenching, cave rescue, rigging, search-and-rescue techniques for inside structures and outside, and taking command at an incident. Also included are vehicle extrication and a complete section on rescue tools. The book covers all the information called for by the rescue sections of NFPA 1001 for Fire Fighter I, II, and III, and is profusely illustrated.

**THE FIRE DEPARTMENT COMPANY OFFICER**
This manual focuses on the basic principles of fire department organization, working relationships, and personnel management. For the firefighter aspiring to become a company officer and the company officer who wishes to improve management skills this manual will be invaluable. This manual will help individuals develop and improve the necessary traits to effectively manage the fire company.

**FIRE CAUSE DETERMINATION**
Covers need for determination, finding origin and cause, documenting evidence, interviewing witnesses, courtroom demeanor, and more. Ideal text for company officers, firefighters, inspectors, investigators, insurance and industrial personnel.

**PRIVATE FIRE PROTECTION & DETECTION**
Automatic sprinkler systems, special extinguishing systems, standpipes, detection, and alarm systems. Includes how to test sprinkler systems for the firefighter to meet NFPA 1001.

**INDUSTRIAL FIRE PROTECTION**
Devastating fires in industrial plants do occur at a rate of 145 fires every day. *Industrial Fire Protection* is the single source document designed for training and managing industrial fire brigades.

This text is a must for all industrial sites, large and small, to meet the requirements of the Occupational Safety and Health Administration's (OSHA) regulation 29 CFR part 1910, Subpart L, concerning incipient industrial fire fighting.

**CHIEF OFFICER**
This text has been designed for the chief officer and the firefighter who wishes to become a chief officer. With over 220 pages of text, *Chief Officer* provides an overview of the skills needed by today's chief officer. Included are coordination of emergency medical services, master planning, planning for possible disasters, budgeting, information management, dealing with labor relations, and passage of legislation.

The role of the fire service has changed from solely fire suppression to functioning as part of a fire control and emergency response system that includes public education, emergency medical services, hazardous materials control, and fire suppression. This text addresses each of these areas.

Where appropriate, chapters are referenced to NFPA Standard 1021, Fire Fighter Professional Qualifications, for levels V and VI.

**SI CHIEF OFFICER**
This manual assists those reading the text in retaining the principles and concepts necessary to be a skilled chief officer. It includes structured questions and answers, exercises, and a new supplemental section on Resolution by Objectives. It will serve as a review of the text and assist in promotional exam preparation.

**HAZ MAT TEAM LEAK & SPILL GUIDE**
A brief, practical treatise that reviews operations at spills and leaks. Sample S.O.P. and command recommendations along with a decontamination guide.

**FIRE SERVICE INSTRUCTOR**
Characteristics of a good instructor; determining training requirements and what to teach; types, principles, and procedures for teaching and learning; training aids and devices; conference leadership

**PUBLIC FIRE EDUCATION**
Public fire education planning, target audiences, seasonal fire problems, smoke detectors, working with the media, burn injuries, and resource exchange.

**WATER SUPPLIES FOR FIRE PROTECTION**
Importance, basic components, adequacy, reliability, and carrying capacity of water systems; specifications, installation, maintenance, and distribution of fire hydrants; flow test and control valves; sprinkler and standpipe systems.

**FIRE APPARATUS PRACTICES**
Various types of fire apparatus classified by functions; driving and operating apparatus including pumpers, aerial ladders, and elevating platforms; maintenance and testing of apparatus.

**FIRE STREAM PRACTICES**
Characteristics, requirements, and principles of fire streams; developing, computing, and applying various types of streams to operational situations; formulas for application of hydraulics; actions and reactions created by applying streams under different circumstances.

**FIRE PROTECTION ADMINISTRATION**
A reprint of the Illinois Department of Commerce and Community Affairs publication. A manual for trustees, municipal officials, and fire chiefs of fire districts and small communities. Subjects covered include officials' duties and responsibilities, organization and management, personnel management and training, budgeting and finance, annexation and disconnection.

**BUILDING CONSTRUCTION**
This 170-page manual covers building construction features vital to developing fire fighting tactics in a structure. Subjects include construction principles, assemblies and their fire resistance, building services, door and window assemblies, and special types of structures.

**FIREFIGHTER SAFETY**
Basic concepts and philosophy of accident prevention; essentials of a safety program and training for safety; station house facility safety; hazards en route and at the emergency scene; personal protective equipment; special hazards, including chemicals, electricity, and radioactive materials; inspection safety; health considerations.

**AIRCRAFT FIRE PROTECTION AND RESCUE PROCEDURES**
Aircraft types, engines, and systems, conventional and specialized fire fighting apparatus, tools, clothing, extinguishing agents, dangerous materials, communications, pre-fire planning, and airfield operations.

**GROUND COVER FIRE FIGHTING PRACTICES**
Ground cover fire apparatus, equipment, extinguishing agents, and fireground safety; organization and planning for ground cover fire; authority, jurisdiction, and mutual aid, techniques and procedures used for combating ground cover fire.

**FIRE SERVICE PRACTICES FOR VOLUNTEER AND SMALL COMMUNITY FIRE DEPARTMENTS**
A general overview of material covered in detail in *Forcible Entry, Ladders, Hose, Salvage and Overhaul, Fire Streams, Apparatus, Ventilation, Rescue, Inspection,* and *Self-Contained Breathing Apparatus, and Public Fire Education*.

**SELF-INSTRUCTION FOR ESSENTIALS**
Over 260 pages of structured questions and answers for studying the *Essentials of Fire Fighting*. This self-instruction book will help you to learn many of the important topics and review the basic text.

Each unit begins with the NFPA Standard No. 1001. required performance objectives. This *Self-Instruction for Essentials* will reinforce and guide your learning toward what you will need to know for certification and your fire service career.

**TRANSPARENCIES**
Multicolored overhead transparencies to augment *Essentials of Fire Fighting*. Since costs and availability vary with different chapters, contact IFSTA Headquarters for details. Units available:

Fire Behavior, Portable Extinguishers, Ropes and Knots, Hose Tools and Appliances, Handling Hose, Handling Ground Ladders, Ventilation, Fire Streams, Ladder Carries and Raises, Forcible Entry, Salvage and Overhaul, Prevention and Identification, Ground Cover Fires, Communications, Water Supply, Automatic Sprinkler Systems, Rescue, Protective Breathing Apparatus.

**FIREFIGHTER VIDEOTAPE SERIES**
Video programs for reinforcement of basic skills and knowledge on a variety of fire fighting topics. Excellent for use with *Essentials* or *Volunteer* to review and emphasize subjects. Titles available: The Anatomy and Behavior of Fire, Fire Safety, Protective Breathing Apparatus, Fire Hose and Nozzles — Part 1, Fire Hose and Nozzles — Part 2, Fire Streams, Ventilation, Sprinklers, Ladders, Forcible Entry, Rescue, Ropes and Knots, Salvage, Fire Alarm and Communications, General Qualifications, First Aid, Inspection — Part 1, and Inspection — Part 2.

**FIREFIGHTER II/III VIDEOTAPE SERIES**
These video programs for the advanced firefighter build on the basic skills presented in the Firefighter Videotape Series (Firefighter I). Titles available are: Fireground Operations, Using and Maintaining SCBAs, Advanced Rescue Techniques, Water Distribution Systems, Testing Water Systems, Developing Fire Flow-Hydraulics, Selecting and Applying Fire Streams, Portable Extinguishers, Power Tools and Forcible Entry, Salvage and Overhaul Operations, Ladders and Aerial Apparatus, Advanced Ventilation Techniques, Pre-Fire Planning, Fire Company Inspection, Inspecting and Testing Sprinkler Systems, First Aid for Burns and Fractures.

**SLIDES**
2-inch by 2-inch slides that can be used in any 35 mm slide projector; supplements to respective manuals and sprinkler guide sets.

**Sprinklers**
Module 1: Introduction to Automatic Sprinkler Protection
Module 2: Types of Sprinkler Systems
Module 3: Maintenance and Inspection of Sprinkler Systems
Module 4: Components of Water Supply Systems
Module 5: Testing and Analysis of Water Supply Systems
Module 6: Factors Affecting the Adequacy of Sprinkler and Water Systems

**Smoke Detectors Can Save Your Life**
**Matches Aren't For Children**
**Public Relations for the Fire Service**
**Public Fire Education Specialist (Slide/Tape)**

**MANUAL HOLDER**
The fast, efficient way to organize your IFSTA manuals. These attractive heavy-duty vinyl holders have specially designed side panels that allow easy access to all of your IFSTA manuals. Manual holders stand unsupported and will hold up to eight manuals.

**IFSTA BINDERS**
Heavy-duty three ring binders that will allow you to organize and protect your IFSTA manuals. Available in two sizes, 1½ inch and 3 inch.

**WATER FLOW TEST SUMMARY SHEETS**
50 summary sheets and instructions on how to use; logarithmic scale to simplify the process of determining the available water in an area.

**PERSONNEL RECORD FOLDERS**
Personnel record folders should be used by the training officer for each member of the department. Such data as IFSTA training, technical training (seminars), and college work can be recorded in the file, along with other valuable information. Letter size or legal size.

Ship to: Date ____________

Name ____________ Account Number ____________

Signature ____________ Phone ____________

Street Address (We Ship UPS!!) ____________

City ____________ State ____________ Zip ____________

(**NOTE: Order can not be processed without signature.)**

Send to
**Fire Protection Publications**
**Oklahoma State University**
**Stillwater, Oklahoma 74078**
**800-654-4055**
**Or Contact Your Local Distributor**

# ORDER FORM

## IFSTA MANUALS

### WRITE THE NUMBER OF COPIES OF EACH MANUAL NEXT TO ITS TITLE

| Title | No. of Each |
|---|---|
| Indoctrination | ______ |
| First Aid | ______ |
| First Responder | ______ |
| Essentials | ______ |
| 500 Competencies for Essentials | ______ |
| Self-Instruction for Essentials | ______ |
| Ladders | ______ |
| Salvage and Overhaul | ______ |
| Forcible Entry | ______ |
| Self-Contained Breathing Apparatus | ______ |
| Ventilation | ______ |
| Rescue | ______ |
| Company Officer | ______ |

| Title | No. of Each |
|---|---|
| Fire Cause Determination | ______ |
| Private Fire Protection | ______ |
| Industrial Fire Protection | ______ |
| Chief Officer | ______ |
| SI Chief Officer | ______ |
| Haz Mat Leak and Spill Guide | ______ |
| Instructor | ______ |
| Public Fire Education | ______ |
| Water Supplies | ______ |
| Fire Streams | ______ |
| Apparatus Practices | ______ |
| Fire Protection Administration | ______ |
| Building Construction | ______ |

| Title | No. Of Each |
|---|---|
| Safety | ______ |
| Aircraft | ______ |
| High-Rise | ______ |
| Volunteer | ______ |
| Ground Cover | ______ |
| Manual Binder | |
| 1½ inch | ______ |
| 3 inch | ______ |
| **SLIDES** | |
| Public Fire Education Specialists | ______ |
| Smoke Detectors Can Save Your Life | ______ |
| Matches Aren't For Children | ______ |

| Title | No. of Each |
|---|---|
| Public Relations for the Fire Service | ______ |

**VISUAL AIDS**
Multicolored overhead transparencies to augment each chapter of *Essentials of Fire Fighting* are now available. Also available are slide programs for each of the major fire pump manufacturers and slides for sprinkler systems. A new addition, The firefighter videotape series is available for both Beta II and VHS, and ¾" formats. Since costs and availability vary with different sets, contact Fire Protection Publications for details.

**CATALOG**
Write or call for a free catalog, for information on other items distributed by Fire Protection Publications.

### OTHER MANUALS AND MATERIALS MAY BE ORDERED BELOW:

| QUANTITY | TITLE | LIST PRICE | TOTAL |
|---|---|---|---|
| | | | |
| | | | |
| | | | |
| | | | |
| | | | |
| | | | |
| | | | |
| | | | |
| | | | |

All Foreign Orders must be prepaid in U.S. currency and include 20% shipping and handling charges.

Obtain postage and prices from current IFSTA Catalog or they will be inserted by Customer Services.

Note: Payment with your order saves you postage and handling charges when ordering from Fire Protection Publications.

Payment Enclosed ☐ Bill Me Later ☐

Allow 4 to 6 weeks for delivery.

**SUBTOTAL** ____________

**Discount, if applicable** ____________

**Postage and Handling, if applicable** ____________

**TOTAL** ____________

**FOR ORDERS**
**TOLL FREE NUMBER — 800-654-4055**

**Oklahoma, Hawaii, and Alaska call 405-624-5723.**

Ship to: Date ______________

Name ______________ Account Number ______________

Signature ______________ Phone ______________

Street Address (We Ship UPS!!) ______________

City ______________ State ______________ Zip ______________

(**NOTE: Order can not be processed without signature.)**


Send to
**Fire Protection Publications**
**Oklahoma State University**
**Stillwater, Oklahoma 74078**
**800-654-4055**
**Or Contact Your Local Distributor**


# ORDER FORM

# IFSTA MANUALS

## WRITE THE NUMBER OF COPIES OF EACH MANUAL NEXT TO ITS TITLE

| | No. of Each |
|---|---|
| Indoctrination | ______ |
| First Aid | ______ |
| First Responder | ______ |
| Essentials | ______ |
| 500 Competencies for Essentials | ______ |
| Self-Instruction for Essentials | ______ |
| Ladders | ______ |
| Salvage and Overhaul | ______ |
| Forcible Entry | ______ |
| Self-Contained Breathing Apparatus | ______ |
| Ventilation | ______ |
| Rescue | ______ |
| Company Officer | ______ |

| | No. of Each |
|---|---|
| Fire Cause Determination | ______ |
| Private Fire Protection | ______ |
| Industrial Fire Protection | ______ |
| Chief Officer | ______ |
| SI Chief Officer | ______ |
| Haz Mat Leak and Spill Guide | ______ |
| Instructor | ______ |
| Public Fire Education | ______ |
| Water Supplies | ______ |
| Fire Streams | ______ |
| Apparatus Practices | ______ |
| Fire Protection Administration | ______ |
| Building Construction | ______ |

| | No. Of Each |
|---|---|
| Safety | ______ |
| Aircraft | ______ |
| High-Rise | ______ |
| Volunteer | ______ |
| Ground Cover | ______ |
| Manual Binder | |
| 1½ inch | ______ |
| 3 inch | ______ |
| **SLIDES** | |
| Public Fire Education Specialists | ______ |
| Smoke Detectors Can Save Your Life | ______ |
| Matches Aren't For Children | ______ |

| | No. of Each |
|---|---|
| Public Relations for the Fire Service | ______ |

**VISUAL AIDS**

Multicolored overhead transparencies to augment each chapter of *Essentials of Fire Fighting* are now available. Also available are slide programs for each of the major fire pump manufacturers and slides for sprinkler systems. A new addition, The firefighter videotape series is available for both Beta II and VHS, and ¾" formats. Since costs and availability vary with different sets, contact Fire Protection Publications for details.

**CATALOG**

Write or call for a free catalog, for information on other items distributed by Fire Protection Publications.

## OTHER MANUALS AND MATERIALS MAY BE ORDERED BELOW:

| QUANTITY | TITLE | LIST PRICE | TOTAL |
|---|---|---|---|
| | | | |
| | | | |
| | | | |
| | | | |
| | | | |
| | | | |
| | | | |
| | | | |
| | | | |

All Foreign Orders must be prepaid in U.S. currency and include 20% shipping and handling charges.

Obtain postage and prices from current IFSTA Catalog or they will be inserted by Customer Services.

Note: Payment with your order saves you postage and handling charges when ordering from Fire Protection Publications.

Payment Enclosed ☐ Bill Me Later ☐

Allow 4 to 6 weeks for delivery.

**SUBTOTAL** ______________

**Discount, if applicable** ______________

**Postage and Handling, if applicable** ______________

**TOTAL** ______________

**FOR ORDERS**

**TOLL FREE NUMBER — 800-654-4055**

**Oklahoma, Hawaii, and Alaska call 405-624-5723.**

**COMMENT SHEET** **FIRST RESPONDER**

DATE ______________________ NAME ______________________________________

ADDRESS ____________________________________________________________

ORGANIZATION REPRESENTED ____________________________________________

CHAPTER TITLE _____________________________________ NUMBER _________

SECTION/PARAGRAPH/FIGURE ____________________________ PAGE _________

1. Proposal (include proposed wording, or identification of wording to be deleted), OR PROPOSED FIGURE:

2. Statement of Problem and Substantiation for Proposal:

RETURN TO: IFSTA Editor
Fire Protection Publications
Oklahoma State University
Stillwater, OK 74078

SIGNATURE ______________________

Use this sheet to make any suggestions, recommendations, or comments. We need your input to make the manuals the most up to date as possible. Your help is appreciated. Use additional pages if necessary.